Bottom Line's

HEALTH BREAKTHROUGHS 2015

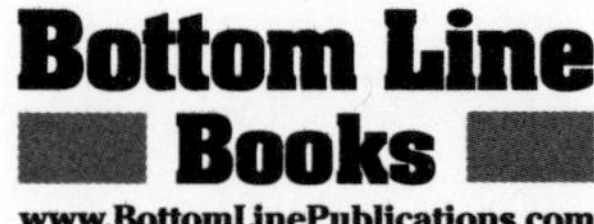

10 9 8 7 6 5 4 3 2 1

ISBN 0-88723-715-0

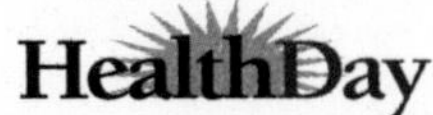

Articles in this book were written by reporters for HealthDay, an award-winning international daily consumer health news service, headquartered in Norwalk, Connecticut.

Bottom Line Books® is a registered trademark of Boardroom® Inc.
281 Tresser Boulevard, Stamford, Connecticut 06901

www.bottomlinepublications.com

Bottom Line Books® is an imprint of Boardroom® Inc., publisher of print periodicals, e-letters and books. We are dedicated to bringing you the best information from the most knowledgeable sources in the world. Our goal is to help you gain greater wealth, better health, more wisdom, extra time and increased happiness.

Printed in the United States of America

Contents

5 • CHOLESTEROL & BLOOD PRESSURE

6 • CONSUMER HEALTH ALERTS

7 • DIABETES

8 • DIET, FITNESS & NUTRITION

9 • DIGESTIVE DISORDERS

10 • EMOTIONAL WELL-BEING

11 • FAMILY MATTERS

12 • HEART & STROKE

13 • INFECTIOUS DISEASES

14 • LONGEVITY & OPTIMUM AGING

15 • MEDICAL NEWSMAKERS

16 • MEDICATION SMARTS

17 • MEN'S HEALTH

Preface

We are proud to bring you the all-new *Bottom Line's Health Breakthroughs 2015*. This collection represents a year's worth of the latest health news and scientific discoveries in a broad spectrum of fields.

When you choose a Bottom Line book, you are turning to a stellar group of experts in a wide range of specialties—medical doctors, alternative practitioners, renowned nutrition experts, research scientists and consumer-health advocates, to name a few.

We go to great lengths to interview the foremost health experts. Whether it's cancer prevention, breakthrough arthritis treatments or cutting-edge nutritional advice, our editors talk to the true innovators in health care.

How do we find all these top-notch professionals? Over the past 20 years, we have built a network of leading physicians in both alternative and conventional medicine. They are affiliated with the world's premier medical institutions. We follow the medical research, and with the help of our partner HealthDay, an award-winning service that reports on evidence-based health news, we bring the latest information to our readers. We also regularly talk with our advisers in teaching hospitals, private practices and government health agencies.

Bottom Line's Health Breakthroughs 2015 is a result of our ongoing research and contact with these experts, and is a distillation of their latest findings and advice. We hope that you will enjoy the presentation and glean helpful information about the health topics that concern you and your family.

As a reader of a Bottom Line book, please be assured that you are receiving reliable and well-researched information from a trusted source. But, please use prudence in health matters. Always speak to your physician before taking vitamins, supplements or over-the-counter medication...changing your diet...or beginning an exercise program. If you experience side effects from any regimen, contact your doctor immediately.

The Editors, Bottom Line Books, Stamford, Connecticut.

Allergies, Asthma & Respiratory Conditions

Is It a Cold, Flu, Allergies... or Something Else?

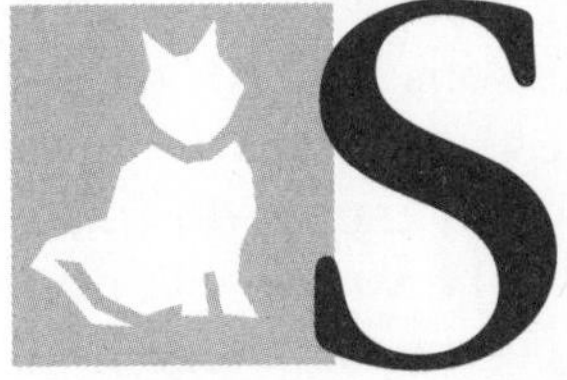

Sniffling, sneezing and wiping your eyes? You might assume you have a cold...but not so fast. These symptoms also can come from the flu or allergies...from something that's similar to an allergy...and even from something else entirely—sinusitis!

Telling these five conditions apart can be tricky—even for doctors and for people who may have developed allergies later in life. *But knowing the difference is the key to getting the most effective treatment...*

COLDS

Colds are caused by more than 100 different viruses. Your symptoms will depend on the specific virus you are infected with.

Telltale signs: In addition to common cold symptoms, such as sneezing, a sore throat, congestion and/or a cough, you may also have a low-grade fever, mild body aches and aching, swollen sinuses. Symptoms usually last a week or two.

My favorite cold remedies: Get into bed and rest. Also, have chicken soup and decaffeinated green tea with lemon and honey. Chicken soup and green tea have anti-inflammatory properties that help fight infection. If you can, watch a funny movie. Research shows that laughing promotes healing. If you need help sleeping, try 25 mg to 50 mg of *diphenhydramine* (Benadryl).

For an immune-boosting herbal cough syrup: Mix one-half teaspoon each of cayenne pepper and freshly grated gingerroot... two tablespoons each of honey and apple cider vinegar...and four tablespoons of water. Take one teaspoon every few waking hours.

Murray Grossan, MD, an otolaryngologist and head and neck surgeon with the Tower Ear, Nose and Throat Clinic at Cedars-Sinai Medical Center in Los Angeles and the founder of the Web-based Grossan Sinus & Health Institute. He is author of *Free Yourself from Sinus and Allergy Problems Permanently* (Basic Health). *GrossanInstitute.com*

THE FLU

The flu will make you feel awful.

Telltale signs: Symptoms can be the same as a cold, but you'll have significant body aches and probably a fever. Also, the flu comes on more suddenly than a cold.

My advice: Get a flu shot. If you still come down with the flu, stay home for at least 24 hours after any fever is gone so you won't spread the virus. Adults over age 65 and those with any chronic health problem should take an antiviral drug, such as *oseltamivir* (Tamiflu), to avoid flu complications, including pneumonia. Antivirals work best if taken within 48 hours of starting to feel sick. (For more information on the flu shot, see page 237.)

ALLERGIES

Allergic rhinitis (nasal allergy) is caused by a hypersensitive immune system that identifies an innocuous substance as harmful, then attacks it, causing symptoms.

Telltale signs: Nasal allergies can cause symptoms that are nearly indistinguishable from a cold—congestion, sneezing, red and runny eyes, scratchy throat, etc.—but allergies do not cause the mild fever or achiness of a cold. With seasonal allergies, you get symptoms from exposure to pollen (trees in spring, grass in summer and weeds in fall). Allergies to pet dander, dust, etc., tend to occur year-round.

Helpful: Use a diary to track your symptoms and the times they occur. It will help you distinguish allergies from other conditions.

My advice: Prescription nasal sprays, like *fluticasone propionate* (Flonase) or *azelastine* (Astelin), work for most people with less risk for side effects than antihistamine pills. Also, avoid spicy foods, which can worsen nasal allergies.

NONALLERGIC RHINITIS (VASOMOTOR RHINITIS)

This condition causes virtually the same symptoms as allergies, but it's not a true allergy that involves the immune system. Rather, it's triggered by specific irritants, such as certain odors, smoke and exhaust—or even changes in the weather.

Natural Remedies for All Sinus Problems

Nasal cilia (tiny, hairlike strands) help clear mucus from the nasal cavity. Slow-moving cilia can lead to nasal and sinus irritation and congestion. To stimulate cilia...

- **Hum.** It may sound far-fetched, but the vibrations from humming break up and thin accumulated mucus. Patients of mine who hum for a few minutes several times a day tend to get fewer sinus infections.
- **Keep the nose moist by using a preservative-free saline nasal spray** such as Simply Saline, available in drugstores. Avoid daily irrigation with a neti pot—the neti pot can easily get contaminated with bacteria, and irrigation can wash away protective elements in the nose.
- **Stay warm and drink hot tea.** Cold temperatures can slow the movement of nasal cilia, so wear a jacket, hat and scarf to keep warm. Additionally, avoid cold beverages and drink hot green or black tea—both contain L-theanine, an amino acid that increases ciliary activity. The excess fluid also will help thin and clear mucus, speeding recovery.

Telltale signs: With nonallergic rhinitis, standard allergy medications fail to relieve symptoms, and allergy tests are negative. Postnasal drip, an irritating flow of mucus down the back of the throat, tends to be worse with nonallergic rhinitis than with seasonal allergies.

My advice: Avoid irritants that you're sensitive to...and consider using the prescription drug *ipratropium bromide* (Atrovent), available as a nasal spray. It helps relax and open nasal passages. This drug can cause side effects, including dizziness, so use it only when needed and at the lowest dose possible.

SINUSITIS

Sinusitis is tough to diagnose because it often occurs in conjunction with colds and allergies.

Reason: The excess mucus from congestion provides an optimal breeding ground for bacteria and viruses.

Telltale signs: Congestion with tenderness and a feeling of pressure around the eyes, cheeks or forehead. Also, when you blow your nose, the mucus will usually have a yellow or greenish color. Fever may be present as well. Symptoms can last for several weeks (acute) or even longer (chronic).

My advice: The prescription nasal sprays mentioned under "Allergies" help open the airways. *Acetaminophen* (Tylenol) or *naproxen* (Aleve) work for sinus pain. Bromelain (from pineapple) and papain (from papaya) also help reduce pain. Antibiotics are not always needed for acute sinusitis—a virus is sometimes the cause.

Herbs, Home Remedies and Other Natural Treatments for Allergies

Joan Wilen and Lydia Wilen, health investigators based in New York City who have spent decades collecting "cures from the cupboard," traditional remedies that have been successfully used by millions of people worldwide. Their most recent book is *Bottom Line's Treasury of Home Remedies & Natural Cures* (Bottom Line Books).

Attention hay fever sufferers, help is here! Natural remedies can reduce symptoms and/or improve the ability of your immune system to resist the seasonal (or perpetual) onslaughts.

Hay fever, also called *allergic rhinitis,* is a catchall term for both seasonal and perennial rhinitis—and it's the most common immune system disorder in the US, affecting about 35 million Americans. Seasonal triggers include ragweed pollen (common in the fall), tree pollen (common in the spring) and grass pollen (common in the late spring and early summer). Year-round hay fever triggers include dust mites and cockroaches, spores from fungi and molds, and dander from pets.

Symptoms include runny nose, watery/itchy eyes, sneezing and/or coughing. You can treat the symptoms with antihistamines or other medications, but they're often expensive and may cause side effects.

Here are our favorite natural remedies. Try one or two at a time to see which one(s) work for you.

Caution: Always check with your doctor before starting or stopping any medications or supplements.

BEE POLLEN

Research has shown that bee pollen (which is made by honeybees and is the food of the young bee) may inhibit the activity of mast cells, a class of immune system cells that release histamine, the substance that causes itchy eyes, nasal congestion and other allergy symptoms.

To use: Start taking bee pollen about four months before the start of your typical hay fever season. For the first few days, take just a few granules at a time. Then slowly increase the amount every day for a month, until you're taking about one teaspoon a day. Follow the same slow progression for the second and third months, until you're taking a total of three teaspoons a day. You have to go slowly because taking too much bee pollen too quickly could cause an allergic reaction of its own, with symptoms such as stomach pain, hives and a fast heart rate.

Caution: If you have an insect allergy—especially to bees—steer clear of bee pollen, which can contain bee saliva.

FENUGREEK TEA

Fenugreek is the herb that gives curries their slightly peppery flavor. As with bee pollen, you can use it to desensitize your immune system prior to allergy season. It's also a mucolytic that naturally loosens phlegm and reduces coughing and sneezing.

To use: About three months before your allergy season, start drinking a daily cup of fenugreek tea. You can buy bags of this tea in health-food stores. Or you can buy the whole seeds...put about one teaspoon in a tea strainer...cover with just-boiled water...and steep for 10 to 15 minutes. Continue to drink it throughout your allergy season.

HONEYCOMB

Honeycomb is a natural antihistamine. When hay fever is flaring, chew a one-inch square of honeycomb. Swallow the honey, and keep chewing the waxy portion for about 10 minutes, then spit it out and discard. You probably will notice the difference right away.

You can buy honeycomb in most health-food stores, but try to find honeycomb that is produced in your area. You want it to contain trace amounts of the same pollens that, in larger amounts, trigger your symptoms.

Caution: If you are allergic to bees, stay away from honeycomb.

GARLIC AND HORSERADISH

Potent chemical compounds in both garlic and horseradish thin mucus and make it more watery. They will help reduce sneezing, congestion and other hay fever symptoms.

To use: Finely mince a clove of raw garlic, and add it to water, orange juice or applesauce. Then add one-quarter teaspoon of horseradish to vegetable juice—or sprinkle it on a salad—and consume that. Both the aromas and the strong flavors of these pungent herbs will clear nasal congestion in seconds.

To prevent nausea, make sure that you have food in your stomach before swallowing raw garlic.

NETTLE

Also known as stinging nettle (because the leaves and stems have hairlike barbs that sting the skin), it's a traditional allergy remedy. When taken orally, it blocks the body's production of histamine and reduces inflammation and congestion.

To use: You can drink a tea made from nettle, but it is easier to take a freeze-dried extract. The typical dose is one or two capsules every two to four hours during allergy flare-ups.

LAVENDER OIL

Lavender can be used as aromatherapy to relieve congestion and other allergy symptoms. The scent-filled molecules act as natural antihistamines and reduce inflammation and congestion in the nasal passages.

To use: Put a drop or two of lavender oil on a handkerchief. Take a deep sniff every few minutes when your allergies are flaring.

QUERCETIN

Every time you eat an apple or add onion to a recipe, you're getting small amounts of quercetin, a bioflavonoid that reduces inflammation. In large enough doses, it inhibits the effects of histamine and reduces nasal congestion. But you can't get adequate amounts of quercetin from foods to control allergies.

To use: When you are having allergy symptoms, take 300 milligrams (mg) to 600 mg of a quercetin supplement daily.

FISH OIL

The omega-3 fatty acids in fish and fish oil have been shown to reduce inflammation throughout the body. Cardiologists often recommend fish oil to lower triglycerides and prevent heart disease and stroke. It also can lessen allergy symptoms by reducing inflammation and swelling in the nasal passages.

To use: Take 2,000 mg daily.

Look for a fish-oil product that says "purified" or "mercury-free" on the label. It should contain at least 500 mg of EPA and 250 mg of DHA per capsule. You can find the capsules online or in health-food stores.

Caution: Check with your doctor, especially if you also are taking a blood-thinning medication such as warfarin. Using both together could increase the risk of bleeding.

No More Allergy Shots

According to recent research, putting allergens under the tongue in a water solution, called sublingual immunotherapy, improved asthma symptoms by more than 40%, including runny nose and eye inflammation. In April 2014, the Food and Drug Administration approved Oralair, the first sublingual immunotherapy available in the US.

Meta-analysis of 5,131 patients, ages four to 74, by researchers at Johns Hopkins University, Baltimore, published in *The Journal of the American Medical Association.*

A RAZOR

Men, this one's for you—your allergies might be originating right under your nose.

It's common for grains of pollen to get trapped in mustaches and beards. Every time you inhale, the featherweight grains waft upward and into the nostrils, triggering allergies.

Helpful: If you would prefer not to shave off your mustache or beard, get into the habit of shampooing it after you've spent time outdoors during your allergy season.

Nasal Allergies and Hay Fever Are Linked to Migraine Frequency

A recent study shows that people with migraine headaches who also have allergies such as hay fever were 33% more likely to have frequent migraines than people who had no allergies.

Theory: Treating allergy symptoms may relieve migraine symptoms. Talk to your doctor.

Vincent Martin, MD, professor of medicine and codirector of the Headache and Facial Pain Program at University of Cincinnati, is the lead author of a study based on questionnaires from 6,000 people with migraines, published in *Cephalalgia*.

Take Infection Precautions When Using Nasal-Rinsing Products

U.S. Food and Drug Administration, news release.

Neti pots and other nasal-rinsing devices are generally safe and useful products, but they must be used and cleaned properly to reduce the risk of infection, according to the U.S. Food and Drug Administration.

These products are used to rinse the nasal passages with a salt-based solution and are a popular treatment for congested sinuses, colds and allergies, and for moistening nasal passages exposed to dry indoor air.

The most important factor in the safe use of nasal-rinsing devices is the water source. Tap water that is not filtered, treated or processed in specific ways is unsafe because it may contain bacteria or other organisms that can cause infections.

In 2011, two people in Louisiana died of a rare brain infection that may have been caused by improper use of neti pots, the FDA said in a consumer update reviewed by the agency.

Water that is safe to use in nasal-rinsing devices includes distilled or sterile water, which can be bought in stores. Or you can boil tap water for three to five minutes and then allow it to cool until it is lukewarm. You can store previously boiled water in a clean, closed container for use within 24 hours.

Another option is to pass water through a filter with an absolute pore size of 1 micron or smaller, which traps potentially infectious organisms. You can buy these filters online or at hardware stores. The U.S. Centers for Disease Control and Prevention has information about choosing a filter.

Wash and dry your hands before using a nasal-rinsing device, and check that it is clean and completely dry. Follow the manufacturer's directions for use. When you're done, wash the device with distilled, sterile or boiled and cooled tap water, and then dry the inside with a paper towel or let it air dry, the FDA recommends.

If a doctor recommends it, nasal-rinsing devices can be used on children as young as age two, according to the agency. Very young children, however, might not tolerate the procedure as well.

Before using a nasal-rinsing device, talk to your doctor to determine if it will be safe and effective for your condition. If your symptoms worsen or do not improve, go back to your doctor, especially if you experience fever, nosebleed or headache while using a nasal-rinsing device, the FDA advised.

info For more information on sinus problems, visit the American Academy of Otolaryngology—Head & Neck Surgery website at *http://www.entnet.org/HealthInformation/sinuses.cfm.*

Memory Loss from Antihistamines

Malaz Boustani, MD, MPH, associate director, Indiana University Center for Aging Research, Indianapolis.

Drug-induced memory loss may occur after just 60 days of antihistamine use. These anticholinergic drugs are in a class of medication that also includes many blood thinners, antidepressants and medications used for overactive bladder, heart disease and chronic obstructive pulmonary disease.

In a recent study of 3,690 adults, those who took a daily dose of a strong anticholinergic drug, such as *diphenhydramine* (Benadryl), for 60 days had mild cognitive impairment, including memory loss.

If you regularly take an anticholinergic: Talk to your doctor about switching to a different drug. *Cetirizine* (Zyrtec) has far fewer anticholinergic side effects and can be used for allergies.

Children in the US Are More Prone to Allergies Than Those Outside the US

American children born outside the US are 48% less likely to have asthma, eczema, hay fever, food allergies and other allergic conditions than American children born in the US.

And: Foreign-born children who live in the US for 10 years or more are more than three times as likely to have allergies as similar children living in the US for two years or less.

Study of 80,000 children by researchers at St. Luke's-Roosevelt Hospital Center, New York City, published online in *JAMA Pediatrics*.

How to Survive an Asthma Attack Without an Inhaler

Richard Firshein, DO, board-certified in family medicine and certified medical acupuncturist and founder and director of The Firshein Center for Comprehensive Medicine, New York City. He is author of *Reversing Asthma: Breathe Easier with This Revolutionary New Program* (Grand Central Publishing).

If you have asthma, then you know how scary it can be when you have an attack and have trouble breathing for anywhere from a few minutes to a few days, depending on its severity.

So you're probably careful to keep your rescue inhaler with you at all times—in case of an emergency.

But what happens if an attack starts and you discover that your inhaler is empty or you don't actually have it?

How can you lessen the severity of an asthma attack and/or stop it altogether without your trusty inhaler?

To find out, we spoke with Richard Firshein, DO, director and founder of The Firshein Center for Comprehensive Medicine in New York City and author of *Reversing Asthma: Breathe Easier with This Revolutionary New Program. And he had some very interesting advice...*

DO YOU NEED TO GO TO THE ER?

First off, quickly determine whether you're in immediate danger, said Dr. Firshein. If you have a peak-flow meter—a device that measures how much air you can expel from your lungs and that many asthmatics keep around the house—use it. If you're less than 25% off your normal mark, go on to the following steps, but if your number is off by more, get to an emergency room, he said, because this indicates that there is a serious problem—one that could be life-threatening, he said. If you don't have a peak-flow meter, then think about your symptoms. For example, if your lips or fingernails turn blue...if you can't stop coughing...if you feel soreness or tightness around the ribs...if you feel like you're having a panic attack...or if you're so exhausted from the effort of breathing that you can't finish a short sentence or stand up, then you need help fast—get to an ER.

HOW TO BREATHE EASIER

If you're not in immediate danger, try the following tricks from Dr. Firshein. Some of these techniques may help within minutes, while others may take a few hours to kick in, but since it's possible for an attack to last for days, try all of them to play it safe. During a typical asthma attack, the airways are constricted, muscles all over your body become tense and your body produces extra mucus—all of those things make it harder to breathe. So Dr. Firshein's advice addresses all of those problems. You know your body best, so if you try all of these tips but your attack still gets worse, go to a hospital.

- **Change your location.** Asthma is typically triggered by an irritant—either an allergen or toxin—that inflames the airways. So remove yourself from the environment that contains the trigger (if you know what it is) as fast as you can. If you're reacting to dust, pets, mold or smoke, for example, get away from it...or at the very least, breathe through a sleeve, a scarf or your jacket collar to reduce your exposure.

- **Tell someone.** Talking to someone may reduce your anxiety, and that's especially helpful, because anxiety can make your asthma attack worse. Also, if your asthma attack becomes more severe later on, you may need a ride to the hospital, so it's always good to keep someone else in the loop.

Also consider taking an over-the-counter decongestant (such as *pseudoephedrine*/Sudafed) and/or an expectorant (such as *guaifenesin*/Mucinex) or a drug that's a combination of the two (*ephedrine+guaifenesin*/Primatene Asthma), because these loosen mucus and make coughs more productive so you can rid your body of more phlegm.

- **Sip hot coffee or nonherbal tea.** Have one or two cups right away (but no more than that in one sitting, or your heart rate might spike too high—this is true among all people, not just asthmatics). Caffeine is metabolized into *theophylline,* which is also a drug that's used to prevent and treat asthma by relaxing the airways and decreasing the lungs' response to irritants. Getting caffeine from any source (a soda, an energy drink, a supplement, etc.) will likely help, but tea and coffee have other compounds that act similarly to caffeine (plus, liquids—especially hot liquids—help loosen mucus), so getting your caffeine in this form is best.

- **Practice breathing exercises.** Many people panic when they have an asthma attack and start breathing quickly, but that only restricts the amount of oxygen that the lungs get—in other words, it makes the attack worse. So breathe in through your nose to the count of four and then out to the count of six. Pursing your lips as you exhale will help slow the exhalation and keep the airways open longer. Continue breathing this way for as long as you need.

- **Press on some acupressure points.** The front parts of your inner shoulders (just above the armpits) and the outer edges of the creases of your elbows (when your elbows are bent) are "lung points." Pressing on one area at a time for a few consecutive minutes may relax muscles that have tightened up.

- **Steam things up.** Take a hot shower or stay in the bathroom with the hot water running from the showerhead or tub or sink faucet. Steam or warm moisture is better than cold moisture because it loosens mucus, so using a cool-air humidifier, although helpful, is not ideal.

- **Ask your doctor about taking magnesium and vitamin C.** Taking 500 milligrams (mg) of magnesium and 1,000 mg of vitamin C during an asthma attack may help if you're an adult. (Children ages 10 to 17 should take half the doses and children between the ages of five and nine should take one-third of the doses.) Magnesium is a bronchodilator that relaxes the

Pollen Will Nearly Double

By the year 2040, the amount of environmental pollen will nearly double.

Also: Pollen production will begin and peak earlier each year due to climate change.

Study by researchers in the department of environmental prediction at Rutgers School of Environmental and Biological Sciences, New Brunswick, New Jersey, presented at a recent meeting of the American College of Allergy, Asthma & Immunology in Anaheim, California.

breathing tubes, and vitamin C has a slight antihistamine effect.

•**Take medications.** The prescription corticosteroid *prednisone*, available in pill form, is used only for acute problems, such as during an attack, because it helps reduce inflammation—so if your doctor has already prescribed it to you and you have it on hand, use it. "This medication will not work as quickly as an inhaler, but it may prevent the problem from getting out of hand if you're having a lengthy attack," said Dr. Firshein. Just call your doctor and let him or her know that you're taking it, so your doctor can supervise your dosing.

Fight Colds the Way Performers Do

Len Horovitz, MD, an internist, a pulmonary specialist and director of Carnegie Medical PC, a private practice in New York City. *New York Magazine* has included him among "The Best Doctors in New York" for both pulmonary and internal medicine. He is a contributor to the medical anthology *The Singer's Guide to Complete Health* (Oxford University).

When you catch a cold, the sneezing, runny nose, sore throat and coughing will most likely make you feel miserable for a week or so, yet you probably manage to go about your business.

But what if you were an opera singer or a Broadway actor and started sniffling a few days before opening night? Or a politician or a preacher? For these so-called "voice professionals" (individuals whose jobs require the use of their voices), a cold wreaks havoc on their ability to work. They can take cortisone (an anti-inflammatory steroid) to quickly relieve laryngitis, but congestion and other symptoms don't give up so easily.

As it turns out, there are a number of effective, unique therapies that voice pros use to prevent and treat colds and related illnesses...

COLDS

The average American catches two to four colds a year. Avoiding the common cold involves well-known precautions such as getting enough rest, drinking plenty of fluids, eating a nutritious diet and frequent hand-washing. But these don't always work.

For voice pros, if a cold or related illness does develop, they must deal with it before it gets bad enough to affect their ability to work.

Their secrets...

•**Slippery elm tea.** Derived from the inner bark of the slippery elm tree, this traditional remedy eases coughs and sore throat pain. The bark contains mucilage, a substance that becomes slick and gel-like when mixed with water. It's a highly effective remedy for coating and soothing the throat.

To make this tea: Pour two cups of boiling water over about two tablespoons of powdered bark. Steep for five minutes and drink. Do this several times a day.

Or try slippery elm lozenges.

•**Lots of black pepper.** It's an expectorant that quickly thins mucus to reduce congestion. Add generous amounts to your meals whenever possible until you've gotten over your stuffy nose.

•**Fruit smoothies.** These tasty drinks will replenish lost fluids, and the antioxidants may even help you recover from a cold more quickly.

What to do: Once or twice a day, blend fruits—such as pineapple, blueberries and/or bananas—with a cup or two of fruit juice and

---

Caffeine Can Stop Mild Asthma

Mild asthma symptoms sometimes can be relieved by drinking coffee, cola or other caffeinated beverages. The drinks may produce a modest improvement in lung function that lasts up to four hours. Caffeinated beverages may not work as quickly as albuterol or other rapid-acting medications—but they are less likely to cause anxiety or other side effects.

Caution: If you experience severe tightness or wheezing, don't rely on caffeine. Use your inhaler instead.

Stephen J. Apaliski, MD, allergist and immunologist, Allergy & Asthma Centres of the Metroplex, Arlington, Texas, and author of *Beating Asthma: Seven Simple Principles* (Salveo Media).

A Surprising Cause of Hoarseness

If you're hoarse, but it's not due to a cold or overuse of your voice (as is often the case with singers, politicians, preachers and sports fans), there may be another cause—and it's often overlooked. Laryngopharyngeal reflux (LPR) is a condition in which stomach acid backs up into the larynx or throat (pharynx). It's similar to what happens with heartburn—but without the typical "burn" in the chest. *What to do...*

• **Follow heartburn-prevention strategies.** The same steps that you follow to prevent heartburn—eating smaller meals... avoiding greasy, fatty foods...not eating within a few hours of going to bed...and raising the head of the bed a few inches—will also help prevent LPR.

• **Neutralize stomach acid.** Alginate is a compound that neutralizes acid and helps prevent it from surging out of the stomach. It is an active ingredient in heartburn products such as Gaviscon.

• **Try DGL.** Taken in pill or powder form before meals when you're feeling hoarse, deglycyrrhizinated licorice (DGL) helps prevent stomach acid from damaging the larynx. Drugs such as Prilosec have a similar effect, but they increase osteoporosis risk. DGL is a safer remedy.

some ice. Do not add anything else—the key is to get a potent shot of antioxidants and a lot of liquid. (If you have diabetes, be sure to check with your doctor before using this remedy, since fruit contains high amounts of natural sugar.)

• **Zinc.** Used within 24 hours after symptoms start, zinc lozenges can shorten the duration of a cold by at least a day. Use the lozenges until the cold is gone, but don't take more than four lozenges a day.

• **Vitamin C.** Throughout cold season, take 500 mg of vitamin C twice a day to prevent colds...or 1,000 mg twice a day to recover from a cold more quickly. (If you get diarrhea from this dose, reduce the amount you take accordingly.)

LARYNGITIS

Most colds clear up in a week or so, but they're sometimes followed by laryngitis, inflammation of the larynx (voice box) that can last for several weeks.

In addition to resting your voice as much as possible, try this...

• **Steam with eucalyptus oil.** Few remedies are better than steam and eucalyptus, a powerful decongestant, for quick relief of laryngitis.

What to do: After boiling a couple of cups of water in a saucepan, turn off the heat and add a few drops of eucalyptus oil (available at health-food stores). Lean over the pan with a towel draped over your head to trap the steam. Being careful not to burn yourself, breathe the steam for a few minutes, two to three times a day.

SORE THROAT

A sore throat is usually due to a viral infection. If the pain is not severe—and the soreness starts to go away within a few days—you probably won't need medical treatment. If the pain doesn't go away, or it seems to be getting worse, see your doctor to check for strep throat.

For a simple sore throat...

• **Gargle.** Use a salt–baking soda solution. The salt draws fluids from the tissues and reduces swelling and pain. Baking soda makes the gargle more soothing.

What to do: Add about one-half teaspoon each of salt and baking soda to one cup of warm water...and gargle for 30 to 60 seconds.

Important: Do not gargle with commercial antiseptic mouthwash. Even though it temporarily reduces bacteria in the mouth, it may damage mucous membranes in the throat and increase the risk for infection.

4 Secrets to Easier Breathing

Gerard J. Criner, MD, a professor of medicine and director of pulmonary and critical care medicine at Temple Lung Center at Temple University School of Medicine in Philadelphia. He is codirector of the Center for Inflammation, Translational and Clinical Lung Research.

If you find it difficult to breathe, walking, climbing stairs or simply carrying on a conversation can be a challenge.

When breathing is a struggle, you wouldn't think that exercise is the answer. But it can be a solution for people with chronic obstructive pulmonary disease (COPD) or heart failure or even for healthy people who occasionally become short of breath.*

Four better-breathing techniques that really help...

PURSED-LIP BREATHING

When you're feeling short of breath, inhale through your nose for two seconds, then pucker your lips as if you were going to whistle or blow out a candle. Exhale through pursed lips for four seconds.

How it helps: It prolongs the respiratory cycle and gives you more time to empty your lungs. This is particularly important if you have emphysema. With emphysema, air gets trapped in the lungs. The trapped air causes the lungs to overinflate, which reduces the amount of force that they're able to generate. This results in a buildup of carbon dioxide that makes it difficult to breathe.

You may need to do this only when you're more active than usual and short of breath. Or you may breathe better when you do it often.

CHANGING POSITIONS

Simply changing how you stand or sit can improve breathing when you're feeling winded.

*If you don't have COPD, you should see a doctor if you have shortness of breath after only slight activity or while resting, or if shortness of breath wakes you up at night or requires you to sleep propped up to breathe.

When to Get Breathing Help from a Professional

You can do many breathing exercises on your own without the help of a health professional. For the techniques below, however, it's best to first consult a respiratory therapist (ask your doctor for a referral) to ensure that you know how to do the exercise properly. You can then continue on your own.

- **Paced breathing for endurance.** This technique is useful for people who have COPD and/or heart failure, since it improves lung capacity and heart function.

How it helps: With practice, this technique can increase your cardiorespiratory endurance by 30% to 40%. To perform the exercise, a metronome is set at a rate that's faster than your usual respiratory rate. Your therapist will encourage you to breathe as hard and as fast as you can for, say, about 15 minutes. (Beginners might do it for only a few minutes at a time.)

Example: The metronome may be set for 20 breaths per minute to start, and you may eventually work up to 40 breaths per minute.

You'll notice that breathing becomes easier when you're doing various activities—for instance, when you're exercising, climbing stairs or taking brisk walks.

- **Inspiratory muscle training.** Think of this as a workout for your breathing muscles. It is especially helpful for people with COPD or other lung diseases and those recovering from respiratory failure. People who strengthen these muscles can improve their breathing efficiency by 25% to 30%.

How it helps: For this breathing exercise, you'll use a device known as an inspiratory muscle trainer, which includes a mouthpiece, a one-way valve and resistance settings. When you inhale, the one-way valve closes. You're forced to use effort to breathe against resistance. Then, the valve opens so that you can exhale normally. This breathing exercise is typically performed for 15 minutes twice a day. You can buy these devices online.

Good choice: The Threshold Inspiratory Muscle Trainer, available at FitnessMart.com for $47.50.

How it helps: Certain positions (see below) help muscles around the diaphragm work more efficiently to promote easier breathing.

Examples: While sitting, lean your chest forward...rest your elbows on your knees...and relax your upper-body muscles. When standing, bend forward at the waist and rest your hands on a table or the back of a chair. Or back up to a wall...support yourself with your hips...and lean forward and put your hands on your thighs.

CONTROLLED COUGHING

Your lungs produce excessive mucus when you have COPD. The congestion makes it harder to breathe. It also increases the risk for pneumonia and other lung infections. A normal, explosive cough is not effective at removing mucus. In fact, out-of-control coughing can cause airways to collapse and trap even more mucus. A controlled cough is more effective (and requires less oxygen and energy). You also can use this technique to help clear mucus from the lungs when you have a cold.

How to do it: Sit on a chair or the edge of your bed with both feet on the floor. Fold your arms around your midsection...breathe in slowly through your nose...then lean forward while pressing your arms against your abdomen. Lightly cough two or three times. Repeat as needed.

Important: Taking slow, gentle breaths through your nose while using this technique will prevent mucus from moving back into the airways.

COLD-AIR ASSISTANCE

This is a quick way to breathe better. When you are short of breath—or doing an activity that you know will lead to breathlessness, such as walking on a treadmill—position a fan so that it blows cool air on your face. You also can splash your face with cold water if you become short of breath.

How it helps: Cool air and water stimulate the trigeminal nerve in the face, which slows respiration and helps ease shortness of breath. That's why the treadmills and exercise bikes used in respiratory-rehabilitation facilities are often equipped with small fans.

New Device Reduces Lung Congestion

The FDA has approved the Lung Flute, which can be used by people with chronic obstructive pulmonary disease (COPD) or asthma to help clear mucus from the airways.

How it works: When the patient blows into the flute, sound waves travel down the airway, mobilizing mucus and making it easier to expel. The sound is inaudible, but patients see the reed flap and hear it hit the interior of the flute. The device should be used for five to 15 minutes twice daily.

If you suffer from COPD or asthma: Ask your doctor about the Lung Flute. Some insurance providers will cover the $45 cost.

Sanjay Sethi, MD, professor of medicine, University at Buffalo School of Medicine and Biomedical Sciences, New York.

COPD-Linked Brain Danger

Lies Lahousse, PhD, PharmD, researcher, Ghent University Hospital, Belgium.

Among 810 people over age 55, those with the common condition chronic obstructive pulmonary disease (COPD) were nearly 45% more likely to have cerebral microbleeds, or episodes of bleeding in the brain, than those with normal lung function. Damage in small brain vessels can lead to cognitive decline and disability.

Theory: The increased inflammation and/or reduced oxygen in COPD patients may cause blood vessel damage.

If you have COPD: Talk to your doctor about lowering your risk for microbleeds with steps such as reducing hypertension.

Long-Term Use of Antibiotic May Help Those With COPD

Victoria Richards, PhD, assistant professor, medical sciences, Frank H. Netter, MD, School of Medicine, Quinnipiac University, Hamden, Connecticut.

Len Horovitz, MD, pulmonary specialist, Lenox Hill Hospital, New York City.

Fernando Martinez, MD, MS, director of pulmonary diagnostic services, University of Michigan Health System, Ann Arbor.

News release, American Thoracic Society annual meeting, Philadelphia.

Thousands of Americans, many of them smokers or ex-smokers, suffer from the lung condition known as chronic obstructive pulmonary disease (COPD). Now a recent study finds that patients placed on the common antibiotic *azithromycin* may be able to cut down on hospitalizations due to flare-ups of the disease.

COPD is a progressive disease involving bronchitis and emphysema that affects the ability to breathe. The condition is often associated with smoking.

"Given that exacerbations of COPD can be life-threatening, prevention of such events is critical," said Victoria Richards, PhD, assistant professor of medical science at Quinnipiac University in Hamden, Connecticut. Use of the antibiotic might also cut down on the need for doctor's office visits and boost patients' quality of life, said Dr. Richards, who was not involved in the study.

STUDY DETAILS

In the recent study, researchers compared how patients fared on a 12-month regimen of the drug versus patients who were given a dummy medication.

"COPD patients who have been hospitalized for a respiratory event are at particularly high risk for re-hospitalization," said lead study author Fernando Martinez, MD, MS, in a meeting news release.

"We wanted to examine whether chronic azithromycin therapy might provide a benefit in these patients," said Dr. Martinez, who is director of pulmonary diagnostic services at the University of Michigan Health System, in Ann Arbor.

To assess treatment effectiveness, the researchers looked at data from a prior study conducted by the COPD Clinical Research Network.

Patients in that study had either suffered a so-called "acute exacerbation" of COPD in the year leading up to the study or were using supplemental oxygen at the beginning of the study.

For one year the patients randomly were assigned to receive either a daily dose of 250 milligrams of azithromycin or a placebo.

The result: Compared with the placebo group, patients taking the antibiotic were able to benefit from longer gaps between hospitalizations.

"We found that there was a significant delay from the first respiratory-related hospitalization to the next one among those treated with azithromycin," Dr. Martinez said. He said the finding also held for re-hospitalizations that were due to any cause, not just respiratory issues.

The research was presented at the annual meeting of the American Thoracic Society in Philadelphia.

EXPERT RESPONSE

One expert said the findings warrant further investigation, but pointed out that the history of

You Don't Have to Be Overweight to Have Sleep Apnea

The chronic condition—which involves shallow or missed breaths during sleep—is most common in people whose airways are partially blocked by fat tissue.

However: It can occur in thin people who have narrow jaws or throats, as well as women in midlife whose throat muscles have weakened. If you suspect sleep apnea, talk to your doctor. Sleep apnea is associated with heart problems and other complications.

Julia Schlam Edelman, MD, clinical instructor at Harvard Medical School, Boston, and a gynecologist in private practice in Middleboro, Massachusetts. She is author of *Successful Sleep Strategies for Women* (Harvard Health).

antibiotic use in people with respiratory disease has had its ups and downs.

"A number of years ago, it was reported that Ketak, an antibiotic in the erythromycin family, was helpful in reducing exacerbations in asthma," said Len Horovitz, MD, a pulmonary specialist at Lenox Hill Hospital in New York City. "[However], there were other problems with this antibiotic, and it was discontinued."

He called the recent findings with azithromycin "promising," but added a caveat—"It was recently found that azithromycin is contraindicated in patients with cardiac arrhythmia, which [can] occur in COPD, so these factors must be viewed with caution."

For his part, Dr. Martinez said more research will need to be done to confirm the study results, and experts note that findings presented at medical meetings are typically considered preliminary until published in a peer-reviewed journal.

info Find out more information about COPD at the U.S. National Heart, Lung, and Blood Institute website at *http://www.nhlbi.nih.gov/health/health-topics/topics/copd/.*

Chest Implant Might Help With Hard-to-Treat Sleep Apnea

Patrick Strollo, MD, co-director, Sleep Medicine Institute, University of Pittsburgh, and director, UPMC Sleep Medicine Center.

Ryan Soose, MD, director, division of sleep surgery, UPMC.

William Kohler, MD, medical director, Florida Sleep Institute, Spring Hill, Florida.

New England Journal of Medicine

A new kind of implant may offer people suffering from sleep apnea an alternative to wearing an air mask while they snooze, researchers report.

With the implant, a pacemaker delivers electrical impulses to a nerve that controls the tongue and maintains the muscle tone of a sleeping person's upper airway, according to a study published in the *New England Journal of Medicine.*

These impulses reduced nightly sleep apnea events by about 68%, according to the results of the one-year clinical trial. Not surprisingly, patients reported a 40% improvement in their ability to stay awake during the day, the researchers added.

BACKGROUND ON SLEEP APNEA

Sleep apnea is a disorder in which a person's breathing pauses or grows shallow while they are asleep. The most common type is obstructive sleep apnea, in which the person's airway collapses or becomes blocked during sleep, according to the U.S. National Heart, Lung, and Blood Institute.

Left untreated, the condition disrupts sleep and causes a person to feel drowsy during the day. Long-term health consequences can include heart disease, insulin resistance and high cholesterol, said study author Patrick Strollo, MD, co-director of the Sleep Medicine Institute at the University of Pittsburgh and director of the university's Sleep Medicine Center.

Doctors most often treat obstructive sleep apnea by asking patients to use a continuous positive airway pressure (CPAP) machine while they sleep, said Dr. Strollo.

With CPAP, patients wear a nose and mouth mask attached to a pump, and the mild air

---

How CPAP Makes You Sexy

Adults with sleep apnea were assessed using precise 3-D facial analysis technology before and two months after consistent treatment with a continuous positive airway pressure (CPAP) device at night.

Result: Observers found that most participants looked more attractive (with less redness and puffiness), youthful and alert after CPAP treatment—probably because of improved cardiac function, which may help reduce excess fluid buildup at night.

If you look and feel tired during the day: Ask your doctor if you should be tested for sleep apnea.

Ronald Chervin, MD, director, University of Michigan Sleep Disorders Center, Ann Arbor.

---

pressure maintained by the pump keeps their airway from collapsing—much in the way that an air pump keeps an inflatable holiday lawn decoration from flopping over.

However, some patients can't sleep with the CPAP mask on or they find the air pressure uncomfortable, Dr. Strollo said.

"We always struggle in the field of sleep apnea to be able to effectively treat patients and present them with options," he said. "This represents a different option for patients that cannot tolerate CPAP."

STUDY DETAILS

In the clinical trial, 124 patients at 22 different hospitals in the United States and Europe were fitted with a pacemaker in their chest. The study was supported by the pacemaker's manufacturer, Inspire Medical Systems. The company also helped design the study alongside the researchers and regulators from the U.S. Food and Drug Administration.

With the device, an electrode runs from the pacemaker to the hypoglossal nerve located under the tongue. Another lead wire runs down to the muscles between the ribs of the chest and keeps track of the person's breathing.

The surgery is minimally invasive, and patients typically were back to regular activity within a day or two, said study coauthor Ryan Soose, MD, director of the division of sleep surgery at UPMC.

"It's a unique and promising new treatment," Dr. Soose said.

As the patient breathes in and out, the pacemaker sends electrical impulses to the nerve, which causes the person's tongue to move slightly forward and their upper airway to contract open. Both movements keep the airway from collapsing.

Patients only used the pacemaker during sleep, turning it on and off by waving a magnet over the implant.

"We found there was a very robust effect on sleep apnea," Dr. Strollo said. Patients experienced much fewer episodes of sleep apnea and received much more oxygen in their blood as a result.

The researchers also found that sleep apnea returned when patients were taken off the pacemaker treatment.

The technology also appears safe. It did no permanent damage to the patients' tongues, Dr. Strollo said, although two out of five patients did report some discomfort associated with the electrical stimulation.

A Food and Drug Administration panel reviewed findings from the clinical trial in February 2014. Inspire Therapy was approved by the FDA in May 2014.

EXPERT COMMENTARY

In an accompanying journal editorial, Atul Malhotra, MD, director of Sleep Medicine at the University of California, San Diego, noted that while the pacemaker appeared to reduce sleep apnea, it didn't eliminate it. He pointed out that the study lacked a comparison group, and that the results could have been due to other factors such as participants' diet or exercise.

A number of teams have been researching this technology, said William Kohler, MD, medical director of the Florida Sleep Institute. He was not involved with the recent study.

Dr. Kohler sees the pacemaker technology as an alternative to CPAP, rather than something that will supplant the air mask.

Blood Pressure Drugs Are Linked to Severe Oral Allergy Symptoms

Oral allergy syndrome is characterized by itching and/or swelling of the lips, mouth and throat after eating tree nuts, raw fruits or raw vegetables.

Problem: *Lisinopril* (Zestril), *quinapril* (Accupril) and other ACE inhibitor blood pressure drugs may trigger symptoms such as extreme facial swelling and/or difficulty breathing. See your doctor immediately. Do not stop taking the drug on your own.

Sunit Jariwala, MD, assistant professor of medicine at Albert Einstein College of Medicine, the Bronx, New York.

"This needs to be investigated as a treatment not in the first line, but if other treatments fail," Dr. Kohler said. "The more therapies we have out there, the better. But we need more experience with it to really see where it's going to fit as far as the overall treatment for sleep apnea goes."

info To learn more about sleep apnea, visit the U.S. National Heart, Lung, and Blood Institute at its website *http://www.nhlbi.nih.gov/health/health-topics/topics/sleepapnea/.*

Treating Sleep Apnea Helps Golfers

Journal of Clinical Sleep Medicine, news release.

Treating their sleep apnea improved middle-aged men's golf games, according to a small recent study.

"The degree of improvement was most substantial in the better golfers who have done a superior job of managing the technical and mechanical aspects of golf," said study lead author Marc Benton, MD, medical director of SleepWell Centers of New Jersey, in Madison.

According to the researchers, most avid golfers in the United States are men aged 40 to 70, which is a group with a high rate of sleep apnea.

STUDY DETAILS

Researchers looked at 12 men with an average age of 55 who had moderate to severe obstructive sleep apnea. The disorder is characterized by frequent episodes of disrupted breathing during sleep.

Their golf performance was assessed before and after up to six months of a sleep apnea treatment called continuous positive airway pressure (CPAP), which helps keep a person's airway open by providing a steady stream of air during sleep.

The therapy led to less daytime sleepiness and improved sleep-related quality of life. The men also had a significant 11% drop in their average golf handicap index, a formula used to estimate a player's skill level.

Among better golfers who had a handicap of 12 or less at the start of the study, the average handicap fell by almost 32% after CPAP treatment, according to the study, which was published in the *Journal of Clinical Sleep Medicine.*

The men attributed their improved golf performance to factors such as improved concentration, endurance and decision making.

info For more information on sleep apnea, visit the U.S. National Heart, Lung, and Blood Institute website, at *www.nhlbi.nih.gov/health/health-topics/topics/sleepapnea/.*

2 Bottom Line's HEALTH BREAKTHROUGHS

Brain Health

Best New Brain Boosters—Your Brain Can Improve at Any Age

Expecting crossword puzzles or any particular activity to give your brain a full workout is a bit like expecting bicep curls to tone your entire body. Our bodies need specific types of exercise to optimize results—and so do our brains.

Newest thinking: Researchers are now discovering that one of the most effective ways to maintain (or even improve) your brainpower is to tailor specific workouts to your age.

To find out more about the best ways to stay mentally sharp, we spoke with one of the country's leading neuroscientists, Sandra Bond Chapman, PhD.

DON'T DWELL ON YOUR MEMORY

When I talk to people about mental fitness, they almost always say that their main goal is to improve their memory. But virtually everyone is surprised to learn that the ability to remember facts has almost nothing to do with brain efficiency.

The ability to understand big ideas, extrapolate meaning and make sound decisions in real-life contexts is far more vital to effective brain performance than maintaining a repository of data. Unnecessary memorization wastes brain energy, depleting reserves better served for higher-order thinking. Fortunately, increasing higher-order thinking ability may naturally help improve your memory.

MENTAL FITNESS FOR LIFE

What exactly can you do to improve your mental fitness? Here are some regimens that are geared toward the changes your brain is undergoing as it ages.

Sandra Bond Chapman, PhD, a cognitive neuroscientist, founder and chief director of the Center for Brain Health and the Dee Wyly Distinguished University Chair at The University of Texas at Dallas. She is coauthor, with Shelly Kirkland, of *Make Your Brain Smarter: Increase Your Brain's Creativity, Energy, and Focus* (Simon & Schuster). *BrainHealth.utdallas.edu*

AGES 46 TO 65

Beginning in one's mid-40s, it's common to start losing the capacity to quickly process new information and store and retrieve data (such as a person's name). However, most people in the 46-to-65 age group are more adept at sorting through information efficiently and accurately discerning critical points to more quickly weigh facts than younger counterparts.

Best brain-boosting strategies if you're age 46 to 65...

•**Narrow your focus.** Multitasking isn't recommended for anyone, but particularly not for people in this age group. As you age, the capacity to rapidly switch from task to task (as occurs with multitasking) slows, adding to brain fatigue and reducing efficiency.

To keep the mind sharp: Pick one job—such as answering e-mails or planning a report—and take your time doing it. Making an effort to create meaningful responses and original content not only increases work quality and productivity but also flexes your brain.

•**Synthesize.** Not every detail is important, so don't let yourself get lost in a sea of information.

To keep the mind sharp: Gather enough information for the task at hand, then focus mainly on the key meanings. Applying internally generated novel ideas to affect an outcome boosts brain health.

Note: Don't feel insecure because your grasp of details may not be what it used to be. This can be a strength—it means that you're more likely to see the bigger picture.

AGES 66 AND OLDER

You may notice increasing incidences of memory glitches, but it is probably not as dramatic as you think. People tend to notice when they forget a few minor details, such as the name of the movie they saw last month. They don't consider the tens of thousands of details that they didn't forget.*

Try to nourish your brain by putting accumulated knowledge and wisdom to work. Deep thinking and disciplined use of brainpower helps fine-tune brain resources for optimal performance.

*If problems with memory or decision-making begin to interfere with daily life, such as completing household tasks, consult your doctor.

Best brain-boosting strategies if you're age 66 or older...

•**Get off autopilot.** At this age, you are especially at risk for slipping into autopilot—a dangerous state, since a bored brain is going backward.

To keep the mind sharp: Continue to push yourself to learn something new, especially if it's related to technology, which can help build new connections in the brain. You will feel energized as you go from being a novice to an expert in an area of interest.

•**Stay challenged.** The problem with crossword puzzles and other brain teasers is that they get easier with practice. People who do crosswords get better mainly at crosswords, and the gains generally don't translate into other high-level mental areas.

To keep the mind sharp: Take on real challenges that you are motivated to master. Forcing yourself to learn a new language just to exercise your brain will not produce the same far-reaching cognitive benefits as honing a foreign language for practical use, such as for a trip. The brain expands and develops new pathways when it's pushed to explore unfamiliar areas.

FORTIFYING YOUNGER BRAINS

Adults who are under age 45 tend to be very comfortable with collecting facts—but they often are less confident than they could be when dealing with abstract concepts and making decisions. *How people in this age group can improve their brain performance...*

•**Don't get distracted.** Younger adults have a tremendous ability to memorize, but they're typically poor at choosing what they need to remember. Most people will function just fine if they ignore about 50% of the information that comes their way.

Helpful: Focus on accomplishing your top two or three priorities for the day without letting distractions, such as constant text, e-mail and social media alerts, disrupt your progress.

•**Zoom out.** When every fact in the world is a click away, our brains often get stuck regurgitating facts and blindly following directions.

Helpful: When you're reading for knowledge (not for entertainment), skim the material quickly...find the takeaway message...and then condense it to a succinct thought. Translating new information into your own words increases comprehension and helps you achieve new perspectives that can inspire your brain to generate new ideas and solutions.

Don't Let Your Brain Shrink

Daniel G. Amen, MD, a brain-imaging specialist and assistant clinical professor of psychiatry and human behavior at the University of California, Irvine, School of Medicine. He is the founder, CEO and medical director of The Amen Clinics and author of several books, including *Use Your Brain to Change Your Age: Secrets to Look, Feel, and Think Younger Every Day* (Harmony).

When scientists talk about memory and learning, the hippocampus, a small, seahorse-shaped structure located deep inside the brain, gets most of the credit for these vital cognitive functions.

What you don't hear much about: The prefrontal cortex (PFC), a much larger part of the brain located just behind and slightly beneath the forehead. Known as the "executive" part of the brain because it controls judgment, insights and impulse control, the PFC is just as important when it comes to staying sharp mentally, learning new information and controlling processes involved in memory.

Unfortunately, millions of Americans don't follow simple lifestyle habits that promote optimal functioning of the PFC.

Result: Lapses in judgment (such as making risky maneuvers when driving)...disorganized thinking (including an inability to prioritize tasks)...shorter attention spans (resulting in difficulty with reading and other activities that require focus)...and impairments in learning and memory.

IMPROVE YOUR BRAIN—LIVE LONGER

The PFC needs good "fuel" to thrive. That's why people with healthful habits tend to have a larger PFC than those who don't take good care of themselves. As a result, they're more likely to live longer (because their judgment about risks is better), and they're less likely to develop Alzheimer's disease.

Important findings: A 2007 study of Catholic nuns and priests found that those who had the most self-discipline were 89% less likely to develop Alzheimer's disease. Self-discipline is one of the traits that is enhanced when you have a robust PFC.

POWER UP YOUR "WIRING"

People with healthful habits have less damage to myelin, the fatty coating on brain cells, than people who are less conscientious about their health. Brain cells that are sheathed in myelin work 10 to 100 times faster than unmyelinated cells. People with healthful habits also tend to have better blood circulation in the brain, which improves thinking as well as memory.

To protect your PFC—and other key parts of the brain...

•**Rethink your alcohol intake.** Millions of Americans drink a glass or two of red wine a day because it's good for the heart. But the cardio-protective properties of alcohol—it raises HDL "good" cholesterol and reduces clots, thus reducing the risk for a heart attack—may be offset by the damage it can do to the brain. Alcohol decreases the size and functioning of the PFC. What's more, even moderate drinking (two drinks daily for men and one for women) can impair brain circulation.

My advice: If your doctor agrees that you can forgo the cardiovascular benefits of drinking wine, limit your intake to no more than two or three alcoholic beverages per week.

•**"Water" your brain.** The brain is 80% water. People who don't drink enough water or who drink a lot of dehydrating liquids, such as alcohol or caffeinated coffee or tea, often have impairments in cognition and judgment, which can occur when the PFC is damaged.

My advice: Drink plenty of water—eight glasses (64 ounces) of water every day is typically sufficient. If you like, add a splash of lemon or lime juice for flavor.

•**Slow down on the omega-6s.** Most Americans get far too many inflammation-promoting omega-6 essential fatty acids in their diets—primarily from cooking oils (such as corn and vegetable), fatty red meats and processed foods—that are harmful to the brain. That's why a plant-based, anti-inflammatory diet is among the most effective ways to reduce damage to the PFC and other areas of the brain.

My advice: Eat lots of greens—including salads—along with vegetables, fruit, whole grains and legumes. Approximately three servings of lean protein daily will help balance blood sugar and keep you feeling sharp. Also, eat at least three servings weekly of cold-water fish such as salmon, mackerel and sardines. The omega-3s in these fish have potent anti-inflammatory effects. Fish oil supplements (1 g to 3 g daily) are also helpful. Check with your doctor first if you use a blood thinner.

Aim to change your diet so that your intake of omega-6 fatty acids is no more than three times higher than your intake of omega-3s.

Good rule of thumb: A plant-based diet that's high in fish provides the ideal 3:1 (or lower) ratio of omega-6s to omega-3s.

•**Try green tea and rhodiola.** Distractibility, disorganization and poor impulse control are commonly associated with children who may be suffering from attention-deficit/hyperactivity disorder (ADHD), but many adults (who may or may not have ADHD) also struggle with such symptoms.

Often linked to low activity in the PFC, these symptoms can be reversed, in part, with green tea and rhodiola, a plant-based supplement frequently used as an energy booster. In one study, researchers at my clinic did brain scans before and after giving patients green tea and rhodiola. Two months later, scans showed a significant increase in circulation in the PFC.

How it helps: Green tea appears to benefit the PFC by increasing the availability of dopamine, a brain chemical that controls the brain's reward and pleasure centers. It also helps regulate emotional responses, such as the motivation to take positive actions. Rhodiola is an "adaptogen," a substance that normalizes the body's functions by boosting blood flow to the brain and raising dopamine and serotonin levels.

My advice: Take 200 mg of rhodiola and drink two to three cups of green tea daily (avoid drinking it in the evening since the tea's caffeine can interfere with sleep...or drink decaffeinated green tea).

•**Keep your BMI in check.** People who are overweight—with a body mass index (BMI) of 25 or higher—have less circulation in the PFC than those of normal weights. Excess body weight is associated with atherosclerosis, diabetes and other conditions that impede circulation throughout the body.

Danger: A high BMI can cause the brain to shrink. Research has shown that people who are obese typically have about 8% less brain tissue than normal-weight adults.

My advice: At least once a year, check your BMI by using an online calculator, such as the National Heart, Lung and Blood Institute's *www.nhlbi.nih.gov/guidelines/obesity/BMI/bmicalc.htm.* A BMI of 18.5 to 24.9 is considered normal. If your BMI is 25 or higher, you need to lose weight.

•**Don't ignore sleep problems.** An estimated 18 million Americans have sleep apnea, a condition in which breathing intermittently stops during sleep. Unfortunately, the condition is undiagnosed in most of these people.

Why does this matter? Scans on patients with sleep apnea show brain changes that resemble early Alzheimer's disease. Poor sleep decreases blood flow to the PFC and other parts of the brain. Snoring, daytime fatigue and morning headaches are common symptoms of sleep apnea. Your doctor may recommend tests in a sleep laboratory.

My advice: If you're overweight, sleep apnea can often be reduced or even eliminated with weight loss. Many patients also benefit from continuous positive airway pressure (CPAP) units, which help keep the airways open during sleep.

Also important: Avoid sleepless nights. Patients with chronic insomnia have a higher risk for cognitive declines than people who sleep well. To prevent insomnia, follow the tried-and-true strategies—relax in a warm bath before bed...reduce arousal by not watching TV or using a computer in the hour before bedtime... and go to bed and wake up at the same times every day.

Also helpful: Melatonin. The standard dose of this sleep hormone supplement is 1 mg to 6 mg taken a half hour before bed. Start with the lower dose and increase it over a period of weeks, if necessary.

Check with your doctor first if you take an antidepressant, blood pressure medication, blood thinner, steroid or nonsteroidal anti-inflammatory drug—melatonin may interact with these medications.

Get These Minerals Out of Your Brain!

Neal D. Barnard, MD, president of the nonprofit Physicians Committee for Responsible Medicine, a Washington, DC–based group that promotes preventive medicine. He is author of *Power Foods for the Brain: An Effective 3-Step Plan to Protect Your Mind and Strengthen Your Memory* (Grand Central Life & Style). *PCRM.org*

Chances are you're doing everything that you can to eat plenty of "superfoods"—blueberries, walnuts and other nutritious and antioxidant-rich wonders—that many scientists believe help reduce risk for a variety of chronic health problems, including Alzheimer's disease.

The missing part of the story: What you may not know is that most people get too much of certain nutrients—even those found in some superfoods—that have long been considered an important part of a nutritious diet.

Iron, copper and zinc, which are widely recognized as key nutrients, actually are metallic minerals. They are common in many of the foods you may be eating, the water you drink—and even in some of the supplements you may be taking to improve your health.

What researchers are now discovering: Excessive amounts of iron, copper and zinc can produce free radicals that impair memory.

In fact, scientists have discovered that these metals are more prevalent in the brains of Alzheimer's patients than in people without the disease. Even in healthy adults, high levels appear to interfere with normal brain functions.

THREE NEWLY DISCOVERED DANGERS

Your body does need iron, copper and zinc, but only in miniscule amounts. If you exceed these levels, your brain is at risk. *What to watch out for...*

•**Iron.** Unless you have been diagnosed with a condition that requires supplemental iron, such as anemia, you probably don't need more than you're already getting from your diet—and even that might be too much.

Compelling evidence: In a study of 793 adults, those who had the most iron in their blood did worse on cognitive tests than those with normal levels.

In a study of 881 adults, those with high hemoglobin levels (a measure of iron in the blood) were three times more likely to develop Alzheimer's disease than those with normal levels. Hemoglobin levels above 13.7 g/dL were associated with increased Alzheimer's risk. Those whose iron levels are too low are also at risk for Alzheimer's.

My advice: Emphasize plant-based foods in your diet. These foods contain as much or more iron than what's found in meat—but our bodies are better able to regulate our intake of the type of iron found in plant-based foods, such as spinach, dried apricots, lima beans and wheat germ. Your body absorbs more of this nonheme iron when you need it and absorbs less when you don't.

In contrast, the heme iron in meats, poultry, fish and shellfish (particularly oysters) is absorbed whether you need it or not. Because of this, a high-meat diet is a main cause of iron overload, which potentially damages not only your brain but also your heart.

Other smart steps...

•Don't use iron cookware. A significant amount of iron leaches from uncoated cast-iron pots, pans and skillets into foods—particularly acidic foods, such as tomatoes.

•Choose an iron-free product if you take a daily multisupplement.

What About Aluminum?

This ubiquitous metal has never been considered a nutrient—it plays no role in the body. While questions have persisted for several years about whether aluminum interferes with brain health, recent studies suggest that the risk is real.

In the UK, researchers found that Alzheimer's cases occurred 50% more often in counties with high aluminum levels in the water. Other studies have had similar results.

My advice: While researchers search for definitive findings on aluminum, err on the side of caution...

- **Don't buy foods that contain aluminum.** Check food labels. Cheese products (such as the cheese on frozen pizza) often contain aluminum. So do baking powders and the baked goods that include them. You can buy an aluminum-free baking powder, such as the Rumford brand.
- **Don't take aluminum antacids.** Use an aluminum-free product, such as Tums. Other drugs, such as buffered aspirin, may also contain aluminum. Check the label.
- **Cook with steel-clad or porcelain-coated pots...**use wax paper instead of aluminum foil...and don't consume foods or beverages that come in aluminum cans.
- **Check your tap water.** If it's high in aluminum or other metals, use bottled water or a reverse osmosis filter. You can use the EPA Web site, *EPA.gov/enviro/facts/sdwis/*, to get information about the water sources in your area.
- **Avoid antiperspirants with aluminum.** Labels may say aluminum or alum to indicate an aluminum-containing ingredient.

- Read cereal labels. Many breakfast cereals are fortified with iron. You don't need it.

Amount of iron you need in your diet: 8 mg per day for men age 19 and older and women age 51 and older. Women age 19 to 50 need 18 mg per day. (In general, women should get the lower amount of iron when they stop menstruating.)

- **Copper.** At proper levels, copper is essential for enzyme function and helps promote heart health and bone strength. At excess levels, copper—like iron—triggers the production of free radicals that can damage brain cells.

Important finding: A study of 1,451 people in southern California found that those who had the least copper in their blood were mentally sharper and had fewer problems with long- and short-term memory than those whose levels were high.

How copper may promote almost 20 years of aging: When high copper levels are combined with excess saturated fat in the diet—another risk factor for brain problems—the effect is particularly detrimental. Data from the Chicago Health and Aging Project found that high copper/saturated fat caused a loss of mental function that was the equivalent of 19 years of aging.

My advice: Don't take any supplement that contains copper. If you have copper plumbing, it's fine to use tap water for doing dishes and washing but not for cooking or drinking. It is better to use bottled water or water filtered with an activated carbon filter (such as those found in Brita pitchers).

You are unlikely to get too much copper from plant foods that are rich in the mineral such as whole grains, nuts and beans because they also contain natural compounds called *phytates* that limit copper absorption.

Amount of copper you need: 0.9 mg daily.

- **Zinc.** Our bodies need adequate zinc levels for key functions such as immunity, skin health and sexual function. Excessive amounts, however, are thought to promote the clumping of beta-amyloid proteins in the brain—the hallmark of Alzheimer's disease.

Much of the excess zinc in the American diet comes from supplements. If you take a multivitamin-mineral supplement and also eat fortified cereals or other foods that include zinc, such as oysters, pumpkin seeds or cocoa, you could be getting too much.

Amount of zinc you need: 11 mg daily for men and 8 mg for women.

TAKEAWAY ON MINERALS

Testing is not needed to check levels of iron, copper and zinc in your blood. It is wise to simply avoid the mineral sources in this article.

If you are getting too much of these minerals, your levels will gradually decline when you avoid excessive intakes.

Important: Avoid multivitamin-mineral supplements.

Better choices: "Vitamin only" supplements such as No Minerals Multi-Vitamin by Nature's Blend or Vitamins Only by Solgar.

5 Best Brain-Boosting Drinks

David Grotto, RD, a registered dietitian and founder and president of Nutrition Housecall, LLC, an Elmhurst, Illinois–based nutrition consulting firm. He is an adviser to *Fitness* magazine and blogs for the Real Life Nutrition community featured on WebMD. He is author of *The Best Things You Can Eat* (Da Capo Lifelong).

Some of the easiest-to-prepare brain foods—meaning foods that can preserve and even improve your memory and other cognitive functions—are actually delicious drinks.

You probably already know about green tea, which is high in epigallocatechin-3-gallate (EGCG), a potent compound that appears to protect neurons from age-related damage. *But the following five drinks are scientifically proven to help your brain, too...*

BEET JUICE

Beets are a nutritional powerhouse—and so is the juice. It increases levels of nitric oxide, a blood gas that improves blood flow. How does that help your brain? Your brain needs good blood flow to function optimally.

A recent study looked at brain scans of participants before and after they drank beet juice. The post-beverage scans showed an increase in circulation to the brain's white matter in the frontal lobes—a part of the brain that's often damaged in people with dementia.

You can buy ready-made beet juice at health-food stores, although it's much less expensive to make your own with fresh beets (include the root and greens, which are nutritious as well).

Beet juice has a naturally sweet taste, but you may want to add a little apple juice or another fruit juice—both for flavor and to make the mixture more pourable.

BERRY SMOOTHIES

Acai, a South American fruit that reduces inflammation, is ranked near the top of brain-healthy foods because it dilates blood vessels and increases blood flow.

Its juice has a pleasant taste—something like a cross between raspberry and cocoa—but it's very expensive (typically $30 or more for a quart).

What I recommend: Blend a variety of everyday frozen berries that have been shown to boost brain health—raspberries, blueberries and strawberries, for example—along with a little acai juice (and a bit of any other fruit juice, if you wish) to make an easy, delicious smoothie.

Why use frozen berries? They retain the nutritional benefit of fresh berries—and they're easy to buy and last a long time in the freezer...they give your smoothie a nice texture, which you can vary by adding more or less juice...and they're less expensive than fresh berries if you buy large bags.

CARROT JUICE

The old adage is that carrots are good for the eyes (indeed they are)—but we now know that carrot juice is absolutely great for the brain. Like other deeply colored vegetables (sweet potatoes, kale, red peppers, etc.), carrots are high in beta-carotene, an antioxidant that reduces inflammation—believed to be a factor in brain deterioration.

If you have tried carrot juice but didn't like the taste (it's surprisingly sweet), that's no problem. It is a very good "base" for multivegetable juices. (Some choices that are good for covering up the

An Eye Check Could Someday Help Determine Brain Health

Wider-than-average blood vessels in the eyes (which are similar to vessels in the brain and could serve as a marker for cognitive health) are often seen in patients with low IQs and cognitive deficits.

Psychological Science

carrot flavor include kale, spinach and other dark greens.)

COCOA

A Harvard/Brigham and Women's Hospital study found that adults who drank two daily cups of cocoa did better on memory tests than those who didn't drink it.

The flavanols (a class of antioxidants) in cocoa relax the endothelial linings of blood vessels and help reduce blood pressure. High blood pressure is a leading risk factor for dementia. The antioxidants in cocoa also reduce the cell-damaging effects of free radicals—this may improve long-term brain health.

Important: Do not go overboard with sugar, though—sugar is not good for your brain (and the jury is still out on artificial sweeteners).

Here's my advice: Buy a brand of unsweetened cocoa powder that is processed to remain high in flavanols. You don't have to buy an expensive specialty brand to get the brain-protecting effects. Most major brands of cocoa powder have respectable levels of cocoa flavanols. I advise against using milk chocolate or chocolate syrup—they typically have the least amount of flavanols and the most sugar.

At first, make your hot cocoa with your usual amount of sugar...then slowly cut back. You'll grow to appreciate the deep and pleasantly bitter true taste of the cocoa itself as less and less sugar stops masking it. As for using milk or water for your cocoa, that's your choice.

RED WINE

Everyone knows that red wine promotes cardiovascular health (easy does it). What you might not know is that red wine has been linked to a lower risk for dementia.

One reason is that people who drink moderate amounts of red wine—up to two glasses a day for men or one glass for women—have an increase in HDL "good" cholesterol. Research from Columbia University has found that people with the highest levels of HDL were less likely to develop dementia than those with the lowest levels.

Want to supercharge the brain-boosting power of your red wine? Make delicious Sangria! You'll get the wine's benefits and extra antioxidants and other nutrients from the fruit.

Sangria is typically made by steeping pieces of fresh fruit—lemon, orange, apple and just about any other fruit you like—in a rich red wine such as Merlot or Cabernet Sauvignon (or a Spanish red if you want to be autentico) and adding sugar and another liquor, such as brandy or rum.

My advice: Skip the sugar and extra liquor, but go ahead and add some orange juice to dilute the wine a bit and add some sweetness.

Best Juice Machines

Here, a juicer and two blenders that I recommend for quality and affordability...

- **Green Star GS-1000 Juice Extractor** uses a low-speed, low-heat system to preserve nutrients from produce. $485, *GreenStar.com*.
- **Ninja Professional Blender** has a powerful 1,000-watt motor and six blades to pulverize produce for drinks with lots of pulp. $100, *NinjaKitchen.com*.
- **Vitamix 5200** is a multipurpose blender that also chops and churns veggies and fruits into smoothies. Easy 30-second self-cleaning. $449, *Vitamix.com*.

Fish Oil Might Guard Against Loss of Brain Cells

James Pottala, PhD, assistant professor, department of internal medicine, University of South Dakota Sanford School of Medicine.

Gregory Cole, MD, professor, medicine and neurology, and associate director, Mary S. Easton Center for Alzheimer's Disease Research, University of California, Los Angeles.

JoAnn Manson, MD, chief, division of preventive medicine, Brigham and Women's Hospital, Boston.

Neurology, online.

The more you consume the omega-3 fatty acids found in fish oils, the less likely you are to lose as many precious brain cells as you age, a recent study suggests.

More research is needed, however, to understand both why this happens and how much of the nutrient brings about the most benefit, the researchers said.

"Our findings support the idea that a higher omega-3 status from fish or supplements is good for brain health," said study author James Pottala, PhD, assistant professor in the department of internal medicine at the University of South Dakota's Sanford School of Medicine.

STUDY DETAILS

According to the study, which was published online in the journal *Neurology*, the researchers tested levels of omega-3 fatty acids in the red blood cells of more than 1,000 older women. Eight years later, the women had MRI scans that measured their brain volumes. At the time of the scans, the women were an average of 78 years old.

Participants whose omega-3 levels were twice as high had a 0.7% higher brain volume. "The results suggest that the effect on brain volume is the equivalent of delaying the normal loss of brain cells that comes with aging by one to two years," Dr. Pottala said.

Higher omega-3 levels also were associated with greater volume in the hippocampus, the region of the brain in which the memory-robbing disease Alzheimer's first attacks.

EXPERT COMMENTS

The study offers valuable information, said Gregory Cole, MD, associate director of the Mary S. Easton Center for Alzheimer's Disease Research at the University of California Los Angeles.

"[The study] has a large number of subjects with an objective measure—the measure of brain volume," Dr. Cole said. "Studies that measure things like [memory and thinking] are not as concrete. People have good days and bad days, but when you measure brain volume you get a pretty repeatable measure."

It's also a plus that the participants are all the same gender, so there is no gender variation in brain size to factor in, Dr. Cole said.

The study's findings are intriguing, said JoAnn Manson, MD, chief of the division of preventive medicine at Brigham and Women's Hospital in Boston. "[But] the results should be interpreted cautiously because it's an observational study and not a randomized clinical trial looking at the relationship between omega-3 intake and changes in brain volume," she said.

Although the study showed an association between omega-3 intake and improved brain volume, it didn't necessarily prove a cause-and-effect link.

Dr. Manson is the principal investigator in a study involving more than 20,000 adults across the United States looking at whether taking daily dietary supplements of vitamin D or omega-3 fatty acids reduces the risk for certain diseases.

The study involves memory testing as well, Dr. Manson said. "We'll have some more information in another two to three years, and I think that will be important to see if increasing supplementation with omega-3s is having a clinical impact on [brain] function," she said.

Dr. Cole said clinical trials are the only way to find out if high omega-3 consumption really increases brain volume and reduces the risk for dementia.

"This is pretty believable. This is a solid finding," he said. "The question is: How can you translate this into [effectiveness] in people? Will it really work to protect peoples' brains?"

FISH REALLY IS BRAIN FOOD

In the meantime, people who want to boost their omega-3 intake can eat nonfried "fatty" fish such as salmon, herring, tuna and sardines. The American Heart Association recommends eating at least two servings of fish a week.

White Wine Is Good for Your Brain

Red wine has more heart-healthy polyphenols, which provide antioxidant protection and ease inflammation, than white wine, but white has more brain-saving compounds called hydroxycinnamates than red.

Caution: Men should have no more than two five-ounce glasses of wine a day...women should have no more than one glass a day.

Men's Health. MensHealth.com

Find out more about omega-3 fatty acids at the American Heart Association website at *http://www.heart.org/* (search "Fish and Omega 3 Fatty Acids").

High-Frequency Noise Boosts Math Skills in Study

Roi Cohen Kadosh, PhD, cognitive neuroscientist, University of Oxford, England
Colleen Loo, MD, professo.r of psychiatry, University of New South Wales, Sydney.
Current Biology

Could you someday zap your way to a smarter brain? Preliminary new research suggests that it's a possibility. Scientists report that they were able to improve the math-calculation skills of college students by buzzing their brains with doses of random high-frequency noise.

But don't go searching for a brain zapper at Walmart just yet. It's not clear why "transcranial random noise stimulation" might boost thinking skills, and the necessary equipment isn't sitting on the shelves at your local hardware store. The treatment is considered to be harmless but has only been studied for a few years, and the study findings aren't definitive.

For now, though, the results of the recent study are promising, said author Roi Cohen Kadosh, PhD, a cognitive neuroscientist at the University of Oxford, in England. "We can enhance one of the most complicated high-level cognitive [mental] functions and improve brain response after just five days of training, with a long-lasting effect six months later."

Scientists have only been studying transcranial random noise stimulation for about five years, Dr. Cohen Kadosh said. Researchers use the technique to stimulate the brain's cortex by putting electrodes on the scalp and delivering random bits of electrical noise. "It is non-invasive, painless—the level of current is generated by home batteries, and is very low—and relatively cheap," he said.

Transcranial random noise stimulation is considered to be harmless, and several studies haven't mentioned any adverse effects in those who have been zapped. Researchers are interested in one possible positive effect, though: changes in how the brain processes things.

"The brain is working on electricity, and in some cases poor behavior and cognitive [thinking] abilities appear when there's less activation of regions that are otherwise active," Dr. Cohen Kadosh said. "We thought that if we can make it easier for neurons to fire, it will allow an improved performance."

STUDY DETAILS

In the study, researchers recruited 51 Oxford students and gave them five days of training and testing as they performed arithmetic tasks. The tasks tested their ability to remember math facts (like 4 x 8 = 32) and make calculations (like 32 - 17 + 5 = 20).

Some of the participants received transcranial random noise stimulation when they performed the math tasks. Those participants were two to five times better at learning the equations, Dr. Cohen Kadosh said. And, six months after the stimulation, they were 28% better at making calculations than the other participants.

Scientists aren't sure why the stimulation treatment may boost learning and thinking, but Dr. Cohen Kadosh said it may have something to do with activating neurons in the brain.

The study appeared in the journal *Current Biology*.

WHY ZAP THE BRAIN?

Why might brain-zapping be a good thing? "We all want to improve our learning and to make it faster if possible, and we also want to help those who have problems in learning" due to disease, developmental problems or aging, Dr. Cohen Kadosh said. Also, "around 20% of the population finds math challenging."

EXPERT CAUTION

However, don't try this at home, advised Colleen Loo, MD, a brain researcher and professor of psychiatry at the University of New South Wales in Australia, who called the research "promising."

"If the electrodes are not correctly applied, it could cause scalp burns," Dr. Loo said. "Also, the exact placement of the positive and negative electrodes is essential, otherwise you could create quite different brain effects, including negative effects. There is still a lot more we need to know about this technology."

What's next? "There is a way to go, but this shows that it is feasible to improve human cognition and brain function in a long-lasting fashion," Dr. Cohen Kadosh said, "and this will hopefully trigger further research that will have more validity."

info For more information about the brain, visit Harvard Medical School's Whole Brain Atlas at *http://www.med.harvard.edu/aanlib/*.

How to Have an "Einstein Brain"

Rudolph E. Tanzi, PhD, Joseph P. and Rose F. Kennedy Professor of Neurology at Harvard Medical School and director of the Genetics and Aging Research Unit at Massachusetts General Hospital, both in Boston. He is coauthor, with Deepak Chopra, MD, of *Super Brain* (Harmony). He also has a special on PBS, *Super Brain with Dr. Rudy Tanzi.*

Albert Einstein was a genius, but sheer intelligence was not all that he had. The man who cracked secrets of the universe also knew the secret of using his own brain for maximum effect. But unlike Einstein, most people fail to actively use the brain in order to heighten its powers.

The first step to changing this is to recognize the various parts of the brain and how each functions...

• **Brain stem.** Sometimes referred to as the "reptilian brain," the brain stem generates instinctive drives for survival and reproduction. The fight-or-flight response to threat comes from the reptilian brain, as does stress and lust.

• **Limbic system.** Situated on top of the brain stem, the limbic system filters the instinctive drives of the reptilian brain through a network of past experiences, producing emotions such as fear, desire and jealousy.

• **Frontal cortex.** Located behind the forehead, the frontal cortex is known as the "thinking brain." It allows us to plan, create and find meaning and purpose in life.

A 10-SECOND EXERCISE

Much of the time, one part of the brain dominates. Uncontrolled rage, ravenous hunger or the health-eroding grind of stress takes over when the reptilian brain is in charge. If the limbic system is leading the way, we're filled with confidence or self-doubt, longing or delight. When the frontal cortex dominates, we plan and judge, seek knowledge and weigh costs against benefits.

The brain actually is at its best when all three parts work together.

Examples: You're falling into the grip of reptilian drives when you become furious after receiving unfair criticism from your spouse. Or perhaps you've had two slices of pizza but a powerful craving for a third is about to take over. *To restore balance to your brain functions, think of the acronym STOP...*

Stop what you're doing.

Take three deep breaths, then force yourself to "feel" a smile all through your body.

Observe yourself. How do you feel now? Paying attention to your whole body takes you out of purely reptilian mode, bringing the limbic circuit and frontal cortex into the game. Think about what you're doing—and the consequences for your health and well-being.

Proceed with full awareness of yourself and those around you. This simple 10-second process allows you to take charge of your brain.

WATCH OUT FOR THE "LOOPS"

Whatever has happened in your life has left its traces in your memory, regardless of whether you have conscious access to these thoughts.

The patterns, or "feedback loops," created by intricate connections within the brain are what shape the attitudes, beliefs, fears and desires we bring to new experiences. The limbic system takes over, and that's why if you were criticized regularly by parents for coming home with poor grades, a situation where you will be judged today is likely to activate old feelings

Better Brain Health Found in Bookworms

Memory and thinking tests given to approximately 300 adults revealed that those who participated in reading, writing and similar activities throughout their lives had a 32% lower rate of memory decline than those who did not. Reading helps strengthen circuits in the cerebral cortex, making them more resilient. The brain needs exercise just like other body parts, so keep it in shape at any age with mentally challenging activities, such as reading and/or writing.

Robert Wilson, PhD, senior neuropsychologist, Rush Alzheimer's Disease Center, Chicago.

of inadequacy and arouse fear and anxiety. You may see work demands as a trial, not a challenge. Or you may not try a new type of exercise for fear of failure.

Surprisingly, even positive feedback loops have a downside. When something feels good, you want to do it again and again. Unchecked, the limbic reward circuit can cause overindulgence that leads to health problems or even addiction.

What to do: Become aware of feedback loops—both positive and negative. Ask yourself where the feeling is coming from and how past associations are shaping present feelings.

Simply observing and recognizing the source of these unproductive feelings will give your brain the new input it needs to begin changing the self-defeating circuits and start "rewiring" it with healthier connections and associations.

LET YOUR THOUGHTS RUN WILD

Einstein opened up his mind to all possibilities, which allowed his brain to form new neural connections that dramatically boosted his mental capacities.

You can do the same thing. When faced with a task or situation in which previous solutions have been unsatisfactory, the logical frontal cortex is likely to take over in an attempt to "figure out" an answer.

What to do: Instead of approaching such situations with logic alone, let your brain activity run wild—allow associations that might seem far-fetched, nonsensical or even outlandish to pop up. Step back and observe what emerges without judgment or fear of being foolish.

Then put your thinking brain to work in sifting through the creative work that the other part of your brain has done. You may very well discover interesting ideas, solutions to vexing problems and refreshing approaches.

Yoga Improves Brain Power More Than Aerobic Exercise

Edward McAuley, PhD, professor, University of Illinois at Urbana-Champaign, Urbana, Illinois. This study was published in *Journal of Physical Activity and Health.*

A good workout can help your brain as much as your body, you've no doubt heard. That's one reason why so many people go for a run when they want to clear their heads. But did you know that, when it comes to boosting your mental prowess, you're probably better off striking a yoga pose than hitting the track or treadmill? *A recent study shows why...*

Participants included 30 adults who did not regularly practice yoga or any similar type of mind-body based exercise (such as tai chi). Each came to the study center on three separate days and took tests designed to measure various aspects of cognitive function.

On one day, they did no exercise prior to taking the tests. On another day, they did 20 minutes of yoga poses, focusing on their breathing and ending with a brief seated meditation, then immediately took the cognitive tests. And on yet another day, they ran on a treadmill for 20 minutes (getting their heart rates up to 60% to 70% of maximum) and then took the same cognitive tests.

The results were surprising—because the participants scored significantly higher after doing yoga than after an aerobic workout or after no exercise. *Specifically...*

• **One test measured inhibitory control,** the ability to ignore irrelevant information and maintain focus on relevant items. On a computer screen, the participants saw numerous rows of arrows facing left or right and had to press the arrow on the keyboard that corresponded to the direction of the arrows in a certain "target" position.

Results: The average score for correct responses after yoga was 90%...but just 83% after running, which was about the same as after no exercise.

• **Another test looked at working memory** (which is responsible for creating and storing memories and retrieving information), with the participants having to remember ever-changing sequences of shapes and respond as quickly as possible.

Results: The average score was 87% after yoga...but just 77% after running and 78% after no exercise. Response time also was faster after yoga—an average of 0.55 seconds, compared with 0.64 seconds after running and 0.60 seconds after no exercise.

Explanation: The researchers offered several possible reasons why yoga boosts brain power. Other studies have shown that yoga improves mood, and better mood is associated with better cognitive function. Yoga also reduces the anxiety that can get in the way of tasks that require full attention. In addition, yoga's emphasis on body awareness and breath control may help enhance the ability to concentrate.

Some questions remain, of course. This study did not demonstrate how long the mental performance-enhancing benefits of yoga might last, given that the participants took their cognitive tests within five minutes after finishing their yoga sessions. And the participants in this study were all women, so we can't say for sure whether men would benefit similarly (though it makes sense that they would).

Still, provided you have your doctor's go-ahead to do yoga, there's certainly no harm—and potentially much to be gained—in doing some yoga poses whenever you feel in need of a brain boost or are about to tackle some challenging mental task.

For inspiration and pose illustrations: Check out the *Yoga Journal* website, *yogajournal.com*

9 Risk Factors Point to Dementia

Early-onset dementia is linked to nine risk factors, many occurring during a person's teens. The most significant risk factor linked to dementia that occurs before the age of 65 is alcohol abuse. The other factors are use of antipsychotic drugs, depression, drug abuse, a father with dementia, poor mental function as a teen, being short, having high blood pressure and stroke. Taken together, these factors accounted for 68% of cases of early-onset dementia.

Study of 488,484 Swedish men by researchers at Umeå University, Sweden, published in *JAMA Internal Medicine*.

Forgetting a Famous Face Could Mean Dementia

Emily J. Rogalski, PhD, research assistant professor, Northwestern University Feinberg School of Medicine, Chicago.

Nearly 60 adults ages 40 to 65 (half of whom had a form of early-onset dementia) were asked to identify pictures of 20 famous people, including John F. Kennedy, Bill Gates and Elvis Presley.

Result: Only 46% of those with dementia could name all the faces (although nearly 80% recognized them). In participants with normal brain function, more than 90% could name the faces.

Explanation: Naming and recognition abilities decline with loss of brain tissue.

If you're having trouble identifying people you once knew: See a neurologist for an evaluation.

Vitamin B Slows Brain Decline

Gwenaëlle Douaud, PhD, Medical Research Council UK Research Fellow, Functional MRI of the Brain Centre, Nuffield Department of Clinical Neurosciences, University of Oxford, UK. Her study was published in *Proceedings of the National Academy of Sciences.*

Imagine your most cherished memories fading away as your mental powers decline, stolen by dementia. It's a distressingly common scenario, given that dementia affects about 5% to 8% of Americans over age 65...and as many as half of those over age 85.

There are many different types of dementia, the most common of which is Alzheimer's disease. Scientists are still struggling to figure out what sets off the degenerative process of Alzheimer's, but they do know that once it has begun, deterioration increases as plaque is deposited in the brain...neurons lose their ability to function and eventually die...and the brain shrinks considerably, actually losing volume.

It would be ideal if we could figure out a way to prevent dementia from ever getting started, but learning how to slow down its progress would also be good news. In that regard, we've just taken a big step forward—because even though seemingly promising drugs have failed in clinical trials, researchers have discovered that a common vitamin could hold the key to slowing down dementia's progress.

DELVING DEEPER

The study participants included 156 seniors age 70 and up who had mild cognitive impairment (MCI). More than just the typical age-related memory problems, such as forgetting where you left the car keys, MCI is characterized by trouble recalling information that previously would have been easily remembered, such as appointments or conversations...and/or difficulty making sound decisions or completing complex tasks. People with MCI are at increased risk for eventually developing Alzheimer's disease or some other type of dementia.

Researchers measured the size of each participant's brain using MRI images. They also measured blood levels of a protein called homocysteine, elevated levels of which have been linked to increased dementia risk in many earlier studies. Then half the participants were given a daily high-dose vitamin-B supplement—consisting of 0.5 milligrams (mg) of vitamin B-12...20 mg of vitamin B-6...and 0.8 mg of folic acid (vitamin B-9)—while the other half received a placebo.

After two years, the MRIs and blood tests were repeated.

Results: People in the vitamin-B group had homocysteine levels that were 29.4% lower than those in the placebo group...and they showed less loss of brain volume (atrophy). By further analyzing the MRI images using 3D reconstructions, the researchers determined that the vitamin B group had significantly less atrophy than the placebo group in key parts of the brain related to memory and cognitive decline—parts that are most affected by MCI and Alzheimer's. What's more, an important type of brain tissue called gray matter (which contains nerve cell bodies) shrank in these brain regions by just 0.5% in the vitamin-B group, compared with a 3.7% loss in the placebo group. This was a very significant difference!

For their next analysis, the researchers divided the study participants into two groups according to their homocysteine levels at the start of the study, comparing those whose measurements were below the median against those whose measurements were above the median.

What they found: Among people who had high homocysteine levels, those taking the placebo lost 5.2% of their gray matter...while those taking vitamin B lost just 0.6% of their gray matter in the brain regions that showed significant benefit from vitamin-B supplementation. For those who already had low homocysteine levels, there was no difference in gray matter loss among placebo users versus vitamin-B users—meaning that taking vitamin B was beneficial only for people with high homocysteine. The researchers concluded that taking vitamin B (particularly vitamin B-12) was as protective as having low homocysteine levels.

In addition, the researchers conducted tests of memory and cognitive function—and they found, as expected, that people who lost less gray matter did significantly better than those whose brains had suffered more atrophy. For example, among the high-homocysteine group, people who received the vitamin-B treatment were 69% more likely than placebo users to be able to correctly remember a list of 12 words.

To B or not to B: It's too early to suggest that everyone should be supplementing with B vitamins, the researchers noted. For one thing, in this study the vitamin-B combination was protective only for people who had high homocysteine levels. For another thing, consuming too much of the B vitamins could create problems—for instance, excess folic acid has been linked to cancer cell stimulation, while excess vitamin B-6 has been linked to nerve damage. Finally (and unfortunately), an earlier study found that people who already had moderate-to-severe Alzheimer's disease did not benefit from taking vitamin-B supplements.

Still, it's worth talking with a doctor who is knowledgeable about nutrition to see whether vitamin-B supplementation might be appropriate for you, particularly if blood tests show that you are deficient in B vitamins or have a high level of homocysteine and/or if you already have signs of mild cognitive impairment. And there's certainly no harm in increasing your consumption of vitamin-B-rich foods, such as clams, fish, liver, milk and spinach.

Alzheimer's: Is It "Type 3" Diabetes?—Here's What You Can Do...

Isaac Eliaz, MD, LAc, an integrative physician and medical director of the Amitabha Medical Clinic & Healing Center in Santa Rosa, California, an integrative health center specializing in chronic conditions. Dr. Eliaz is a licensed acupuncturist and homeopath and an expert in mind/body medicine. He has coauthored dozens of peer-reviewed scientific papers on natural healing. *DrEliaz.org*

For years, scientists from around the world have investigated various causes of Alzheimer's disease. Cardiovascular disease factors, such as hypertension, stroke and heart failure...other neurological diseases, such as Parkinson's disease...accumulated toxins and heavy metals, such as aluminum, lead and mercury...nutrient deficiencies, including vitamins B and E...infections, such as the herpes virus and the stomach bacterium H. pylori...and head injuries each have been considered at one time or another to be a possible contributor to the development of this mind-robbing disease.

However, as researchers continue to piece together the results of literally thousands of studies, one particular theory is now emerging as perhaps the most plausible and convincing of them all in explaining why some people—and not others—develop Alzheimer's disease.

A PATTERN EMERGES

Five million Americans are now living with Alzheimer's, and the number of cases is skyrocketing. Interestingly, so are the rates of obesity, diabetes and metabolic syndrome (a constellation of risk factors including elevated blood sugar, high blood pressure, abnormal cholesterol levels and abdominal fat).

What's the potential link? Doctors have long suspected that diabetes increases risk for Alzheimer's. The exact mechanism is not known, but many experts believe that people with diabetes are more likely to develop Alzheimer's because their bodies don't properly use blood sugar (glucose) and the blood sugar–regulating hormone insulin.

Now research shows increased dementia risk in people with high blood sugar—even if they do not have diabetes. A problem with insulin appears to be the cause. How does insulin dysfunction affect the brain? Neurons are starved of energy, and there's an increase in brain cell death, DNA damage, inflammation and the formation of plaques in the brain—a main characteristic of Alzheimer's disease.

AN ALZHEIMER'S-FIGHTING REGIMEN

Even though experimental treatments with antidiabetes drugs that improve insulin function have been shown to reduce symptoms of early Alzheimer's disease, it is my belief, as an integrative physician, that targeted nondrug therapies are preferable in preventing the brain degeneration that leads to Alzheimer's and fuels its progression. These approaches won't necessarily reverse Alzheimer's, but they may help protect your brain if you are not currently fighting this disease...or help slow the progression of early-stage Alzheimer's.

My advice includes...

• **Follow a low-glycemic (low sugar) diet.** This is essential for maintaining healthy glucose and insulin function as well as supporting brain and overall health. An effective way to maintain a low-sugar diet is to use the glycemic index (GI), a scale that ranks foods according to how quickly they raise blood sugar levels.

Here's what happens: High-GI foods (such as white rice, white potatoes and refined sugars) are rapidly digested and absorbed. As a result, these foods cause dangerous spikes in blood sugar levels.

Low-GI foods (such as green vegetables...fiber-rich foods including whole grains...and plant proteins including legumes, nuts and seeds) are digested slowly, so they gradually raise blood sugar and insulin levels. This is critical for maintaining glucose and insulin function and controlling inflammation.

Helpful: *GlycemicIndex.com* gives glucose ratings of common foods and recipes.

• **Consider trying brain-supporting nutrients and herbs.*** These supplements, which help promote insulin function, can be used alone or taken together for better results (dosages may be lower if supplements are combined due to the ingredients' synergistic effects)...

• Alpha-lipoic acid (ALA) is an antioxidant shown to support insulin sensitivity and protect neurons from inflammation-related damage. *Typical dosage*: 500 mg to 1,000 mg per day.

• Chromium improves glucose regulation. *Typical dosage*: 350 micrograms (mcg) to 700 mcg per day.

*Consult your doctor before trying these supplements, especially if you take any medications or have a chronic health condition, such as liver or kidney disease. If he/she is not well-versed in the use of these therapies, consider seeing an integrative physician. To find one near you, consult The Institute for Functional Medicine, *FunctionalMedicine.org*

Blood Pressure Medication May Reduce Alzheimer's Risk

Patients who took medication for high blood pressure—specifically, diuretics, angiotensin receptor blockers (ARBs) or angiotensin-converting-enzyme (ACE) inhibitors—had 50% lower risk for Alzheimer's. Patients who took other blood pressure medications did not show this benefit. Hypertension is a known risk factor for Alzheimer's, so talk to your doctor about the right medication for you.

Sevil Yasar, MD, PhD, assistant professor of medicine at The Johns Hopkins University School of Medicine, Baltimore, and leader of a study of 2,200 people, published in *Neurology.*

• Alginates from seaweed help reduce glucose spikes and crashes. *Typical dosage*: 250 mg to 1,000 mg before meals.

• L-Taurine, an amino acid, helps maintain healthy glucose and lipid (blood fat) levels. *Typical dosage*: 1,000 mg to 2,000 mg per day.

KICK UP YOUR HEELS!

Regular exercise, such as walking, swimming and tennis, is known to improve insulin function and support cognitive health by increasing circulation to the brain. Dancing, however, may be the ultimate brain-protective exercise. Why might dancing be better than other brain-body coordination exercises, such as tennis? Because dancing is mainly noncompetitive, there isn't the added stress of contending with an opponent, which increases risk for temporary cognitive impairment.

Best: Aerobic dances with a social component, such as Latin, swing or ballroom, performed at least three times weekly for 90 minutes each session. (Dancing for less time also provides some brain benefits.) If you don't like dancing, brisk walking for 30 minutes a day, five days a week, is also shown to help protect the brain against dementia.

Free courses: In addition to getting regular physical activity, it's helpful to learn challenging new material to "exercise" the brain. For 750 free online lectures provided by professors at top universities such as Stanford and Johns Hopkins, go to *OpenCulture.com/freeonlinecourses.* Subjects include art history, geography, international relations and biology.

Fluorescent Scans May Have Potential to Track Alzheimer's Progression

Neuron, news release

Newly developed fluorescent compounds may help doctors track Alzheimer's disease as it advances in living patients, a recent study reveals.

Tests showed that these compounds highlighted so-called *tau protein clusters* on PET scans of the brains of people with Alzheimer's disease.

The study was published in the journal *Neuron*.

In the brains of Alzheimer's disease patients, tau proteins clump together and become tangled. These tau tangles are an important marker of brain deterioration in people with the disease. Until now, it was difficult to monitor tau tangles while patients are still alive.

These new fluorescent compounds may help doctors track the processes that occur in the brain during the development and progression of Alzheimer's disease, according to a journal news release.

This ability could prove helpful in diagnosing the disease, monitoring the effectiveness of treatments, and testing new drugs to prevent and treat the disease, according to study senior author Dr. Makoto Higuchi, of the National Institute of Radiological Sciences in Japan, and colleagues.

Tau tangles also play a role in other types of dementias and movement disorders. These new fluorescent compounds could also help doctors diagnose, monitor and treat these diseases, the researchers noted.

Another protein called amyloid beta accumulates into plaques in the brains of people with Alzheimer's disease. Imaging technologies have also been developed to observe the spread of amyloid beta plaques in patients' brains.

The U.S. National Institute on Aging has more about Alzheimer's disease at its website *http://www.nia.nih.gov/alzheimers/topics/alzheimers-basics.*

Alzheimer's Patients Mimic Emotions of Those Around Them

Virginia Sturm, PhD, assistant professor, department of neurology, University of California, San Francisco.
Sam Gandy, MD, associate director, Mount Sinai Alzheimer's Disease Research Center, New York City.
Proceedings of the National Academy of Sciences, online

People with Alzheimer's disease or early thinking and memory problems tend to mirror the emotions of those around them, researchers find.

This transfer of emotions, known as emotional contagion, appears heightened in people with Alzheimer's and related mental decline, according to the University of California, San Francisco (UCSF) team. And it can be important in the management of these patients, they added.

"Calm begets calm," said Sam Gandy, MD, associate director of the Mount Sinai Alzheimer's Disease Research Center in New York City, who was not involved in the study.

Emotional contagion is a rudimentary form of empathy, enabling people to share and experience other people's emotions, said lead researcher Virginia Sturm, PhD, an assistant professor in the UCSF department of neurology.

"It's a way by which emotions travel across people quickly and even without awareness," explained Dr. Sturm. This process can shape behaviors and cause changes in the brain, she added.

In the early stages of Alzheimer's disease and in people with mild thinking and memory problems, emotional contagion increases, the researchers found. It is even more apparent in people with dementia, they noted.

"In Alzheimer's disease and other dementia we think some people may have an increased sensitivity to other people's emotions," Dr. Sturm said.

"As their memory and thinking abilities decline, it seems this is accompanied by the enhancement of other emotional processes," she said.

This means that if caregivers are anxious or angry, their patients will pick up and copy these emotions.

On the other hand, if the caregiver is calm and happy, patients will emulate these positive emotions, Dr. Sturm said.

"This is a way Alzheimer's patients connect with others, even though they don't have an understanding of the social situation," she said. "In order to manage patients, it might be that the caregivers being calm and happy would go a long way in keeping their patient calm and happy."

Alzheimer's disease is an age-related brain disorder that begins slowly and gradually robs people of their ability to lead their everyday lives. In the United States, one-third of the nation's seniors die with Alzheimer's or another type of dementia, according to the Alzheimer's Association.

STUDY DETAILS

The study, published online in the *Proceedings of the National Academy of Sciences*, involved 237 adults. Sixty-two patients had mild memory and thinking problems and 64 had Alzheimer's disease. The others were mentally healthy.

Participants took tests to identify depression and other mental health problems and also underwent MRI scans to identify changes in the brain related to emotional contagion.

The researchers found higher emotional contagion in those with mild mental impairment and Alzheimer's disease, compared with those who did not have these conditions.

This growth of emotional contagion paralleled the increase in damage to the right temporal lobe of the brain, reflecting biological changes in the neural system, the study found.

"The right temporal lobe is important for different aspects of emotion and social behavior," Dr. Sturm said.

Depression was also greater among those with mild mental impairment and Alzheimer's disease, the study found.

EXPERT COMMENT

From a neurologist's perspective, "it is extraordinary that something so complex as emotional perception can be controlled by such a localized part of the brain," Dr. Gandy said.

"Also, classically it has been the frontal lobe damage that leads to emotional disturbance," Dr. Gandy added. "Now we know the temporal lobes can play similar roles."

info For more information on Alzheimer's disease, visit the Alzheimer's Association website at *http://www.alz.org/*.

Vitamin E Slows Alzheimer's Symptoms

When people with mild-to-moderate Alzheimer's took a high dose of vitamin E—2,000 international units (IU) daily—they had slower declines in activities of daily living, such as dressing and bathing without help, than people who didn't take the vitamin or took the Alzheimer's drug *memantine* (Namenda). Vitamin E provided just over a six-month delay in the disease's progression over a two-year period.

Note: A doctor should be consulted before this therapy is tried—it may increase risk for bleeding and/or interact with medications.

Maurice Dysken, MD, geriatric psychiatrist, Minneapolis VA Health Care System, Minnesota.

Statin Drugs May Fight Parkinson's

Chia-Hsuin Chang, MD, ScD, attending physician and assistant professor of internal medicine, National Taiwan University Hospital, Douliou City.

An analysis of nearly 44,000 adults found that those who stopped taking lipophilic (fat-soluble) statin drugs, such as *simvastatin* (Zocor) and *atorvastatin* (Lipitor), after reaching their LDL "bad" cholesterol target were 58% more likely to develop Parkinson's disease than those who continued to take the drugs.

Theory: Lipophilic statins have anti-inflammatory properties that may help prevent or delay the degeneration of brain cells that occurs in Parkinson's patients.

If you're considering going off statins: Talk with your doctor about your risk for Parkinson's.

Aphasia—Finally, There's Hope for People With This Communication Problem

Susan Wortman-Jutt, MS, CCC-SLP, a certified speech-language pathologist in the outpatient speech department at the Burke Rehabilitation Hospital in White Plains, New York. Active in both patient care and clinical research, Ms. Wortman-Jutt coauthored and recently presented research at the National Convention of the American Speech-Language-Hearing Association.

Aphasia (pronounced uh-FAY-zhuh) sounds more like the name of a fancy perfume than a chronic and frustrating neurological condition. But approximately one million people in the US—about one in 250—have some form of aphasia. That's more than twice the toll taken by multiple sclerosis, a much better-known condition.

Aphasia is a disorder that affects a person's ability to communicate with words. It occurs when stroke, severe head injury or a brain tumor damages the brain in an area that governs communication.

How does aphasia affect one's ability to communicate? Depending on the location and severity of the damage to the brain, a person may have difficulty speaking, reading or writing and/or comprehending the speech of others. In mild or moderate cases, reading or writing may be preserved. In some severe cases, aphasia may lead to near total loss of verbal and written language skills.

Good news: With more and more research being done on neuroplasticity—the ability of the brain to form new pathways—there's increasing evidence that many people with aphasia can improve even years after their brain damage has occurred. This fact, combined with exciting advances in the development of therapies that stimulate the brain with electrical currents, gives aphasia patients more opportunity to improve than ever before.

NEWER AND BETTER THERAPIES

Until recently, treatment for aphasia was conducted only one-on-one with a speech-language therapist.

Now: New technologies and cut-backs in the amount of therapy covered by most health insurers have led to innovations that give aphasia patients options to receive therapy in their homes...

- **Computerized treatment.** Instead of weekly one-hour sessions with a therapist (or as an adjunct to that treatment), people with aphasia can work at home with a "virtual therapist" via a computer program.

Typically, the human therapist programs the computer with scripted sessions tailored to specific needs—such as 10 phrases that need to be repeated—which the patient can take home and play back on the computer. Some programs use pictures instead of printed words, which is helpful for those who have difficulty reading.

With some programs—for example, Vast by Speak in Motion (SpeakinMotion.com)—a close-up video of a mouth making clear lip and tongue movements provides cues for the patient to follow. A human therapist is needed to periodically evaluate the patient's progress, but computerized treatment gives the sights and sounds of an actual therapist in the home and the opportunity to practice saying words. This type of virtual therapy is particularly helpful for people who don't have easy access to speech-therapy centers.

- **Apps.** There also are several apps available for the iPad, iPod Touch, iPhone and Android devices that can help aphasia patients.

One user-friendly app is Language TherAppy by Tactus Therapy Solutions (TactusTherapy.com). This four-in-one app for people with aphasia includes lessons in comprehension, naming, reading and writing. In addition, the app can track data from sessions and send e-mails to your therapist, so your progress can be professionally monitored. The app costs $60. There is a free sample version—Language TherAppy Lite—that can be downloaded from the iTunes App Store. Another company that provides simple but effective apps for aphasia in the App Store is VirtualSpeechCenter.com. Costs range from $10 to $35.

• **Social media.** It used to be that if you wanted the benefit of a support group, you attended a meeting that might be held once a week. With social media, you have access 24/7. One of the best such options is a Facebook group called "Living Successfully with Aphasia."

Part support group and part information resource, it allows individuals with aphasia at any level of impairment to check in any time and communicate with other aphasia patients.

EXCITING NEW ADVANCES

The single most exciting advancement being studied in aphasia treatment is noninvasive brain stimulation. With this therapy, an electrical current is used to stimulate or inhibit the areas of the brain responsible for the aphasia. It may prime the brain for traditional therapy and may increase the rate of language improvement over traditional speech therapy alone. *Two forms of brain stimulation now being tested for use with aphasia...*

• **Transcranial magnetic stimulation (TMS).** With TMS, which is FDA approved as a treatment for depression, a magnetic coil is placed lightly against the patient's forehead and delivers a current to the desired area.

• **Transcranial direct current stimulation (tDCS).** With tDCS, small electrodes that supply the current are placed on the top of the scalp. A patient who undergoes this therapy also can receive speech therapy while the brain is being stimulated. This form of brain stimulation is administered on equipment that is portable and less costly than that used for TMS. However, tDCS targets more general areas of the brain, so it may be less useful when a specific area needs treatment.

Patients who are interested in these therapies can find a medical research center doing clinical trials at *ClinicalTrials.gov.*

THE BEST SUPPORT

Despite all the technologies and advances, research shows that the single best predictor of success with aphasia treatment is support from family and friends.

Not only can family members and friends provide moral support, but they also can help the person with aphasia practice his/her communication skills. For example, language "exercises" provided by a therapist can be performed by the patient in a workbook or on a computer—the activities may include repeating words or phrases...practicing writing...or answering simple questions.

A supportive family environment also helps by simply exposing the person with aphasia to lots of different types of communication—listening to and being included in conversation... and feeling comfortable making "mistakes."

info For more information, consult the National Aphasia Association at *Aphasia.org* or 800-922-4622.

Both Sides of Brain Involved in Speech, Study Finds

New York University, news release.

Speech involves the use of both sides of the brain, according to a study that may overturn the widely held belief that only one side of the brain is used for this task.

The findings improve understanding of how speech is generated in the brain and could help lead to new ways to treat speech problems, the researchers said.

They noted that previous conclusions about speech were from studies that relied on indirect measurements of brain activity. This recent study directly examined the link between speech and brain activity. Patients in the study had specialized electrodes implanted directly inside and on the surface of the brain.

The researchers focused on parts of the brain used during speech. The participants were asked to repeat two "non-words"—"kig" and "pob." Using non-words to trigger brain activity enabled the researchers to isolate speech from language.

The results showed that the participants used both sides of the brain for speech, according to the study published in the journal *Nature*.

"Now that we have greater insights into the connection between the brain and speech, we can begin to develop new ways to aid those trying to regain the ability to speak after a stroke or injuries resulting in brain damage," study senior author Bijan Pesaran, an associate professor in New York University's Center for Neural Science, said in a university news release.

"With this greater understanding of the speech process, we can retool rehabilitation methods in ways that isolate speech recovery and that don't involve language," he added.

info For more information, the U.S. National Library of Medicine has more about speech and communication disorders.

Autoimmune Encephalitis: The Brain Disease That Makes People Seem Crazy

Souhel Najjar, MD, associate professor of neurology, director, electroencephalogram laboratory, NYU Langone Medical Center, New York City, and director, Neuroscience Center, Staten Island University Hospital, New York. His role in diagnosing and saving a patient stricken with anti-NMDA receptor autoimmune encephalitis is described in the book by Susannah Cahalan, *Brain on Fire: My Month of Madness* (Simon & Schuster).

"Ricki," had it all—a great job, great little Manhattan apartment, great life. Only in her early 20s, she already had accomplished much in the fashion world.

But over the course of barely more than a month, all that blew up as Ricki developed increasingly weird and worrisome behaviors.

First, there were memory problems. She couldn't recall simple things, such as where she normally kept her car keys or the names of her coworkers. The following week, her speech slowed, her body felt numb and her movements became awkward. Soon after, Ricki began hallucinating and a psychiatrist put her on medication.

A week later, she had a seizure and was hospitalized. A huge battery of tests, including a spinal tap and brain MRIs, revealed nothing except a little inflammation...doctors were stumped.

Then Ricki began having violent spells, leaping at nurses and orderlies. Said to be psychotic, she was transferred to a psychiatric hospital. And there she might have stayed for the rest of her life—if not for a stroke of luck.

Ricki's father, a retired physician, did not believe that the daughter who had always been so sweet, smart and sane could have become, in a matter of weeks, seriously and irrevocably mentally ill. So he diligently researched her symptoms and discussed her condition with his doctor friends. Fortunately, one of the father's colleagues suggested consulting Souhel Najjar, MD, a neurologist at NYU Langone Medical Center in New York City.

Dr. Najjar gave the young woman a thorough examination, including a special blood test that revealed antibodies targeting certain receptors in the brain—and within days, he had made the diagnosis. Ricki was suffering from a rare autoimmune disorder called anti-NMDA receptor encephalitis.

DEADLY "DEMONIC" DISEASE

Encephalitis, or inflammation of the brain, usually is the result of a viral infection, but it also can be caused by bacteria, fungi or parasites—or, as doctors now realize, by an autoimmune disorder.

In the case of anti-NMDA receptor encephalitis, severe brain inflammation occurs when the immune system attacks special proteins on the surface of nerve cells in the brain called NMDA receptors. These receptors control various cognitive functions, mood, behavior and personality traits—so when they are compromised, the brain malfunctions.

The resulting symptoms include mood and personality changes, violent outbursts, paranoia, psychosis, memory loss, speech problems, numbness, seizures, involuntary movements, increased heart rate, irregular heart rhythm, slowed breathing and/or decreased levels of consciousness. Patients sometimes sink into an unresponsive catatonic state that may last for weeks. Some experts even suspect that anti-NMDA receptor encephalitis is the true cause underlying many cases of "demonic possession" described in the Bible and in a number of popular movies.

This disease is largely unknown, having first been reported in the medical literature only six years ago. It typically strikes in early adulthood, but it has been diagnosed in children as young as one and in seniors as old as 85. It can strike both genders, though more than 75% of those affected are female.

We spoke with Dr. Najjar to learn more about this disturbing and devastating disease. He said that, though considered rare, anti-NMDA receptor encephalitis may be more common than is currently recognized, with many patients being misdiagnosed with severe psychiatric disorders. "These patients act aggressive, belligerent, violent, psychotic and paranoid. Yet now that we know what the real problem is, we have to wonder how many people have been locked up in psychiatric units for years after they were misdiagnosed," Dr. Najjar said.

Sadly, some patients with anti-NMDA receptor encephalitis die from medical and neurological complications related to irregular heart rhythm, very low blood pressure, slowed breathing, prolonged convulsions and/or persistent coma.

BRAIN-SAVING TREATMENT

The earlier that anti-NMDA receptor encephalitis is diagnosed and treated, the better the outcome tends to be. Treatment includes immunotherapy—a heavy-duty dose of steroids and other drugs aimed at suppressing the body's attack on itself. Typically, Dr. Najjar said, the treatment is effective, and most severe symptoms improve within three to four weeks after treatment begins. However, patients often need physical, occupational and/or cognitive therapies to regain their ability to walk, talk and function normally, and full recovery may take up to two years.

What causes this disease? That's not entirely clear. As with other autoimmune disorders, such as lupus or rheumatoid arthritis, a genetic predisposition may contribute to an individual's risk, Dr. Najjar said.

A certain type of ovarian tumor called a teratoma appears to play a key role, particularly in females of childbearing age. Bizarrely, teratomas often contain skin, hair, tooth and/or brainlike cells. A recent study from the University of Pennsylvania found that up to 55% of female patients under 18 years of age who had anti-NMDA receptor encephalitis also had teratomas in their ovaries. The body's immune system may be provoked into producing antibodies that attack the abnormal brainlike cells in the tumor, Dr. Najjar explained. Since the antibodies don't distinguish between the brainlike cells in the tumor and cells in the brain itself, the patient's brain becomes a battlefield. If a teratoma is found in a patient's ovary, the ovary needs to be surgically removed.

What's puzzling is that anti-NMDA receptor encephalitis also can develop in patients who do not have teratomas. Such cases may be the result of some kind of virus that damages the blood/brain barrier, allowing antibodies to enter the brain, Dr. Najjar said. These patients are at greater risk for recurrence, even many years after the initial episode. For instance, the University of Pennsylvania researchers reported that, of the 20% of anti-NMDA receptor encephalitis patients who experienced a relapse, most had not had teratomas.

Lucky lady: Ricki is recovering nicely, thanks to timely intervention. But here's what all of us should remember from her story...

If a loved one suddenly starts exhibiting psychiatric symptoms that are way out of character, Dr. Najjar said, it is vital to consult a neurologist and ask whether anti-NMDA receptor encephalitis could be the culprit.

Antiviral Drug May Extend Brain Cancer Survival, Researchers Say

Cecilia Soderberg-Naucler, MD, PhD, professor, medicine, Karolinska Institute, Stockholm, Sweden.

David Reardon, MD, director, Center for Neuro-Oncology, Dana-Farber Cancer Institute, Boston.

Chang-Hyuk Kwon, PhD, assistant professor, neurological surgery, Ohio State University Comprehensive Cancer Center, Columbus.

New England Journal of Medicine

A drug used against a common virus may lengthen the lives of people with a deadly form of brain cancer, a preliminary study suggests.

Writing in the *New England Journal of Medicine*, researchers reported on 50 patients who were given the antiviral drug *valganciclovir* (Valcyte) to help treat glioblastoma, the most common form of brain tumor in adults. The tumor carries a dismal prognosis—with a typical survival of just over a year.

These 50 patients, however, fared far better, researchers found.

After two years, 62% were still alive. Of the 25 who took the antiviral continuously, 90% were still alive. That compared with just 18% of patients who received most of the same treatments—including surgery and chemotherapy—but did not take Valcyte.

"These data are by far the best ever seen for these patients," said lead researcher Cecilia Soderberg-Naucler, MD, PhD, of the Karolinska Institute in Stockholm, Sweden.

Glioblastoma is diagnosed in two or three people per 100,000 in the United States and Europe, according to the National Brain Tumor Society. No one is sure what causes the cancer, but it is more common in men and in people older than 50.

A brain cancer expert not involved in the research also voiced enthusiasm. "These are very exciting data," said David Reardon, MD, director of neuro-oncology at the Dana-Farber Cancer Institute in Boston.

But he also urged caution because there are many unknowns, and the findings need to be verified in a controlled clinical trial—in which patients would be randomly assigned to take Valcyte or not, and then followed over time.

Valcyte is a pill used to treat cytomegalovirus (CMV) eye infections in people with AIDS. CMV is a very common virus—up to 80% of adults contract it by age 40—and it usually causes no harm in someone with a healthy immune system.

Researchers have found, however, that CMV dwells in the tumor cells of most people with glioblastoma, which suggests that the virus contributes to the cancer in some way.

One recent lab study found that when certain cancer-promoting gene mutations are present, CMV might speed the growth of glioblastoma.

"It appears that the virus alone is not sufficient to cause any human tumors," said Chang-Hyuk Kwon, PhD, one of the researchers on that study.

Instead, it seems that CMV "cooperates with human cancer gene alterations to accelerate development and growth of the cancer," said Dr. Kwon, assistant professor, neurological surgery, Ohio State University Comprehensive Cancer Center in Columbus.

As Dr. Reardon put it, "For some reason, these [glioblastoma] cells are a place where CMV likes to proliferate."

That has been known for several years, he said. The news here is that an anti-CMV drug might extend people's survival.

STUDY DETAILS

Still, there are questions, Dr. Reardon said. The study, which was funded partly by Valcyte maker Hoffman-La Roche, included 50 patients from a single hospital. Many were given the antiviral drug as part of a "compassionate use" program at the hospital.

The researchers then compared them with 137 patients who were treated for glioblastoma at the same hospital around the same time, but were not given Valcyte. All patients in both groups received standard treatment, which typically meant surgery, chemotherapy and, in many cases, radiation.

Dr. Reardon said the problem with that type of study is that there's a risk of bias. Patients who were chosen to receive Valcyte may have been younger, in better overall health and more likely to respond to treatment.

On the other hand, he said, the survival figures for the Valcyte patients were "so far above average, it's hard to imagine they're just the result of cherry-picking the patients."

Dr. Reardon said more work is needed to see what drug dose is optimal, and whether patients have to take it indefinitely.

CAN BE PRESCRIBED OFF-LABEL

Doctors could prescribe Valcyte for glioblastoma patients, Dr. Reardon said. But since it's not specifically approved for the cancer, insurers may not pay—a big obstacle, since the drug costs a couple thousand dollars a month.

MORE QUESTIONS AND CONCERNS

Another question, Dr. Kwon said, is whether the drug treatment actually reduced CMV levels in the patients' tumors, or if the virus was still lurking.

Plus, there's a risk of side effects with Valcyte, Dr. Kwon said, including [illegible], vomiting and [illegible] kidney or liver [illegible]

[illegible] aid, given the [illegible] na, "anti-CMV [illegible] nsidered."

[illegible] r Society has [illegible] website, *www.* [illegible] *mation/*

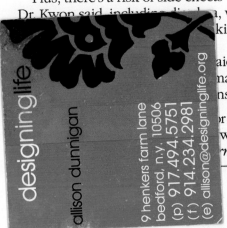

Breast Cancer

New Clarity on Breast Cancer Screening

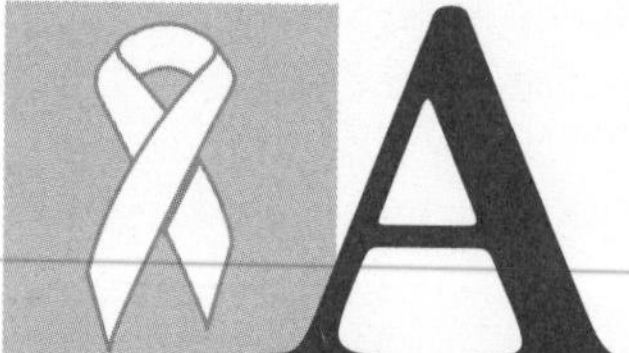

A recent study from Harvard has reignited the controversy surrounding which women should and should not have routine mammograms...how often those tests should be done...and the ages at which screening should start and stop. Since this new research contradicts the Task Force recommendations, women are left wondering, Whom should we listen to? *So we went after the answer...*

THE CRUX OF THE CONTROVERSY

Two aspects of the Task Force recommendations sparked outrage among many women (and many doctors, too)—the idea that women in their 40s did not need routine mammograms...and that screening should take place every other year rather than yearly. When challenged, the Task Force defended its position, asserting that "although the benefit of screening seems equivalent for women aged 40 to 49 years and 50 to 59 years, the incidence of breast cancer and the consequences differ." It further claimed that the test's "harms"—such as inconvenience, discomfort and the risk for false-positive results—outweighed its benefits for women under age 50 and warranted the less-frequent screening schedule for older women.

However, the Harvard researchers now contend that the previous studies on which the Task Force recommendations were based had gone about their calculations all wrong—and that lives would be saved if women were screened more frequently and at a younger age.

BIGGER BENEFIT FOR YOUNGER WOMEN

The recent study is of a type called a failure analysis. Such analyses look backward from death to discover correlations at diagnosis,

Blake Cady, MD, professor of surgery (emeritus), Harvard Medical School, Boston. His study was published in *Cancer.*

rather than looking forward from the beginning of a randomized trial—a technique that eliminates problems of noncompliance and "contamination biases" that can skew results.

Researchers from two major academic teaching hospitals in Boston reviewed their records for women who were diagnosed with potentially curable (stage I, II or III) invasive breast cancer between 1990 and 1999 and followed through 2007. They found 7,301 such patients...and of those, 609 died from breast cancer during the follow-up period.

The researchers analyzed these 609 confirmed breast cancer deaths, comparing screened women (those who had had a mammogram at least every two years in the absence of symptoms) with unscreened women (those who never had a mammogram or hadn't had one within two years of their cancer diagnoses). *What they found...*

The vast majority of deaths, or 71%, were among unscreened women—even though unscreened women accounted for only 20% of the total patient population in the study. Of the women who died, 65% had never had a screening mammogram...and 6% had not had a mammogram for at least two years prior to their diagnoses. Only 29% of the deaths were among screened women. The fact that most of the women who died were not participating in screening clearly supports the importance of early detection through mammography, the researchers said.

Of all breast cancer deaths, a startlingly high 50% were in women younger than 50—the very same age group that, under the current Task Force guidelines, would not be expected to benefit from screening mammograms!

Among patients younger than age 50, the breast cancer death rate was 13%—nearly double the 7.6% death rate for the patients between ages 50 and 74.

Likely reason: The Harvard researchers pointed out that the biological nature of breast cancer in young women is more aggressive than in older women.

Interval cancers are those that are detected when they cause actual symptoms in the interval between a normal, negative mammogram and a woman's next regularly scheduled mammogram. Among screened women who were diagnosed in their 40s, 47% of those who died had interval cancers...whereas among screened women who were diagnosed in their 60s, only 24% of those who died had interval cancers. These findings, the researchers said, suggest that it's appropriate to do more frequent screening in women younger than 50 and less frequent screening in women age 60 and up.

Bottom line on breast cancer screening: By definition, screening refers only to people who have no signs or symptoms of a disease. If you do have possible symptoms of breast cancer (a lump, thickening of tissue, nipple discharge, inverted nipple, dimpling or other skin changes), it is vital that you get a diagnostic mammogram to start the process that can determine whether or not your symptoms are caused by cancer.

It's also important to note that screening recommendations apply to the public in general. Women at increased risk for breast cancer often are advised to begin screening earlier, to screen more often and/or to screen with other technologies (such as ultrasound or MRI) in addition to mammography. So if you have a family history of breast cancer, had a previous biopsy with high-risk though benign results or have tested positive for the BRCA1 or BRCA2 gene, ask your doctor to provide details on the most appropriate screening schedule and methods for you.

Absent such risk factors, however, the researchers from this recent study suggested that,

Better Breast Cancer Detection

Mammograms using digital radiography (DR) are slightly more effective than computer radiography (CR) mammograms.

Recent finding: DR detected 4.9 cancers per 1,000 mammograms, while CR detected 3.4.

Study of 816,000 mammograms carried out on 688,000 women, ages 50 to 74, by researchers at several cancer care centers in Ontario, Canada, published in *Radiology*.

in general, "a screening sequence that corresponds to the biological behavior of breast cancer" would be for women to get mammograms every six to 12 months in their 40s...every year in their 50s...every two years in their 60s...and every two to three years from age 70 onward until life expectancy is less than 10 years.

The researchers put it this way: Participating in mammography is like buying home owners' insurance. You pay a premium even though you're unlikely to ever need to file a claim—but in the event of disaster, you are protected from ruin. With breast cancer, the disaster of death is largely avoided due to early detection.

Women Who Test Negative for the Breast Cancer Gene Still May Be at Risk

It was originally thought that women who come from families with BRCA mutations but who test negative for any BRCA mutations had the same risk for breast cancer as the general population.

Recent finding: Women from such families with negative BRCA2 mutation had four times the risk for breast cancer as the general population.

Gareth Evans, MD, is honorary professor of medical genetics and a cancer epidemiologist at The University of Manchester in England and lead author of a study of 800 families, published in *Cancer Epidemiology, Biomarkers & Prevention.*

Best Cancer-Screening Tests for Women With Dense Breasts

Margarita Zuley MD, associate professor of radiology, University of Pittsburgh, and medical director of breast imaging, Magee-Womens Hospital, both in Pittsburgh.

Have you ever been told that you have dense breasts? It's an important piece of information because women who have them are at increased risk for breast cancer...and because mammograms don't do a very good job of detecting cancer in dense breasts.

That's why several states (including California, Connecticut, New York, Texas, Virginia, Nevada, North Carolina and Oregon) now have laws requiring mammography clinics to inform women if they have dense breasts. Similar legislation is currently being considered in other states, as well as in Congress.

No matter where you live, though, if your doctor doesn't bring up the subject of breast density, you should ask about it, said Margarita Zuley, MD, an associate professor of radiology at the University of Pittsburgh and medical director of breast imaging at Magee-Womens Hospital. Ask, too, whether you need additional screening tests for breast cancer, as many dense-breasted women do...and also discuss the best timing for those tests.

Why it matters: Breasts are made up of ducts, glands, fibrous connective tissue and fatty tissue. Dense breasts have a higher percentage of fibrous and glandular tissues and less fatty tissue. Younger women are most likely to have dense breasts because breasts typically become more fatty with age, but even so, as many as 25% of postmenopausal women have dense breasts.

Concern: Women with dense breasts are two to six times more likely to develop breast cancer—perhaps because dense breasts have more milk ducts and lobes, and the majority of breast cancers form in such tissues.

What's more, tumors are harder to detect in dense breasts because, on a mammogram, dense tissue looks white...and so do cancers. That's why looking for cancer in a dense breast is like looking for a polar bear in the snow. Fatty tissue looks darker, so it provides more contrast compared with any cancer that might be present. When a radiologist looks at your mammogram and compares it with your mammograms from previous years, he or she is looking for areas that once appeared dark and now look whiter, Dr. Zuley said. If you have dense breasts, little cancers buried between glandular breast tissues can easily go undetected.

The only way to know whether you have dense breasts is by having a mammogram.

Your doctor cannot tell just by doing a manual breast exam.

TRIO OF TESTS

Dense-breasted women still do need regular mammograms because the test does spot some tumors in dense breasts, including ones that other tests miss. However, the best odds of detecting cancer in dense breasts occur when mammography is combined with an additional screening test. *If you have dense breasts, discuss these options with your doctor...*

•**Ultrasound.** The most commonly used supplemental breast-screening test, ultrasound often picks up cancers in dense-breasted women that mammography misses. It's also noninvasive, relatively inexpensive (about $100) and doesn't involve radiation. Dr. Zuley said that ultrasound is generally considered an appropriate add-on test for dense-breasted women who are at average or intermediate risk for breast cancer.

The downside is that ultrasound has a high rate of false-positive results. Dr. Zuley explained that breast ultrasounds reveal a lot of abnormalities, such as fibroadenomas (solid, benign, glandular breast tumors), which must be biopsied to see whether they are cancerous but which ultimately turn out to be benign. False-positives involve unnecessary anxiety, inconvenience and expense.

Number crunch: Studies show that, for every 1,000 women screened, the addition of ultrasound spots three to five cancers that mammograms miss...however, to find three tumors, 63 biopsies or other invasive procedures are done.

•**Magnetic resonance imaging.** MRI is better at detecting breast cancer than other screening methods are. However, it is generally used only for women who are at high risk for breast cancer because they carry the breast cancer gene or because one or more of their first-degree relatives (parent, sibling) had the disease.

Why isn't MRI used for all dense-breasted women? Because compared with ultrasound, breast MRI is much more costly (upwards of $700)...more invasive, as it requires the injection of an intravenous contrast dye...and has an even higher rate of false-positives.

•**Tomosynthesis (3D mammography).** With regular 2D mammography, a single image is taken each time the breast is compressed—which means that tissues overlap and details are obscured. With tomosynthesis, however, the arm of the X-ray machine rotates in an arc above the breast, taking many separate images. Those are then processed on a computer to create a 3D image that the radiologist can manipulate to view 50 to 60 individual millimeter-thin "slices" of breast tissue, making it easier to spot tumors hiding in dense tissue.

Recent studies show that radiologists who had access to both 2D and 3D mammograms detected 40% more cases of invasive breast cancer than those who saw only the 2D mammograms...and that the combination of 2D and 3D images reduced false-positive results by 39%. Due to the 3D test's higher rate of detection of invasive breast cancer, Dr. Zuley recommends tomosynthesis for all women, whether dense-breasted or not. The 3D scan uses about the same amount of radiation as the 2D scan, so getting both tests doubles your radiation exposure. Still, the total radiation dose for the combined tests is well below three milligray, which is the FDA limit for a single mammogram.

A QUESTION OF TIMING

Because tomosynthesis is relatively new, it is currently FDA-approved for use only in addition to, not instead of, regular 2D mammography. So

Vitamin D Protects Against Breast Cancer

In a recent study, women with the lowest blood levels of vitamin D in the three months before a diagnosis of premenopausal breast cancer had three times as high a risk for the disease as women with the highest vitamin D levels. Women should take at least 1,000 international units (IU) of vitamin D-3 daily.

Cedric F. Garland, DrPH, an adjunct professor in the department of family and preventive medicine at University of California, San Diego, and leader of a study of 1,200 women, published online in *Cancer Causes & Control*.

Exercise Update

A Walk a Day Lowers Breast Cancer Risk

Postmenopausal women who walk an hour a day have a 14% lower risk of breast cancer compared with their inactive counterparts. And women who do at least one hour of strenuous physical activity daily have 25% lower risk for breast cancer. Physical activity is thought to lower risk by reducing hormones...improving weight control, glucose metabolism and insulin sensitivity...and lowering inflammation.

Alpa Patel, PhD, strategic director of the Cancer Prevention Study-3 (CPS-3) for the American Cancer Society, Atlanta, and leader of a study of 73,615 postmenopausal women, reported in *Cancer Epidemiology, Biomarkers & Prevention*.

Exercise—at Any Age—Cuts Risk for Breast Cancer

In a study of more than 3,000 women (both premenopausal and postmenopausal), those who did 10 hours of moderate exercise a week—including walking and gardening—had a 30% lower risk for breast cancer than those who were sedentary.

Theory: Besides reducing body fat, exercise may increase antioxidant capacity and enhance cell repair.

Lauren McCullough, PhD, epidemiologist, The University of North Carolina at Chapel Hill.

even if your doctor recommends that you get a 3D mammogram, he or she will still tell you that you need the 2D test as well—at least until additional studies lead to FDA approval of tomosynthesis as a stand-alone mammography technique. Since both types of mammograms can be performed on the same equipment in rapid succession, both tests generally are done at the same time.

No matter whether a woman gets just a 2D mammogram or a 3D mammogram as well, if her doctor also wants her to get an ultrasound or MRI, the question of timing arises. That issue is currently being debated in the radiology community.

Some doctors believe it is best for a woman to have her regular annual mammography screening and then, six months later, to have her breast ultrasound or MRI. This way, if she has a fast-growing tumor, it will be detected sooner because she will never go longer than six months before having some kind of imaging test.

However, Dr. Zuley and many other experts prefer to do the annual mammography screening and the ultrasound or MRI on the same day. That's because the six-month alternating schedule has not been shown to increase detection rates, she said...and because comparing the two test results at the same time helps reduce the rate of false-positives, avoiding a lot of unnecessary anxiety and biopsying of tissues that turn out to be fine.

Some health insurance policies cover the cost of the additional screening tests for dense-breasted women, but some do not—so check with your insurer.

For Breast Cancer Radiation, Facedown Position May Be Safer

Silvia C. Formenti, MD, chair, department of radiation oncology, New York University Langone Medical Center, New York City. Her study was published in *JAMA*.

A woman with breast cancer who has had a lumpectomy also may have radiation to improve her odds of beating the disease. However, her heart and lungs wind up being exposed to the radiation, too, which increases her long-term risk of developing potentially deadly heart problems or lung cancer. Recent research suggests a simple way to reduce this risk—just have the woman roll over. *Here's the idea...*

Usually, a woman receiving radiation lies on her back to give access to the breast tissue being targeted. Researchers wondered what would happen if she were instead to lie on her stomach, on a table that has an opening so that the affected breast is hanging down and not squished beneath her.

The study included 400 breast cancer patients. Half had had a lumpectomy in the right breast and the other half had had a lumpectomy in the left breast. Normally, prior to radiation, a CT scan is done to pinpoint the location of the breast tissue being targeted. For this study, each participant had two CT scans—one lying faceup and the other lying facedown—so that researchers could compare the amount of lung and heart tissue that would be within the radiation field in each position. (The amount of radiation from the extra CT scan was nowhere near as potentially harmful as the radiation used in actual cancer treatments.)

Results: In all patients, the facedown position vastly reduced the lung volume that was exposed to radiation, as compared with the faceup position. For women with left breast cancer, it was a whopping 91% reduction...for women with right breast cancer, it was an 86% reduction.

To gauge the effects on the heart, researchers looked only at the women who had had cancer in the left breast (since the heart risk is much smaller when the right breast receives radiation). Among these patients, the facedown position reduced the amount of heart tissue within the field of radiation by 86%, on average, as compared with the faceup position. However, for 15% of these women—most of whom had relatively small breasts—the faceup position was either the same or slightly better for reducing heart exposure.

Keep in mind that this is a preliminary study. The researchers did not actually compare the long-term effects of faceup versus facedown radiation treatment, so there's no way yet to quantify how a patient's position would affect her odds of developing heart or lung problems from radiation. Still, the data in radiation oncology suggest that keeping normal tissue out of the radiation field drastically reduces the risk for treatment complications.

More studies will come. In the meantime, if you or a woman you love ever needs radiation for breast cancer, talk to your oncologist about the possible advantages of the facedown position. Some radiation centers already provide facedown breast radiation, with the dose coming from below or from the side rather than from above—so ask your doctor for a referral. Why take chances with your heart or lungs if you might be able to avoid it just by rolling over?

Implants May Delay Breast Cancer Detection, Raise Death Risk

Eric Lavigne, PhD, graduate in epidemiology, faculty of medicine, University Laval, Quebec City.

Stephanie Bernik, MD, chief of surgical oncology, Lenox Hill Hospital, New York City.

BMJ, online

Women with breast implants could run the risk of having breast cancer diagnosed at later stages, when survival might be worse, according to Canadian researchers.

Breast implants can make it more difficult to diagnose breast cancer early because they block some areas of the breast on mammograms, experts say.

"Women who currently have breast implants and those considering breast augmentation should be aware of the possible long-term health effects of cosmetic breast implants," said lead author Eric Lavigne, a PhD graduate in epidemiology with the faculty of medicine at University Laval, in Quebec City.

"They should also be reassured that physicians and other health professionals will continue to offer the best medical practices to these women," he added.

RESEARCH DETAILS

To see whether breast implants had an effect on breast cancer diagnosis and survival, Dr. Lavigne's team reviewed studies published after 1993. This process, known as a meta-analysis, attempts to find a consistent pattern from different studies. In many cases, these patterns aren't the focus of or apparent from each individual study, but emerge only after the data are combined.

In this case, by analyzing 12 studies, the researchers found that women with breast implants had a 26% increased risk of being diagnosed with late-stage breast cancer compared with women without implants.

When Dr. Lavigne's group looked at another five studies, they found that women with breast implants had a 38% increased risk of dying from breast cancer than women without implants.

This finding "may be explained by the advanced breast cancer diagnosis received," Dr. Lavigne said.

These results, however, need to be interpreted with caution since only a small number of studies were included in this summary, and many factors in each study can affect the overall results, he said.

Although the analysis linked breast implants to later-stage breast cancer diagnoses, it did not establish a cause-and-effect relationship.

The report was published online in the journal *BMJ*.

EXPERT RESPONSE

Stephanie Bernik, MD, chief of surgical oncology at Lenox Hill Hospital in New York City, said she will be more cautious with patients.

"Patients ask if it's OK to do implants," Dr. Bernik said. "We don't tell them not to, but they have to understand that it comes with a risk of obscuring some of the breast tissue."

If someone has a family history of breast cancer, they should be cautious, Dr. Bernik said. "Everybody should be informed that there is this problem," she said. "It will limit the ability for cancer detection with mammography."

Dr. Bernik suggested that women with breast implants also have an ultrasound or MRI to get around the problem of the implant hiding breast tissue during a mammogram. She said, however, that for this purpose MRIs aren't covered by insurance.

info To learn more about breast cancer, visit the American Cancer Society at *http://www.cancer.org/cancer/breastcancer.*

Hypertension Medication May Increase Breast Cancer Risk

Blood pressure medication may increase risk for breast cancer. According to a recent finding, women who took calcium-channel blockers for 10 years or longer had more than double the risk for breast cancer, compared with women who did not take these medications. No risk was found for short-term use of the drug (less than 10 years) or for any other antihypertensive medication.

Christopher Li, MD, PhD, an epidemiologist specializing in breast cancer at Fred Hutchinson Cancer Research Center, Seattle, and lead author of a study of nearly 3,000 women, published in *JAMA Internal Medicine.*

Drug Lowers Risk for Breast Cancer in Older, High-Risk Women

Jack Cuzick, PhD, head, Cancer Research U.K. Centre for Cancer Prevention and director, Wolfson Institute of Preventive Medicine, Queen Mary University of London.

Amy Tiersten, MD, associate professor of medicine, division of hematology and oncology, Icahn School of Medicine at Mount Sinai, New York City.

Stephanie Bernik, MD, chief of surgical oncology, Lenox Hill Hospital, New York City.

American Association for Cancer Research, news release

The drug *anastrozole* (Arimidex) reduces the risk of developing breast cancer by more than 50% among postmenopausal women at high risk for the disease, according to a recent study.

The finding, presented at the San Antonio Breast Cancer Symposium in Texas, and published in the journal *The Lancet,* adds hope that Arimidex might be a valuable new preventive option for some women.

BACKGROUND

"Two other antihormone therapies, *tamoxifen* and *raloxifene*, are used by some women to prevent breast cancer, but these drugs are not as effective and can have adverse side effects, which limit their use," said study lead author Jack Cuzick, PhD.

"Hopefully, our findings will lead to an alternative prevention therapy with fewer side effects for postmenopausal women at high risk for developing breast cancer," said Dr. Cuzick, head of the Cancer Research U.K. Centre for

Cancer Prevention and director of the Wolfson Institute of Preventive Medicine at Queen Mary University of London.

HOW ARIMIDEX WORKS

About 80% of US breast cancer patients have tumors with high levels of hormone receptors, and these tumors are fueled by the hormone estrogen. Arimidex prevents the body from making estrogen and is therefore used to treat postmenopausal women with hormone receptor-positive breast cancer.

STUDY DETAILS

The study included more than 3,800 postmenopausal women at increased risk for breast cancer due to having two or more blood relatives with breast cancer, having a mother or sister who developed breast cancer before age 50, or having a mother or sister who had breast cancer in both breasts.

About half the women took Arimidex for five years while the others took a placebo, or dummy drug. Those who took the drug were 53% less likely to develop breast cancer than those who took the placebo.

Side effects among the women taking the drug included hot flashes and small increases in muscle aches and pains.

The study received funding from the drug companies AstraZeneca and Sanofi-Aventis, and Dr. Cuzick is on the speaker's bureau for AstraZeneca.

EXPERTS OPTIMISTIC

"This is very exciting information," said Amy Tiersten, MD, associate professor of medicine at the Icahn School of Medicine at Mount Sinai, in New York City. She said that although tamoxifen and raloxifene can also cut a woman's odds for breast cancer, "these medications can slightly increase the risk of blood clots and uterine cancer."

"It is great to have a less toxic option to offer patients in the preventative arena," she said of Arimidex.

Stephanie Bernik, MD, chief of surgical oncology at Lenox Hill Hospital in New York City, agreed. "It is with open arms that we can add [Arimidex] to the medications that can be offered to postmenopausal women that are at high risk of developing breast cancer," she said.

"Because [Arimidex] has less side effects, more women are likely to undergo preventive treatment," Dr. Bernik said. "This will eventually help decrease the incidence of breast cancer in women in this category."

"We are planning to continue following the study participants for at least 10 years, and hopefully much longer," study author Dr. Cuzick said. "We want to determine if [Arimidex] has a continued impact on cancer incidence even after stopping treatment, if it reduces deaths from breast cancer, and to ensure that there are no long-term adverse side effects."

The U.S. National Cancer Institute has more about breast cancer prevention at *www.cancer.gov/cancertopics/pdq/prevention/breast/Patient/.*

Expanded DNA Testing Might Allow Personalized Breast Cancer Treatment

Fabrice Andre, MD, PhD, researcher, Gustave Roussy Institute, Villejuif, France.

Claudine Isaacs, MD, professor of oncology, Georgetown Lombardi Comprehensive Cancer Center, Washington, DC.

George Somlo, MD, professor of medical oncology and therapeutics research, City of Hope Comprehensive Cancer Center, Duarte, CA.

The Lancet Oncology

Testing the entire genetic makeup—or all the DNA—of tumor cells from women with advanced breast cancer may help identify patients who could be helped by specific treatments, according to recent research.

The approach is considered the wave of the future by both the French researchers who conducted the study and US experts.

"It is possible to deliver personalized medicine," said study researcher Fabrice Andre, MD, PhD, of the GustaveRoussy Institute in Villejuif, France. "Until now, we could [test] one gene in a large number of patients, or larger numbers of genes in a few patients."

RECENT RESEARCH

In the recent study, the researchers evaluated the whole genome—the entire collection of a person's genes—of more than 400 patients. The approach is much more extensive than testing for mutations in specific genes, such as the BRCA1 and BRCA2 genetic mutations known to raise the risk of breast cancer.

From 2011 to 2012, Andre's team evaluated the women from 18 centers in France, all of whom had breast cancer that had spread. First they took biopsy samples. Then they conducted the whole-genome analysis to see if they could find unique characteristics and abnormal genes that could then be targeted for treatment in clinical trials.

Nearly half of the patients were found to have a genetic alteration that could be addressed with targeted treatment. Another 39% of women had rare alterations, many of which don't have treatments currently available, the researchers said.

Next, the researchers matched 55 of the women with new treatments being tested in clinical trials, targeting them to the women's specific genetic alteration. Of those, 43 women received the targeted treatments. And of those, four women had a response and nine others had stable disease for more than 16 weeks, the researchers said.

The study findings were published in the journal *The Lancet Oncology*.

EXPERT REACTION

Some of the larger cancer centers in the United States are also working on the whole-genome approach, said George Somlo, MD, a professor of medical oncology and therapeutics research at the City of Hope Comprehensive Cancer Center, in Duarte, California. He reviewed the findings but was not involved in the study.

"It is very expensive, very labor intensive," he said. "In the United States, the approach is evolving."

The cost of whole-genome testing varies greatly, but some laboratories offer it for less than $10,000. Experts say the cost will drop more in the future.

Claudine Isaacs, MD, a professor of oncology at the Georgetown Lombardi Comprehensive Cancer Center, in Washington, D.C., said the approach has advantages.

"The advantage of screening the tumor either for a large battery of mutations or doing whole-genome analysis is that it gives a much broader analysis and understanding of possible patient- or tumor-specific molecular 'drivers' for that particular tumor," said Dr. Isaacs, who also reviewed the findings. "It will pick up both suspected and unsuspected [genetic] alterations."

"I do think this is the wave of the future," she said. "The hope of such an approach is to better provide our patients with a personalized approach to their care."

As promising as the approach is, Dr. Somlo said, it's important to realize that "not every tumor needs to have whole-genome testing." It's already known that some specific mutations or changes in genetic activity will result in particular breast cancer patients benefiting from targeted therapy, he said.

For instance, he said, the drug *trastuzumab* (Herceptin) is used as a targeted therapy for women found to be over-activating the protein known as HER2 (human epidermal growth factor receptor).

For breast cancer patients, the difficulty of finding an effective treatment increases when the disease spreads, Dr. Somlo said.

"There are multiple mutations and the curability of those patients is very low," he said. Obtaining the genetic information in these cases would

Less Invasive Breast Cancer Treatment May Be Better for Some Women

Over a 14-year study period, early-stage breast cancer patients 50 years old and older who chose a lumpectomy plus radiation were 13% less likely to die from breast cancer and 19% less likely to die from any cause than similar women who had more invasive mastectomies.

Study of 112,154 women by researchers at Duke Cancer Institute, Durham, North Carolina, and the Cancer Prevention Institute of California, Fremont, published in *Cancer*.

best be done as soon as possible after the cancer's spread is detected, he said.

info To learn more about human genomes, visit the U.S. National Institutes of Health website at *www.genome.gov/12011238*.

Anesthesia Technique May Affect Survival After Breast Cancer Surgery

Palle Steen Carlsson, MD, PhD, researcher, Aarhus University Hospital, Denmark.

Michael Lew, MD, professor and chairman of anesthesiology, City of Hope Comprehensive Cancer Center, Duarte, CA.

American Society of Anesthesiology annual meeting, San Francisco.

The anesthesia technique used during breast cancer surgery may affect cancer recurrence and survival, Danish researchers report.

In a small study that followed 77 breast cancer patients, researchers found the combination of a general anesthetic plus injections of a nerve block resulted in increased survival and fewer recurrences, said Palle Steen Carlsson, MD, PhD, a researcher at the Aarhus University Hospital in Denmark.

A six-year follow-up found that 13% of patients who got the combination had their cancer recur versus 37% of those who got anesthesia alone. And 10% of those in the combination group died compared with 32% of those given anesthesia alone.

Dr. Carlsson reported her findings at the American Society of Anesthesiologists' annual meeting in San Francisco.

HOW SURGERY AFFECTS CANCER CELLS

During cancer surgery, tumor cells released into the blood can implant in lymph nodes and other organs, she said. The immune system kicks in to fight these cells, but surgery and anesthesia can impair the immune system.

STUDY DETAILS

In the study, Dr. Carlsson randomly assigned the 77 patients to general anesthesia plus injections of saline or general anesthesia plus injections of local anesthetic (this is called a paravertebral block) about an inch from the middle of the spine.

Besides differences in recurrence and survival, medical records six years later showed the women who got the combination approach needed fewer opioids for pain relief.

In an earlier study, researchers found that the combination of general anesthesia and regional anesthesia reduced recurrences and the spread of breast cancer four-fold, but that study looked back at medical records. Dr. Carlsson said her study is believed to be the first to follow patients forward.

POSSIBLE EXPLANATION

Dr. Carlsson can't say for sure why women who got the nerve block plus anesthesia tended to fare better. One theory is that better pain relief during and after surgery reduces the stress response to the procedure, she said. Or perhaps the need for fewer narcotic painkillers after surgery reduces the risk of cancer spreading.

The idea that the anesthesia technique used during breast cancer surgery affects results is evolving, anesthesiologists say, and needs more study. Dr. Carlsson found a link between the two, but her study didn't show a direct cause-and-effect relationship.

Dr. Carlsson acknowledged the study's limitations. "The weakness of our study is the size," she said.

EXPERT COMMENTARY

The concept has been a hot topic for several years among anesthesiologists, said Michael Lew, MD, professor and chairman of anesthesiology at the City of Hope Comprehensive Cancer Center in Duarte, California. Dr. Lew was not involved in the study.

"[This study] is exciting and a step in the right direction," he said. "However, [Carlsson] is correct in saying there needs to be more numbers."

More information is expected soon, Dr. Lew said, citing a clinical trial under way at the Cleveland Clinic and elsewhere. It will compare different anesthesia approaches used in more than 1,100 breast cancer patients over five years and evaluate differences in outcomes.

ADVICE

Until more findings are in, Dr. Lew suggests that women facing breast cancer surgery tell their surgeon they want a general anesthetic with as few opioids as possible. "The opioids inhibit natural killer cells [that attack roaming cancer cells]," he said.

Dr. Lew said he sometimes gives a general anesthetic plus intravenous anti-inflammatory medicine to combat pain.

info To learn more about breast cancer, visit the American Cancer Society website, *www.cancer.org/cancer/breastcancer/index.*

New Guidelines Might Limit Need for Lymph Node Removal for Breast Cancer

Stephanie Bernik, MD, chief, surgical oncology, Lenox Hill Hospital, New York City.

Debra Patt, MD, medical director, Pathways Task Force and Healthcare Informatics, US Oncology Network.

American Society of Clinical Oncology.

Biopsies of so-called "sentinel" lymph nodes under the arms should become more widespread among breast cancer patients, according to updated guidelines from the American Society of Clinical Oncology (ASCO).

The group, which represents cancer specialists, said the new recommendations should also restrict the number of women who will require further removal of multiple nodes after biopsy, cutting down on painful side effects.

SENTINEL VERSUS AXILLARY LYMPH NODES

In sentinel lymph node biopsy, a few lymph nodes are removed and checked for signs of cancer—hence the name "sentinel." Usually, if these lymph nodes have no cancer, it means the remaining, unchecked lymph nodes should also be cancer-free.

The new ASCO recommendations expand eligibility for sentinel node biopsy and will reduce the number of patients who undergo a more invasive procedure called axillary—underarm—lymph node dissection, which carries a higher risk of complications, the group said.

In axillary lymph node dissection, most lymph nodes under the arm on the same side as the breast tumor are removed and examined for cancer. This procedure can cause long-term side effects, such as pain and numbness in the arm and swelling due to a build-up of lymph fluid.

NEW GUIDELINES

The new guidelines state that for women whose sentinel lymph nodes show no signs of cancer, removal of more underarm lymph nodes is not recommended.

The guidelines also addressed the case of women who undergo lumpectomy instead of full mastectomy and are also scheduled for whole-breast radiation therapy to help "mop up" residual cancer. If these patients have signs of cancer in only one or two sentinel lymph nodes upon biopsy, they too may opt to avoid further node removal, the ASCO experts said.

Women who have undergone mastectomy but show signs of cancer's spread in sentinel lymph nodes should be offered further node removal, the guidelines reaffirmed.

High Cholesterol Increases the Severity of Breast Cancer

The molecule 27HC, a derivative of cholesterol, mimics estrogen, a hormone that increases breast cancer risk and reduces the effectiveness of anti-estrogen treatments for breast cancer such as aromatase inhibitors and *tamoxifen*. Women with breast cancer and high cholesterol should talk to their doctors about lowering cholesterol with statins and/or dietary changes.

Donald McDonnell, PhD, chairman of the department of pharmacology and cancer biology at Duke University School of Medicine, Durham, North Carolina. He is lead author of a study published in *Science*.

The ASCO also said women who are diagnosed with certain breast cancers while pregnant can skip sentinel node biopsy.

The ASCO issued initial guidelines on sentinel node biopsy in 2005. The new guidelines, published in the *Journal of Clinical Oncology*, are based on the findings of a panel of experts who reviewed studies published between 2004 and 2013.

"The updated guideline incorporates new evidence from more recent studies—nine randomized controlled trials and 13 cohort studies since 2005," said panel co-chairman Armando Giuliano, MD.

"Based on these studies, we're saying more patients can safely get sentinel node biopsy without axillary lymph node [removal]," he said. "These guidelines help determine for whom sentinel node biopsy is appropriate."

Panel co-chairman Gary Lyman, MD, MPH, said, "We strongly encourage patients to talk with their surgeon and other members of their multidisciplinary team to understand their options and make sure everybody is on the same page."

"The most critical determinant of breast cancer prognosis is still the presence and extent of lymph node involvement," he said. "Therefore, the lymph nodes need to be evaluated so we can understand the extent of the disease."

EXPERT REACTION

"Over the past few years, there has been a movement to limit the amount of axillary [lymph node] surgery in patients undergoing breast conservation," said Stephanie Bernik, MD, chief of surgical oncology at Lenox Hill Hospital in New York City.

Dr. Bernik said the new guidelines are important because some doctors have been reluctant to move away from further underarm node removal when a patient has even one affected sentinel node. "This update will give surgeons the confidence to tell patients that a sentinel lymph node biopsy may be enough, even if there is evidence of spread, in patients undergoing [lumpectomy and radiation]," Dr. Bernik said.

"However, it is still important for surgeons to discuss the pros and cons with a patient, as not all [real-world] patients fit the study criteria," she said. "Furthermore, it needs to be stressed that the more limited surgery does not apply to women undergoing mastectomies."

Debra Patt, MD, is the medical director of an expert panel that assesses cancer care guidelines for the US Oncology Network. She said she was "thrilled" at the new ASCO guidelines because they seem to echo the results of recent studies.

"In 2010, a study presented at the ASCO annual meeting showed that women undergoing breast-conservation surgery with clinically node-negative small breast cancers could safely avoid removing all the lymph nodes from under the arm in most cases," Dr. Patt said.

info The American Academy of Family Physicians has more information on breast cancer at *http://familydoctor.org*. Search "breast cancer."

Key to Preventing Lymphedema After Breast Cancer

Suzanne Miller, PhD, professor and director of the Psychosocial and Biobehavioral Medicine Program, Fox Chase Cancer Center, Philadelphia. Her study was presented at the American Association for Cancer Research San Antonio Breast Cancer Symposium.

After breast cancer treatment, about half of patients develop a distressing and potentially disfiguring complication called lymphedema. The condition involves mild to extreme swelling of the arm closest to the affected breast due to buildup of fluid in the nearby tissues—a result of the removal of lymph nodes and scarring that damage the normal function of the lymph system. This fluid buildup can cause significant pain and loss of arm function. Symptoms may develop soon after surgery or may appear months or even years later. Once lymphedema arises, it can be treated but not cured, which means that prevention is crucial.

Certain steps can help—for instance, guarding against injury to the arm, not constricting the arm and controlling weight. Yet many breast cancer survivors do not follow this advice or take the other precautions that would reduce their risk for lymphedema. Why don't they?

Insights from a recent study: Researchers met with 103 women immediately after their breast cancer surgery to discuss lymphedema and distribute recommendations from the American Cancer Society on how to reduce their risk. The recommendations included moisturizing the arm several times daily...using an electric shaver instead of a razor on the underarm and wearing gloves when doing housework or physical activity to guard against cuts and infection...avoiding tight jewelry and restrictive clothes...protecting the arm from being jostled or squeezed...and not carrying heavy objects.

Six months later, the researchers checked in with the patients—and discovered that only half of them had followed the advice. The biggest stumbling blocks were a lack of confidence in their own ability to make these lifestyle changes...and a lack of effective strategies for coping with stress. How does stress enter into the equation? The researchers explained that, for patients, the behavioral changes needed to reduce lymphedema risk can serve as daily reminders of their breast cancer—reminders that increase anxiety and stress. *More on stress-reducing strategies...*

The researchers suggested several ways that survivors can boost confidence and reduce stress after breast cancer...

- **Develop a system for keeping track of when you do and don't follow the lymphedema prevention guidelines.** When you do comply with them, reward yourself—for instance, by buying that new CD you've been wanting or phoning a friend to say, "I did it—celebrate with me!"

- **Talk to your family about specific ways they can support your efforts**—for example, by taking over tasks (such as those involving heavy lifting) that are not safe for you.

- **With your doctor or a therapist,** discuss stress-reducing strategies and relaxation techniques that you can use when feeling overwhelmed.

- **Join a local or Web-based breast cancer support group or online chat room.** These are invaluable resources for emotional support as well as practical tips on preventing lymphedema. You can find support groups through the National Lymphedema Network...Susan G. Komen...and BreastCancer.org.

Also helpful: Other research suggests that timely physical therapy reduces the odds of developing lymphedema.

Additional information on lymphedema is available from the National Lymphedema Network. You also can download a PDF from the American Cancer Society called "Lymphedema: What Every Woman With Breast Cancer Should Know."

Unfounded Fear Prompts Unnecessary Mastectomies

Shoshana Rosenberg, ScD, MPH, postdoctoral research fellow, Harvard School of Public Health and Dana-Farber Cancer Institute, Boston.

Sarah Hawley, PhD, associate professor of internal medicine, University of Michigan Health System, Ann Arbor, Michigan.

Stephanie Bernik, MD, chief, surgical oncology, Lenox Hill Hospital, New York City.

Annals of Internal Medicine

Young women with breast cancer tend to overestimate their risk for getting cancer in the opposite, healthy breast—sometimes driving them to have that breast removed, according to recent research.

Researchers polled 123 young women two years after they chose double mastectomy for breast cancer at age 40 and younger, asking how they made the decision to have the opposite breast removed and how they estimated the cancer risk in the healthy breast.

"Most women who were considered average risk actually overestimated their risk of having contralateral [opposite breast] breast cancer," said study researcher Shoshana Rosenberg, ScD, MPH, a research fellow at Harvard School of Public Health and Dana-Farber Cancer Institute.

Despite evidence that having the procedure—called contralateral prophylactic mastectomy—does not improve survival rates, growing numbers of women treated for early stage breast cancer decide to have it, the study authors said.

While about 6% of women with early stage cancers had the procedure in the 1990s, now up to one-fourth do.

Dr. Rosenberg and her colleagues wanted to look more closely at the patients' decision-making process. The research was published in the *Annals of Internal Medicine.*

In the survey, 98% of women who opted for contralateral prophylactic mastectomy said they wanted to avoid getting cancer in the opposite breast and 94% said they wanted to improve survival, although only 18% believed that the procedure actually improved survival.

About one-quarter of the women were genetically at higher risk of cancer, due to having a BRCA gene mutation. Of participants who did not have the gene mutation, patients estimated that 10% would get cancer in the opposite breast within five years without the preventive surgery, although the actual risk is about 2% to 4% over the five years, according to Dr. Rosenberg.

"Risk perception is very complex," Dr. Rosenberg said. "It could be that their doctor is not communicating it effectively." In addition, this is a very anxiety-provoking time period. "There are lots of decisions to make, and concerns about recurrence," she noted.

"We are not telling women what surgery to have," Dr. Rosenberg said. "We want to be sure they are making an informed decision."

Women should talk over the pros and cons with their physicians, she suggested. While 80% of the women said they spoke with their doctor about the reasons for having contralateral mastectomy, only 51% reported that their doctors talked about reasons not to have the surgery.

EXPERTS COMMENT

The findings echo some previous research, according to Sarah Hawley, PhD, an associate professor of internal medicine at the University of Michigan Health System, in Ann Arbor. In her study, presented last year at a medical meeting, Dr. Hawley found that nearly 70% of women choosing the contralateral prophylactic mastectomy actually had a low risk of developing cancer in the healthy breast.

"Their findings are consistent with ours, in that desire to prevent cancer in the non-affected breast is a big reason patients reported for getting [contralateral prophylactic mastectomy]," Dr. Hawley said.

Better communication is needed to be sure women know the risks and benefits, and lack of benefit of getting the preventive surgery, Dr. Hawley pointed out. Better strategies to help patients manage anxiety and worry would help, too, she added.

Women choose to have contralateral prophylactic mastectomy for a number of reasons, said Stephanie Bernik, MD, chief of surgical oncology at Lenox Hill Hospital, in New York City. She reviewed the findings.

"Although there may be no survival benefit, many women are concerned that they want to move on with their lives and want to reduce the chance of developing a cancer on the opposite breast in the future," Dr. Bernik said. They may be trying, understandably, to avoid another round of treatment in the future.

Women need to decide what is right for them, Dr. Bernik stated. "It is clear that with breast cancer surgery, one size does not fit all."

Better Odds for Beating Breast Cancer

Breast cancer survivors have a one in six chance of developing cancer in the other breast.

Recent animal study: A moderate dose of radiation delivered to the unaffected breast reduces the cancer risk by threefold.

PLOS ONE

Exercise May Help Breast Cancer Survivors Battle Bone Loss

American Institute for Cancer Research, news release.

Aerobics and strength-training exercises may help reduce bone loss and the risk of fractures in breast cancer survivors, a recent study suggests.

BREAST CANCER SURVIVORS AT RISK FOR BONE LOSS

Bone loss is a serious problem for breast cancer survivors. Medications, such as aromatase inhibitors, block the production of estrogen, a hormone that fuels the growth of many breast cancers. Estrogen, however, is needed for bone formation.

The researchers also said chemotherapy can trigger early menopause, resulting in low estrogen levels and bone loss.

STUDY DETAILS

This 12-month study included breast cancer survivors who had recently completed treatment. About half of them took part in an aerobic/resistance exercise program three times a week at a fitness center. The other women were assigned to a control group and given recommendations of 30 minutes of moderate-intensity exercise most days of the week.

By the end of the study, the women in the intervention group had more physical endurance, greater muscle mass and lower fat mass than those in the control group, according to the study, which was presented at the annual meeting of the American Institute for Cancer Research, in Bethesda, Maryland.

"Women who are completing cancer therapy should be getting a strong prescription for health promotion, which includes aerobic-resistance exercise," said study author M. Tish Knobf, PhD, RN, a professor at the Yale School of Nursing. "Routine exercise improves muscle strength, balance, quality of life, mood, functional ability and cardiovascular status, and may minimize the risk of bone loss."

LOW LEVELS OF VITAMIN D LINKED TO BREAST CANCER

Another study presented at the same meeting found that many survivors of breast cancer and other cancers are at risk for low levels of vitamin D, and many will need to take vitamin D supplements. The vitamin helps promote bone health.

"Patients with breast cancer and several other cancers are at increased risk of rapid bone loss and fractures," said Bess Dawson-Hughes, MD, director of the Bone Metabolism Laboratory at Tufts University. "While not sufficient to prevent bone loss when taken alone, calcium and vitamin D are very important components of any pharmacologic regimen to minimize bone loss."

info The Hormone Health Network has more information about breast cancer and bone loss at *www.hormone.org/questions-and-answers/2010/breast-cancer-and-bone-loss.*

Cancer Breakthroughs

Starve Cancer to Death With the Ketogenic Diet

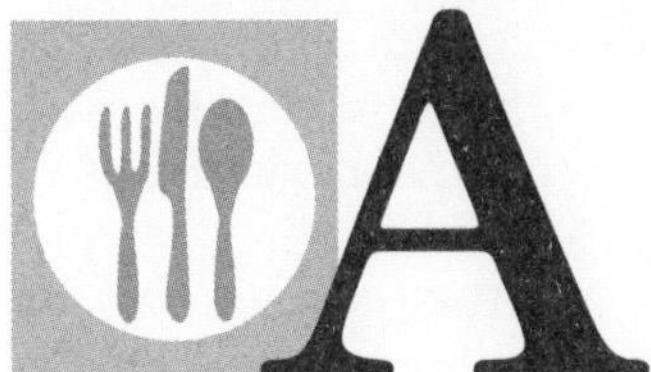

A 65-year-old woman with brain cancer had surgery to remove the tumor, but the operation couldn't remove it all. The woman started following the ketogenic diet—a diet very high in fat, moderate in protein and very low in carbohydrate. She also had chemotherapy and radiation. After six weeks on the diet, a brain scan showed that the tumor had disappeared. A brain scan five months later showed it was still gone. However, the patient stopped the diet—and a scan three months later showed that the tumor had returned.

Yes, a special diet called the ketogenic diet can fight cancer. It is being used to manage brain cancer and advanced (metastatic) cancer, which is when the disease has spread beyond the original tumor to other parts of the body (such as breast cancer that spreads to the liver and bones). It may be effective in fighting most, if not all, cancers, but it must be done under the supervision of an experienced oncological nutritionist.

Here, what you need to know about this little-known therapy for cancer...

HOW IT WORKS

The ketogenic diet is very high in fat—the ratio is four grams of fat to one gram of protein/carbohydrate. It has long been used to control epilepsy and is offered as an epilepsy treatment at hundreds of hospitals and clinics around the world, including The Johns Hopkins Epilepsy Center, Mayo Clinic and Mattel Children's Hospital at UCLA.

It eases epilepsy by stabilizing neurons (brain cells). It does so by reducing glucose (blood

---

Thomas N. Seyfried, PhD, a professor of biology at Boston College and author of *Cancer as a Metabolic Disease: On the Origin, Management, and Prevention of Cancer* (Wiley). His numerous scientific articles have appeared in *Nature Medicine, Science, The Lancet Oncology, Proceedings of the National Academy of Sciences, Journal of Oncology, Cancer Letters, Journal of Neurochemistry* and many other medical and scientific journals.

sugar), the main fuel used by neurons, and increasing ketones (beta-hydroxybutyric acid and acetoacetic acid), a by-product of fat metabolism used by neurons when glucose levels are low. Reducing glucose and increasing ketones play key roles in fighting cancer as well.

The typical American diet is about 50% to 60% carbohydrate (fruits, vegetables, breads, cereals, milk and milk products, and added sugars in sweetened foods and beverages). The body turns carbohydrate into glucose, which is used for energy.

Cancer cells gorge on glucose. Eating a ketogenic diet deprives them of this primary fuel, starving the cells, which stop growing or die. Also, ketones are a fuel usable by normal cells but not by cancer cells, so this, too, helps stop cancer growth. *In addition, the diet...*

- **Puts you into a metabolic state similar to that of fasting**—and fasting has repeatedly been shown to arrest cancer.
- **Lowers levels of insulin (the glucose-regulating hormone) and insulin-like growth factor**—both of which drive tumor growth.

CASE HISTORIES

The first case report about the ketogenic diet for cancer appeared in *Journal of the American College of Nutrition* in 1995. The ketogenic diet was used by two children with advanced, inoperable brain cancer who had undergone extensive, life-threatening radiation and chemotherapy. They both responded remarkably well to the diet.

Can the Diet Prevent Cancer?

Cancer survivors and people with a family history of cancer may wonder if they should go on the ketogenic diet as a preventive measure. It is not necessary for people to follow the diet if they do not have cancer. A six-to-seven-day water-only fast done once or twice a year—under a doctor's supervision—can be effective in reducing the risk for recurrent cancer in survivors and in those individuals with a family history of cancer. Fasting reduces glucose and elevates ketones.

A case report that I coauthored, published in *Nutrition & Metabolism* in 2010, told the story (see beginning of this article) of the 65-year-old woman with glioblastoma multiforme—the most common and most aggressive type of brain tumor, with a median survival of only about 12 months after diagnosis. Standard treatment—surgery to remove as much of the tumor as possible, plus radiation and/or chemotherapy—extends average survival time only a few months beyond that of people who aren't treated.

My viewpoint: In animal research, the ketogenic diet is the only therapeutic approach that deprives tumors of their primary fuel...stops tumor cells from invading other areas...stops the process of angiogenesis (blood supply to tumors)...and reduces inflammation, which drives cancer. The diet also could reduce the need for anticonvulsant and anti-inflammatory medications in brain cancer patients.

Considering how ineffective the current standard of care is for brain cancer (and for metastatic cancer), the ketogenic diet could be an attractive option for many cancer patients.

WORKING WITH AN EXPERT

The ketogenic diet for cancer is not a diet you should undertake on your own after reading a book or other self-help materials. It requires the assistance of an oncological nutritionist or other health professional who is familiar with the use of the regimen in cancer patients. Ask your oncologist for a referral.

Important aspects of the ketogenic diet include...

- **Measuring glucose and ketone levels.** For the management of cancer, blood glucose levels should fall between 55 mg/dL and 65 mg/dL, and ketone levels between 3 mmol and 5 mmol. In order to monitor those levels—and adjust your diet accordingly—you need to use methods similar to those used by patients with diabetes. These methods include glucose testing several times a day with a finger stick and glucose strip...daily urine testing for ketones...and (more accurate) home blood testing for ketones, perhaps done weekly.
- **Starting with a water-only fast.** If you are in relatively good health (aside from the cancer, of course), it is best to start the ketogenic

diet with a water-only fast for 48 to 72 hours, which will quickly put you in ketosis—the production of a therapeutic level of ketones. This fast should be guided by a health professional.

If you are fragile or in poor health, you can skip the water fast and initiate ketosis with the ketogenic diet, reducing carbohydrates to less than 12 grams a day. This should produce ketosis within two or three weeks.

•**Macronutrient ratios and recipes.** Working with a nutritionist, you will find the fat/protein/carbohydrate ratio that works best for you to lower glucose and increase ketones…and the recipes and meal plan that consistently deliver those ratios. A food diary, a food scale and the use of a "KetoCalculator" (available on websites such as *www.KetoCalculator.com/ketocalc/diet.asp*) are necessary tools to implement the ketogenic diet.

Helpful: The oncological nutritionist Miriam Kalamian, EdM, MS, CNS, managed her own son's brain tumor with the ketogenic diet, and she counsels cancer patients around the world in the implementation of the diet. You can find more information on her website, DietaryTherapies.com.

CLINICAL TRIALS

Currently, there are several clinical trials being conducted using the ketogenic diet for cancer.

•**Brain cancer.** There are trials at Michigan State University and in Germany and Israel testing the diet's efficacy as a complementary treatment with radiation for recurrent glioblastoma…and by itself to improve the quality of life and survival time in patients with brain cancer. Michigan State University currently is recruiting patients for its trial.

Contact: Ken Schwartz, MD, 517-975-9500, e-mail: *ken.schwartz@hc.msu.edu.*

•**Pancreatic cancer.** A trial at Holden Comprehensive Cancer Center at University of Iowa is recruiting patients with pancreatic cancer for a trial using the ketogenic diet along with radiation and chemotherapy.

Contact: Sandy Vollstedt, RN, BSN, 319-353-7143, e-mail: *sandy-vollstedt@uiowa.edu.*

•**Lung cancer.** The University of Iowa also is recruiting lung cancer patients for a similar trial. The contact information is the same as for the trial on pancreatic cancer.

•**Metastatic cancer.** The VA Pittsburgh Healthcare System is recruiting patients with metastatic cancer for a study of the effect of the ketogenic diet on quality of life, tumor growth and survival.

Contact: Jocelyn Tan, MD, 412-360-6178, e-mail: *jocelyn.tan@va.gov.*

info You can find out more about these trials at *ClinicalTrials.gov.* Enter "Ketogenic Diet" into the search engine at the site for a complete listing of cancer trials and trials testing the ketogenic diet for other conditions, including epilepsy, amyotrophic lateral sclerosis (ALS), Lafora disease (a severe neurological disease), Parkinson's disease and obesity.

Frozen Broccoli—How to Restore Its Cancer-Fighting Power

Elizabeth Jeffery, PhD, professor, department of food science and human nutrition, College of Agricultural, Consumer, and Environmental Sciences, University of Illinois, Urbana-Champaign. Her study was published in *Journal of Food Sciences.*

Broccoli got a bum rap when President George H.W. Bush declared that he didn't like it and never again wanted to see it served in the White House or on Air Force One. Hopefully you don't share his aversion, because broccoli is super-healthful. It's high in fiber, folate, vitamin C and antioxidants…and because it contains a cancer-fighting compound called sulforaphane, eating just a few servings per week can reduce your cancer risk.

But: If you buy your broccoli frozen, you don't get the full benefits—because the pre-freeze processing and typical cooking method destroy the vegetable's anticancer properties.

Cool new discovery: There's a simple trick you can use to restore frozen broccoli's super powers, a recent study reveals.

A DELICATE BALANCE

You know the pungent odor that fills your kitchen when you grind up broccoli scraps in your disposal? That smell comes from all the sulfur compounds, one of which is the sulforaphane responsible for broccoli's ability to combat cancer. When you eat fresh broccoli, you get lots of sulforaphane, provided you eat it raw or nearly raw (for instance, steamed for no more than three to five minutes). But when broccoli is frozen, the sulforaphane is lost. *Here's why...*

Sulforaphane is created when another compound found in broccoli, glucoraphanin, comes in contact with one of broccoli's enzymes, myrosinase. This contact occurs when broccoli is chewed or chopped. Typically, before broccoli is frozen, commercial vegetable processors extend its shelf life by blanching it at a very high temperature (typically above 200°F) to inactivate its peroxidase, an enzyme thought to cause broccoli to degrade over time. Unfortunately, this high heat also inactivates the myrosinase—thus rendering the glucoraphanin incapable of creating sulforaphane.

Researchers at the University of Illinois tried to get around this problem by blanching broccoli at a lower temperature before freezing it. They discovered that blanching at 169°F did preserve most of the myrosinase. Yet after this blanched broccoli was frozen and then cooked, the researchers found that no sulforaphane formed. They realized that this is because the typical instructions for cooking frozen broccoli are to microwave it—which again raises the temperature too high and/or for too long. In other words, the myrosinase in frozen broccoli gets hit with a double whammie from both the blanching and the microwaving. (Note that, even with fresh broccoli, cooking the vegetable too long inactivates the myrosinase.)

So then the researchers took a different approach. Instead of worrying about blanching temperatures or cooking methods, they instead added an outside source of myrosinase—a bit of ground freeze-dried daikon radish (a mild-flavored radish that looks sort of like a fat white carrot)—while the frozen broccoli was being cooked. The amount of radish powder the researchers added was too little to change the taste or appearance of the broccoli, but it provided enough myrosinase to allow the interaction with glucoraphanin, triggering the formation of sulforaphane. Thus the frozen broccoli's cancer-fighting properties were restored!

TRY THIS AT HOME

Hopefully, commercial food processors will catch on to this new technique for preserving frozen broccoli's full nutritional punch and start sprinkling on some daikon powder at the processing plant. Until that happens, though, you can easily perform this bit of food magic yourself at home.

Simply add some freeze-dried daikon (comparable to the amount of salt you'd normally add) to your frozen broccoli either before or after cooking it. You can find daikon radish (also called white radish) at Asian grocery stores, Whole Foods stores or online.

Another option: Whenever you eat broccoli that has been frozen, in the same meal include another outside source of myrosinase, such as raw red radishes, cabbage slaw or watercress...or eat one-quarter teaspoon of horseradish, wasabi or mustard along with your serving of broccoli.

Five Supplements That Help Prevent Cancer Recurrence

Lise N. Alschuler, ND, board-certified naturopathic oncologist in practice at Naturopathic Specialists in Scottsdale, Arizona. A breast cancer survivor, she is coauthor of *The Definitive Guide to Thriving After Cancer: A Five-Step Integrative Plan to Reduce the Risk of Recurrence and Build Lifelong Health* (Ten Speed). *DrLise.net*

It's a top question on the minds of many cancer survivors—What will help keep the cancer from coming back? Unfortunately, conventional medicine often doesn't have much of an answer beyond, "Take care of yourself, and try not to worry." Naturopathic medicine, however, does have some specific recommendations for cancer survivors—and dietary supplements play a key role.

The reason: "Dietary supplements are able to fit into the 'nooks and crannies' of our biochemical pathways, creating specific changes that influence our bodies on a cellular level," said Lise Alschuler, ND, a breast cancer survivor and coauthor of *The Definitive Guide to Thriving After Cancer.*

The five supplements listed below comprise what Dr. Alschuler calls a "foundational supplement plan" for just about every cancer survivor—and for just about every person who wants to reduce the odds of ever getting cancer in the first place. *Each of the five supplements helps reduce cancer risk through five key pathways...*

- **Boosting immune system function.**
- **Reducing inflammation.**
- **Improving insulin sensitivity.**
- **Supporting digestion and detoxification.**
- **Reducing stress-induced hormone imbalances.**

Although dietary supplements are available over-the-counter, before you start taking them, it is essential to check with a naturopathic doctor (ideally one with additional board certification in naturopathic oncology) or an integrative medical doctor with specific expertise in integrative cancer care. These providers have training in nutritional biochemistry as it relates to cancer. They can confirm that the following supplements are appropriate for you and determine the dosages and the specific brands that will best suit your needs.

For her own post-cancer patients, Dr. Alschuler typically prescribes all five of the following supplements, to be taken daily starting as soon as conventional treatment is completed. "Some patients may be advised to start taking some of these supplements during their conventional treatment, but that should be done only under the guidance of an integrative health-care physician," she said.

The top five cancer fighters include...

- **Omega-3 fatty acids.** These essential fatty acids—found in supplements of fish oil, flaxseed oil and algae-based oil—positively influence all five of the key pathways mentioned above. However, they are especially important for reducing chronic inflammation, which is one of the precursors of cancer. "Think of inflammation as a burning ember in your body that can change your tissues in ways that favor the growth of abnormal cells. Omega-3s quench that fire," Dr. Alschuler said.

Though omega-3s are helpful for survivors of all types of cancer, studies show particular benefits for patients who have battled colon, prostate, breast or lung cancer. A typical daily dosage is 1,000 mg to 3,000 mg of omega-3 oil.

Caveat: Omega-3s can increase bleeding, so it's vital to get your doctor's OK before taking omega-3s if you are on blood-thinning medication or are anticipating any surgery.

- **Probiotics.** Beneficial bacteria in the intestinal tract help metabolize nutrients, bind waste products for removal in stool and regulate immunity. When beneficial bacteria are depleted, the digestive tract is overrun with harmful bacteria and a condition called dysbiosis develops. This contributes to an increased risk for cancer recurrence. Studies have shown that supplementing with beneficial intestinal bacteria called probiotics can reduce the risk for infection after surgery and improve the immune system's response.

You can get some probiotics from eating yogurt and fermented foods such as fresh sauerkraut, miso, tempeh and kefir. However, to fully support her patients' beneficial digestive bacteria, Dr. Alschuler typically prescribes a supplement that combines several types of probiotics at a dosage of at least one billion colony-forming units (CFU) daily.

Vitamin B-12 and Cancer

A recent study found that people with elevated vitamin B-12 levels (above 800 pg/mL) had an increased risk for such cancers as leukemia and malignancies of the lung or bladder. None of the study participants were taking B-12 supplements.

Theory: Elevated B-12 levels may result from some not-yet-identified cancer-related process.

If your blood work consistently indicates higher-than-normal levels of vitamin B-12: Discuss your cancer risk with your doctor.

Johan Arendt, researcher, Aarhus University Hospital, Denmark.

Better Screening for Lung Cancer

According to recent research, risk-calculating software that was used when reading the CT scans of nearly 2,700 current or former smokers predicted with more than 90% accuracy which nodules were benign or malignant.

Implication: After an initial CT scan, doctors can now better determine what type of follow-up is needed—a second CT scan, biopsy or surgery.

If you need a CT scan to screen for lung cancer: Your doctor can use the risk-calculating spreadsheet at *Brocku.ca/Lung-Cancer-Risk-Calculator.*

Stephen Lam, MD, professor of medicine, The University of British Columbia, Vancouver, Canada.

Caution: Probiotics are not appropriate for people whose white blood cell count is below normal—some evidence suggests that probiotics can increase the risk for blood infection in those individuals.

•**Polyphenols.** Healthful, colorful fruits and vegetables get their rainbow hues from the naturally occurring plant compounds called polyphenols (also referred to as flavonoids). According to Dr. Alschuler, three polyphenols are particularly important in the fight against cancer...

- Green tea catechins, which may lower the risk for cancers of the digestive tract, breast, bladder, lung, blood and prostate.
- Curcumin, the bright yellow flavonoid found in turmeric root, which appears to inhibit cancer formation in a variety of ways, helping protect against the majority of cancer types.
- Resveratrol, which gives color to red grapes and some berries, has shown promise against breast, colorectal and liver cancers by activating tumor suppressor genes and increasing the rate of apoptosis (normal programmed cell death).

Your doctor may prescribe a combination supplement that contains all three of these polyphenols, or you may take each one separately. "Many high-quality brands also include other polyphenols. But watch out for what I call 'window-dressing' supplements that list 20 to 30 different polyphenols—because the amount of each one will be so small that you might as well just eat a salad," Dr. Alschuler said.

•**Antioxidants.** "Look at metal that's been exposed to rain and sunlight—it starts to rust because it's being oxidized. That's essentially what happens to our bodies from exposure to 'free radicals,' or oxidative toxins," Dr. Alschuler said. Antioxidants guard against this by binding to oxidative toxins so they can be eliminated (but see next article for a specific caution concerning lung cancer and antioxidants)...and they also stimulate cell repair and normal apoptosis. Cancer treatment can deplete your antioxidant capacity because cancer drugs themselves exert their cancer-killing effects via oxidation. A plant-based diet provides antioxidants, but cancer survivors should get additional support by taking...

- Glutathione, the body's "master antioxidant," which is critical for the elimination of environmental toxins. A typical dosage is 250 mg to 500 mg daily.
- Coenzyme Q10 (CoQ10), which is associated with decreased risk for breast and thyroid cancer, as well as melanoma, studies show. A typical daily dosage is 30 mg to 100 mg.

•**Vitamin D.** Numerous studies have shown the cancer-preventing potential of this vitamin, which promotes proper cell maturation and regulates inflammation, among other activities. "Without adequate levels of vitamin D, it's hard for our bodies to maintain good blood sugar control or reduce inflammation," said Dr. Alschuler.

Although it's often called the sunshine vitamin, many people in the northern hemisphere cannot get enough vitamin D just from being outdoors, especially during cooler seasons. Ask your doctor to measure your blood level of vitamin D—that information will help determine the right dosage for you.

Caution: If you take the heart medication digoxin, be especially sure to talk with your doctor before taking vitamin D because the combination could lead to abnormal heart rhythms.

Important: "Dietary supplements are called 'supplements' for a reason—they are meant to supplement the diet, not to replace healthy eating," Dr. Alschuler said. "Over time, they provide targeted molecular support that gently but radically alters the terrain in your body, creating an environment that impedes cancer recurrence…so you can get back to the business of living your life."

Could Antioxidants Speed Up Cancer Progression?

Martin Bergo, MD, PhD, codirector, Sahlgrenska Cancer Center, University of Gothenburg, Sweden.
Per Lindahl, professor of biochemistry and cell biology, University of Gothenburg, Sweden.
Peter Campbell, PhD, director, Tumor Repository, American Cancer Society, Atlanta.
Science Translational Medicine

Smokers and other people at high risk for lung cancer could make matters worse if they take antioxidant supplements, a recent study of rodents suggests.

Antioxidants appear to accelerate cancer progression by short-circuiting one of the body's key immune responses to malignant cells, researchers from Sweden report.

STUDY DETAILS

Normal doses of vitamin E and smaller doses of the antioxidant supplement acetylcysteine increased the growth of tumors in mice with early lung cancer, the researchers reported in *Science Translational Medicine.*

"We found that antioxidants caused a threefold increase in the number of tumors, and caused tumors to become more aggressive," said senior author Martin Bergo MD, PhD, "Antioxidants caused the mice to die twice as fast, and the effect was dose-dependent. If we gave a small dose, tumors grew a little. If we gave a high dose, tumors grew a lot."

Dr. Bergo, codirector of the Sahlgrenska Cancer Center at the University of Gothenburg, said the findings are particularly concerning because acetylcysteine is used to improve breathing in patients with chronic obstructive pulmonary disease, or COPD. Most people who have COPD are current or former smokers.

HOW ANTIOXIDANTS AFFECT CANCER GROWTH

Antioxidants are supposed to protect the body from disease by preventing cell damage caused by molecules called free radicals. "These radicals can damage almost anything inside the cell, including DNA, and DNA damage can lead to cancer," Dr. Bergo said.

But this protection backfires in people who already have cancerous or precancerous cells, the researchers said.

When the body detects cellular DNA damage that can lead to cancer, it releases a key tumor-suppressing protein called p53.

In laboratory tests with mouse and human cancer cells, researchers found that antioxidants suppress the release of p53 by halting DNA damage done to cancer cells by free radicals.

"By reducing the DNA damage, the antioxidant actually helps the cancer cells escape detection," said coauthor Per Lindahl, a professor of biochemistry and cell biology at the University of Gothenburg.

IMPLICATIONS

The findings suggest that people carrying small, undiagnosed tumors in their lungs should avoid taking extra antioxidants, the study concludes.

"If you have lung cancer, or if you have an increased risk of developing lung cancer, then taking extra antioxidants may be harmful and

Coffee: More Good News

An analysis of more than 3,000 adults found that drinking one to three cups of caffeinated coffee daily reduced liver cancer risk by at least 40%.

Theory: Coffee has been shown to reduce the risk for diabetes, which has been linked to liver cancer.

Carlo La Vecchia, MD, head of epidemiology, Istituto di Ricerche Farmacologiche Mario Negri, Milan, Italy.

Two Blood Tests Favor Early Detection of Lung Cancer

One test checks for serum-free fatty acids, which are much higher in people with lung cancer and prostate cancer. The test accurately identified cancer patients 70% of the time.

Study of 95 cancer patients by researchers at Cleveland Clinic, Ohio, presented at the annual meeting of the American Society of Anesthesiologists in San Francisco.

Another study conducted by researchers in China found that people with lung cancer have high levels of the so-called "biomarker," isocitrate dehydrogenase (IDH1). Lung cancer is rarely diagnosed in the earliest stages. The new test looks for IDH1, a protein that rises when tumors are present.

Clinical Cancer Research

it could speed up the growth of a tumor," Dr. Bergo said.

While studies involving animals can be useful, they may fail to produce similar results in humans.

CORROBORATES PREVIOUS RESEARCH

However, this isn't the first study to indicate that antioxidants are bad for cancer patients, said Peter Campbell, PhD, director of the Tumor Repository at the American Cancer Society in Atlanta.

Human trials conducted in the 1980s and 1990s found that the antioxidants beta-carotene, vitamin A and vitamin E substantially increased the incidence of lung cancer in smokers, he said.

"This study doesn't stick out like a sore thumb," Dr. Campbell said. "We've known for some time that some of these agents tend to backfire. It's nice to have laboratory evidence to corroborate what we've seen in human populations."

The human body creates its own antioxidants, and is built to use additional antioxidants gained from the food a person eats, Dr. Campbell said. By taking antioxidant supplements, people could be defeating the body's ability to fight cancer and disease.

"There is a food supplement industry that has done a really good job marketing itself, suggesting that if we take these molecules normally found in food we will have better health and, well, a little is good so a whole lot would be better," Dr. Campbell said. "There are very intricate, complicated pathways that are supposed to sense and signal and destroy these precancerous cells. When our body doesn't turn that system on, these cancerous cells can proliferate."

ADVICE

However, the Swedish researchers stopped short of saying that no one should take antioxidants.

"If I had a patient with lung cancer, I would probably recommend they do not take extra antioxidants," Dr. Bergo said. "Would I make that recommendation with healthy people? Absolutely not."

info For more about antioxidants and cancer, visit the National Cancer Institute website, *www.cancer.gov*, and search "antioxidants and cancer prevention."

Raw Garlic Protects Against Lung Cancer

Jin-Kou Zhao, MD, PhD, professor of epidemiology, Jiangsu Provincial Center for Disease Control and Prevention, Nanjing, China. His study was published in *Cancer Prevention Research*.

Though smoking tops the list of risk factors that increase the odds of developing lung cancer, nonsmokers get it, too. That's why we all need to do what we can to guard against this terrible disease.

Good news: Now there's a specific, real-life strategy we all can follow that may reduce our lung cancer risk. According to a recent study, the key is garlic—but you have to eat a certain amount of it, and in a certain way...

BAD FOR BREATH BUT GOOD FOR LUNGS

For the study, researchers recruited 1,424 lung cancer patients, then matched those patients by age and gender with 4,543 healthy adults who lived in the same areas. All participants were interviewed extensively and asked specific questions about factors that can increase or decrease lung cancer risk—smoking, exposure to pollution, alcohol consumption, weight, exercise, family history, dietary habits, etc.

What hurt: Not surprisingly, smoking was confirmed as a strong risk factor, increasing lung cancer risk by 2.5 times. Risk also rose with environmental exposure to nearby factories, family history of lung cancer and frequent consumption of fried foods.

What helped: Drinking green tea and getting regular exercise were associated with a 15% and 18% reduction in lung cancer risk, respectively. But the big winner was eating raw garlic. Compared with people who never consumed raw garlic, those who ate it twice or more per week, on average—consuming about 33 grams weekly (about 10 to 30 cloves per week, depending on size)—had a 44% lower risk for lung cancer. That is a huge reduction in risk! The "twice or more per week" part seemed very important, because eating raw garlic just once per week on average was associated with only an 8% reduction in risk.

Even smokers reaped the benefits! Smokers who ate raw garlic at least twice a week had a 30% lower risk for lung cancer than smokers who did not eat it.

GARLIC'S POWERS

Garlic's medicinal powers are thought to be related to several sulfur compounds that are formed when garlic is crushed or chopped. When raw garlic is chewed and swallowed, the volatile oils that contain the beneficial compounds are breathed in and then mostly excreted via the lungs—which is really interesting and unusual!—and this could explain why garlic may protect against lung cancer specifically. In addition, earlier studies done in laboratories have shown that garlic's compounds, including allicin, can kill human liver, colon and gastric cancer cells...and animal studies suggest that garlic also provides some protection against breast cancer and lymphoma.

This recent study did not examine the effects of eating cooked garlic or taking garlic supplements, and earlier studies that looked at those forms of garlic had inconsistent results. So for now, the evidence suggests that raw garlic is the way to go. Fortunately, there are many simple and tasty ways to incorporate fresh, raw garlic into your diet by adding it to other healthful foods. For example, you can put chopped raw garlic in fresh salsa and bruschetta, which also include nutritious tomatoes...in guacamole, which also is rich in healthful avocado oils...and in hummus, a good source of plant protein.

Even easier: You also can add chopped raw garlic to salad dressings—homemade or store-bought—just before serving and get an automatic "dose" to help protect your lungs every time you enjoy a salad.

Lung Cancer Breakthroughs—Prevention and Detection

Peter Bach, MD, epidemiologist and lung cancer specialist, Memorial Sloan-Kettering Cancer Center, New York City. He has done extensive research and development on lung cancer prediction models and has authored numerous articles on lung cancer for medical journals.

Men worry about prostate cancer...women worry about breast cancer...everybody worries about colon cancer, skin cancer and brain cancer. But there's another cancer that claims more Americans' lives than those five other types combined. It's lung cancer, the number-one cancer killer in the country, responsible for more than 157,000 deaths each year.

The good news: Recent advances in prevention and detection are helping in the battle against this fearsome disease. For instance, there's a new screening tool that can cut the

> **Early Stomach Cancer Diagnosis**
>
> Stomach cancer could be diagnosed before it turns deadly, according to researchers who recently identified glycans (sugars attached to proteins) that are found only in these cancer patients.
>
> *Cancer Prevention Research*

odds of dying from lung cancer by 20%. Is it right for you or for someone you love? For answers to that question and more, we turned to Peter Bach, MD, an epidemiologist and lung cancer specialist at Memorial Sloan-Kettering Cancer Center in New York City.

OVERDUE PREVENTION TACTIC

Not all cases of lung cancer are caused by cigarette smoking, but up to 90% are. The percentage of Americans who smoke has declined significantly over the past few decades, from 42% in 1965 to 19% in 2011...but it's still way too high.

Public education campaigns and high cigarette taxes do help reduce smoking, but now the FDA is exploring a new tactic—regulating or even banning menthol cigarettes. The reason? Because menthol may make it easier to become addicted to smoking and harder to quit.

Why it has taken the FDA so long to consider regulating menthol is a mystery. Back in 2009, when the FDA banned the candy, clove and fruit flavorings that made cigarettes more palatable to young smokers, it also called for an investigation on the impact of mentholated cigarettes on public health. Two years later, the FDA's advisory committee concluded that it is "biologically plausible" that adding menthol to cigarettes makes them more addictive, and that removing menthol from cigarettes would improve public health.

Menthol's allure: The addition of menthol is a trick used by tobacco companies—in fact, the flavoring is added to all cigarettes, not just those not marketed as menthol. Menthol-flavored cigarettes have about 10 times more added menthol than regular cigarettes, but even at the lower levels, the menthol helps mask the harshness of tobacco and the irritation associated with nicotine. Without the added menthol, the harshness and irritation could be turnoffs for new smokers—making them less likely to stick with the dangerous habit.

Menthol works by stimulating the cold receptors on nerve endings in the mouth, nose and skin, creating a cooling sensation. When menthol is added at higher levels, the cooling sensation also is felt in the lungs. At the same time, menthol contains substances that enhance nicotine's "bite," a sensation that smokers seem to crave, further reinforcing smoking behavior.

The FDA is considering banning menthol because it lures smokers and keeps them, but other studies suggest that menthol also makes cigarettes more harmful. Last year, we reported that smokers of menthol cigarettes had more than twice the risk for stroke as smokers of regular cigarettes. People who smoke menthol cigarettes also show decreased elasticity and increased stiffness of the carotid arteries (the main arteries feeding the brain) compared with smokers of regular cigarettes. In addition, menthol's cooling action slows respiration, increasing breath-holding time and, in turn, leading to greater exposure to the cigarette's toxins. What's more, the cilia (tiny hairlike structures in the airway that move things along) slow down when exposed to menthol, impairing clearance of toxins from the airway.

Our opinion: It's way past time for menthol to be banned from cigarettes.

LIFESAVING SCREENING: FOR WHOM?

Lung cancer has one of the lowest five-year survival rates of all cancers mainly because it usually is diagnosed too late to be cured. About 90% of people who get lung cancer die because of it.

Recently, the US Preventive Services Task Force, an independent panel of experts in prevention and evidence-based medicine, sought to update its previous determination against routine lung cancer screening for smokers. The task force reviewed relevant studies, relying most heavily on the National Lung Screening Trial (NLST).

The NLST included more than 53,000 smokers who were randomly assigned to undergo three annual exams with either chest x-rays or low-dose CT scans.

Findings: In each of the three rounds of screening, CT exams found more cancers than x-rays. In the first round alone, CT scans identified 270 people with lung cancer, compared with 136 in the x-ray group. CT screening reduced lung cancer deaths by 20%.

Based on these findings, a task force recommendation now in draft form advises annual

CT screening for people at high risk—those between the ages of 55 and 79 who have a smoking history of at least 30 pack-years. (A pack-year is an average of one pack per day for one year. So, for example, if you smoked two packs each day for 15 years, you have a 30-pack-year history.) The recommendation applies even to ex-smokers who have quit smoking within the past 15 years. (The NLST did not look at ex-smokers who quit more than 15 years ago.)

If you fall in to the high-risk category, should you go get a CT scan? Probably—but there are several factors to consider first, Dr. Bach said, because the benefits to you may not be quite as great as the NLST findings suggest. The NLST was conducted at 33 academic medical centers around the country, all with expertise in diagnosing and managing lung cancer—whereas the same high-quality results may not be found outside of a top-notch academic community. Also, Dr. Bach believes that the task force's estimate of 20,000 lives saved every year from annual CT screening is overly optimistic. He explained that his institution's analysis of the data, using different statistical methods, estimates about 4,000 lives saved each year.

Why does it matter whether the true benefits are somewhat less than the NLST suggests? Because CT scans are not without risk. Although low-dose CT exposes you to much less radiation than a standard chest CT, it's still much higher than the exposure you'd get from a regular chest x-ray. CT scans also may result in false-positive findings or incidental findings (abnormalities that don't cause harm), both of which can lead to unnecessary invasive testing and anxiety.

Bottom line: If you clearly fall into the high-risk category (age 55 to 79 with a smoking history of at least 30 pack-years and less than 15 years since you quit), you should be aware of the screening option and seriously consider the trade-offs of benefits versus risks. "The most aggressive we should be is to suggest that such patients discuss screening with a doctor who is disinterested—meaning someone who is not the owner of a CT scanner or radiology center," Dr. Bach said.

Lower-risk people should not be offered screening, in his opinion. "Outside of the high-risk group, the potential danger of radiation vastly exceeds the possible benefits of screening. That's even more true for women than for men because the radiation also can contribute to breast cancer risk."

GENDER EQUALITY?

Speaking of women, let's consider the issue of gender as it relates to lung cancer risk. Lung cancer used to be considered primarily a man's disease. But several years ago, the pendulum swung in the opposite direction when some studies suggested that female smokers were more susceptible to the harms of cigarettes than male smokers...and that women who had never smoked were more likely to get lung cancer than men who had never smoked.

However, those theories did not hold up in more rigorous studies. Most experts agree, Dr. Bach said, that lung cancer is neither predominantly a man's disease nor a woman's disease. Women and men have the same risk of developing lung cancer and dying from it...and it is the leading cause of cancer death for both men and women in the US.

HELP FOR SMOKERS AND EX-SMOKERS

If you smoke or used to smoke, visit these three important websites...

- **The CDC's Tips from Former Smokers** public service campaign has been instrumental in convincing more than 100,000 smokers to drop their smoking habit.
- **Go to *http://smokingpackyears.com/calculate* to calculate your pack-years**—an important number when considering whether CT screening is appropriate for you.
- **Memorial Sloan-Kettering Cancer Center**, one of the nation's top cancer hospitals, has developed its own online tool (*http://www.mskcc.org/cancer-care/adult/lung/screening-decision-tool*) that can help you decide whether you should be screened. The criteria used are slightly different than those developed by the task force—so it will be helpful to discuss the guidelines with your own doctor.

New Personalized, Precision Approach to Lung Cancer Treatment

Peter Bach, MD, epidemiologist and lung cancer specialist, Memorial Sloan-Kettering Cancer Center, New York City. He has done extensive research and development on lung cancer prediction models and has authored numerous articles on lung cancer for medical journals.

Prasad Adusumilli, MD, thoracic surgeon and researcher, Memorial Sloan-Kettering Cancer Center, New York City. He has researched and published extensively on lung cancer topics, including the personalization of lung cancer surgical resection procedures.

Despite the grim survival rate still reported with lung cancer, exciting advances are happening in the treatment of this terrible disease.

Yes, the odds of surviving lung cancer admittedly still aren't great, but these days a lung cancer diagnosis is not an automatic death sentence—even in the case of late-stage cancer. We have many more options for treating the disease than we did just a decade ago...and treatment today is more personalized and precise than ever.

For instance, doctors now can look at the individual characteristics of a tumor, including particular cell patterns and genetic mutations. This information helps them to set treatment plans that are more likely to work—and to avoid recommending treatments with low chances of success. In fact, Peter Bach, MD, an epidemiologist and pulmonologist at Memorial Sloan-Kettering Cancer Center in New York City, explained that he is "extremely enthusiastic" about the progress that's been made over the past decade.

The problem: Despite the remarkable advances, not all hospitals have the needed tools in their arsenals...and not all doctors understand which patients will benefit from such a personalized approach.

SECRETS FOUND IN CELL PATTERNS

The term lung cancer actually is misleading because the disease is not just one entity. Rather, there are two major types of lung cancer, each with different risk factors, probable prognoses and treatments. And then even within one of those types, different tumors can have different characteristics that affect how aggressive the cancer may be and which treatment may work.

The majority of lung cancers fall into the non–small cell category. Adenocarcinoma is the most common non–small cell cancer, accounting for about half of all lung cancers. It's the type found most often in current and former smokers—and also in people who never smoked.

When adenocarcinoma is detected before it has had a chance to spread, it's treated surgically. Most of the time, the surgeon performs a lobectomy by removing the entire lobe that has the cancer in it (a pair of lungs has five lobes, three on the right side and two on the left). In some cases, the surgeon does a limited resection, removing just part of the affected lobe.

Tricky: The decision about which procedure to do can be a tough one, according to Prasad Adusumilli, MD, a thoracic surgeon and scientist at Memorial Sloan-Kettering Cancer Center. That's because the surgeon wants to remove enough lung tissue to prevent a cancer recurrence, but at the same time leave enough tissue to preserve lung function. Until now, there hasn't been an evidence-based system to guide surgeons, so the size and location of the tumor (for example, how far the tumor is from the edge of the lung) often have been used as criteria in deciding how much to remove.

Breakthrough: Surgeons at Memorial Sloan-Kettering perform about 1,000 of these operations each year. With all the data they have accumulated over the years, Dr. Adusumilli and his research team have developed an algorithm to help surgeons decide which operation is best for patients with adenocarcinoma.

The research that led to the new algorithm was complicated, but basically the researchers performed microscopic examinations of many hundreds of samples of early-stage adenocarcinoma, classifying each according to the proportion of the five major cell patterns (acinar, papillary, lepidic, micropapillary and solid) seen in the tumor. Then they analyzed the follow-up data to determine the chances of cancer recurrence based on the cell pattern and the type of surgery that was done.

Overall, the five-year incidence of cancer recurrence was 21% for patients who had a limited resection and 15% for patients who had a lobectomy. When the specific cell patterns were analyzed, though, it became clear that tumors with a higher percentage of cells showing a micropapillary pattern had a much higher risk for recurrence within the same lobe if patients underwent limited resection.

Bottom line: Doctors can now use this knowledge about cell patterns to opt for the tissue-sparing limited resection procedure in patients whose tumors do not have the aggressive micropapillary pattern...and save the more extensive lobectomy for patients whose cell pattern indicates a high risk for recurrence.

Only a limited number of hospitals have the expertise needed to determine a lung tumor's cell pattern right on the spot, in the operating room, at the time of the actual surgery. "This requires expert pathological experience and a large volume of tumors for the pathologists to get experienced," Dr. Adusumilli explained. At hospitals that do not currently have this ability, some patients who get a limited resection may end up needing another operation later if their cancer subsequently is found to have the micropapillary pattern...or, worse, they may have a cancer recurrence.

Hopefully, that will change soon. Dr. Adusumilli and his team of researchers are now trying to develop tools that can more easily determine the cell's pattern—preferably before surgery—sparing patients the need to go under the knife a second time.

SECRETS FOUND IN GENETIC MUTATIONS

When lung cancer is diagnosed after it has spread to the lymph nodes or beyond, as it is most of the time, treatment involves more than just surgery—it also requires medication. Now, in what Dr. Bach refers to as a "very exciting" development, the particular medications that will work best often can be determined based on specific genetic mutations in the tumors.

How it started: About 10 years ago, during clinical trials for two new lung cancer drugs, doctors observed that some people receiving the drugs *gefitinib* (Iressa) and *erlotinib* (Tarceva) had a much better response than others—even though all the patients had advanced adenocarcinoma. This led to the discovery that the patients who responded well had tumors that showed a specific mutation in the epidermal growth factor receptor (EGFR) gene. People with the mutation survived nearly twice as long on the drug regimen as those without it. It turns out that the mutation is present in about 20% of people diagnosed with advanced adenocarcinoma.

A few years later, researchers discovered another mutation on the anaplastic lymphoma kinase (ALK) gene, which is present in 7% of people with adenocarcinoma. A drug that inhibits ALK activity, called *crizotinib* (Xalkori), is very effective in people who have that particular mutation.

All three of these drugs have been approved, and the required genetic testing is available. Many experts now recommend that all patients with advanced adenocarcinoma have their tumors analyzed for mutations of EGFR and ALK—including patients who have mixed cancer types, even with just a small component of adenocarcinoma. Referring to molecular testing in its entirety, not just for EGFR and ALK, Dr. Bach said, "Now, 60% to 70% of adenocarcinomas have important molecular information that affects therapeutic choices. That's huge! Lung cancer might be the poster child for this kind of precision, personalized medicine."

If you are diagnosed with lung cancer: If at all possible, see an oncologist at a hospital associated with a university, Dr. Bach advised. Academic medical centers usually have the technology and expertise to take advantage of these new tests and procedures. If you live too far away to see a doctor there regularly, consider having a consultation with an appropriate expert at such a facility—that person can advise you and your doctor on the best treatment for you.

Could an Antidepressant Combat Lethal Lung Cancer?

Stanford University, news release

An older and little-used class of antidepressants may help combat a particularly deadly form of lung cancer, according to a recent study.

Using a unique computer program, researchers from the Stanford University School of Medicine identified tricyclic antidepressants as a potential treatment for small cell lung cancer. This class of drugs was introduced decades ago and is still approved for use in the US, but has been supplanted by newer antidepressants with fewer side effects.

Follow-up experiments showed that the tricyclic antidepressant called *imipramine* (Tofranil) was effective against human small cell lung cancer cells grown in the laboratory and growing as tumors in mice. The drug activated a self-destruction pathway in the cancer cells and slowed or blocked the spread of cancer in mice.

Imipramine maintained its effectiveness regardless of whether the cancer cells had previously been exposed, and become resistant, to traditional chemotherapy treatments, according to the study, which was published online in the journal *Cancer Discovery*.

HUMAN TRIALS TO MOVE QUICKLY

Because tricyclic antidepressants already have U.S. Food and Drug Administration approval for use in people, the Stanford team was quickly able to launch a clinical trial to test imipramine in patients with small cell lung cancer and certain other types of cancer.

"We are cutting down the decade or more and the $1 billion it can typically take to translate a laboratory finding into a successful drug treatment to about one to two years and spending about $100,000," study co-senior author Atul Butte, MD, director of the Center for Pediatric Bioinformatics at Lucile Packard Children's Hospital at Stanford, said in a university news release.

STOPPING A HIGH DEATH RATE

"The five-year survival for small cell lung cancer is only 5%," study co-senior author Julien Sage, PhD, an associate professor of pediatrics at Stanford University, said in the news release. "There has not been a single efficient therapy developed in the last 30 years. But when we began to test these drugs in human cancer cells grown in a dish and in a mouse model, they worked, and they worked, and they worked."

Another drug, an antihistamine called *promethazine* (Phenergan), also exhibited the ability to kill cancer cells, according to the researchers.

info For more information on small cell lung cancer, visit the website of The U.S. National Cancer Institute at *http://www.cancer.gov/cancertopics/pdq/treatment/small-cell-lung/patient/*.

Better Way to Prevent Esophageal Cancer

Barrett's esophagus, often caused by severe, chronic heartburn, can lead to abnormal changes in cells of the esophagus that can develop into cancer. In a new study of 136 patients with low-grade Barrett's esophagus, those who underwent radiofrequency ablation—in which the abnormal cells were destroyed with electricity applied through an endoscope—had a 7.4% lower risk for cancer than those who had no treatment. Radiofrequency ablation was shown earlier to also improve outcomes for those with more severe forms of Barrett's esophagus.

Jacques Bergman, MD, PhD, professor of gastrointestinal endoscopy, University of Amsterdam, the Netherlands.

Intravenous Vitamin C May Boost Chemo's Cancer-Fighting Power

Jeanne Drisko, MD, endowed professor and director, integrative medicine, University of Kansas Medical Center, Kansas City.

Stephanie Bernik, MD, chief, surgical oncology, Lenox Hill Hospital, New York City.

Michael Seiden, MD, chief medical officer, The US Oncology Network, The Woodlands, TX.

Science Translational Medicine

Large doses of intravenous (IV) vitamin C have the potential to boost chemotherapy's ability to kill cancer cells, according to recent laboratory research involving human cells and mice.

Vitamin C delivered directly to human and mouse ovarian cancer cells helped kill off those cells while leaving normal cells unharmed, University of Kansas researchers report.

"In cell tissue and animal models of cancer, we saw when you add IV vitamin C it seems to augment the killing effect of chemotherapy drugs on cancer cells," said study coauthor Jeanne Drisko, MD, director of integrative medicine at the University of Kansas Medical Center.

In follow-up human trials, a handful of cervical cancer patients given intravenous vitamin C along with their chemotherapy reported fewer toxic side effects from their cancer treatment, according to the study published in *Science Translational Medicine.*

"In those patients, we didn't see any ill effects and we noticed they had fewer effects from the chemotherapy," Dr. Drisko said. "It seemed to be protecting the healthy cells while killing the cancer cells."

BACKGROUND

Intravenous vitamin C has been considered an integrative medical therapy for cancer since the 1970s, Dr. Drisko noted.

But vitamin C's cancer-killing potential hasn't been taken seriously by mainstream medicine ever since clinical trials performed by the Mayo Clinic with oral vitamin C in the late 1970s and early 1980s found no anti-cancer effects, she explained.

Researchers have since argued that those trials were flawed because vitamin C taken orally is absorbed by the gut and excreted by the kidneys before its levels can build up in the bloodstream.

But it's been hard to attract funding for further research. There's no reason for pharmaceutical companies to fund vitamin C research, and federal officials have been uninterested in investing research dollars into the effort since the Mayo research was published, Dr. Drisko said.

RECENT RESEARCH

This latest investigation began with researchers exposing human ovarian cancer cells to vitamin C in the lab. They found that the cells suffered DNA damage and died off, while normal cells were left unharmed.

The researchers then tested vitamin C on mice with induced ovarian cancer. The vitamin appeared to help chemotherapy drugs either inhibit the growth of tumors or help shrink them.

Finally, the team conducted a pilot phase clinical trial involving 27 patients with stage III or stage IV ovarian cancer.

The patients who received intravenous vitamin C along with their chemotherapy reported less toxicity of the brain, bone marrow and major organs, the investigators found.

These patients also appeared to add nearly 8.75 months to the time before their disease relapsed and progressed, compared with people who only received chemotherapy. The researchers did note that the study was not designed to test the statistical significance of that finding.

HOW VITAMIN C WORKS AGAINST CANCER

Vitamin C in the bloodstream helps kill cancer cells because it chemically converts into hydrogen peroxide when it interacts with tumors, Dr. Drisko said.

"If you can get your blood levels of vitamin C very high, it gets driven into the space around the cancer cells," she explained. "In that space, it's converted into hydrogen peroxide. It's very similar to what our white blood cells do. They create hydrogen peroxide to fight infection."

EXPERT COMMENTARY

Stephanie Bernik, MD, chief of surgical oncology at Lenox Hill Hospital in New York City, said intravenous vitamin C therapy is not unheard of among cancer doctors.

"I've had patients come in and say they were doing vitamin C intravenous therapy," Dr. Bernik said. "I always tell them we don't know enough to know whether it is good or bad."

This recent research raises interesting possibilities, but until larger clinical trials are conducted Dr. Bernik says her advice to patients will not change.

"You have to do a bigger study with patients and look at outcomes. You also have to make sure these treatments don't interfere with the treatments we're giving currently," she said. "There may be some efficacy in what they're doing. It just needs to be proven. This is just the start of more studies looking at this in-depth."

Michael Seiden, MD, chief medical officer for The US Oncology Network, based in The Woodlands, Texas, agreed.

"It is important to emphasize that many vitamin therapies have shown interesting results when applied to cancer cells in test tubes yet, to date, these approaches typically are not effective and occasionally prove harmful in human studies," he said. "At this time, there is still no evidence that high-dose vitamin C should be part of the treatment for women with ovarian cancer."

While she agreed that larger trials need to be conducted, Dr. Drisko was not as hesitant.

"It's safe. It's inexpensive. There's a plausible mechanism we're investigating for why it works," she said. "We should be using this in patients, rather than dragging our feet and worrying about using it at all."

info For more information on vitamin C and cancer, visit the National Cancer Institute website at *http://cam.cancer.gov/newsletter/2009-spring/6.html.*

Carbon Monoxide for Cancer

This deadly gas was found in animal studies to both prevent tumor growth and increase the effectiveness of chemotherapy 1,000-fold. Researchers hope that this finding will lead to therapies that improve chemo results in humans.

Cancer Research

Getting Radiation at the Right Time of Day May Minimize Hair Loss for Cancer Patients

Satchidananda Panda, PhD, associate professor, Salk Institute for Biological Studies, La Jolla, California. His study was published in *Proceedings of the National Academy of Sciences* (PNAS).

Am I going to lose my hair? That's a question many cancer patients ask when they find out that they need radiation.

Such treatment can save lives, but the hair loss that often accompanies it can be quite upsetting. True, compared with battling the cancer itself, losing hair is a relatively minor issue—but it's one more source of distress at a time that's already overwhelmingly stressful. So wouldn't it be nice if that side effect could be avoided?

Maybe it can, an encouraging recent study shows, simply by altering one minor aspect of treatment—the time of day when radiation is given. *Here's why...*

SPLITTING HAIRS

Radiation kills cancer cells, but it also damages nearby healthy tissue, including hair follicles. When radiation is delivered to the head or neck area—to treat cancer of the brain, mouth, throat, thyroid, etc.—partial hair loss or total baldness can result. (With radiation, hair loss occurs only at the part of the body that is being treated. Chemotherapy, which wasn't included in this study, can lead to hair loss all over the body.) Sometimes the hair eventually grows back...sometimes it doesn't.

Researchers wondered whether the time of day at which radiation was given would affect the subsequent amount of hair loss. Why did they think there might be a connection? Because hair is constantly undergoing a complex cycle of growth and restoration that relies on circadian rhythm. (You probably think of circadian rhythm in terms of the 24-hour "master clock" in the brain that governs sleep and certain other biological functions. However, scientists now know that various tissues, including hair follicles, have their own "local" circadian clocks that orchestrate rhythms for their particular functions. The local clock for hair also operates on a 24-hour cycle.)

First, the researchers confirmed that there were many more mitotic cells (cells in the process of dividing and proliferating) within hair follicles in the morning...and that the mitotic cells decrease by 50% to 70% in the evening. As a consequence, hair grows faster in the morning...whereas in the evening, follicles are busy repairing whatever DNA damage was done during the growing time. Just think of a man's beard—shaving in the morning leads to a 5:00 (pm) shadow in the early evening...but shaving in the evening does not lead to a 5:00 (am) shadow in the early morning.

During the mitotic phase of the cells' cycle, hair is particularly vulnerable to damage from any sort of stress—and radiation is especially harmful because the extreme levels of energy damage the cells' DNA (which is why it works on killing cancer cells). So researchers designed an experiment using mice to measure the effects of scheduling radiation at different times of day.

Fascinating findings: Radiation delivered at 9 am resulted in nearly bald mice, with 85% of their hair lost...but when the same amount of the same type of radiation was delivered at 5 pm, the mice kept most of their hair, with only 17% being lost! This same connection between radiation timing and the amount of hair lost was seen at all levels of radiation except for the very highest dose tested, where hair loss was extensive no matter what time of day it was given. (With human patients, radiation doses do vary depending on the type and severity of the cancer—but the doses used in this animal study corresponded to the dosage range used in humans.)

To confirm the connection, the researchers also did the experiment on mice that were circadian deficient (missing the master clock that sets the circadian rhythm). In those mice, hair loss was the same regardless of the time of day when radiation was given.

DOES IT WORK IN HUMANS?

The researchers theorize that, in the evening, when hair follicles are in the restoration part of the cycle, they are already primed to repair damage from normal sources and can more easily handle the additional stress from the radiation.

Think of it this way: Adding one more wrinkled shirt to the pile isn't a big deal when you're already ironing the weekly laundry...but having to deal with a wrinkled shirt the next day, after the ironing board is put away, is a bigger hassle.

Cancer cells, which are constantly dividing, do not have circadian clocks. This means that altering the time of day at which radiation treatment is given would not make the therapy any less effective at combating the cancer.

We don't yet know for sure whether scheduling radiation therapy for a certain time of day would reduce hair loss in humans—studies on people rather than animals are needed to explore that—but the researchers think that it's

New Urine Test Predicts Bladder Cancer Recurrence

A urine test that measures genetic biomarkers was 80% successful in predicting when bladder cancer would return in a recent study of 90 cancer survivors. Current tests, which include biopsy and cystoscopy, are 15% to 35% successful in predicting cancer recurrence. The new urine test may become available in the next year or two. To participate in a clinical trial for this urine test, go to *ClinicalTrials.gov.*

Gangning Liang, PhD, associate professor of urology, USC Norris Comprehensive Cancer Center, Los Angeles.

Better Melanoma Treatment

A commonly used dye (PV-10) stimulates the immune system and could treat melanoma. In animal studies, a single injection of the dye reduced tumor size and helped prevent the cancer from spreading.

Moffitt Cancer Center, *moffitt.org*

likely. In fact, they suspect that other tissues with similar circadian cycles, such as bone marrow and the gastrointestinal tract lining, also might be spared from collateral damage if radiation therapy is timed appropriately.

The researchers stopped short of suggesting that cancer patients schedule their radiation appointments for late in the afternoon rather than first thing in the morning, citing the need for additional research. But in the meantime, cancer patients might want to aim for those afternoon sessions...and hope that the strategy will help them keep their hair during the battle against cancer.

Mushroom Extract May Hold Key to Pancreatic Cancer Cure

Daniel Sliva, PhD, senior investigator, Cancer Research Laboratory, Methodist Research Institute, Indiana University Health, Indianapolis. His study was published in *International Journal of Oncology*.

Michael Landon, Luciano Pavarotti, Sally Ride, Jack Benny, Patrick Swayze. Those are familiar names of people who have died from pancreatic cancer. You probably know someone who has succumbed to it as well, given that it is the fourth-leading cause of cancer-related deaths in the US.

Pancreatic cancer moves fast—many of its victims die within months of being diagnosed, and the five-year survival rate is dismal, not even reaching 5%. That's why any good news about pancreatic cancer is most welcome. So it's heartening to learn that a traditional Asian remedy made from mushrooms may hold the key to winning the battle against this dreaded disease, according to a recent laboratory study.

MAGIC MUSHROOMS?

Poria cocos is a type of mushroom that grows on pine trees. Among practitioners of traditional Asian medicine, the mushroom has been used for many years as a sedative, diuretic and stomach settler. Recent studies suggested that bioactive compounds in mushrooms might protect against breast and skin cancer...so researchers set out to discover whether they also might hold promise against pancreatic cancer, for which there is no known cure.

For the recent study, normal pancreatic cells and pancreatic cancer cells were laid out in culture trays in a laboratory, then treated with extracts from the Poria cocos mushroom to see how the cells would react.

Exciting: Within just one day, the mushroom extract inhibited several different mechanisms by which pancreatic cancer proliferates—so that the cancer cells acted less aggressively and didn't multiply as rapidly as they usually would. For instance, the mushroom extract seemed to silence one particular gene, MMP-7, that is overactive in pancreatic cancer cells. Importantly, the mushroom extract had minimal effect on the normal pancreatic cells.

Of course, these findings do not mean that pancreatic cancer patients can be cured by eating pine tree mushrooms. But scientists are already working on the next phase of research to determine exactly how the mushroom extract turns down the MMP-7 gene...and whether the extract has the same effects in real life as it does in the lab.

Cause for hope: The potent drugs morphine, penicillin and *paclitaxel* (Taxol, which is used to treat lung, breast and ovarian cancers) were derived from poppy plants, mold and Pacific yew tree bark, respectively. So it's not at all far-fetched that a mushroom might eventually prove to play a pivotal role in curing deadly pancreatic cancer.

Look Beyond the Sun for Skin Cancer Culprits, Doctors Warn

Alan Fleischer, MD, professor, dermatology, Wake Forest Baptist Medical Center, Winston-Salem, North Carolina.

Sherrif Ibrahim, MD, assistant professor, department of dermatology, University of Rochester Medical Center, Rochester, New York.

Think "skin cancer" and blame immediately goes to the sun. Justifiably so—though not totally, skin doctors say.

"Hands down, sun exposure is the biggest risk factor for skin cancer," said Sherrif Ibrahim, MD, assistant professor of dermatology at the University of Rochester Medical Center in New York. "And it's a cumulative risk. The more exposure you've gotten, the bigger the risk. The skin doesn't know if you're out one time for an hour or 12 times for 5 minutes at a time. Your skin keeps a running meter."

SKIN CANCER—IT'S NOT JUST THE SUN'S FAULT

Each year, more than 3.5 million basal and squamous cell skin cancers, known as non-melanoma cancers, are diagnosed in the United States, according to the American Cancer Society. These types of skin cancer aren't as deadly as melanoma, which affects about 75,000 US residents annually. About 9,000 people die from melanomas and 2,000 from non-melanoma skin cancers each year, according to the society.

However, the sun isn't the only thing that can be problematic. Tattoos, certain chemicals, other diseases and possibly even those better-for-the-environment light bulbs all have been linked to skin cancer.

And people who think tanning beds are safer than soaking up the sun should think again, Dr. Ibrahim said.

"There's an unquestionable link between tanning booths and skin cancer," Dr. Ibrahim said. "There's been an enormous surge in the popularity of tanning booths, and with it the average age of people with melanomas is much lower. I had a 22-year-old patient just the other day."

Better Lymphoma Care

According to recent research, cancer patients with chemotherapy-resistant, large B-cell lymphoma who were treated with *azacitidine* (Vidaza)—a DNA methyltransferase (DNMT) inhibitor—responded to chemo after taking the drug and then went into remission.

Possible reason: DNMT inhibitors genetically reprogram cancer cells, which seems to help chemo drugs work better. Larger studies are under way to see if DNMT is effective for other cancers.

Leandro Cerchietti, MD, assistant professor of medicine, Weill Cornell Medical College, New York City.

This is because it doesn't matter if the ultraviolet light comes from the sun or from an artificial source. Alan Fleischer, MD, dermatology professor at Wake Forest Baptist Medical Center in Winston-Salem, North Carolina, explained that "the kind of light produced by tanning beds isn't better or worse than natural sunshine, but people may get more and longer exposure, especially in areas where outdoors, they might display more modesty."

Even getting a manicure can expose you to ultraviolet light.

"Ultraviolet nail treatment units do produce UV light, but the risk is quite small," said Dr. Fleischer. The lights are used to help set or harden nail treatments.

Even things that seem unrelated to UV light—such as getting an organ transplant or a tattoo, or having an autoimmune disease—have been linked to skin cancer diagnoses.

People who've had an organ transplant have an extremely elevated risk for skin cancer—up to 200 times higher than others, according to Dr. Ibrahim.

This stems from the medications that must be taken after a transplant to suppress the immune system. As a result, the immune system, which normally fights off growing cancer cells, may not be strong enough to do its job.

Like people who've had an organ transplant, those with autoimmune diseases often take medications that suppress their immune system. These drugs can also increase their chances of developing skin cancer, Dr. Fleischer said.

The experts also pointed out other potential sources of skin cancer risk, including...

- **Compact fluorescent bulbs—**These "eco-friendly" lightbulbs emit ultraviolet light, which normally isn't a problem because of a coating on the bulbs. However, if there's a crack in the coating, UV light can come through. A study in the journal *Photochemistry and Photobiology* showed that these bulbs can emit some UV light, but no one has yet shown a link to skin cancer.
- **Previous radiation—**Areas of skin that have been exposed to radiation, such as that used for treatment of other types of cancer, have an increased risk for skin cancer, according to the American Cancer Society.
- **Parkinson's disease—**A study in the *Archives of Neurology* found an increased risk for melanoma in people with Parkinson's disease. The authors, whose research was published in September 2012, suspect that some of the genes that cause Parkinson's disease may also give rise to skin cancers.
- **Smoking—**Researchers also suspect a link between cigarette smoking and skin cancer. Two studies—one published in June 2012 in the *Archives of Dermatology* and the other in December 2011 in the journal *Cancer Causes and Control*—found that squamous cell cancer was more common in smokers than in nonsmokers.

Cotton Shirts Don't Offer Sufficient Protection from the Sun

They have an ultraviolet protection factor (UPF)—the equivalent of SPF—of no more than eight. That drops to two if the shirt gets wet. Do not rely on clothing for sun protection unless it is made for that purpose. Some long-sleeved shirts made of a spandex-and-nylon mix have a UPF rating of 50+. Use sunscreen, and reapply it often.

Health. www.Health.com

- **Chemical exposure—**Workplace exposure to certain chemicals can increase the risk of non-melanoma skin cancers, according to the American Cancer Society. These chemicals include arsenic, which is found naturally in well water and is used in the manufacture of some pesticides, as well as tar, coal, paraffin and some types of oil.
- **Driving—**Dr. Fleischer said that in the US, skin cancers are much more common on the left side of the body because of the time spent driving. In Europe, more cancers occur on the right side. And, though he said he hasn't seen any studies on it, he suspects that people who regularly drive convertibles probably have higher rates of skin cancer because of increased exposure.

WHAT THE EXPERTS RECOMMEND

Organ transplant recipients should talk to a dermatologist to get an idea of their baseline risk for skin cancer and find out how often they need to be screened. Dr. Ibrahim said that some high-risk people who've had organ transplants need screening every three to four weeks.

Although tattoos aren't known to increase the risk for skin cancer, tattoos can make it harder to detect cancer-related changes in moles. If you're considering a tattoo, make sure there aren't any moles in the area you're thinking about inking, according to experts from the American Academy of Dermatology.

Despite the low risk at the nail salon, the American Academy of Dermatology still recommends putting sunscreen on your hands before you get a manicure.

Both Dr. Fleischer and Dr. Ibrahim recommended wearing sunscreen regularly (applying liberally and reapplying often), avoiding the midday sun, seeking shade, wearing a wide-brimmed hat outside and covering up as much of your body as possible to lessen your sun exposure.

Though other factors can and do increase risk, "there's no question that the sun is the biggest risk factor for all types of skin cancer," Dr. Fleischer said.

info The American Academy of Dermatology has more about skin cancer at its website, *www.aad.org*.

At-Home Stool Test for Colon Cancer Accurate, But Not Foolproof

Elizabeth Liles, MD, MCR, Kaiser Permanente Center for Health Research, Portland, Oregon.
Andrew Chan, MD, MPH, director, gastroenterology training program, Massachusetts General Hospital, Boston.
Annals of Internal Medicine

A newer type of test that looks for hidden blood in the stool is an effective way to screen for colon cancer, a research review suggests.

The tests, called fecal immunochemical tests (FITs), are done at home and detect tiny amounts of blood in the stool—a possible sign of colon cancer. In a recent review, researchers found that across 19 studies, FITs caught more than three-quarters of colon tumors, and were very good at ruling out the cancer.

Experts said the findings give "reassurance" that an already commonly used test performs well.

"FIT testing continues to have very good potential as a screening tool," said Elizabeth Liles, MD, of the Kaiser Permanente Center for Health Research in Portland, Oregon.

COLON CANCER STATISTICS

In the United States, the average lifetime risk of colon cancer is about one in 20, according to the American Cancer Society. In each of the past several years, more than 50,000 Americans have died of the disease—but the death rate has been declining for a couple decades, partly because of screening, the cancer society said.

Still, many people aren't getting screened, Dr. Liles said.

In November 2013, a federal report said that more than one-third of Americans aged 50 to 75 were not up to date with their colon cancer screening. That included 28% who had never had any type of screening test.

CURRENT COLON CANCER TEST OPTIONS

Experts currently recommend that people at average risk of colon cancer start getting screened at age 50. And they can choose from several options, including yearly stool tests followed by a colonoscopy if the result is positive, a colonoscopy done every 10 years or sigmoidoscopy every five years. Colonoscopy and sigmoidoscopy are both invasive procedures that inspect the interior of the colon, but sigmoidoscopy is less thorough—looking only at the lower portion of the colon.

Colonoscopy is widely considered the "gold standard" for screening, because it allows the doctor to visually inspect the interior of the colon—and, if necessary, remove precancerous growths called polyps.

In recent years, more doctors have been using FITs instead of the traditional fecal occult blood test, because they're better at picking up cancer and they're easier for people to use.

Still, individual studies have had a fairly wide range of findings on the FIT tests' sensitivity—that is, their likelihood of giving a positive result when a person has colon cancer.

STUDY DETAILS

For the recent review, Dr. Liles and her colleagues analyzed 19 studies done since 1996, looking at eight different brands of FIT tests. They found that the tests' sensitivity did vary from study to study, but the discrepancy narrowed when the researchers excluded tests that are no longer on the market.

On average, the review found that FITs catch about 79% of colon cancers, and their specificity

Blood Pressure Medicines Can Cause Lip Cancer

Some common blood pressure drugs, including the diuretic *hydrochlorothiazide*, the calcium channel blocker *nifedipine* and the ACE inhibitor *lisinopril*, increase sun sensitivity and can make users more likely to develop lip cancer. But lip cancer is rare, curable and rarely spreads—in most cases, the drugs' benefits outweigh the risk.

Study comparing 712 patients with lip cancer who were taking blood pressure drugs with 22,904 people who did not have lip cancer by researchers at Kaiser Permanente Northern California Division of Research, published in *Archives of Internal Medicine*.

consistently tops 90%. That means the tests accurately give a negative result to more than 90% of people who do not have colon cancer.

One surprise, Dr. Liles said, was that FITs that require two or three stool samples performed no better than single-sample tests. That matters, she said, because people might be more willing to do the test if it's simpler.

The U.S. National Institute of Diabetes and Digestive and Kidney Diseases and the National Cancer Institute provided much of the funding for the review. Dr. Liles and her colleagues reported their findings in the journal *Annals of Internal Medicine*.

EXPERT COMMENT

The new study gives a clearer idea of how the tests perform on average, according to a colon cancer expert who was not involved in the research.

"It gives some very valuable information," said Andrew Chan, MD, a gastroenterologist at Massachusetts General Hospital in Boston.

But there are still bigger questions, Dr. Chan said. Experts still don't know which screening test is most effective at preventing deaths from colon cancer.

Dr. Chan said it's not yet clear how FIT and colonoscopy compare when it comes to cutting people's risk of dying from colon cancer.

There are studies under way, though. A large US government trial is randomly assigning people to have either a colonoscopy or an annual FIT screening, then following their rates of death from colon cancer over 10 years. (In the United States, colonoscopy is the most common screening method, followed by stool testing. Few doctors perform sigmoidoscopy.)

HOW TO USE FIT

FIT screening is already fairly easy. Like older stool tests, they're done with a take-home kit: You use a brush to get a stool sample, and then mail it to a lab. But unlike older tests, FITs don't require any diet or medication restrictions in the days before the test.

The simplicity of the stool test is an obvious advantage over colonoscopy screening, Dr. Liles said. But she agreed that more research is needed to know which screening test is more effective at saving lives.

WHICH TEST IS RIGHT FOR YOU?

So which exam should you choose? "That decision is between you and your doctor," Dr. Chan said. What matters most, he added, is that "some form of screening is done."

Dr. Liles agreed. "It's said that the best screening test is the one that you'll actually get done," she said.

info The U.S. Centers for Disease Control and Prevention has more on colon cancer screening at its website, *http://www.cdc.gov/cancer/colorectal/basic_info/screening/index.htm.*

Prepping for a Colonoscopy—Why It's a Necessary Evil

Pankaj Vashi, MD, lead national medical director and national clinical director of gastroenterology and nutrition, Cancer Treatment Centers of America, Chicago.
Grant Hutchins, MD, gastroenterologist and director of endoscopy, Nebraska Medical Center, and assistant professor of gastroenterology, University of Nebraska, Omaha.
Gastrointestinal Endoscopy, online
Exact Sciences, Madison, Wisconsin, news release.

Let's face it—the very mention of the word "colonoscopy" is enough to make many people shudder, at least a bit. But, colonoscopy is an extremely effective cancer screening tool, and it's the only cancer screening that can actually prevent cancer from developing in the first place because doctors can remove precancerous polyps during the test.

Most people who've had a colonoscopy say the test itself is no big deal. It doesn't take a lot of time, and you're sedated.

What people really don't like, however, is the colon-cleansing preparation that's required before the test. People who've had a colonoscopy often say that the prep is the worst part of the whole procedure.

However, it's a crucial part of the procedure. If the bowel isn't thoroughly cleaned out, doctors might miss a pre-cancerous polyp during the colonoscopy because they simply can't see it.

"I've had patients tell me the prep was cruel and unusual punishment, but it clears the colon wall so we can identify polyps," said Grant Hutchins, MD, a gastroenterologist at the Nebraska Medical Center in Omaha.

Pankaj Vashi, MD, the national clinical director of gastroenterology and nutrition at the Cancer Treatment Centers of America in Chicago, agreed. "We're looking for very small lesions, from 3 millimeters to 1 centimeter," he said. "If the colon isn't completely cleaned out, we can potentially miss small polyps. It's a crucial thing to have a cleaned-out colon."

A recent study from the journal *Gastrointestinal Endoscopy* found that as many as a third of polyps are missed when people fail to adequately prepare for their colonoscopy.

So, why are some people short-changing their bowel preparation?

Some find that the necessary volume of liquid is difficult to drink, and some people balk at the taste of some of the preparation solutions, according to Dr. Hutchins.

In the past, colonoscopy preparation required drinking an entire gallon of a salty solution the night before the procedure. Today, most preparations require half that volume, Dr. Vashi said. Dr. Hutchins noted that minor flavoring has been added to some preparation solutions to make them more palatable.

Pills are now an option, though they must be consumed with liquids, and the standard prep relies on taking 32 pills, according to Dr. Vashi. Researchers are working on developing options with fewer tablets.

Another option is to take the over-the-counter laxative MiraLAX, along with 64 ounces of a sports drink, such as Gatorade. It's also possible to split the preparation, doing half the night before and half in the morning, five hours or so before the colonoscopy.

Most doctors have a method that they prefer and will recommend. But if you've tried a particular method in the past and know you don't like it, ask your doctor what other options are available.

Whatever method of preparation is used, the goal is to induce diarrhea to clean out your bowels. So, plan to spend a lot of time in the bathroom. And to make the process as comfortable as possible, it's a good idea to buy flushable moist wipes.

Preparation also requires that you fast the day before the procedure, consuming only a clear liquid diet that doesn't contain any red or purple coloring, according to Dr. Hutchins. Examples of liquids that are OK to consume are water, apple juice, ginger ale, Jell-o and clear broth.

NO ESCAPE WITH A VIRTUAL COLONOSCOPY

People hoping to avoid the preparation by having a virtual colonoscopy—a test that uses CT scanning technology to capture images of the bowel—are out of luck. The virtual colonoscopy still requires bowel preparation, though researchers at the Mayo Clinic have come up with a new technique that requires just four cleansing tablets before a virtual colonoscopy. Also, Harvard researchers have developed a preparation that involves putting a contrast medium into low-fiber foods and snacks for two days before the test. The contrast agent makes fecal matter stand out on the scan, making it easy to remove from the image.

The drawback to virtual colonoscopy, however, is that if a polyp is found, you'll still need to undergo a regular colonoscopy.

Colon Cancer Alert

According to a recent study, using current screening guidelines, about one in 10 colon malignancies was missed among people with a family history of advanced colon polyps (precursors of colon cancer).

If you have a first-degree relative (a parent, sibling or child) who had advanced polyps diagnosed at any age: Talk to your doctor about getting screened more often than the current recommendation (once every five years beginning at age 40).

N. Jewel Samadder, MD, assistant professor of medicine, Huntsman Cancer Institute, University of Utah, Salt Lake City.

Some researchers are hoping to develop screening tests that can bypass the colonoscopy altogether. A company called Exact Sciences has indicated that it intends to seek U.S. Food and Drug Administration approval for a noninvasive, DNA-based stool test it has developed. It's designed to detect changes in DNA that indicate cancerous or pre-cancerous changes. Of course, if cancerous changes were detected, you'd still need to have a colonoscopy.

Both Drs. Hutchins and Vashi said that cleaning out the bowel before colonoscopy will probably be a necessary part of the procedure for some time to come.

"We've come a long way already, and while we do keep on trying to make it easier for patients, we don't want to compromise the quality of the bowel preparation and the colonoscopy," Dr. Vashi said.

info The American College of Gastroenterology has more about bowel preparation and the colonoscopy procedure at its website, *http://patients.gi.org/topics/colonoscopy/.*

Cancer Survivors: How to Get the Care You Need

Sheetal Kircher, MD, an oncologist and clinical director of the Cancer Survivorship Institute at the Robert H. Lurie Comprehensive Cancer Center of Northwestern University in Chicago. Dr. Kircher's research focuses on improving cancer care and cancer survivorship.

You beat cancer. Now what? For the 14 million cancer survivors in the US, this is no small question.

Latest development: Cancer survivors have traditionally lacked coordinated follow-up care by their physicians after completing their treatments. But there's now a new option for getting specialized aftercare. Hospitals and cancer centers across the US are offering *survivorship-care programs** that give patients state-of-the-art methods for keeping tabs on their health and reclaiming their emotional equilibrium after battling cancer.

GETTING ON WITH YOUR LIFE

At a cancer-survivorship program, a team of medical doctors, physical therapists, psychologists, nutritionists and other health professionals focus exclusively on the individual needs of each cancer patient. This includes monitoring for complications that can result from cancer treatment. *Among the most important to watch for...*

• **Heart damage.** Chemotherapy and radiation can harm any organ, notably the heart. It doesn't necessarily happen right away—a potent class of drugs called *anthracyclines,* commonly used to treat some lymphomas, breast cancer and certain rare types of cancer like sarcoma, can cause cardiomyopathy (weakening of the heart) decades after treatment is completed.

Radiation that reaches the heart, as often occurs, for example, with lung cancer, can cause damage, too. Similarly, a study appearing in the *Journal of Clinical Oncology* attributed up to 25% of the deaths of former Hodgkin's disease patients to heart disease caused in some part by radiation.

Best self-defense: Depending on the treatment you received, your doctor may recommend one or more tests, such as MRI, ultrasound and/or electrocardiogram, to closely monitor your heart health.

• **Infection.** Chemo, radiation and stem cell transplants used to treat cancer suppress the immune system, increasing risk for infection.

Best self-defense: Vaccines must be used carefully in cancer survivors. For example, "live" vaccines (such as Zostavax for shingles) should not be used in cancer patients with weakened immunity—they are at increased risk of contracting the infectious disease from the live organism in the vaccine. Cancer patients should talk to their doctors about the vaccines they need.

• **Fatigue.** Up to 82% of cancer survivors are affected by persistent fatigue, brought on by chemo and/or radiation or as a result of stress or chronic pain.

*To find a cancer-survivorship program near you, go to the National Cancer Institute (NCI) website, *CancerCenters.Cancer.gov.* Cancer-survivor programs are often used in conjunction with care from one's primary care doctor and are covered by most health insurers.

Best self-defense: It's common for individuals who have received chemo and/or radiation to suffer mild to moderate fatigue for up to a year. However, other conditions not directly related to the cancer itself—for example, an underactive thyroid, anemia, arthritis or insomnia—or even the use of pain medication may be partially to blame.

If these possibilities are ruled out, the best defense is often a carefully designed exercise program. A physical therapist on staff at a cancer-survivorship program will be knowledgeable about the issues that cancer survivors confront.

For best results: Pace yourself! Start with just 20 minutes of brisk walking and/or resistance training one to three days a week...and gradually increase to 20 to 60 minutes up to five days a week.

•Pain. More than one-third of cancer survivors experience chronic pain—often due to chemotherapy, radiation or surgery.

Best self-defense: Don't rely on just one pain-fighting strategy. A combination of approaches, such as physical therapy, exercise, oral painkillers, lidocaine (injections, creams or patches) and massage, may be recommended.

•Depression. This is also common after cancer treatment.

Best self-defense: Don't shrug off worrisome symptoms, such as trouble sleeping, an inability to focus, lingering feelings of sadness and anger or an overwhelming sense of isolation or fear. These are all red flags that depression may have taken hold.

The psychologists, social workers and other mental health professionals at survivorship programs are trained to identify and treat cancer-related complications, such as fatigue and pain, that may contribute to depression. In addition, therapy and/or medication may be needed to treat the depression.

•Additional postcancer issues. Cancer-survivorship programs also treat sexual dysfunction...cognitive decline...and sleep problems.

RISKS FOR RECURRENCE

Up to 70% of cancer survivors report having significant fear of a cancer recurrence. If you have survived cancer, the best way to catch a recurrence early—when the malignancy would be most treatable—is to stay on top of follow-up visits to your doctors.

How often? Follow-up visits are generally recommended every three to four months for the first few years following treatment and once or twice annually after that. However, the exact schedule depends on such factors as the type of cancer you had, the treatments you received and your age.

Which tests? It's crucial to have an after-cancer screening plan that may include specific tests (such as blood tests and MRI and/or CT scans) that are sometimes used to help detect cancer recurrences.

Best resource: Guidelines from the National Comprehensive Cancer Network. Go to *NCCN.org/default.aspx.* Under "NCCN Guidelines," click on "NCCN Guidelines for Patients."

Cholesterol & Blood Pressure

The Big Statin Question—Here's How to Decide Whether You Need One...

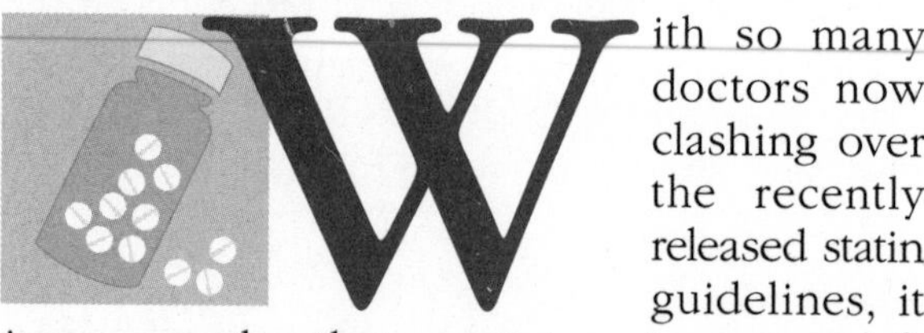

With so many doctors now clashing over the recently released statin guidelines, it is no wonder that most Americans are left with lots of unanswered questions about their heart health.

Some medical experts say that the new guidelines, which include a controversial online risk calculator, overestimate risk and recommend statin drugs for too many people. Other authorities argue that the new guidelines represent a state-of-the-art upgrade.

What you need now are clear answers, not just claims and counterclaims from medical honchos. To provide some real perspective on the guidelines, we turned to Harlan M. Krumholz, MD, one of the most respected cardiologists in the country and a leading "quality-of-care" researcher. He was not involved in the creation of the new statin guidelines. *Four steps that he uses to advise his patients on statins...*

Step 1: Don't ignore cholesterol levels. The most fundamental change in the new guidelines is that they now suggest the use of statin therapy for certain groups of people—for example, those with existing cardiovascular disease or diabetes—rather than focusing on very specific cholesterol targets when prescribing statins. However, even though targets have been largely abandoned, the guidelines do still indicate that everyone with very high LDL "bad" cholesterol levels should strongly consider taking a statin.

Harlan M. Krumholz, MD, the Harold H. Hines Jr. professor of medicine (cardiology) and professor of investigative medicine and of public health (health policy) at the Yale School of Medicine in New Haven, Connecticut. Dr. Krumholz is also codirector of the Clinical Scholars Program and director of the Yale-New Haven Hospital Center for Outcomes Research and Evaluation.

What this means for you: Knowing your cholesterol level is still vital in assessing your risk for cardiovascular disease and whether you would likely benefit from a statin. Therefore, a cholesterol test should be part of your initial evaluation. If you're not put on a statin, you can also retest every five years.

Step 2: Forget about keeping score. Until now, the generally accepted goal of cholesterol-lowering drug treatment was to bring LDL below a target level—100 mg/dL to 130 mg/dL for most people...and 70 mg/dL for those at very high risk for heart disease. If cholesterol failed to drop sufficiently, the statin dose was often increased or other drugs were added.

Why the targets? For years, doctors assumed that because higher LDL cholesterol means more risk for heart attack, reducing these levels with medication would mean fewer heart attacks. But research now shows that this isn't necessarily so.

Key Points of the New Statin Guidelines

According to new guidelines issued by the American Heart Association and American College of Cardiology, statins are recommended for people who have...

- **Cardiovascular disease.** This includes those with a history of heart attack, angina, stroke or transient ischemic attack or anyone who has undergone a procedure, such as angioplasty, to widen arteries.
- **Extremely high LDL "bad" cholesterol levels** (190 mg/dL or above).
- **Type 2 diabetes and are ages 40 to 75.**
- **An estimated 10-year risk for cardiovascular disease of 7.5% or higher,** based on the online calculator, and are ages 40 to 75.*

*Visit *https://www.heart.org/gglRisk/main_en_US.html* to access the online risk calculator.

What this means for you: If you start taking a statin, think of the medication not just as a cholesterol-lowering drug, but as a heart-protecting drug, since it will reduce risk regardless of your cholesterol level.

Once you're on a statin, there's no reason to measure your cholesterol levels. It would be useful only if you want to reconsider this decision, which might make sense if you're overweight but then lose weight, start exercising or make other lifestyle changes.

Step 3: Start with nondrug approaches. By shifting away from cholesterol targets, the new guidelines focus more on other factors affecting heart health.

What this means for you: Before you consider whether to use a statin, talk to your doctor about active steps you can take to reduce your risk with a healthier lifestyle...

- **If you smoke, stop!**
- **Improve your diet by curbing saturated fats...** and boosting "good" fats like those in olive oil and nuts.
- **Get regular exercise.**
- **Control your blood pressure.** If diet, weight loss, exercise and stress control do not bring your readings below 140/90 mmHg, talk to your doctor about blood pressure medication.
- **Lose weight if you need to.** Excess body weight not only raises your risk for heart disease but also makes you more vulnerable to diabetes—a major risk factor for heart attack and stroke in its own right.

Step 4: Remember to think for yourself. At best, guidelines can provide information about your risk of having a heart attack, stroke or dying and suggest strategies to modify it. But remember, the risk calculator provides no more than an estimate of your risk and should be used as only part of your assessment.

What's more, guidelines cannot say whether the benefit of taking medication is worth the risk to you. Statins can have side effects, including muscle damage and increased risk for diabetes.

Important: There's little convincing evidence that the newer cholesterol-lowering drugs, including the higher-priced option *ezetimibe* (Zetia), are as effective as statins. So don't take them unless you can't use statins because of side effects and until you have had a thorough discussion with your doctor.

Also, guidelines don't factor in your feelings about taking a drug simply on the chance—not with a guarantee—that it will make you healthier and perhaps live longer. Given the same facts, one person will choose treatment and another will not, and they can both be right based on their preferences and goals.

What it means for you: Use the guidelines as the starting point for a conversation with your doctor about treatment—not as the answer. Ultimately, the decision is yours.

Some Doctors Challenge New Statin Guidelines

Donald Lloyd-Jones, MD, ScM, chair, department of preventive medicine, Northwestern University's Feinberg School of Medicine, Chicago.

Neil Stone, MD, chair, American Heart Association's cholesterol guideline committee and professor, preventive cardiology, Northwestern's Feinberg School of Medicine.

Kevin Marzo, MD, chief of cardiology, Winthrop-University Hospital, Mineola, New York.

David Goff, MD, PhD, FACP, FAHA, dean, School of Public Health, University of Colorado-Denver.

Steven Nissen, MD, chief of cardiovascular medicine at the Cleveland Clinic.

Sidney Smith, MD, cardiologist, University of North Carolina at Chapel Hill and past president American Heart Association.

The New York Times

A new online cholesterol risk calculator produced by two leading U.S. heart organizations is flawed and overstates a person's risk of heart disease, a pair of Harvard Medical School professors say. The calculator coincides with the release of new cholesterol-lowering guidelines.

The professors contend that this flaw could lead the calculator to mistakenly suggest that millions of people should be taking cholesterol-lowering statin drugs, according to *The New York Times*.

Key officials with the American Heart Association (AHA) and the American College of Cardiology (ACC) support the calculator. The two heart groups unveiled the calculator in November 2013 along with aggressive new guidelines for combating high cholesterol. Those guidelines call for the use of statins to treat more people.

Previously, doctors adhered to rigid clinical guidelines to prescribe a statin when cholesterol levels reached a certain threshold.

Under the new guidelines, people will be advised to take statins based on a number of different health risk factors. These risk factors include if they already have heart disease, if their bad (LDL) cholesterol is extremely high (190 milligrams per deciliter of blood or more) or if they're middle-aged with type 2 diabetes.

In addition, people between 40 and 75 years of age with an estimated 10-year risk of heart disease of 7.5% or more are advised to take a statin. Experts say this new rule could greatly alter the number of patients who will now be advised to take such a drug.

Harvard professors Paul Ridker, MD, and Nancy Cook, PhD, reportedly pointed out problems with the calculator in 2012, saying that it did not seem to work accurately when they tested it using patient data, the *Times* reported.

When the online calculator went live late in 2013, Dr. Ridker and Dr. Cook again tested it and reported serious flaws that could overestimate a person's risk of heart disease by 75% to 150%, the newspaper reported. Their findings were published in the medical journal *The Lancet.*

TWO MAIN HEART GROUPS SUPPORT GUIDELINES

AHA and ACC officials said that the Harvard professors' analysis of the calculator relied on patient data from three heart studies involving people both younger and healthier than the average American.

"These people exist in the US population, but it's a very healthy, skewed group," said Donald Lloyd-Jones, MD, ScM, chair of the department of preventive medicine at Northwestern University's Feinberg School of Medicine.

The two heart-health groups said they created the calculator—as well as a set of aggressive new cholesterol-lowering guidelines—using a broad range of patient data that allowed them to incorporate factors that hadn't been included in previous risk assessments. For example, prior attempts did not include calculations for

African-American populations, and did not attempt to include stroke risk.

"The truth is, the risk equations work exactly the way we asked them to," said Dr. Lloyd-Jones, who worked on the guideline committee for the AHA.

CALCULATORS ARE MEANT TO PROMPT DISCUSSION WITH DOCTOR

Officials from both heart groups added that just because the calculator suggests some people would benefit from statins doesn't mean they absolutely have to take them.

Instead, the calculator should prompt a conversation with their doctor about whether they need to take statins or undertake other lifestyle changes to lower their cholesterol.

"We're acknowledging the unique judgment of a physician when he looks at the patient's specific condition," said Neil Stone, MD, chair of the AHA's cholesterol guideline committee and a professor of preventive cardiology at Northwestern's Feinberg School of Medicine.

MORE EXPERTS COMMENT

Cardiologists are concerned that the confusion surrounding the calculator and new cholesterol treatment guidelines could cause patients to refuse to take statins.

"I fear that the confusion is going to shake the public's confidence in these lifesaving drugs," said Kevin Marzo, MD, chief of cardiology at Winthrop-University Hospital in Mineola, New York. "It is my hope that the guideline writers will revise the online calculator so that any deficiencies created will be quickly corrected."

"We've come up with an approach that calls for treating about a third of adults between 40 and 75 years of age with statins for primary prevention," said David Goff, MD, PhD, co-chair of the risk assessment working group for the guidelines and dean of the Colorado School of Public Health at the University of Colorado-Denver.

"I think it sounds about right," given that one out of three adults in America die from heart disease and stroke, Dr. Goff said.

The alleged problems with the calculator prompted at least one prominent cardiologist to tell the *Times* that implementation of the new cholesterol treatment guidelines should be delayed.

"It's stunning," Steven Nissen, MD, chief of cardiovascular medicine at the Cleveland Clinic, told the *Times*. "We need a pause to further evaluate this approach before it is implemented on a widespread basis."

Dr. Sidney Smith, a cardiologist at the University of North Carolina at Chapel Hill and a past AHA president, said that would not happen.

"We intend to move forward with these guidelines and develop effective strategies to implement them," Dr. Smith said.

info For more on statins visit the U.S. National Library of Medicine at its website, *http://www.nlm.nih.gov/medlineplus/statins.html.*

If You Don't Want to Take a Statin...Natural Ways to Lower Your Cholesterol

Allan Magaziner, DO, an osteopathic physician and the founder and director of the Magaziner Center for Wellness in Cherry Hill, New Jersey. One of the country's top specialists in nutritional and preventive medicine, Dr. Magaziner is coauthor of *The All-Natural Cardio Cure: A Drug-Free Cholesterol and Cardiac Inflammation Reduction Program* (Avery). *DrMagaziner.com*

As the controversial new guidelines on statins begin to kick into use in doctors' offices around the country, the number of Americans for whom these drugs will be recommended is expected to double. But plenty of people don't like to take any type of prescription medication if they can avoid it.

Most integrative physicians, who prescribe natural therapies (and drugs when needed), agree that the majority of people who take statins—and most of those who will be recommended to do so under the new guidelines—could get many of the same benefits, such as lower cholesterol and inflammation levels, with fewer risks, by relying on targeted food choices (see examples in box on page 84) and supplements. Exercise—ideally, about 30 minutes at least five days a week—should also be part of a healthy-heart regimen.*

The natural regimen that I've fine-tuned over the past 25 years for my patients...

THE BEST CHOLESTEROL-LOWERING SUPPLEMENTS

• **Fish oil.** (*Typical daily dose*: 1,000 mg total of EPA and DHA). Fish oil fights inflammation, lowers LDL "bad" cholesterol and is part of most good heart-protective regimens.** In addition, I recommend using the first supplement below and adding the other three supplements if total cholesterol levels don't drop below 200 mg/dL...

• **Red yeast rice.** You have probably heard of this rice, which is fermented to produce monacolins, chemical compounds with statinlike effects. It can lower LDL cholesterol by roughly 30%.

Red yeast rice can be a good alternative for people who can't tolerate statins due to side effects such as muscle aches and increased risk for diabetes. Red yeast rice also has other natural protective substances, such as isoflavones, fatty acids and sterols, not found in statins.

Typical dosage: 1.2 g to 2.4 g daily. I advise starting with 1.2 g daily. The dose can be increased as needed, based on your physician's advice.

What I tell my patients: Unfortunately, red yeast rice has gotten a bad rap because of the way some products were labeled. The supplements that I recommend are manufactured with high standards of quality control and contain therapeutic levels of active ingredients.

Good products: Choleast by Thorne Research, Thorne.com...and High Performance Formulas' Cholestene, HPFonline.com.

When taking red yeast rice, some people have heartburn, gastrointestinal (GI) upset or mild headache—these effects usually are eliminated by taking the supplement with food.

• **Niacin.** Few doctors recommend niacin routinely even though it's one of the most effective cholesterol remedies. Although a recent study questioned the effectiveness of niacin, most research finds it beneficial. It may lower LDL by about 10% and increase HDL "good" cholesterol by 15% to 35%. It can lower levels of triglycerides and Lp(a), a sticky cholesterol particle that causes atherosclerosis.

Typical dosage: 1 g to 3 g of time-released niacin daily, divided into two doses and taken with food.

What I tell my patients: Start with 250 mg daily, and increase the dose by 250 mg every two weeks until you are taking the amount recommended by your doctor. People who take high doses of niacin too quickly often have uncomfortable facial flushing and sometimes stomach upset or other GI disturbances. "Flush-free" niacin is available, but it doesn't lower cholesterol as effectively as the regular version.

• **Pantethine.** You may not be familiar with this supplement, a form of pantothenic acid (vitamin B-5). Recent studies show that it raises HDL cholesterol—and it prevents LDL from oxidizing, the process that causes it to cling to arteries.

Yummy Cholesterol Fighters

For years, oat bran and oatmeal were touted as the best foods for high cholesterol. Rich in soluble fiber, these foods help prevent cholesterol from getting into the bloodstream. A daily serving of oats, for example, can lower LDL by 20%. Other good foods rich in soluble fiber include barley, beans, pears and prunes. But research has now gone beyond these old standby food choices. *Here are some other fiber-rich foods that have been found to give cholesterol the heave-ho...*

• **All nuts.** Walnuts and almonds are great cholesterol fighters, but so are pistachios, peanuts, pecans, hazelnuts and other nuts, according to recent research. Eat a handful (1.5 ounces) of nuts daily.

• **Popcorn actually contains more fiber per ounce than whole-wheat bread.** Just go easy on the salt and butter, and stay away from store-bought microwave popcorn (it can contain harmful chemicals).

Smart idea: Put one-quarter cup of organic plain popcorn in a lunch-size brown paper bag, and pop in the microwave. It's delicious—and there's no cleanup.

*Talk to your doctor before taking any of these supplements—they may interact with medications or affect certain chronic health conditions. ** A recent study linking fish oil to increased risk for prostate cancer is not supported by other medical research, so most men can take fish oil supplements under a doctor's supervision.

Typical dosage: 900 mg, divided into two or three doses daily. Good pantethine products are made by Jarrow, Jarrow.com...and NOW Foods, NOWFoods.com.

What I tell my patients: Take pantethine with meals to reduce the risk for indigestion and to aid absorption.

•**Sterols and stanols.** These cholesterol-lowering plant compounds are found in small amounts in many fruits, vegetables and grains. But sterol and stanol supplements are much more powerful. In supplement form, the plant compounds reduce LDL by about 14% and cause no side effects.

Typical dosage: Take 3 g of a sterol/stanol supplement daily. Pure Encapsulations makes a good product, PureEncapsulations.com.

Most integrative physicians are very knowledgeable about natural remedies. To find one in your area, consult the American College for Advancement in Medicine at ACAM.org.

Statins May Cause Delirium

Statin drugs, which reduce cholesterol, are associated with a 30% increase in risk for postsurgical delirium in people age 65 and older. The result can be long-lasting or even permanent cognitive impairment in the oldest and sickest patients. Factors typically associated with surgery—including general anesthesia, reduced blood pressure and opioids for pain control—may cause statins to raise delirium risk.

Self-defense: Most patients can safely stop taking statins about two days before surgery, then resume taking them the first day after surgery—but always get your doctor's approval.

Donald A. Redelmeier, MD, director of the clinical epidemiology unit at Sunnybrook Health Sciences Centre, University of Toronto, and leader of a study published in *Canadian Medical Association Journal.*

Cholesterol Drugs Linked to Muscle and Joint Problems

Ishak Mansi, MD, VA North Texas Health Care System, Dallas.
JAMA Internal Medicine, online

People taking statin drugs to lower their cholesterol may slightly increase their risk for muscle and joint diseases as well as strains and sprains, a recent study suggests.

Statins, such as Zocor and Lipitor, are widely used to reduce cholesterol levels and help prevent heart disease. But they're also thought to contribute to muscle weakness, muscle cramps and tendon problems.

This recent study, based on nearly 14,000 US active-duty soldiers and veterans, confirmed an association between the drugs' use and musculoskeletal injuries and diseases. But the findings need to be replicated in other types of studies and should not deter people at risk of heart disease from taking the medications, said lead researcher Ishak Mansi, MD, from the VA North Texas Health Care System in Dallas.

"Do not stop taking statins; these medications have been life-savers for some patients," Dr. Mansi said. "But talk to your doctor about the benefit-risk ratio for you."

Whether statins should be prescribed universally in people without risk factors for heart disease, as some in the health care field suggest, is another matter, Dr. Mansi said.

"The side effects of statins are not totally known yet," Dr. Mansi said. "Advocating widespread use, specifically for primary prevention in otherwise healthy subjects, is unsound."

STUDY DETAILS

The researchers matched nearly 7,000 statin users with a similar number of nonusers to assess the risk of musculoskeletal problems associated with statin use.

They found that people taking statins had a 19% greater risk of having musculoskeletal problems compared with nonusers. Specifically, statin users were 13% more likely to suffer dislocations, strains or sprains. They were only 0.7% more likely to develop osteoarthritis or other joint problems, which was not considered statistically significant, the researchers found.

In the study, three-quarters of the participants were taking *simvastatin* (brand name Zocor) and about 20% were taking *atorvastatin* (Lipitor). Smaller numbers were prescribed *pravastatin* (Pravachol), *rosuvastatin* (Crestor), *fluvastatin* (Lescol) or *lovastatin* (Mevacor).

The greater likelihood of strains, sprains and dislocations with statin use has not been previously reported, the researchers said. The findings might have implications for physically active people, such as members of the military.

The results were published online in the journal *JAMA Internal Medicine*.

info For more information on statins, visit the website of the U.S. National Library of Medicine at *http://www.nlm.nih.gov/medlineplus/statins.html.*

Statins Plus Certain Antibiotics May Set Off a Toxic Reaction

Amit Garg, MD, PhD, professor, department of epidemiology and biostatistics, University of Western Ontario, London, Ontario, Canada.

Gregg Fonarow, MD, professor, cardiology, University of California, Los Angeles, and spokesman, American Heart Association.

Annals of Internal Medicine

Doctors should avoid ordering certain antibiotics for older patients who take cholesterol-lowering statin drugs, such as Lipitor, Canadian researchers say.

Statins, which are taken by many millions of people, don't mix well with the antibiotics *clarithromycin* or *erythromycin*, according to a study, published in the *Annals of Internal Medicine*.

These two commonly used antibiotics inhibit the metabolism of statins and increase statin concentration in the blood, which can cause muscle or kidney damage, and even death, the researchers said.

"These drugs do interact and cause difficulties for patients," said lead researcher Amit Garg, MD, PhD, a professor in the department of epidemiology and biostatistics at the University of Western Ontario in London, Ontario.

These adverse reactions are rare, Dr. Garg added. "Most people will be fine," he said. "But at a population level, hundreds of preventable hospitalizations are occurring."

STUDY DETAILS

The study of more than 144,000 statin users over the age of 65 compared those prescribed clarithromycin or erythromycin with those taking *azithromycin*.

The study data included more than 73,000 patients prescribed clarithromycin, about 3,200 prescribed erythromycin and more than 68,000 people who took azithromycin. Almost three-quarters of the statin users were taking *atorvastatin* (Lipitor). The other commonly used statins were *simvastatin* (Zocor) and *lovastatin* (Altoprev, Mevacor).

In terms of absolute risk, the odds of kidney damage increased 26% among people over 65 who took clarithromycin or erythromycin and statins compared with patients who took azithromycin with statins.

Also, hospitalizations for muscle damage (a condition called rhabdomyolysis) and deaths were slightly higher—0.02% and 0.25%, respectively—in the clarithromycin or erythromycin groups compared with the azithromycin group, the study authors found.

The study authors noted that younger patients are less likely than older adults to experience serious side effects from drug interactions.

RESEARCH PRESENTS ALTERNATIVES

For someone taking a statin, the study suggests that substituting a different antibiotic—azithromycin—is safer because it doesn't interfere with the metabolism of statins.

Another strategy is to stop the statin until the antibiotic course is finished, Dr. Garg said.

EXPERT RESPONSE

Gregg Fonarow, MD, a spokesman for the American Heart Association, said patients should not stop taking statins, which are known to prevent heart disease. Instead, doctors should prescribe another antibiotic, he suggested.

"It is well documented that certain medications that inhibit the liver enzyme cytochrome P450 isoenzyme 3A4 can increase the drug level of statin medications," said Dr. Fonarow, a professor of cardiology at the University of California, Los Angeles. "Nevertheless, large-scale randomized clinical trials and clinical effectiveness studies have demonstrated [that] the benefits of statin therapy in reducing fatal and nonfatal cardiovascular events outweigh the potential risks."

Clarithromycin and erythromycin are often prescribed for respiratory illness such as pneumonia. Previously, the U.S. Food and Drug Administration had warned that statins don't interact well with these and certain other drugs used to treat HIV and hepatitis.

info For more information on statins, visit the website of the U.S. National Library of Medicine at *http://www.nlm.nih.gov/medlineplus/statins.html.*

Statins May Hamper Workout Results

John P. Thyfault, PhD, associate professor, Clinical Research Center, University of Missouri School of Medicine.

Robert H. Eckel, MD, professor of medicine, University of Colorado School of Medicine, and past president, American Heart Association.

Journal of the American College of Cardiology, online

Statins are drugs taken by millions to lower their cholesterol, but the medications also could hamper heart patients' ability to improve their cardiovascular health through exercise, researchers say.

A small group of overweight or obese people were unable to make any significant fitness gains while taking a 40 milligram daily dose of *simvastatin*, while another group not on the drug but undergoing the same exercise regimen did show improvement, according to a study published in the *Journal of the American College of Cardiology*.

"If you exercise a group of people, they are going to have an increase in their fitness," said study author John Thyfault, PhD, associate professor at the Clinical Research Center in the University of Missouri School of Medicine. "In our group who was only taking statins, the improvements were blocked or did not occur."

This finding could drastically affect the way physicians treat heart patients, particularly if it is found that other types of statin medications have the same negative effect on exercise benefits, Dr. Thyfault said.

People at risk for heart disease or metabolic syndrome (a cluster of factors that raise the risk for coronary artery disease, stroke and diabetes) often are prescribed statins to lower their blood cholesterol and at the same time advised to exercise more, he said. Both statins and exercise have been independently proven to lower cardiovascular disease risk, but may not pair well.

"Statins have saved lives, but I think physicians need to be careful about who they prescribe to, that it should be reserved for the most at-risk patients," Dr. Thyfault said. "We need to rethink it. Not like a lot of people used to say, that statins should be put in the water supply."

STUDY DETAILS

In the study, 19 people at risk for cardiovascular disease were placed on a 12-week exercise regimen in which they walked or jogged on a treadmill for 45 minutes, five days a week. Another 18 people were placed on the same exercise regimen but also were prescribed a daily dose of *simvastatin*, sold commercially under the brand name Zocor.

The people assigned exercise alone ended up experiencing a 10% improvement in their cardiorespiratory fitness, while those taking simvastatin only enjoyed a 1.5% increase in fitness, the researchers found.

Statins Are Associated With a Higher Risk for Cataracts

The cholesterol-lowering drugs may interfere with cell regeneration in the eye's lens, which requires cholesterol to maintain transparency. But people with certain risk factors, such as a family history of heart disease, may need statins despite the risk.

Ishak Mansi, MD, staff internist at VA North Texas Health System and professor of medicine at University of Texas Southwestern, both in Dallas. He led a study published online in *JAMA Ophthalmology.*

Additionally, people in the exercise-only group experienced a 13% increase in "skeletal muscle mitochondrial content," meaning that their muscle cells became more efficient in converting glucose and oxygen into energy. People taking simvastatin had a 4.5% decrease—their muscles actually became less capable of using energy.

At the same time, the drug did help reduce cholesterol for those taking it. Total cholesterol decreased by 29% and "bad" LDL cholesterol decreased by 38% in the exercise-plus-statin group, while there were no significant changes in total cholesterol or LDL in the exercise-only group.

EXPERT RESPONSE

This study should prompt more research into whether other types of statins have the same effect and whether a lighter dosage would make a difference, said Robert Eckel, MD, a professor of medicine at the University of Colorado School of Medicine and past president of the American Heart Association. He was not involved with the study.

"I'm not totally surprised by this. The idea of exercise and statins and the interactions between the two of them has been known for some time," Dr. Eckel said. "The new wrinkle here is the idea that fitness is modified in terms of the training effect."

Dr. Eckel said it is also very likely that other statins will have the same effect, given that they all work in much the same way.

At the same time, it is too soon for heart patients to toss away their medication in favor of exercise, he continued.

"It's hard to refute a large amount of data that supports the benefit of statins in preventing heart disease," Dr. Eckel said.

info Visit the American Heart Association website at *http://www.heart.org/HEARTORG/GettingHealthy/PhysicalActivity/* for advice on exercise and heart health.

Cholesterol-Lowering Drugs May Help Reduce Risk for Parkinson's

Study of 43,810 statin users from 2001 to 2008 by researchers at National Taiwan University Hospital, Taipei, published in *Neurology.*

In a recent finding, people who stopped taking fat-soluble statins were almost 58% more likely to suffer from Parkinson's disease than people who kept taking them.

Theory: Fat-soluble statins, such as *simvastatin* (Zocor) or *atorvastatin* (Lipitor), reduce inflammation and alter dopamine pathways in the brain that are linked to Parkinson's. Water-soluble statins, such as *rosuvastatin* (Crestor) and *pravastatin* (Pravachol), do not provide the same benefit. People taking water-soluble statins develop Parkinson's at about twice the rate as people taking fat-soluble statins.

Self-defense: If you are taking a statin and have a family history of Parkinson's, ask your doctor if you should be taking a fat-soluble statin.

Could Vaccines Someday Improve Heart Health?

Hiroshi Koriyama, MD, Osaka University, Japan.
Barbara V. Howard, PhD, senior scientist, MedStar Health Research Institute, and professor, Georgetown University Hospital, Washington, DC.
James Howard, MD, spokesperson, American Heart Association, and endocrinologist and internist, MedStar Washington Hospital Center, Washington, DC.
American Heart Association annual meeting, Dallas.

People routinely get vaccinations to ward off the flu or prevent infectious diseases such as measles and whooping cough. Could there be a vaccine in the future that would prevent a heart attack?

Two animal studies suggest that vaccines might someday be used to reduce high cholesterol levels and lower blood pressure, according to findings presented in 2013 at the American Heart Association (AHA) annual meeting in Dallas.

In both cases, the vaccines interrupt processes in the body that, if left alone, can lead to high cholesterol and elevated blood pressure.

STUDY #1

The first study, out of Vienna, found that mice and rats had lower cholesterol levels for a year following treatment with a vaccine that protects a cell's ability to remove "bad" LDL cholesterol from the bloodstream.

"This is one of the most exciting things that's now under development in the controllability of cholesterol," said James Howard, MD, an AHA spokesperson and an endocrinologist and internist at MedStar Washington Hospital Center in Washington, DC.

The vaccine targets an enzyme called PCSK9. This enzyme causes cells to become less able to yank LDL cholesterol from the bloodstream and convert it into hormones or other useful products, Dr. Howard said.

"When you make an antibody to it, it just can't function," he said of PCSK9.

By reducing the amount of active PCSK9 in a body, the vaccine also reduces the cholesterol levels as cells become more efficient in using cholesterol.

"It has incredible power to lower LDL cholesterol, and can be taken with statins," Dr. Howard said.

Scientists note that research conducted in animals often fails to provide similar results in humans.

STUDY #2

The second study, this one from Japan, used a different vaccine to lower high blood pressure in laboratory rats for up to six months.

This vaccine interferes with a hormone called angiotensin II, which increases blood pressure by causing blood vessels to constrict. Medications already are widely used to block angiotensin II and control blood pressure, but they have to be taken daily to be effective.

"It's a hormone that increases blood pressure, and many of the common drugs antagonize it and reduce blood pressure," said Barbara Howard, PhD, a senior scientist at MedStar Health Research Institute and a professor at Georgetown University Hospital, in Washington, DC. "The idea is if you can knock out the production, you can have a sustained reduction that will last longer."

There are some concerns about medicines or vaccines that target this hormone, however. "It's part of a very complex network of hormones that regulate sodium balance in your body," she said. "It has to be very tightly regulated, or it can cause damage to the whole vascular system."

In this study, the vaccine reduced the rats' blood pressure for months and reduced damage to the heart and blood vessels associated with

High Blood Pressure Cure?

According to a recent study, blood pressure dropped significantly when tiny nodules (each about the size of a rice grain) found on the carotid arteries were removed. Human trials are now under way.

Nature Communications

high blood pressure. It also did not cause any damage to the kidneys, heart or liver.

While these findings are promising, Dr. Howard said there needs to be more studies before it is ready as a vaccine for humans.

"There's a lot of danger of overshooting and disturbing that sodium balance, and they didn't give any real data in this report," she said.

"It's got to be done in humans, and it's got to be accompanied by many more measures of functional safety. If you lower it enough to affect blood pressure, can you do that without affecting sodium balance?"

At this point, the vaccine is at least five to six years away from human trials, according to study coauthor Hiroshi Koriyama, MD, of Osaka University, in Japan.

There likely will be a similar amount of time needed to bring the cholesterol vaccine to human trials, said Dr. Howard.

However, he noted that human trials now are taking place for another form of the cholesterol vaccine that has to be taken every couple of weeks by injection.

HEALTHY LIFESTYLE RECOMMENDED FOR CHOLESTEROL CONTROL

In the meantime, the AHA recommends eating a heart-healthy diet, getting weekly aerobic and muscle-strengthening activity, and avoiding tobacco smoke as good ways to help control cholesterol.

Because the studies were presented at a medical meeting, the data and conclusions should be viewed as preliminary until published in a peer-reviewed journal.

info For more information on treatment of high cholesterol, visit the website of the American Heart Association at *Heart.org* (search "prevention and treatment of high cholesterol").

Hypertension and Memory Loss

Blood pressure fluctuations may lead to memory loss. In a study of 5,400 adults over age 70, those with the greatest fluctuations in blood pressure performed worse on tests of memory, attention and reaction time than those with more stable levels, even if blood pressure was high. Extreme swings in blood pressure are also associated with brain microbleeds, which may contribute to cognitive decline.

Possible explanation: Unstable blood pressure can disrupt blood flow to the brain, which could lead to dementia over time.

Simon Mooijaart, MD, PhD, director, Institute for Evidence-Based Medicine in Old Age, Leiden University Medical Center, the Netherlands.

Alert! New Hypertension Guidelines and What to Do

Samuel Mann, MD, a hypertension specialist at NewYork-Presbyterian Hospital and author of *Hypertension and You* (Rowman & Littlefield).

For decades, we've been told to keep our blood pressure below 140/90.

Now: New expert guidelines have plenty of doctors crying foul. According to these relaxed recommendations, people over age 60 don't need treatment until systolic (top number) blood pressure rises to 150 or higher (no change was recommended for diastolic pressure). For people under age 60, 140/90 still is the cutoff.

Why the change? The committee that created the guidelines concluded that there isn't enough evidence that the additional blood pressure–lowering prevents heart attacks and strokes. In the absence of benefit, the risk for side effects from medication is not justified. Samuel Mann, MD, a hypertension specialist at NewYork-Presbyterian Hospital and author of *Hypertension and You* (Rowman & Littlefield), disagrees. *He says...*

Most of the studies analyzed by the committee followed patients for only three to five years—not long enough to observe the benefits of lowering systolic pressure to 140 versus 150.

Blood pressure reduction also has other long-term benefits that would not be evident in a three-to-five-year study, such as lower risk for dementia, erectile dysfunction and other vascular-related conditions.

With the many excellent medications available today, we usually can get the systolic pressure under 140 without side effects.

Dr. Mann's takeaway: A target below 140/90 still is best for most adults.

One exception: Adults age 80 and older may do better with systolic pressure of up to 160.

High Blood Pressure May Be Worse for Women

Wake Forest Baptist Medical Center, news release.

High blood pressure might be more dangerous for women than men, a recent study suggests.

As a result, women may need earlier and more aggressive treatment for the condition, the study authors said.

"The medical community thought that high blood pressure was the same for both sexes, and treatment was based on that premise," lead author Carlos Ferrario, MD, a professor of surgery at Wake Forest Baptist Medical Center, said in a medical center news release. "This is the first study to consider sex as an element in the selection of [drugs to treat high blood pressure] or base the choice of a specific drug on the various factors accounting for the elevation in blood pressure."

Although deaths due to heart disease have dropped dramatically among men over the past three decades, the same is not true for women, the researchers noted. On the contrary, heart disease is a leading cause of death among American women, according to the news release.

STUDY DETAILS

The researchers conducted a series of specialized tests on 100 men and women aged 53 and older with untreated high blood pressure but no other medical conditions. Tests measured the forces involved in blood circulation as well as the hormones involved in blood pressure regulation. Their purpose was to determine if the heart or the blood vessels were primarily involved in participants' high blood pressure.

Among women and men with the same level of high blood pressure, the women had 30% to 40% more vascular disease than the men, the study found. Significant physiologic differences were also found in the women's cardiovascular system, including the types and levels of hormones that regulate blood pressure.

The researchers said these differences influence how aggressively the condition needs to be treated.

The study was published in *Therapeutic Advances in Cardiovascular Disease.*

IMPLICATION

"We need to evaluate new protocols—what drugs, in what combination and in what dosage—to treat women with high blood pressure," Dr. Ferrario said.

Watch Out for the "Salty Six"

If your doctor has you on a low-salt diet to help keep your blood pressure in check, you need to look out for hidden salt.

The following foods are notorious for high sodium content—bread, cold cuts, pizza, poultry, canned soups and sandwiches (a combination of bread and cold cuts).

Examples: One slice of white bread may contain 230 mg of salt...three ounces of deli or prepackaged turkey can have 1,050 mg...a four-ounce slice of cheese pizza from a restaurant can contain 760 mg...four ounces of boneless, skinless chicken breast can have 330 mg...one cup of canned chicken noodle soup may contain 940 mg. Eat fewer processed foods and, when possible, read food labels.

Centers for Disease Control and Prevention data, published in *Harvard Health Letter. Health.Harvard.edu*

info For more information about high blood pressure, visit the U.S. National Heart, Lung, and Blood Institute website at *http://www.nhlbi.nih.gov/health/health-topics/topics/hbp/.*

Green Tea May Interfere With a Blood Pressure Medicine

Gregg Fonarow, MD, professor of medicine and associate chief, division of cardiology, University of California, Los Angeles David Geffen School of Medicine.

Suzanne Steinbaum, DO, MD, cardiologist and director of women's heart health, Lenox Hill Hospital, New York City, and spokesperson, Go Red For Women campaign, American Heart Association.

Clinical Pharmacology & Therapeutics, online

Drinking green tea may lessen the effects of the medication *nadolol* (Corgard), used to treat high blood pressure, a recent study suggests.

Nadolol is a type of blood pressure lowering drug known as a beta blocker, used to treat both high blood pressure and angina, the chest pain associated with heart disease.

Beta blockers, in general, work by reducing the heart rate and the heart's workload and reducing the output of blood, thus lowering pressure, according to the American Heart Association.

STUDY DETAILS

Researchers gave 10 volunteers a single dose of 30 milligrams of nadolol after they had consumed either water or about three cups of green tea daily for 14 days.

When researchers tested blood levels of the drug, they were 76 percent lower in the group that drank green tea compared with the water-drinking group.

According to the study's authors, that means that "patients treated with nadolol should avoid taking green tea." They published the findings online in the journal *Clinical Pharmacology & Therapeutics.*

Researchers for this study say ingredients in the green tea could interfere with the absorption of the medication in the intestine. The researchers included Shingen Misaka, PhD, of Fukushima Medical University in Japan and his colleagues from other universities in Germany, Japan and Italy.

EXPERT COMMENTARY

"Individuals who take nadolol and also consume green tea should be aware of this potential interaction and discuss this with their physician," advised Gregg Fonarow, MD, a professor of cardiology at the University of California, Los Angeles, and a spokesman for the American Heart Association. He reviewed the findings but did not take part in the study.

In the United States, nadolol is used less frequently than other beta blockers, Dr. Fonarow said.

"It's not a commonly used beta blocker," agreed Suzanne Steinbaum, DO, MD, cardiologist and director of women's heart health at Lenox Hill Hospital, in New York City, and a spokeswoman for the American Heart Association's Go Red for Women campaign.

Among the recent study's limitations are the small number of patients included, just 10, Dr. Steinbaum said. And she believes that amount of tea consumed would be unusual, at least in the United States. "It is rare to see a patient who drinks more than two cups of green tea a day," she said of her own patients.

Yogurt May Lower Hypertension Risk

Yogurt may lower your risk of developing high blood pressure. People who consumed at least 2% of their daily calories from yogurt were 31% less likely to develop high blood pressure during a 14-year period than those who ate less or no yogurt. The 2% level is the equivalent of at least one six-ounce serving of yogurt every three days.

Study of data on 2,197 adults without high blood pressure, 913 of whom developed it over a 14-year period, by researchers from Jean Mayer USDA Human Nutrition Research Center on Aging, Tufts University, and Massachusetts General Hospital, both in Boston, published in *Hypertension.*

Dr. Fonarow said that the results may apply only to green tea and nadolol. "It is not clear that those receiving other heart medications and drinking green tea need to be concerned, or that these findings apply to black tea," he said.

Nadolol isn't the only drug that interacts with food or beverages. For instance, grapefruit and grapefruit juices can interact with medicines, such as cholesterol-lowering medicines and some blood pressure drugs, according to the U.S. Food and Drug Administration.

Also, although the study showed reduced levels of nadolol in patients who drank green tea, it could not establish a cause-and-effect relationship. The researchers note that larger studies are needed to understand how green tea may react with drugs like nadolol.

The study was funded partially by the Japanese Ministry of Education, Culture, Sports, Science and Technology.

info To learn more about different blood pressure medicines, visit the website of the American Heart Association at *www.heart.org* and search "types of blood pressure medications."

Munch on This for Lower Blood Pressure

Jamey Wallace, ND, a naturopathic physician and chief medical officer at Bastyr Center for Natural Health, the teaching clinic of Bastyr University, in Kenmore, Washington.

If you've got high blood pressure or want to prevent it, you may want to stock up on celery. Why? Celery contains phthalides, chemicals that dilate the blood vessels and act as a diuretic, actions found in certain blood pressure-lowering drugs.

Some risks of high blood pressure are widely known (such as increased risk for heart attack and stroke). But high blood pressure also makes you more likely to develop dementia, kidney disease, eye disease, sleep apnea and sexual dysfunction. Normal blood pressure is less than 120/80.

What to do: For a consistent blood pressure-lowering effect, eat four medium-sized celery stalks per day. One easy way is to cut them into snack-sized pieces to munch on throughout the day—at midmorning, midafternoon and bedtime. (Talk to your doctor, though, if you have sun sensitivity—celery can increase skin reactions.)

Even better: Liven up your celery with other blood pressure-lowering foods—for example, hummus or nut butter (such as almond). People who eat these foods have lower blood pressure—possibly due to the foods' fiber and protein content.

Important: Four stalks of celery a day won't completely control high blood pressure. Use this remedy as part of an overall plan that includes increasing your intake of vegetables and fruits...exercising regularly...controlling your weight...reducing stress...and taking blood pressure medication, if necessary.

Also: Consult a physician familiar with natural therapies, if possible. Or talk with your regular doctor before you try this remedy—celery can interact with some medications.

Yoga May Help Ease High Blood Pressure, Study Finds

David Friedman, MD, chief, heart failure services, North Shore-LIJ Plainview Hospital, Plainview, New York.

Howard Weintraub, MD, associate professor, department of medicine, Leon H. Charney Division of Cardiology, NYU Langone Medical Center, New York City.

American Society of Hypertension, news release.

People who follow the ancient practice of yoga may be getting an added health boost, with a recent study suggesting it can fight high blood pressure—also known as hypertension.

STUDY DETAILS

In the study, researchers led by Debbie Cohen, MD, of the University of Pennsylvania tracked 58 women and men, aged 38 to 62, for six months.

Although the study couldn't prove a cause-and-effect relationship, doing yoga two to three times a week was associated with an average drop in blood pressure readings from 133/80 to 130/77, the researchers said.

In comparison, the average decrease in blood pressure was smaller (134/83 to 132/82) among people who ate a special diet but did not do yoga.

In a bit of a surprise, doing yoga in tandem with a special diet did not outperform doing yoga alone—blood pressure numbers fell only slightly (135/83 to 134/81) among people who ate a special diet and also did yoga, the researchers said.

The small decline in blood pressure among people who ate a special diet and did yoga may be because doing both required a greater amount of time, making it more difficult for participants to stick with their regimens, the authors said.

EXPERT RESPONSE

"This study confirms many people's feelings that exercise may be useful in the control of hypertension," said Howard Weintraub, MD, a cardiologist and associate professor of medicine at NYU Langone Medical Center in New York City. Dr. Weintraub was not connected to the recent study.

Based on the new findings, "yoga would be a useful adjunct in the lowering of blood pressure in certain populations," he said.

Dr. Weintraub said the study shows that "yoga can have a favorable effect" on hypertension. Although the amount of change was small, he said, "some large population studies have suggested that changes of this magnitude could have very significant long-term benefits."

The study did have some limitations, including its relatively short length and the fact that most participants were young and had milder forms of high blood pressure, Dr. Weintraub said.

Another expert agreed that the ancient Indian practice of yoga might ease hypertension.

"Yoga, along with deep breathing exercises, meditation and inner reflection, is a good adjunctive and integrative cardiovascular approach to better health, including lowering blood pressure, as this data suggests," said David Friedman, MD, chief of Heart Failure Services at the North Shore-LIJ Plainview Hospital, in Plainview, New York.

"In addition to proper diet and aerobic physical fitness most days of the week, I recommend that my patients take time each day for the above measures of finding disciplined inner peace, for improved health and well-being," he said.

The findings were presented at the annual scientific meeting of the American Society of Hypertension, in San Francisco. Findings presented at medical meetings typically are considered preliminary until published in a peer-reviewed journal.

info For more information, The American Academy of Family Physicians has more about high blood pressure.

Flaxseed Lowers Blood Pressure

Adults with hypertension who ate muffins or bagels laced with 30 g (about three tablespoons) of flaxseed daily for six months had an average drop in blood pressure of 15 points in the top (systolic) reading and seven points in the bottom (diastolic) number.

Why: Flaxseed has omega-3s, which may help lower blood pressure.

Grant Pierce, MD, executive director of research, St. Boniface Hospital, Winnipeg, Manitoba, Canada

Why Sunlight Is Good for Your Blood Pressure

Martin Feelisch, PhD, professor, experimental medicine and integrative biology, University of Southampton, United Kingdom.

Gregg Fonarow, MD, professor, medicine, and associate chief, division of cardiology, University of California, Los Angeles, David Geffen School of Medicine.

Journal of Investigative Dermatology

Sunlight is known to lower blood pressure, but now a team of British researchers has figured out why.

What they found is that nitric oxide stored in the top layers of the skin reacts to sunlight and causes blood vessels to widen as the oxide moves into the bloodstream. That, in turn, lowers blood pressure.

"This is an unexpected finding, in that the skin has not been considered to be involved in blood pressure regulation," said lead researcher Martin Feelisch, PhD, a professor of experimental medicine and integrative biology at the University of Southampton.

Dr. Feelisch said he thinks—if this finding is confirmed in further research—exposure to ultraviolet light might help reduce the risk for heart disease. "That's where it becomes interesting," he said.

STUDY DETAILS

For the study, Dr. Feelisch and his colleagues exposed 24 people with normal blood pressure to ultraviolet A radiation equal to spending about 30 minutes in the sun.

They found that the exposure widened the blood vessels, which significantly lowered blood pressure and changed the levels of nitric oxide in the blood.

Among people with normal blood pressure, the effect of ultraviolet light is modest—a drop in blood pressure of between 2 and 5 millimeters of mercury (mmHG), Dr. Feelisch said.

"This is a mild effect," he said. "But if you repeat this study in people with high blood pressure, I would predict you will see a more substantial drop."

WHAT DOES THIS MEAN FOR PEOPLE WITH HYPERTENSION?

Avoiding sunlight or using sunblock constantly out of a fear of skin cancer could be a new risk factor for heart disease, Dr. Feelisch said.

He isn't suggesting that people should sunbathe or use tanning beds in hopes of lowering blood pressure, however. What he recommended is spending a moderate amount of time outdoors.

"People are dying of skin cancer, and sunlight is the major risk factor that contributes to skin cancer," Dr. Feelisch said. "We are fully aware of that and don't say everyone should get as much sun as possible. There is a very real risk—but so is the risk for [heart] disease. One of the main contributors to the disease is high blood pressure."

Excessive exposure to sunlight carries the risk of developing skin cancer, Dr. Feelisch said, but too little might increase the risk of heart disease. However, more people die from heart disease than from skin cancer, he said.

Check Your Blood Pressure at Home

Tracking your own blood pressure at home helps control hypertension, according to a recent research review. Self-monitoring includes keeping a record of the readings so that a physician can determine if your blood pressure medicine is working effectively or needs tweaking. Left uncontrolled, high blood pressure can lead to stroke, eye and kidney damage and heart disease.

Ethan Balk, MD, assistant professor of medicine, Tufts Medical Center, Boston, and leader of the study published in *Annals of Internal Medicine*.

"We believe current public health advice, which is dominated by concerns of skin cancer, needs to be carefully reassessed," he said. "It's time to look at the balance of risk for skin cancer and cardiovascular disease."

The report was published in the *Journal of Investigative Dermatology*.

EXPERT RESPONSE

Gregg Fonarow, MD, associate chief of the division of cardiology at the University of California, Los Angeles, David Geffen School of Medicine, said high blood pressure is a major risk factor for stroke and kidney disease, in addition to heart disease.

That blood pressure levels are higher during winter and further away from the equator has been known, but the reasons behind these observations had not been entirely clear, he said.

"This study finds that UV light exposure to the skin induced nitric oxide release and modestly lowered blood pressure, suggesting that this may play a role in modulating blood pressure," said Dr. Fonarow, a spokesman for the American Heart Association.

Further studies are needed to determine the degree to which varying levels of light exposure might play a role in regulating blood pressure and reducing heart risk, he said.

info Visit the website of the American Heart Association at *Heart.org* for more about high blood pressure.

Consumer Health Alerts

Don't Rinse the Chicken...and Other Secrets to Avoiding Food Poisoning

Here's the dilemma—Kale, spinach and other leafy greens are some of the most healthful foods you can eat...but they also are among the most likely sources of food poisoning.

A very real threat: Every year, one in six Americans gets sick after eating contaminated foods. While the symptoms, including upset stomach, abdominal cramps, diarrhea and/or vomiting, usually are not life-threatening, about 3,000 people will die from the illness, according to the Centers for Disease Control and Prevention (CDC).

So how do you get the health benefits of vegetables, fruits and other common foods without running the risk of getting sick? *Here's how you can minimize your risk...*

FRESH PRODUCE

•**Vegetables** account for about one-third of all cases of food poisoning in the US, and leafy greens, such as spinach, lettuce and kale, are the highest-risk produce. That's because leafy greens grow close to the ground and are easily contaminated from irrigation water and livestock runoff. Leafy greens also have shapes and textures that make them harder to clean than other types of produce.

Important: Bagged and prewashed lettuce mixes may be somewhat riskier than "whole" produce because multiple heads of lettuce are used and mixes are handled more during processing. *To minimize risk...*

Richard Besser, MD, chief health and medical editor of ABC News. He has served as the acting director of the Centers for Disease Control and Prevention (CDC) and managed the CDC's public health emergency preparedness and emergency response activities. He is author of *Tell Me the Truth, Doctor: Easy-to-Understand Answers to Your Most Confusing and Critical Health Questions* (Hyperion).

• Get a package from the back of the store's refrigerator when buying precut lettuce. The colder temperature in this location inhibits bacterial growth.

• Check the expiration date. While most people are careful to check the expiration date on dairy, that's not always the case for produce. Packaged fresh produce that's eaten at least five days before the "sell by" date is less likely to cause food poisoning than older produce.

• Rinsing produce, including prewashed lettuces, will remove some harmful organisms, but not all of them. In addition to rinsing, buy the freshest produce possible, keep it refrigerated and, if possible, cook it thoroughly to kill any bacteria.

POULTRY

Most Americans wouldn't think of preparing a chicken or turkey without rinsing the bird first. The common belief is that rinsing washes away Salmonella or other disease-causing microbes. In fact, rinsing poultry is the worst thing you can do. It isn't very effective at removing bacteria—and it sprays potentially contaminated water droplets around the kitchen.

Some harmful organisms can survive for days or even weeks on faucets, countertops, the refrigerator handle, etc. They cause cross-contamination when other foods (or your fingers) touch the invisible hot spots. *To minimize risk...*

• **Always cook poultry** (whether in your kitchen or on the grill) to an internal temperature of 165°F. High temperature—not rinsing—will ensure that the bird is safe.

• **Wash your hands after handling poultry.** Most people remember to wash their hands before handling foods, but it's actually more important to do so afterward to prevent the spread of bacteria.

THE CUTTING BOARD

It's one of the most contaminated surfaces in your kitchen, particularly if you use the same one for all of your food preparation. The bacteria from poultry and other meats are easily transferred to other foods. Wiping a cutting board with a sponge isn't an effective way to remove microbes. Unless it's new or sanitized (put it in the dishwasher or microwave on "high" for one minute), it might actually introduce new organisms.

To minimize risk: Every home should have two cutting boards—one that's used only for poultry/other meats and one that's used only for produce.

Common mistake: Not washing a knife you've used to cut poultry before cutting other foods. Wash it with hot, soapy water or use a clean one.

Plastic or wood? Plastic cutting boards are less porous and easier to clean. Wood boards have natural bacteria-inhibiting properties. Either is acceptable—just keep it clean by using hot, soapy water or sanitize it in the dishwasher.

UNPASTEURIZED DAIRY

According to a CDC study, dairy products (mostly unpasteurized) accounted for 14% of all cases of food poisoning in the US—and the organisms in contaminated dairy are more likely than those in other foods to cause illness that leads to hospitalization.

Some states require all dairy foods to be pasteurized, while others allow the sale of unpasteurized (raw) milk, cheese and other dairy products. *To minimize risk...*

• **Buy only pasteurized milk, cream, cheese and other dairy products.** One study found that unpasteurized dairy was 150 times more likely to cause a food-borne illness than pasteurized versions.

LEFT-OUT LEFTOVERS

Bacteria need just two things—enough time and a high enough temperature—to multiply. *To minimize risk...*

• **Never eat food that was left out overnight.** This guideline applies even if the food was originally cooked at a high temperature or reheated the next day. The risk for contamination is just too high if food was unrefrigerated for that long.

• **Throw out food that you dipped into after the cooking was completed but didn't refrigerate within two hours.** Let's say you prepared a pot of stew or soup, then had seconds or thirds after it was cooked. If this food wasn't refrigerated within two hours, throw it out. By introducing the spoon multiple times into the pot, you could have introduced harmful organisms that may have multiplied. Some bacteria do grow at cold temperatures but at slower rates. For this reason, you should reuse leftovers within a few days.

DON'T FORGET THE SINK

Multiple studies have shown that kitchen sinks, including the faucet handles, have extremely high bacterial loads. *To minimize risk...*

- **Thoroughly wash the sink—and faucet handles.** Use hot, soapy water or a bleach solution—mix one tablespoon of unscented, liquid bleach per one gallon of water, and let stand for five minutes. Rinse well and air dry.

"Sell By" Dates and Other Misleading Labels Cause Terrible Food Waste

Emily Broad Leib, JD, director, Food Law and Policy Division, Harvard Law School, Boston. She is coauthor of a report titled *The Dating Game: How Confusing Food Date Labels Lead to Food Waste in America*, copublished with The Natural Resources Defense Council, an international nonprofit environmental group.

Open your refrigerator or pantry, and pick up a few random jars, bottles, cans or cartons of food—peanut butter, orange juice, cereal, soup or whatever. Most of them probably are stamped with a date that says something like "sell by" or "enjoy by." And if you're like many people, you throw out the food once that date has passed—because you assume that it's no longer safe to consume.

But are those assumptions correct? Typically not. In fact, in many cases those dates are arbitrary and meaningless! This makes it all the more aggravating that "date label confusion" is a significant contributor to the staggering amount of food waste that occurs in this country.

Food waste is bad for our wallets, costing the average American family of four $1,365 to $2,275 per year. What's more, we're suffering a lot of needless anxiety, worrying that what we eat is going to make us sick. A new report from the Harvard Food Law and Policy Clinic explains the problem and offers some solutions...

WASTEFUL NATION, CONFUSED CONSUMERS

In the US, we waste an appalling 160 billion pounds of food per year. If only one-third of what's thrown away somehow could be distributed to the 15% of Americans who don't have enough food, no one would go hungry.

Much of that waste occurs when food is tossed unnecessarily by consumers who are confused by the food date labeling system. Yet it's no wonder they're confused—because terms such as "sell by" and "best before" have no official, standardized definitions. Is the food no longer fit to eat...or do manufacturers just want you to throw out stuff that's been in your pantry for a while so that you'll buy more of their products? Though people often assume that the food cannot be safely consumed after the stamped date, most food label dates indicate only peak freshness and optimal flavor, not an end to any safe window of opportunity for consumption.

The inconsistency problem: Although the FDA and the USDA have the authority to regulate various types of food labeling, they generally do not regulate date-labeling practices, instead leaving this to food manufacturers, states or even local governments. The result is wild inconsistency. For instance, a carton of eggs sold in South Carolina can be stamped with a date that's up to 45 days after the carton is packed, while a carton of eggs sold in Alaska is marked with a date that's not more than 24 days after packing.

The authors of the recent Harvard report point out that it is impossible to provide actual definitions for all the date label terms currently in use because meanings are not legally defined. They vary by state, and there is no consensus about how to apply them to different categories of food products. *However, the terms generally can loosely be interpreted as...*

- **"Production" or "pack" date**—the date on which the food product was manufactured or placed in its final packaging.
- **"Sell by" date or "expiration date"**—information to retailers for stock control, leaving

a reasonable amount of shelf life for the consumer after purchase.

• **"Best if used by" date**—typically an estimate of a date after which food will no longer be at its highest quality.

• **"Use by" date**—also typically a manufacturer's indication of the last date recommended for the use of the product while at peak quality.

• **"Freeze by" date**—a reminder that quality can be maintained much longer by freezing a product.

• **"Enjoy by" date**—essentially useless to consumers.

Is there any term being used that indicates when a product is no longer safe to consume? No! And that's the whole point of the report.

The authors had several recommendations for the food industry that could help cut back on needless waste, including standardizing the labeling system and improving the use of safe-handling instructions so consumers know which foods should be refrigerated or frozen and how long foods last in different conditions.

But until such industry changes are made, consumers can use common sense to waste not, want not. Obviously, you shouldn't eat or drink anything that looks, smells or tastes like it has gone bad. For instance, toss anything with visible mold or discoloration, an "off" odor, changes in texture or flavor or marred packaging (such as a broken seal on a bottle or a misshapen or corroded lid on a can). *Other than that, though...*

• **Remember that the "sell by" date is purely for grocers' inventory-management systems.** If you're in the store and want to compare dates to select the freshest items for your cart, that's fine, as is opting not to buy foods that are past the "sell by" date. But once a food is in your home, don't misinterpret the "sell by" date as an "eat or throw away by" date.

• **With nonperishable items (canned goods, spices, honey) and packaged foods (cereals, crackers), safety isn't really an issue, the researchers said.** However, these foods may taste less flavorful after a long time in storage.

• **Perishable foods**—such as unfrozen shellfish, fish, meat or poultry, and eggs and dairy products—can spoil and make you ill. However, there's so much variability from food to food that it's impossible to give a blanket number of days after the "use by" date within which all products should be consumed. For more information on particular types of foods, check a reputable resource such as Nutrition.gov.

• **Be sure to store each food as the label directs**—for instance, by refrigerating after opening, if so instructed. That's the best way to avoid food waste.

Warning...Your Green Tea Isn't What You Think It Is

Tod Cooperman, MD, president, founder and editor at ConsumerLab.com, a leading independent evaluator of nutritional and vitamin/mineral supplements in White Plains, New York. He is author of *Health, Harm or Rip-off: What's Really in Your Vitamins & Supplements* (Bottom Line).

With voluminous scientific evidence now showing that it protects the heart, helps stave off diabetes and provides other significant health benefits, it's no surprise that green tea is among the most popular health foods in the US.

The disease-fighting punch of green tea is largely due to its high concentration of epigallocatechin gallate (EGCG), a substance with more antioxidant activity than vitamins C and E and other nutritional heavyweights.

The other side of the green tea story: Even if you are consuming green tea, the truth is that you might not be getting what you pay for.

Some bottled green teas and even green tea supplements contain only trace amounts of EGCG. Meanwhile, the amount of EGCG in other green tea–based products can vary by more than 240%. These and other findings, from the scientists at ConsumerLab.com, an independent laboratory that evaluates supplements and other products, show just how important it is to shop wisely for green tea products.

WHY GREEN TEA?

Both green and black teas (they come from the leaves of the same plant) contain catechins, a group of antioxidants that includes EGCG. Green tea is particularly rich in these compounds, with about four times more EGCG than black tea.

Multiple large studies suggest that green tea is good for cardiovascular health. For example, people who drink five or more cups daily are about 20% less likely to develop heart disease than those who don't drink green tea. Green tea drinkers also have lower cholesterol and a lower risk for stroke.

One large analysis, which pooled data from 20 previous studies, found that people who drank three or more cups of green or black tea daily were 16% less likely to develop diabetes. Green tea has also been linked to reduced risk for stomach, lung, breast and other cancers.

While these studies did not examine the brand or exact source of the green teas that were consumed, it stands to reason that if you want to get the health benefits, you want a green tea with a good amount of EGCG.

LABELS THAT LIE

The FDA doesn't test tea or tea-based supplements. Without testing, it's impossible to know how much EGCG is in a particular product. And even when this information is included on the label, it may not be accurate.

ConsumerLab.com purchased dozens of commonly available tea products, including tea leaves, tea bags, bottled beverages and supplements. The products were tested for levels of EGCG, lead contamination and amounts of caffeine, which naturally occurs in green tea. They were also analyzed for cost—how much you have to pay to get 200 mg of EGCG, which is the daily amount that's recommended by many experts. *Key findings...*

TEA LEAVES/TEA BAGS

Labels may or may not include the amount of EGCG per serving. You will obviously get more if you drink more tea or if you increase the strength of the tea by using more than the recommended amount.

Don't forget that green tea does contain caffeine—the amounts range widely from about 20 mg per cup to as much as 85 mg. If caffeine is a problem for you, decaffeinated green tea may be a good option. Some reports have suggested that decaffeinated green tea has less EGCG due to processing than the caffeinated version, but that was not shown to be the case in ConsumerLab.com's analysis.

A variety of products were tested using the serving amounts recommended on the labels. The amounts of EGCG varied widely. A brand of loose-leaf tea, Teavana Gyokuro Green Tea, provided the most EGCG, with 86 mg per one-teaspoon serving. Bigelow Green Tea had the least, with 25 mg per tea bag.

Important: When you brew loose-leaf or bagged teas, steep them for three to five minutes. That's how long it takes to extract the EGCG. Longer steeping times won't extract more EGCG and may make the tea more bitter tasting.

Cost: Lipton Green Tea was the least expensive way to get EGCG due to its low cost (10 cents per bag) and relatively high level of EGCG (71 mg per bag). The most expensive was Teavana Gyokuro Green Tea at 94 cents per serving, despite its high level of EGCG (86 mg).

BOTTLED TEAS

If you are drinking tea mainly for the health benefits (rather than taste), bottled teas may not be the best choice. They are expensive...often contain little EGCG...and tend to be high in sweeteners.

None of the bottled green teas that were tested listed the amount of EGCG on the label, but Honest Honey Green Tea listed the amount of catechins. However, it had only 63% of the catechins listed on the label.

When tested, Harney & Sons Organic Green was found to contain 46.8 mg of EGCG per eight-ounce serving, which is comparable to some brewed teas. Honest Green Tea had 27.2 mg of EGCG, and AriZona Green Tea—Ginseng & Honey had only 5.4 mg. Snapple Diet Green Tea had even less—just 3.5 mg.

Cost: To get 200 mg of EGCG from bottled teas, you would have to spend a lot more per serving than with tea leaves/tea bags. The least expensive was Harney & Sons Organic Green at $4.45. The most expensive by far was Snapple Diet Green Tea. To obtain 200 mg of EGCG, you would have to spend more than $70 and drink 28 16-ounce bottles.

TEA SUPPLEMENTS

Supplements can be an effective way to get large amounts of EGCG. You would have to drink two or more cups of green tea to get the amount that's included in a few supplement capsules. Also, supplements (in terms of their EGCG content) may be less expensive than other forms of green tea.

Here's the problem: Most supplements list the amount of EGCG on the label, but you can't always trust the numbers. For example, Omega Sports Green Tea contained only 38% of the EGCG listed on the label. The amounts of EGCG in other products averaged 188 mg per daily serving (that's typically two capsules).

Cost: Trunature (Costco) Green Tea and NOW EGCG Green Tea Extract were the best value, with a cost of approximately 10 cents for 200 mg of EGCG. One of the more expensive supplements (which ConsumerLab.com didn't approve in its report because of incorrect label information) would cost $3.41 for the same amount of EGCG.

BEWARE OF LEAD

In four tea-leaf products that were tested, small amounts of lead (2 mcg to 5 mcg per serving) were detected. Exposure to lead can lead to brain, nerve and kidney damage, particularly in children, who shouldn't be exposed to more than 6 mcg per day from all sources. Adults can handle more (25 mcg to 70 mcg per day), but it's best to avoid unnecessary lead exposure—it accumulates in the body.

All plants can absorb lead from the environment, but tea absorbs it more readily than other plants. In China, tea that's grown near roadways or industrial areas can accumulate high levels of lead within the leaf and on the leaf surfaces. Fortunately, only about 10% to 20% of the lead that's in tea gets into the liquid portion—most stays trapped within the leaves. If you don't swallow the leaves, your lead exposure will be minimal.

My advice: When brewing tea, use tea bags or a fine strainer to help prevent leaf fragments from getting into the liquid.

Also: Check where the tea originated. When comparing the largest producers of green tea, the teas from Japan are less likely to contain lead than Chinese teas.

Genetically Modified Foods Are Everywhere!

Jayson Calton, PhD, a nutritionist in private practice in Nokomis, Florida. A fellow of the American Association of Integrative Medicine, he is board-certified in integrative health, sports nutrition and alternative medicine and serves on the board of directors of the American Holistic Health Association. He is also author, with Mira Calton, CN, of *Rich Food, Poor Food: The Ultimate Grocery Purchasing System* (Primal Nutrition). *CaltonNutrition.com*

What do most European nations, Australia, New Zealand and about 50 other countries—including China—require of food manufacturers that the US does not? Labeling of genetically modified foods.

While the strictness of these labeling laws varies by country, hundreds of food-safety groups now say that products made with genetically modified organisms (GMOs) should be marked as such in the US.* Lawmakers in more than two dozen states are considering GMO labeling legislation.

What you need to know about GMO foods...

THE DEBATE RAGES ON

For nearly two decades, food manufacturers have increasingly relied on GMOs as a way to, among other things, improve a plant's resistance to pests and tolerance of herbicides, making them more apt to survive weather changes and increasing crop yield. In addition, GMOs are a cheap source of feed, which also reduces the overall cost of food production.

Now: In the US, about 80% of packaged, processed foods—and even some fresh foods, such as certain vegetables and fruits—contain

*The Whole Foods grocery chain recently announced that every GMO product sold in its stores would be labeled by 2018.

GMOs. For example, 90% of corn crops in the US are genetically modified...93% of soy crops, which may include some seemingly healthful foods such as certain edamame (soybeans in the pod) products...and 95% of sugar beets, which are used to produce sweeteners that are then added to thousands of products.

Here's how it works: Today's GMO foods are not just old-fashioned "hybrids" like the ones plant scientists have been breeding for more than 100 years. Instead, to make today's GMO foods, scientists use much more recent technology to insert genetic material from a variety of organisms, including not only plants and animals but also bacteria, viruses and insects, into the foods that we eat every day.

Food manufacturers insist that genetically modified crops are safe because they have not been proven to cause harm or illness in humans. Meanwhile, most food-safety advocates argue that humans are being used as guinea pigs in consuming these products without proof that they are safe.

The fact is, no one knows how safe these foods are. There are no published studies proving that GMOs are safe for human consumption, and results of animal studies are worrisome. Several animal studies suggest significant health risks, including infertility, immune problems and impaired insulin regulation.

PLAY IT SAFE

Because it sometimes takes decades of scientific research to definitively prove harm in humans, play it safe—avoid GMO foods whenever possible.

Even though processed foods are generally known to contain the highest percentage of GMO ingredients, many whole foods—including most of the milk, eggs and meats in the grocery store—may contain ingredients and additives that were produced from GMOs. That's because the animals from which these foods are derived were nourished with genetically modified feeds.

Be a smart shopper: Most people are surprised to learn that even some food products with food labels that say "made with organic ingredients" are allowed to include up to 30% nonorganic ingredients, including GMOs.

Diet Pill Labels Are Misleading

A recent study by the FDA found that nine of 21 diet pill products marketed as all-natural contained *beta-methylphenethylamine*, an amphetamine-like compound that has not been tested on humans.

And: All the products' labels claimed that they included a natural ingredient called *Acacia rigidula* taken from a bushy plant in Texas and Mexico, but researchers could not find the substance in tests of the plant.

Study of 21 diet pills by scientists at the US Food and Drug Administration, Washington, DC, published in *Journal of Pharmaceutical and Biomedical Analysis.*

Best approach: When shopping for multi-ingredient products, such as soups, pastas and sauces, look for the USDA Organic seal on the label. This verifies that the product is 95% certified organic—therefore, these foods will contain few or no GMOs. *To avoid GMOs or reduce your intake of these foods...*

- **Fresh produce.** Most fresh produce is GMO-free, but there are exceptions—zucchini, yellow (crookneck) squash, Hawaiian papaya and sweet corn. These are the only vegetables and fruits in US grocery stores that can be genetically modified—for now. A new apple (brand name: Arctic Apple) has been genetically modified to prevent it from turning brown. It may appear in stores within the next few years.

My advice: Even though there are currently only four vegetables and fruits that can be genetically modified, I recommend opting for organic produce whenever possible because it ensures that no potentially dangerous pesticides or antibiotics (which are sometimes sprayed on fruit trees and vegetable crops to combat disease) have been used.

- **Dairy.** Dairy cows are routinely given GMO soy and corn for cheap feed, so nonorganic milk may contain ingredients and additives from GMOs.

My advice: Whenever possible, purchase dairy that is labeled USDA organic. It comes from animals that were not given GMO feed and ensures that the animals weren't given antibiotics or hormones—both are widely used in the US, even though antibiotics in animals are believed to promote antibiotic resistance in humans and synthetic growth hormone has been linked to various types of cancer.

Examples of milk that's GMO-free: Organic Valley Grassmilk...Traders Point Creamery Creamline Milk. Or try organic nondairy almond or coconut milk.

•**Meat.** Choose beef from animals that were grass-fed and pork and poultry from pasture-raised animals, which ensures that the animals did not consume GMO feed. The meat (and dairy) from grass-fed/pasture-raised animals is higher in essential micronutrients, including omega-3 fatty acids. Grass-fed and pasture-raised animals are also unlikely to have received antibiotics or hormones.

Alternative: Look for the USDA Organic seal to ensure that the animal did not receive GMO feed, antibiotics or hormones.

•**Fish.** About half of the fish that is sold in the US comes from fish farms. Farming makes sense for sedentary mollusks, such as mussels and oysters. However, much of the fish that most Americans eat—such as salmon and tilapia—are raised in overcrowded ponds and given unnatural feed.

Example: One company is seeking to get FDA approval for a genetically modified salmon that will grow twice as fast as its natural, non-GMO counterpart. Even when farm-raised fish are not directly genetically modified, they're routinely fed GMO pellets.

My advice: Eat wild-caught fish—Alaskan salmon, haddock, Atlantic mackerel, etc. Unfortunately, you can't always find wild-caught fish in mainstream supermarkets.

Helpful: Stores that mainly sell farmed fresh fish will sometimes stock wild-caught fish in their frozen-food sections.

•**Breakfast cereals.** Because most of the corn and virtually all of the soy in the American diet have been genetically modified, many breakfast cereals—including whole-grain cereals—contain GMOs.

The more ingredients that you see on a cereal box, the more likely it is to contain GMOs. The recent discovery of GMO wheat in a field in Oregon has raised fears that the US wheat supply could contain GMOs.

My advice: Choose a grain-free breakfast like old-fashioned organic eggs and bacon. If you must eat cereal, choose organic GMO-free cereals that are made only from grains such as oats, rice, quinoa, buckwheat, millet and amaranth.

GMO-free products that are low in sugar include Pocono Cream of Buckwheat...Louise's Grain Free Granola Bites...and Lydia's Organics Sprouted Cinnamon Cereal.

Chemicals May Increase Food Allergies

Chemicals called *dichlorophenols*, used to chlorinate public water and found in insect- and weed-control products, can reduce food tolerance and cause food allergies in some people. Avoiding tap water is likely not enough. Limit your exposure to dichlorophenols by buying organic produce and avoiding areas where pesticides have been applied.

Elina Jerschow, MD, MSc, allergist, American College of Allergy, Asthma and Immunology, and leader of a study of 2,211 participants in the US National Health and Nutrition Examination Survey, published in *Annals of Allergy, Asthma and Immunology.*

Better Labeling on Gluten-Free Foods

Margaret A. Hamburg, MD, FDA Commissioner, Silver Spring, Maryland.

Some foods labeled "gluten-free" have contained enough gluten (a protein found in wheat, barley and rye) to trigger symptoms in sensitive people.

Now: Breads, cereals and other foods with "gluten-free," "no gluten," "free of gluten" and "without gluten" on the label must have less than 20 parts per million of gluten (the smallest amount that can be reliably measured). In people with celiac disease, gluten causes cramping, bloating and diarrhea—and can even lead to osteoporosis, malnutrition and intestinal cancer. The only treatment is to avoid gluten. Millions of people are also gluten-sensitive and suffer intestinal cramping, diarrhea, headaches, fatigue and other symptoms.

Is Your Home Polluted?—These DIY Test Kits Can Help Keep You Healthy

Caroline Blazovsky, president of My Healthy Home, a Whitehouse Station, New Jersey, firm that has advised home owners on indoor air-quality products and services for more than 10 years. A certified indoor environmentalist (CIE) and certified mold remediator (CMR), she is a member of the Indoor Air Quality Association. *HealthyHomeExpert.com*

You probably tested radon levels when you bought your house. But have you retested since then? And what about your drinking water...do you really know what toxins it might contain? Most people aren't sure exactly when to test for such in-home pollution or the best ways to do it. *What you need to know...*

THE DANGER: RADON

Contrary to popular belief, elevated radon levels have been found in homes in all states. And even though it originates underground, this tasteless, odorless, invisible radioactive gas can seep into the house through cracks in the foundation or basement and into the air at any time. Radon exposure is the second-leading cause of lung cancer in the US.

What you need to do: Test for radon every two years. Over time, cracks in the foundation of a home and deteriorating weather stripping can cause radon to seep inside the home. Even if you have a radon mitigation system, it may have been installed improperly or had a mechanical failure. Also, be sure to test for radon following a renovation.

Reason: Your home traps radon inside. When you put in new windows, roofing or siding, for example, you might be trapping more radon indoors than you were prior to the renovation.

What to look for: Short-term and long-term radon tests are available. A short-term test (used for two to four days) offers a quick snapshot of your risk and can indicate whether long-term testing or mitigation is needed. Short-term tests can be used when you need the results quickly, such as before a home sale.

A long-term test remains in place for 90 days to a year. It is more accurate, since it gives an average of the radon in your home over a longer period of time through various ventilation and weather conditions. If you want immediate radon results, you can hire a home inspector or mitigator who has a continuous radon monitor (CRM). This device has a sensor to read radon levels immediately.

Test results, from either the short or long test, of 4 picocuries per liter (pCi/L) or higher are dangerous, according to the EPA. But in 2009, the World Health Organization determined that a dangerous level of radon was considerably lower, 2.7 pCi/L. So, in my opinion, it's a good idea to hire a mitigation expert to install a ventilation system to reduce levels of 2.7 pCi/L or above.

Kits to try: Doctor Home Air by Alpha Energy Laboratories, Short-Term Radon Test, $11.95...and Long-Term Radon Test, $24.95 plus shipping and handling, *DoctorHomeAir.com/radontest.* This company has knowledgeable customer-service reps who can help find radon experts in your state. Or you can use the kits from Air Chek, Inc., Short-Term Radon Test Kit, $14.95...and Alpha Track Long-Term Test, $25.95, both with prepaid shipping, *Radon.com.* Air Chek is an excellent provider of educational material on radon.

THE DANGER: TOXINS IN YOUR WATER

Most people know that there can be hundreds of chemicals in drinking water. That's why home owners with wells have their water tested regularly—and why many of us use water-filtration systems. But your water may still have contaminants.

How to start: To find out if pollutants exceeding health guidelines have been detected in the tap water in your area, go to EWG.org/tap-water and enter your zip code.

What you need to do: If you have well water, conduct a test for total coliform bacteria, nitrates, total dissolved solids and pH levels annually and do a comprehensive test (such as those below) every three years. If you have city water, a comprehensive test every three years should be sufficient. Do additional checks if you notice a change in the color, taste or smell of your water...or if your skin becomes irritated with no obvious explanation.

Kits to try: For well water, Watercheck, $167 plus shipping and handling...or for city water, City-Check Standard, $206 plus shipping and handling, both at *Watercheck.com*. The kits include vials you fill with water to send to a lab for analysis.

If you have elevated radon levels in your air, you may also have elevated levels in your water, especially if you have well water—radon from the soil can seep into your water. If you have high radon levels in your water, a specialist can install filters or aeration devices.

Kit to try: National Testing Laboratories Standard Radiological Test, $150 plus shipping and handling, Watercheck.com. This test measures radon and uranium in well or city water.

Nail Polish Alert!

Connie Engel, PhD, science and education manager, Breast Cancer Fund, San Francisco.

Painted nails are nice. But are those pretty colors harmful? It depends on the brand of polish you're using. In the past, many polishes contained the "toxic trio" of hazardous chemicals—dibutyl phthalate, formaldehyde and toluene—but many manufacturers, including OPI, Orly and Sally Hansen have pledged to remove them.

Look for polishes that are free of the toxic trio by reviewing labels to make sure these ingredients are not present. You also can find water-based polishes that don't contain these chemicals.

To find out if your favorite nail polish and other products are harmful, check the cosmetics database at *EWG.org/skindeep*. You also can check for toxic ingredients with the Think Dirty app for the iPhone (available soon for Android). Scan a polish (or other cosmetic) while shopping, and the app will give you a toxicity score. If it's high, safer alternatives will be suggested.

Always ask the staff at nail salons if their products are "toxic-trio free," or bring your own polish. Choose salons with good ventilation, which helps protect you (and salon workers) from inhaling noxious fumes.

Danger in Your Hair—Deadly Dyes, Straighteners, Sprays and More

Sonya Lunder, MPH, senior analyst with the Environmental Working Group, a nonprofit environmental health research and advocacy organization in Washington, DC. The Environmental Working Group's Skin Deep website offers safety profiles for more than 80,000 cosmetics, haircare products and related items. *EWG.org/skindeep*

Hair-care products generally are not required to pass government safety tests before being sold in stores or used in salons. Some contain ingredients known to be toxic or to trigger potentially severe allergic reactions. This can be true even of hair-care products labeled "natural" or "hypoallergenic" or that salons insist are perfectly safe.

Sonya Lunder, senior analyst with the Environmental Working Group, a nonprofit organization that provides safety ratings for thousands of hair-care products on its Skin Deep website (*ewg.org/skindeep*) shares her important warnings for men and women...

• **Chemical hair straighteners usually contain formaldehyde,** which can cause skin irritation, allergic reactions and even cancer. This is true even of the hair straighteners used at high-end salons.

Example: The makers of the popular hair straightener Brazilian Blowout claimed that this product did not contain formaldehyde, but tests revealed that it did.

Even if a hair straightener truly does not contain formaldehyde, it likely contains chemicals closely related to formaldehyde that have similar health effects...or chemicals that are not technically formaldehyde but that release formaldehyde when heated by a hair dryer. Some hair straighteners also contain lye and other highly caustic chemicals.

What to do: There is no chemical hair straightener that's safe enough to recommend. Chemical-free heat straightening—that is, straightening blown-dry hair with a flat iron—is safer but, of course, not long-lasting.

•**"Gradual-change" hair dyes often contain lead acetate.** Some men's hair dyes are designed to alter hair color slowly over a period of weeks to make the change less jarring. But gradual-change hair dyes often contain lead acetate, which is extremely toxic and can lead to serious health issues including cancer. These hair dyes actually can cause elevated lead levels throughout the homes of people who use them, triggering health issues for other family members, too.

Examples: Grecian Formula for Men and some Youthair hair dyes have been found to contain lead acetate.

What to do: Avoid hair dyes that list lead or lead acetate as an ingredient. Check the safety rating on the Skin Deep website of any hair dye that claims to change hair color gradually.

•**Permanent dark hair dyes frequently contain coal-tar ingredients linked to cancer,** such as aminophenols and/or pheylenediamines. (Other hair dyes sometimes contain potential carcinogens and allergens, too.) The European Union recently banned 181 hair-dye ingredients for health reasons, yet many of these remain in use in the US because the FDA does not have to approve the majority of products used in hair salons.

What to do: Consider using temporary or semipermanent hair dyes rather than permanent dyes, particularly with dark-color dyes. These tend to be safer. If you use a permanent dark dye, do full dye jobs as infrequently as possible—just touch up your roots in between.

Wear plastic gloves when applying hair dyes to limit exposure to your skin. Before using any hair dye, enter its name into the Skin Deep site to find out about any potential health risks.

•**Aerosol hair sprays often are inhaled,** because aerosol cans typically distribute a mist of hair spray throughout the area around your head. Inhalation increases the risk for internal exposure and any associated health consequences. Even natural fragrances could trigger allergic reactions when inhaled.

What to do: Choose a hair spray that comes in a pump bottle rather than one that comes in an aerosol can. The spray from pump bottles tends to be less widely dispersed than that from aerosol cans, decreasing the odds of significant inhalation.

•**Shampoos and conditioners can cause allergies.** Shampoos and conditioners tend to be rinsed off relatively quickly, reducing exposure to any problematic ingredients relative to leave-on products. However, some people are allergic to the ingredients in these products, including the chemicals that add fragrance...preservatives and antibacterials that increase a shampoo's shelf life...and surfactants that, for example, work as an antistatic agent in conditioners.

What to do: If your scalp or neck gets itchy or red, look up your shampoo and conditioner on the Skin Deep site. If you discover that one or both contain ingredients known to cause allergic reactions, try a different shampoo or conditioner that doesn't contain these ingredients and see if the condition improves.

Manufacturers Need to Prove That Antibacterials Are Better Than Regular Soap

Restrictions on antibacterial soaps will require manufacturers to prove that these soaps are safe, effective and better at stopping illness than ordinary soap and water. Products that cannot provide proof will have to be reformulated or relabeled.

Los Angeles Times

How to Take Charge in the ER to Get the Care You Need

Steven Z. Kussin, MD, a gastroenterologist and founder of The Shared Decision Center in Utica, New York. He has taught at Albert Einstein College of Medicine of Yeshiva University and Columbia University College of Physicians and Surgeons, both in New York City. Dr. Kussin is author of *Doctor, Your Patient Will See You Now: Gaining the Upper Hand in Your Medical Care* (Rowman & Littlefield)

Emergency rooms are crowded, chaotic and confusing places. Americans now make about 130 million ER visits each year. It's estimated that about half of all hospital admissions now come from ER referrals.

Problem: Patients who are seen in ERs (or "emergency departments") and/or admitted to the hospital may be subjected to disjointed care, medication errors, misdiagnoses and poor outcomes.

Solution: To protect yourself or a loved one, it's more important than ever to be both assertive and savvy about managing your own care in the ER and/or hospital.

IN THE ER

People have been known to die in ER waiting rooms. It's not uncommon to wait three hours or longer. But if you're really sick and getting sicker, you need to get attention now. *Here's how...*

- **Go to the head of the line.** ER nurses assess each new arrival (this is called triage), and the sickest or most badly hurt patients see doctors first. When you're asked why you're there, don't waffle or give a long-winded reason. Keep to the point. Say something like "chest pain" or "excruciating headache."

- **Stick to your worst symptoms.** Pain and other symptoms tend to cycle from bad to bearable. Don't downplay discomfort. If your pain was severe two hours earlier, focus on that. This is not the time to be stoic. Get their attention.

- **Go over their heads.** If you're not getting triaged or end up sitting for hours after you're put in an examining room, you (or a family member) should check in every 20 minutes or so with the triage nurse. If this doesn't help, ask to see a caseworker. They're responsible for coordinating medical care and making sure that patients get what they need—including a nurse's or doctor's attention.

Important: If your condition is worsening, notify the ER staff immediately.

- **Get your test results.** When you leave the ER, get copies of the results of any tests you received. It might take extra time, but it's worth the wait. Even though you'd assume that the ER would forward this to the proper hospital floor if you're admitted (and to your personal doctor), it's safer to have these test results with you. This ensures that hospital physicians have the information they need to treat you.

IN THE HOSPITAL

If you are admitted to a hospital for any reason, be sure to bring your relevant medical records and the prescription bottles for any medications you're taking. If you aren't able to do this, send a relative to your primary care physician's office to get copies of your records from at least the last year and to your home to get your pill bottles.

Poor communication causes about 40% of all medication errors—one-quarter of which occur when doctors don't get a complete medical history or fail to review your prior medical records. Fortunately, many hospitals now have electronic

---

Enhanced Recovery Program Available to Hospital Patients

Surgery patients can go home sooner if they follow an enhanced recovery program.

Program basics: Non-narcotic painkillers are used instead of intravenous morphine or other opioid drugs.

Also: Patients are encouraged to consume sports drinks up to two hours before surgery. Hydrated patients require less intravenous fluid. Ask your surgeon for details.

Traci Hedrick, MD, colorectal surgeon and assistant professor of surgery, and Robert Thiele, MD, anesthesiologist/intensivist and assistant professor of anesthesiology, both at University of Virginia, Charlottesville.

---

medical records, which allow doctors to easily access most records. *What to do…*

•**Get your doctor on board.** Most hospital care is now managed by hospitalists, doctors who are trained in acute and inpatient care. But a hospitalist will not know you.

Why it matters: Your regular doctor knows your health background, which can affect treatment. The hospitalist will not. If you are the patient, you are likely to be very sick and unable to communicate clearly on your own behalf. If this is the case, try to have a family member—one who isn't afraid to speak up—with you at all times.

Important: Find out which hospitalist is assigned to your case, and let your regular doctor know who it is. Ask your doctor if he/she will drop by every other day to check on things…talk to the hospitalist…and review your test results. Also let the hospitalist know the name of your primary care doctor in case he wants to make contact.

•**Wait for test results.** Hospitals discharge patients much more quickly than they used to—even when all of the tests haven't been completed. One study found that 40% of test results were still pending when patients left hospitals—and some of these tests could have affected treatment options or even the diagnosis.

My advice: When you check into a hospital, ask to meet with the hospitalist and the discharge planner. Tell them that you'd like to have your entire hospital record—including all test results—on the day you're discharged. If the hospital staff says that only a discharge summary can be made available, ask your primary care doctor to follow up within 48 hours for your full hospital record.

•**See your doctor soon after you leave the hospital.** Don't wait more than two weeks—sooner is better. Research has shown that patients who don't schedule follow-up visits with their doctors are up to 10 times more likely to be readmitted to the hospital within 30 days.

GO TO THE RIGHT ER FOR SEVERE INJURIES

Choosing the right ER before an emergency can greatly improve your quality of care…and could save your life. If you've suffered a severe injury (for example, in a serious car accident or a bad fall) and are able to express your preference regarding the hospital you go to, ask to be taken to a Level I trauma center, or if that's not possible, a Level II trauma center. Both types of ERs are always staffed with surgeons, anesthesiologists and other specialists. However, a Level II center, unlike a Level I center, may not have research/training programs. (Such programs may mean that more emergency medicine physicians are likely to be working in the ER.) To find a trauma center near you, go to *FACS.org/trauma/verified.html.*

Important: I don't recommend urgent-care centers or nonhospital-affiliated emergency facilities for serious emergencies. Use them only for problems that you already know aren't too serious—or when they're the only facilities that you can get to in a hurry.

Do You Really Need That Surgery?

Dennis Gottfried, MD, an internist with a private practice in Torrington, Connecticut, and an associate professor of medicine at the University of Connecticut School of Medicine in Farmington. He is also author of *Too Much Medicine: A Doctor's Prescription for Better and More Affordable Health Care* (Paragon House).

Before you agree to undergo a surgical procedure, ask yourself if it really needs to be done. Based on some of the latest research, there's a good chance that it doesn't.

Shocking statistic: Nearly one-third of all health-care dollars are spent on unnecessary medical services, including tens of thousands of surgeries. This alarming statistic is a good reminder that everyone should get a second opinion.

Procedures you should question—and possible alternatives…

NECK SURGERY

It's one of the most commonly performed orthopedic procedures in the US.

Problem: A herniated disk in the neck that presses on a nerve can cause severe pain and sometimes numbness and tingling that extends down an arm and into the hand. However, the bulging or rupturing of a disk herniation usually corrects itself over weeks to months.

Important finding: A recent study found that 23% of patients with neck problems had been advised to have surgery, even though they didn't meet the commonly accepted criteria of MRI or CT evidence of a spinal nerve root with pain and weakness throughout that nerve.

Disk surgery has serious potential risks, including nerve damage, infection and chronic postoperative pain.

Who does need neck surgery: People with persistent, severe pain that interferes significantly with their daily lives...or those with significant muscle weakness in the arm or hand that's caused by pressure on the nerve.

Who doesn't need neck surgery: Individuals whose only symptoms are pain, tingling or numbness. They often do well with nonsurgical measures such as anti-inflammatory medications, physical therapy, localized steroid injections and massages. Symptoms for the majority of people with a ruptured cervical disk will improve in time.

GALLBLADDER SURGERY

About 35% to 40% of older Americans have gallstones, lumps of cholesterol, calcium salts and other substances that can be as small as a grain of salt or as large as a golf ball. In about 90% of cases, the stones cause no symptoms at all.

Problem: Doctors often recommend a cholecystectomy, the removal of the gallbladder, for cholecystitis, an inflammation of the gallbladder characterized by pain in the upper-right quadrant of the abdomen along with fever, nausea and vomiting. Cholecystitis is usually caused by gallstones blocking the outflow from the gallbladder.

Surgery to remove the gallbladder presents risks. The traditional open cholecystectomy and the more commonly done laparoscopic technique carry such risks as infection...peritonitis (inflammation of the peritoneum, the thin tissue that lines the inner wall of the abdomen)...bile leakage...and even death.

Who does need gallbladder surgery: People who have acute cholecystitis with blockage in the pancreatic or common bile duct almost always have surgery. Other people with acute cholecystitis, who are otherwise healthy, usually have their gallbladders removed.

Who doesn't need gallbladder surgery: Twenty percent of Americans have vague abdominal pains. Many of them coincidentally also have gallstones. A cholecystectomy in those people rarely provides any benefit and subjects them to the risks of the procedure.

Isolated acute cholecystitis without involvement of the common bile duct usually resolves in days. However, it may recur months or years later. Although a person who is otherwise healthy usually has his/her gallbladder removed, it may be better not to remove the gallbladder in someone who is not in good health, since acute cholecystitis is often an isolated event.

COLONOSCOPY

This is the most accurate test to detect and prevent cancer of the colon and rectum. Most people are advised to have a colonoscopy every 10 years, starting at age 50. Regular screenings can reduce death from colorectal cancer by about 50%. Colorectal cancer screening is an essential part of cancer prevention.

Problem: A study of Medicare patients who had a colonoscopy found that 46% repeated the test within seven years, and nearly half didn't need a follow-up test that soon.

Colonoscopy is expensive, inconvenient—and sometimes risky. Its major complications are bleeding and perforations. Colonoscopy is technically considered surgery, since anesthesia is used and biopsies are often performed.

Who needs more frequent colonoscopies: Overall, about 30% of Americans over age 50 have colon polyps found during colonoscopy, with polyps coming in different types and sizes.

If you have had polyps, ask the doctor what size and type they were. People with a villous adenoma polyp or multiple and/or large tubular adenoma polyps have an increased risk of developing colon cancer and may need a colonoscopy every three to five years. Those with a parent, sibling or child who had colon cancer (or an adenomatous polyp before age 60) are screened every five years.

Coffee Speeds Recovery After Surgery

Drink three cups of hot black coffee a day, starting as soon after the procedure as your doctor allows. People who drank this amount of coffee had a bowel movement 10 hours sooner than those who drank hot water...spent one day less in the hospital...and were able to return sooner to a diet of solid foods. Major surgery shuts down bowel function, which usually returns two to five days later. Speeding the return of bowel function helps the body resume normal processing of food, which is important for recovery.

Study of 80 patients by researchers at University Hospital, Heidelberg, Germany, published in the *British Journal of Surgery* (BJS).

Who doesn't need frequent colonoscopies: People without any polyps...with one or two small (less than 1 cm) tubular adenoma polyps...or with hyperplastic polyps in the descending colon or rectum are at no increased risk and can be screened every 10 years, unless they have other risk factors.

For people over age 75, the risk of routine colonoscopy outweighs its benefit and no further screening is indicated.

KIDNEY STONE REMOVAL

Many people with kidney stones never have symptoms. Symptoms generally occur when a stone migrates into the ureter, one of the two tubes that carry urine from the kidneys to the bladder. A "passing" stone can cause severe groin or side pain, blood in the urine, a burning sensation when urinating, nausea, vomiting and/or chills.

Problem: Doctors often recommend procedures to remove kidney stones that are causing no problems. Stones passing through the ureter will frequently pass on their own with medication, fluid and time.

Who does need kidney stone removal: People who develop an infection in the kidney from an obstructing ureteral stone. When the blockage is affecting the function of the kidney or the pain is severe and persists for more than two weeks, surgery is recommended.

Typically, the doctor will insert a tube via the urethra into the bladder and then thread a small instrument into the ureter until it reaches the stone. The stone can often be removed or repositioned to be broken up by shock waves (lithotripsy).

Stones in the kidney that are greater than 2 cm can usually be treated with lithotripsy. The procedure requires anesthetic but is done on an outpatient basis.

Who doesn't need kidney stone removal: People whose stones are asymptomatic or those who have only occasional mild pain. Most stones less than 5 mm in diameter may hurt while they pass through the ureter, but they will pass (sometimes it takes weeks). I advise patients not to worry about asymptomatic stones and to give a ureteral stone, if appropriate, time to pass.

Future stone formation can often be prevented, depending on the type of kidney stone, by drinking lots of water, limiting sodium intake and taking medications if indicated by your doctor.

Hospital Patients Need Natural Light

Esther Bernhofer, PhD, RN, nurse researcher at the Cleveland Clinic's Nursing Institute, Cleveland, Ohio, and lead author of a study published in *Journal of Advanced Nursing.*

People need 3,000 lux to 5,000 lux (lux is a unit of illumination) during the day to maintain a proper sleep-wake cycle.

Problem: Most hospital patients get less than 200 lux during the day.

Result: Greater fatigue...increased pain... and sometimes a slower recovery.

Self-defense: If possible, hospital patients should spend at least 30 minutes in the morning and another 30 in the afternoon within two feet of a window.

One in Three Hospitals Now Has an Observation Unit

While patients in these units are physically in the hospital, many end up with hefty bills since Medicare and most private insurers consider services received to be outpatient care. Patients often must pay out-of-pocket for the same services and medications that would be covered if they were formally admitted.

If you go to the hospital: Make sure you know your admission status and financial obligations.

Jason Hockenberry, PhD, assistant professor of health policy and management, Emory University, Atlanta.

Google Steers Online Shoppers to Phony Pharmaceuticals

Jim Hood, attorney general of the state of Mississippi. He leads a group of national attorneys general concerned that Google's search algorithm often puts sites known to sell counterfeit goods at the top of search listings. *AGJimHood.com*

If you use Google.com to search online for prescription pharmaceuticals, you might get scammed. And unlike most Internet scams, this one could cost you more than money—it could cost you your health or even your life.

Online shoppers often trust merchants that appear near the top of Google's rankings when they search for products. But when you enter the name of a prescription pharmaceutical plus the words "buy" or "prescription" into Google, it's likely that some of the sites near the top of the list will sell counterfeit drugs. Also, Google lets sites buy ads that run above the search results, and many counterfeit-prescription-drug merchants take advantage by buying ads.

The dangers: Counterfeit drugs often don't contain the correct dosages. Some don't contain the correct active ingredients at all. And some are not only ineffective but harmful.

Example: FDA investigators purchased the prescription flu drug Tamiflu from an online seller. What they received not only didn't contain Tamiflu's active ingredient *oseltamivir,* it did contain an ingredient not found in genuine Tamiflu that can cause fatal allergic reactions.

When counterfeit drugs are taken to control a serious long-term condition, it might not be obvious that the drugs aren't working until it's too late.

There are financial risks as well—an online merchant unethical enough to sell fake drugs also might misuse its customers' credit card information.

Avoiding fakes: If you wish to fill a prescription online, it's best to do so through the website of a well-known pharmacy chain. *Certainly avoid any pharmacy site that...*

- **Doesn't require a prescription to purchase prescription drugs.**
- **Doesn't have a pharmacist on duty who can be reached by phone.**
- **Doesn't list a physical street address.**

Almost every major prescription pharmaceutical has counterfeit versions, but fakes are particularly common with prescription painkillers and drugs that treat erectile dysfunction and sexually transmitted diseases.

When Medicine Goes "Retail"

Charles B. Inlander, consumer advocate and health-care consultant based in Fogelsville, Pennsylvania. He was the founding president of the nonprofit People's Medical Society, a consumer advocacy organization credited with key improvements in the quality of US health care in the 1980s and 1990s, and is author or coauthor of more than 20 consumer-health books.

The growth of what is called "retail medicine" is one of the most significant changes slipping into today's health-care scene. Retail medicine includes those clinics you now see in pharmacies, grocery stores and "big-box" retailers such as Target and Walmart. Some are open 24 hours a day, seven days a week and are staffed by nurse practitioners and, in some cases, doctors. Just about all are operated by for-profit companies. There are more than 1,400 such clinics in the US, and dozens more are opening every month. With more than six million visits a year (and growing) to these retail medical settings, chances are you might want or need to use one. *Here's what you'll need to know...*

•**The hours are good.** The popularity of retail clinics is largely based on their hours. Even retail clinics that don't see patients 24/7 usually are open at least 12 to 16 hours a day. Many people use them because their doctors' offices are closed or too backed up with appointments. The clinics handle such common problems as upper-respiratory infections, sore throats, inner-ear infections, sprains, minor cuts and more. They will tell you if your problem is an emergency and call an ambulance for you if you can't do it yourself.

•**The care is reliable, and the price is right.** After reviewing two years' worth of medical outcomes and cost data, the respected Rand Health organization reports that the quality of care at retail clinics is generally equal to that in conventional settings, such as a primary care physician's office. The research also found that even though many clinics are located in pharmacies or stores that sell prescription drugs, retail clinics do not overprescribe such products (a concern raised when the clinics first appeared).

Insider alert: Even though retail clinics are primarily for profit, the cost of care per medical episode was found to be substantially lower than equal services performed or initiated at a physician's office, urgent-care center or hospital emergency room (ER). This can mean substantial savings if you have high co-pays or deductibles.

•**Emergency care will cost you.** There's another new kind of medical facility in town—or soon will be. There are now more than 400 non-hospital affiliated, stand-alone, for-profit ERs. Originally opened to serve rural communities, they are sprouting up in major metropolitan areas where hospital ERs are backed up with patients. They differ from so-called urgent-care centers in that they can handle life-threatening conditions, such as heart attack and stroke. But ambulances usually will not take critically ill patients to one of these ERs (under most state laws, ambulance services must take people to hospitals).

Insider alert: Be prepared for sticker shock. Unlike the reasonably priced care of retail clinics, services from a for-profit ER can cost four or five times as much as comparable services from an urgent-care center or clinic. Similarly, for-profit ERs charge more than most hospital ERs, which handle huge volumes and negotiate rates with insurers. Most insurers do pay for care at stand-alone ERs, but some are now challenging their high charges.

Compare Hospitals and Health-Care Providers Using Online Tools

The hospital-comparison tool at *Medicare.gov* shows how a facility rates against state and national averages for readmissions, complications and patient satisfaction—Medicare now is penalizing hospitals with excessive readmissions. Medicare's physician comparison tool is expected to start providing quality measurements this year. Psychiatric facilities and hospices also will be rated with upcoming tools.

Caution: The ratings are not so accurate that you should automatically drop a doctor with a low ranking.

Roundup of experts in online evaluations of health care, reported at *CNNMoney.com*.

5 Questions Doctors Should Ask

Jamison Starbuck, ND, naturopathic physician in family practice and a guest lecturer at the University of Montana, both in Missoula. She is past president of the American Association of Naturopathic Physicians and a contributing editor to *The Alternative Advisor: The Complete Guide to Natural Therapies and Alternative Treatments* (Time Life).

When you see a doctor for the first time or visit your longtime doctor just for a routine checkup, if you're like most people, you probably spend no more than a few minutes talking about yourself or your problem. Chances are, a naturopathic physician—or any doctor who has a holistic (whole-body) approach to practicing medicine—would never settle for that.* Below are five key questions that I routinely ask my new patients. If you see a new doctor who doesn't ask these types of questions or your own doctor has never inquired about such information, give as much of it as possible to him/her anyway. Your answers may well affect your diagnosis and treatment. If the doctor isn't interested in hearing these details, consider replacing him with a doctor who is. *Questions all doctors should ask...*

Question #1: **What's your health time line?** On my intake form for new patients, I ask for a health history that includes significant life events—both emotional (such as marriage, divorce or loss of a loved one) and medical (surgeries, accidents or major illnesses). Besides giving me information I can use as a physician, filling out this form arms patients with self-awareness, so they become better prepared to ask questions and give more pertinent details during our appointments.

Question #2: **How are your diet and digestion?** To help assess digestive function and nutrient status, I ask about patients' eating habits and digestion health. It's also useful to learn what foods they crave, what foods they dislike and what they ate in childhood. I've found that many patients don't really know how to eat a balanced diet, and helping them correct that (with specific dietary goals) can lead to huge strides in overall health.

Question #3: **What's your daily fluid intake?** Sometimes, a seemingly mysterious medical problem is simply due to a person getting too much caffeine, alcohol and/or soda (regular or diet). And some people drink zero ounces of plain water daily. These individuals often are surprised to hear (but later thankful when they start to feel better) that I recommend drinking half of one's body weight in ounces of water daily! Low water intake can be hard on the kidneys and heart, in particular.

Question #4: **How is your sleep?** This includes total hours of sleep time, when they go to bed, when they get up and sleep interruptions. I also want to know where a person sleeps. Surprisingly, many people spend the night in a recliner or in a child's bedroom. Knowing a person's sleep patterns can offer significant clues that help diagnose and treat ailments.

Question #5: **How's your emotional health?** Are you happy, restless, angry, resentful, peaceful, longing for change or generally content? This information gives me a better understanding of how best to treat the person I am caring for—emotional issues can worsen or cause physical symptoms.

*To find a naturopathic physician near you, consult The American Association of Naturopathic Physicians, Naturopathic.org...or for a holistic medical doctor, check with the American Holistic Health Association, *AHHA.org*.

Are You Getting the Most from Your Blood Tests?

James B. LaValle, RPh, CCN, a clinical pharmacist, nutritionist and founder of LaValle Metabolic Institute, an integrated-care practice in Cincinnati. He is author of *Your Blood Never Lies: How to Read a Blood Test for a Longer, Healthier Life* (Square One). *JimLaValle.com*

Unless your doctor tells you there's a problem, you may not give much thought to the blood tests that you receive periodically.

But standard blood tests and certain other blood tests that you may request from your doctor can offer valuable—even lifesaving—clues about your health, including explanations for such vexing conditions as short-term memory loss and fatigue.

What you may not realize: If your doctor says that your test results are "normal," this is not the same as "optimal" or even "good."

For example, a total cholesterol reading of 200 mg/dL is considered normal, even though the risk of developing heart disease is sometimes higher at this level than it would be if your numbers were lower. Always ask your doctor what your target should be.

Blood test results that you should definitely make note of—and certain tests you may want to request...*

•Low potassium. Low potassium (hypokalemia) is worrisome because it can cause fatigue, constipation and general weakness, along with heart palpitations.

Causes: An imbalance of the hormone insulin often causes low potassium. It also can be due to problems with the adrenal glands or a loss of fluids from vomiting and/or diarrhea. A magnesium deficiency or a high-sodium diet can lead to low potassium, too. It is also a common side effect of certain medications, including diuretics, such as *hydrochlorothiazide*...laxatives...and some asthma drugs, such as *albuterol.*

Normal potassium: 3.6 mEq/L to 5.2 mEq/L.

Optimal potassium: 4.5 mEq/L to 5.2 mEq/L.

What to do: If your potassium is not optimal, your doctor will probably recommend that you eat more potassium-rich foods, such as fruits (bananas, oranges, cantaloupe)...vegetables (tomatoes, sweet potatoes)...and whole grains (quinoa, buckwheat). You'll also be advised to reduce your sodium intake to less than 2,300 mg daily—high sodium depletes potassium from the body. Additionally, you may be advised to take a magnesium and potassium supplement.

Also: Keep your stress level low. Chronic stress can lead to a high level of the hormone cortisol—this can overwhelm the adrenal glands and lead to low potassium.

•"Normal" glucose. Most people know that high blood glucose (126 mg/dL or above) is a warning sign of diabetes. But you may not be aware that slight increases in blood sugar—even when it is still within the so-called normal range—also put you at greater risk.

Surprising: Among 46,000 people who were tracked for 10 years, for every one-point rise in fasting blood glucose over 84 mg/dL, the risk of developing diabetes increased by about 6%. Vascular and kidney damage may begin when glucose reaches 90 mg/dL—a level that's within the normal range.

Causes: High blood glucose usually occurs when the body's cells become resistant to the hormone insulin and/or when the pancreas doesn't produce enough insulin. Obesity and genetic factors are among the main causes.

Normal glucose: 65 mg/dL to 99 mg/dL.

Optimal glucose: 70 mg/dL to 84 mg/dL.

What to do: If your fasting glucose isn't optimal or if tests show that it's rising, try to get the numbers down with regular exercise, weight loss and a healthier diet.

Powerful spice: Add one-quarter teaspoon of cinnamon to your food each day. People who take this small dose can lower their blood glucose by 18% to 29%.

Alternative: A standardized cinnamon extract in capsule form (125 mg to 250 mg, two to three times daily).

•High homocysteine. Most doctors recommend a homocysteine test only for patients with existing heart problems. Everyone should get it. High homocysteine may damage arteries and increase the risk for heart disease and stroke.

Causes: Homocysteine rises if you don't get enough B-complex vitamins or if you're unable to properly metabolize methionine, an amino acid that's mainly found in meat, fish and dairy. Vegetarians tend to have higher homocysteine levels. Other causes include a lack of exercise, chronic stress, smoking and too much caffeine.

Normal homocysteine: Less than 15 umol/L.

Optimal homocysteine: 8 umol/L or below.

What to do: If your homocysteine level isn't optimal, take a daily B-complex vitamin supplement that has at least 50 mg of vitamin B-6.

Also helpful: A fish oil supplement to reduce inflammation and protect the arteries. Take 1,000 mg, two to three times daily.**

•Low DHEA. This is a hormone that's used by the body to manufacture both testosterone and estrogen. It's also an antioxidant that supports the immune system and increases insulin

*These blood tests typically are covered by health insurance.

**Check with your doctor before using fish oil, especially if you take a blood thinner—fish oil can interact with it and certain other medications.

sensitivity and the body's ability to metabolize fats. DHEA is not usually measured in standard blood tests, but all adults should request that their levels be tested.

Low DHEA is a common cause of fatigue, weight gain, depression and decreased libido in men and women of all ages. Over time, it can damage the hippocampus, the "memory center" of the brain.

Causes: It's normal for DHEA to slightly decrease with age. Larger deficiencies can indicate an autoimmune disease (such as rheumatoid arthritis) or chronic stress.

Normal DHEA: Levels of this hormone peak in one's late 20s. Normal levels vary widely with age and gender.

Optimal DHEA: The high end of the normal range is optimal—it reflects a reserve of DHEA.

Examples: 200 mcg/dL to 270 mcg/dL for men...and 120 mcg/dL to 180 mcg/dL for women.

What to do: If your DHEA level isn't optimal, managing emotional stress is critical. Get at least eight hours of sleep every night...exercise aerobically for about 30 minutes, three to four times a week...and practice relaxation techniques, such as yoga and meditation.

Also helpful: A daily supplement (25 mg to 50 mg) of DHEA. If you take this supplement, do so only under a doctor's supervision—you'll need regular blood tests to ensure that your DHEA level doesn't get too high.

• **High LDL-P (LDL particle number).** Traditional cholesterol tests look only at triglycerides and total LDL and HDL cholesterol. I advise patients to get a fractionated cholesterol test for a more detailed picture.

Important: Patients with a large number of small LDL particles have an elevated risk for a heart attack even if their overall LDL level is normal. The greater the number of these cholesterol particles, the more likely they are to lodge in the lining of blood vessels and eventually trigger a heart attack.

Causes: Genetics is partly responsible for high LDL and LDL-P. A poor reading can be due to metabolic syndrome, a group of factors that includes abdominal obesity, elevated triglycerides and high blood pressure. A diet high in animal fats and processed foods also can cause an increase in LDL-P.

Normal LDL-P: Less than 1,300 nmol/L.

Optimal LDL-P: Below 1,000 nmol/L on an NMR lipoprofile (this test is the most accurate).

What to do: If your LDL-P level is not optimal (and you have not had a coronary event), I recommend exercise...weight loss...blood pressure and blood sugar management...more antioxidant-rich foods such as vegetables, berries and legumes...and three to five cups of green tea daily—it's a potent antioxidant that minimizes the oxidation of cholesterol molecules, which is important for reducing heart attacks.

Also: Daily supplements of bergamot extract, which has been shown to change the size of cholesterol particles (Earl Grey tea, which is flavored with oil of bergamot, provides a less potent dose)...and aged garlic extract, which has a beneficial effect on multiple cardiovascular risk factors. If these steps do not sufficiently improve your LDL-P level, talk to your doctor about taking a statin and/or niacin.

Now You Can Get Your Own Lab Results

Deven McGraw, director of the Health Privacy Project at the Center for Democracy & Technology, a nonprofit organization, Washington, DC. *CDT.org*

Have you ever gone for a blood test and then had to wait weeks for your doctor to call you back...or maybe you never heard from him/her at all?

Well, now you have direct access to your lab results. A recent federal ruling requires medical labs to provide test results directly to patients who request them. Previously, patients in most states had to wait for labs to send results to their doctors, then for those doctors to contact them.

This ruling could not only help you obtain your lab results faster but also improve the odds that you will get your results at all. A recent study published in *Archives of Internal Medicine* showed that medical providers neglect to inform patients about potentially problematic test results 7% of the time.

Waiting to receive lab results from the doctor may be the best option for you. (Call your doctor if you don't hear back.) It ensures that you have a doctor's help interpreting potentially confusing results.

But for a patient who has a chronic condition that requires frequent tests from the same lab, obtaining results directly from the lab could be an effective way to keep track of a health issue. Many people with chronic conditions have learned to interpret their own lab results.

Labs needed to comply with this new rule no later than October 6, 2014. The federal ruling supersedes existing state rules that previously prohibited labs from providing results directly to patients in 13 states.

When Medical Tests Are Wrong

Charles B. Inlander, consumer advocate and health-care consultant based in Fogelsville, Pennsylvania. He was the founding president of the nonprofit People's Medical Society, a consumer advocacy organization, and is author or coauthor of more than 20 consumer-health books.

Several years ago, my doctor called to tell me that the results of my PSA test (which measures prostate specific antigen to identify possible prostate cancer) showed levels that were three times higher than normal. My doctor quickly suggested that I get retested because the result might have been a "false-positive" (that is, a mistaken finding of disease that is not present). I was retested at another lab, and the results were normal.

False-positive test results are more common than you might think. Over the course of a lifetime, one in four women will get at least one false alarm from a mammogram. Each year, about 3 million women will get Pap smear results suggesting an abnormality in their cells. Yet only one in 1,000 turns out to be malignant. Blood test results, including those for cholesterol, also can be inaccurate.

What often gets overlooked, however, is the fear and panic that patients suffer due to false-positive test results. According to a recent study, a woman's anxiety can equal that of someone who truly does have breast cancer. So what can you do to protect yourself or a loved one? *My advice...*

•**Aim for Monday or Tuesday.** When your doctor orders a test, try to schedule it early in the week. Results from the majority of widely used medical tests can be sent to your doctor within a day. Ask that he/she let you know the results promptly when they are received. If the results suggest a problem, your doctor can order a follow-up or retest by midweek. This eliminates the anxiety of waiting over the weekend or longer if you need to repeat the test or have other follow-up tests.

Helpful: Many hospitals and testing facilities now provide prompt test results (for mammograms, CT scans and MRIs, for example) and follow-up testing if necessary. To save yourself both time and anxiety, check in your area for testing centers, hospitals and labs that offer such services.

•**Follow the rules.** Many false-positive results occur because patients don't follow pretest instructions. Cholesterol test results may come back too high (in the danger zone) because the patient failed to fast 12 hours prior to the test. Other tests report inaccurate results

New Tool Helps Predict Delirium

Up to one in five hospital patients develops delirium, which can lead to severe confusion and disorientation.

Recent study: Upon hospital admission, 374 patients age 50 and older were scored using a tool called AWOL—Age (A)...ability to spell "world" backward (W)...whether they were oriented to their location (O)...and their overall illness severity (L). High scores accurately identified patients at increased risk for delirium, who generally require closer monitoring.

Vanja C. Douglas, MD, assistant clinical professor of neurology, University of California, San Francisco School of Medicine.

because patients didn't stop taking certain medications or supplements before the test. Ask your doctor to carefully go over what you should or shouldn't do in the hours or day(s) before the test.

•**Try not to worry.** Sure, it is easier said than done, but remember, false-positive test results are common. By following the advice above, you can quickly determine if there really is a problem. And most importantly, don't let false-positive test results stop you from getting the medical tests you need. I have continued to have my PSA checked and will do so until a better test comes along!

No More Soreness After Medical Tests

Jamison Starbuck, ND, naturopathic physician in family practice and a guest lecturer at the University of Montana, both in Missoula. She is past president of the American Association of Naturopathic Physicians and a contributing editor to *The Alternative Advisor: The Complete Guide to Natural Therapies and Alternative Treatments* (Time Life).

Invasive medical tests are not fun, but thankfully anesthesia makes most of them manageable. The problem is, many people experience uncomfortable symptoms after the procedures. With a little preparation and help from natural medicine, you don't have to suffer these troubling aftereffects. Here are some general helpful steps I recommend...

•**Drink plenty of water.** I always recommend drinking half your body weight in ounces of water daily to stay well hydrated. This is especially important to do before and after the testing to help support a healthy metabolism.

Important: Just be sure to follow any fluid restrictions given by your doctor.

•**Go easy with the foods you eat.** If the procedure involves your digestive tract or one of your elimination systems, such as the bowels or kidneys, it's wise to limit your diet to fruits, steamed or baked vegetables, small amounts of rice and liquids (such as soup, juice and tea) for two days after the procedure. This will ease your elimination processes and accelerate the healing of any tissues that have been poked or prodded during the test.

•**Get up and at 'em.** While you should avoid vigorous exercise such as running, high-impact aerobics or biking until your increased risk of bleeding has passed (usually five to seven days after a procedure), walking is gentle and promotes good circulation, which helps speed recovery. I suggest a 10-minute walk every two waking hours after an invasive medical procedure, unless your personal circumstances make walking difficult or your doctor advises against it.

Certain botanical medicines also promote recovery from a medical procedure. If you are scheduled to receive one of the tests below, ask your doctor if the natural remedy listed would be all right for you to take.

•**Colonoscopy.** Three cups of peppermint tea per day, consumed 30 minutes away from meals, will reduce intestinal gas and gastrointestinal spasms—common complaints after a colonoscopy.

•**Cystoscopy (bladder study).** Cornsilk—literally silk from the ears of corn—is a soothing diuretic that helps heal urinary tract irritation, which often occurs when a tube is inserted through the ureter for this procedure. The tincture form of cornsilk is best absorbed. A typical dose is one-quarter teaspoon in four ounces of water, taken away from food, four times a day for up to a week after a cystoscopy.

•**Endoscopy.** A sore throat is the most common complaint after this procedure, since the membranes get scratched and irritated when the doctor sticks a tube down your throat. I recommend drinking three daily cups of tea made from licorice root and slippery elm.

One of my favorite premixed sore throat teas: "Throat Coat" by Traditional Medicinals, available at natural-food stores.

Diabetes

The Best Way to Prevent Diabetes—No Drugs Needed

If your doctor ever tells you (or has already told you) that you have prediabetes, you'd be wise to consider it a serious red flag. It means that your blood sugar level is higher than normal—though not yet quite high enough to be classified as diabetes—because your pancreas isn't making enough insulin and/or your cells have become resistant to the action of insulin.

A whopping 35% of American adults now have prediabetes. Nearly one-third of them will go on to develop full-blown diabetes, with all its attendant risks for cardiovascular problems, kidney failure, nerve damage, blindness, amputation and death.

That's why researchers have been working hard to figure out the best way to keep prediabetes from progressing to diabetes. And according to an encouraging recent study, one particular approach involving some fairly quick action has emerged as the winner—slashing prediabetic patients' risk for diabetes by an impressive 85%... without relying on drugs.

NEW LOOK AT THE NUMBERS

The recent study draws on data from the national Diabetes Prevention Program, the largest diabetes prevention study in the US, which began back in 1996. The program included 3,041 adults who had prediabetes and were at least somewhat overweight.

Participants were randomly divided into three groups. One group was given a twice-daily oral placebo and general lifestyle modification recommendations about the importance of healthful eating, losing weight and exercising. A second group was given twice-daily oral *metformin* (a drug that prevents the liver from

---

Nisa M. Maruthur, MD, assistant professor of medicine, The Johns Hopkins School of Medicine and the Welch Center for Prevention, Epidemiology, and Clinical Research, both in Baltimore. Her study was published in *Journal of General Internal Medicine.*

producing too much glucose) and those same lifestyle recommendations. The third group was enrolled in an intensive lifestyle-modification program, with the goal of losing at least 7% of their body weight and exercising at moderate intensity for at least 150 minutes each week.

The original analysis of the data, done after 3.2 years, showed that intensive lifestyle modification reduced diabetes risk by 58% and metformin use reduced diabetes risk by 31%, as compared with the placebo group.

Updated analysis: Researchers wanted to know whether those odds could be improved even further, so they did a new analysis, this time looking specifically at what happened in the first six months after prediabetes patients began treatment and then following up for 10 years. What they found...

- **At the six-month mark,** almost everyone (92%) in the intensive lifestyle-modification group had lost weight...while more than 25% in the metformin group (and nearly 50% in the placebo group) had gained weight. The average percentage of body weight lost in each group was 7.2% in the lifestyle group...2.4% in the metformin group...and 0.4% in the placebo group. Ten years later, most of those in the lifestyle group had maintained their substantial weight loss—quite an accomplishment, given how common it is for lost pounds to be regained.

- **In the intensive lifestyle-modification group,** those who lost 10% or more of their body weight in the first six months reduced their diabetes risk by an impressive 85%. But even those who fell short of the 7% weight-loss goal benefited. For instance, those who lost 5% to 6.9% of their body weight reduced their risk by 54%...and those who lost just 3% to 4.9% reduced their risk by 38%.

If you have prediabetes: Don't assume that diabetes is an inevitable part of your future...and don't assume that you necessarily have to take drugs. By taking action now, you can greatly reduce your risk of developing this deadly disease. So talk with your doctor about joining a program designed to help people with prediabetes adopt healthful dietary and exercise habits that will promote safe, speedy and permanent weight loss. Ask your doctor or health insurer for a referral.

Mediterranean Diet Alone May Lower Diabetes Risk

Connie Diekman, RD, director, university nutrition, Washington University, St. Louis.

Christine Laine, MD, editor-in-chief, *Annals of Internal Medicine,* and associate professor, medicine, Jefferson Medical College, Philadelphia.

Annals of Internal Medicine

Adults at risk for heart disease who eat a Mediterranean diet rich in olive oil can lower their chances of developing diabetes, even without restricting calories or boosting exercise, recent research suggests.

STUDY DETAILS

In the study, Spanish researchers followed more than 3,500 older adults at high risk of heart disease. The researchers assigned them to one of three groups—a Mediterranean diet with extra-virgin olive oil, a Mediterranean diet supplemented with mixed nuts, or a low-fat diet, which served as the comparison. They did not get special instructions on losing weight or increasing their physical activity.

A Mediterranean diet focuses on fruits, vegetables, whole grains and fish, besides the olive oil.

Those in the nut group were allowed about an ounce a day of walnuts, almonds and hazelnuts. Those in the olive oil group were allowed a little more than three tablespoons daily.

The researchers followed the men and women, aged 55 to 80, for about four years, between 2003 and 2010. During the follow-up, 80 in the olive oil group developed type 2 diabetes, while 92 in the nuts group and 101 in the comparison diet group did.

After adjusting for other factors affecting diabetes risk, the researchers found those in the olive oil group reduced diabetes risk by about 40% compared with the comparison diet group.

Catch-Up Sleep Helps Stave Off Diabetes

When a group of 19 nondiabetic men who usually sleep about six hours a night during the week spent three days in a sleep lab where they slept 10 hours every night, their insulin sensitivity improved, lowering their risk for type 2 diabetes. Regular sleep, just like good eating habits, keeps insulin levels balanced.

If you get less than seven hours of sleep a night during the week: Plan to get more sleep every night, but if you can't, get more on weekends.

Peter Liu, MD, PhD, principal investigator, division of endocrinology, metabolism & nutrition, Los Angeles Biomedical Research Institute, Harbor-UCLA Medical Center.

Those in the nuts group reduced risk by 18%, which was not statistically significant.

EXPERT COMMENT

The recent research, published online in the *Annals of Internal Medicine*, is good news, said Christine Laine, MD, editor-in-chief of the journal and an associate professor of medicine at Jefferson Medical College in Philadelphia.

The study "suggests it is possible to reduce the risk of diabetes by changing the composition of your diet. It is another piece of evidence that the Mediterranean diet has health benefits," said Dr. Laine, who was not involved in the research.

She hopes the findings don't discourage people from diet and exercise. Excess weight is a risk factor for type 2 diabetes, she said, and diet and exercise can help control weight. Adding diet and exercise to the Mediterranean diet could theoretically reduce the diabetes risk even more, she noted.

Those at risk for type 2 diabetes, Dr. Laine said, "should work hard to maintain a healthy body weight." However, even if they are not able to do that successfully, she said the recent study suggests—but does not prove—that adding olive oil to their diet may provide some benefit.

The oil's anti-inflammatory and antioxidant properties, among other factors, may explain the link, the researchers said. However, while the finding shows an association between long-term olive oil consumption and reduced risk of diabetes, it doesn't establish a cause-and-effect relationship.

People with diabetes, which has more than doubled in incidence worldwide in the past 30 years, have trouble controlling their blood sugar because they don't produce the hormone insulin or don't use it properly. The disease can lead to blindness, kidney failure and amputation.

The recent study "demonstrates the power of plant foods and an overall healthful diet," said Connie Diekman, director of university nutrition at Washington University in St. Louis.

"The important message from this study is the value of a Mediterranean diet plan to satiety and overall health," Diekman said. "Inclusion of plant foods, including nuts, along with the use of olive oil in place of solid fats provides a wider variety of phytonutrients, which promote health, aid metabolism and provide feelings of fullness, all important aspects of weight control."

The research was funded by the Spanish government's Institute of Health Carlos III. Industry sources provided the olive oil and nuts.

info To learn more about the Mediterranean diet, visit the American Academy of Nutrition and Dietetics website at *http://www.eatright.org.*

Chocolate, Tea, Berries May Cut Diabetes Risk: Study

University of East Anglia, news release.

A diet that includes substances found in chocolate, tea and berries could help protect people against diabetes and other diseases, recent research shows.

The study included nearly 2,000 healthy women in the United Kingdom who completed a food questionnaire and were tested for blood sugar (glucose) regulation, inflammation and insulin resistance.

"Our research looked at the benefits of eating certain sub-groups of flavanoids. We focused on flavones, which are found in herbs and vegetables such as parsley, thyme and celery, and anthocyanins, found in berries, red grapes, wine and other red or blue-colored fruits and vegetables," study leader Aedin Cassidy, of the University of East Anglia in England, said in a university news release.

The investigators found that consuming high levels of flavones and anthocyanins was associated with lower insulin resistance, better blood sugar regulation and lower levels of inflammation. Chronic inflammation is associated with diabetes, obesity, cardiovascular disease and cancer.

The study was published in the *Journal of Nutrition*.

"This is one of the first large-scale human studies to look at how these powerful bioactive compounds might reduce the risk of diabetes," Cassidy said.

Earlier research that took place in laboratories suggested that these types of foods might affect blood sugar, which plays a role in type 2 diabetes risk, she noted. However, it was unknown how regular consumption of these ingredients might affect a person's blood glucose and inflammation levels and insulin resistance, Cassidy said in the news release.

What remains unclear is exactly what amounts of these compounds are needed to reduce the risk of diabetes, the study authors added. Also unclear is how much of a health benefit the compounds really carry—the study found an association between consumption and seemingly better health but not cause-and-effect.

According to study coauthor Tim Spector, of King's College London, "This is an exciting finding that shows that some components of foods that we consider unhealthy like chocolate or wine may contain some beneficial substances. If we can start to identify and separate these substances we can potentially improve healthy eating," he said in the news release.

info The U.S. Department of Health and Human Services outlines how to prevent type 2 diabetes at its website, *http://www.healthfinder.gov/HealthTopics/Category/health-conditions-and-diseases/diabetes/take-steps-to-prevent-type-2-diabetes*.

Brown Rice Lowers Risk for Diabetes

Eating brown rice twice a week can lower risk for type 2 diabetes by 11%. Brown rice has more fiber and magnesium than white rice and does not cause a significant rise in post-meal blood sugar.

If you don't like the taste of brown rice: Try mixing brown and white rice together until you become more accustomed to the taste of brown rice.

Qi Sun, MD, ScD, assistant professor, department of nutrition, Harvard School of Public Health, Boston, and leader of a study of 197,228 people, published in *Archives of Internal Medicine*.

Fish Oil Pills Might Cut Diabetes Risk, Researchers Say

The Endocrine Society, news release.

Fish oil supplements could help reduce the risk for type 2 diabetes, recent research suggests.

The supplements, also known as omega-3 fatty acids, increase levels of a hormone called *adiponectin* that's linked to insulin sensitivity, Harvard researchers found. Higher levels of this hormone in the bloodstream have also been linked to a lower risk for heart disease.

"While prior animal studies found fish oil increased circulating adiponectin, whether similar effects apply in humans is not established," the study's lead author, Jason Wu, PhD, from the Harvard School of Public Health, said in a news release from the Endocrine Society.

STUDY DETAILS

For their study, the researchers conducted a "meta-analysis" of 14 clinical trials. A meta-analysis reviews existing research and attempts to find a consistent pattern. In this case, the studies that were reviewed were all randomized, placebo-controlled trials, which is considered the gold standard in research.

Two Large Meals a Day Are Better for Weight Loss Than Many Small Meals

People with type 2 diabetes lost more weight when they ate two large meals a day (breakfast and lunch—no dinner) than similar people who ate six small meals with the same number of calories.

Study by researchers at Institute for Clinical and Experimental Medicine in Prague, Czech Republic, presented at the 2013 American Diabetes Association Meeting in Chicago.

"By reviewing evidence from existing randomized clinical trials, we found that fish oil supplementation caused modest increases in adiponectin in the blood of humans," Dr. Wu explained.

Overall, the recent study looked at 682 people who took fish oil supplements, and 641 who were given placebos such as sunflower or olive oil.

Among the people treated with fish oil, adiponectin levels increased by 0.37 micrograms per milliliter of blood. This hormone plays a beneficial role in processes that affect metabolism, such as blood sugar regulation and inflammation.

Because the effects of fish oil varied significantly in the studies analyzed, the researchers suggested that omega-3 fatty acids could have a stronger effect in certain groups of people. The investigators concluded that more research is needed to determine which people would benefit most from fish oil supplements.

"Although higher levels of adiponectin in the bloodstream have been linked to lower risk of diabetes and coronary heart disease, whether fish oil influences glucose [blood sugar] metabolism and development of type 2 diabetes remains unclear," Dr. Wu said.

"However, results from our study suggest that higher intake of fish oil may moderately increase blood level of adiponectin, and these results support potential benefits of fish oil consumption on glucose control and fat cell metabolism," he added.

But the association does not prove a cause-and-effect relationship between fish oil supplementation and decreased diabetes risk.

Roughly 37% of adults and 31% of children in the United States take fish oil supplements, according to a 2007 survey by the National Institutes of Health's National Center for Complementary and Alternative Medicine.

The study was published in the *Journal of Clinical Endocrinology & Metabolism.* It was supported by grants from the National Institutes of Health's National Heart, Lung, and Blood Institute.

info The U.S. National Library of Medicine has more about fish oil supplements at its website, *http://www.nlm.nih.gov/medlineplus* (search "fish oil supplements").

Fight Diabetes Naturally—Three Proven Nondrug Remedies

Bill Gottlieb, CHC, a health coach certified by the American Association of Drugless Practitioners. Based in northern California, he is author of *Defeat High Blood Sugar—Naturally! Super-Supplements and Super-Foods Selected by America's Best Alternative Doctors* (Online Publishing & Marketing). *BillGottliebHealth.com*

Scientific research and the experience of doctors and other health professionals show that supplements and superfoods can be even more effective than drugs when it comes to preventing and treating diabetes. I

Eating More Red Meat Raises Diabetes Risk

People who increased their red-meat consumption by more than half a serving a day over a four-year period had a 48% higher risk for type 2 diabetes in the following four years. People who reduced their consumption by at least half a serving daily had a 14% lower risk for type 2 diabetes. Red-meat consumption has been linked to diabetes before, but this is the first study to observe the results of increases or decreases in consumption over time.

Analysis of three studies involving a total of more than 149,000 people by researchers at National University of Singapore, published online by *JAMA Internal Medicine.*

reviewed thousands of scientific studies and talked to more than 60 health professionals about these glucose-controlling natural remedies. One is magnesium. Studies show that magnesium significantly reduces the risk for diabetes. *Here are three more standout natural remedies...*

Caution: If you are taking insulin or other medications to control diabetes, talk to your doctor before taking any supplement or changing your diet.

GYMNEMA

Gymnema has been the standard anti-diabetes recommendation for the past 2,000 years from practitioners of Ayurveda, the ancient system of natural healing from India. Derived from a vine-like plant found in the tropical forests of southern and central India, the herb also is called gurmar, or "sugar destroyer"—if you chew on the leaf of the plant, you temporarily will lose your ability to taste sweets.

Modern science has figured out the molecular interactions underlying this strange phenomenon. The gymnemic acids in the herb have a structure similar to glucose molecules, filling up glucose receptor sites on the taste buds. They also fill up sugar receptors in the intestine, blocking the absorption of glucose. And gymnemic acids stimulate (and even may regenerate) the cells of the pancreas that manufacture insulin, the hormone that ushers glucose out of the bloodstream and into cells.

After-Dinner Walks Best for Lowering Blood Sugar

A group of adults over age 60 who were at risk for diabetes took either a daily 45-minute walk or three 15-minute walks after meals. After one month, researchers found that blood sugar levels were most effectively reduced when walking occurred soon after meals, especially a big evening meal.

Possible explanation: Eating can trigger a sudden spike in blood sugar, which is immediately blunted when a person starts walking.

Loretta DiPietro, PhD, chair of exercise science, The George Washington University School of Public Health and Health Services, Washington, DC.

Standout research: Studies published in *Journal of Ethnopharmacology* showed that three months of using a unique gymnema extract, formulated over several decades by two Indian scientists, reduced fasting blood glucose (a blood sample is taken after an overnight fast) by 23% in people with type 2 diabetes (defined as fasting blood sugar levels of 126 mg/dL or higher). People with prediabetes (defined as those with blood sugar levels of 100 mg/dL to 125 mg/dL) had a 30% reduction.

Important: The newest (and more powerful) version of this extract is called ProBeta, which is available at PharmaTerra.com. A naturopathic physician who uses ProBeta with his patients told me that the supplement can lower fasting glucose in the 200s down to the 120s or 130s after five to six months of use.

Typical daily dose: ProBeta—two capsules, two to three times a day. Other types of gymnema—400 milligrams (mg), three times a day.

APPLE CIDER VINEGAR

Numerous studies have proved that apple cider vinegar works to control type 2 diabetes. Several of the studies were conducted by Carol Johnston, PhD, RD, a professor of nutrition at Arizona State University.

Standout scientific research: Dr. Johnston's studies showed that an intake of apple cider vinegar with a meal lowered insulin resistance (the inability of cells to use insulin) by an average of 64% in people with prediabetes and type 2 diabetes...improved insulin sensitivity (the ability of cells to use insulin) by up to 34%...and lowered postmeal spikes in blood sugar by an average of 20%. Research conducted in Greece, Sweden, Japan and the Middle East has confirmed many of Dr. Johnston's findings.

How it works: The acetic acid in vinegar—the compound that gives vinegar its tart flavor and pungent odor—blunts the activity of disaccharidase enzymes that help break down the type of carbohydrates found in starchy foods such as potatoes, rice, bread and pasta. As a result, those foods are digested and absorbed more slowly, lowering blood glucose and insulin levels.

Supplement Boosts Diabetes Medications

According to a recent study, adults with type 2 diabetes who took 250 mg daily of the polyphenol resveratrol (along with diabetes medications) for three months had a significant improvement in their systolic (top number) blood pressure readings, blood glucose and total cholesterol levels compared with those who took only diabetes medications.

If you have type 2 diabetes: Ask your doctor if a resveratrol supplement is right for you.

MJ Nanjan, PhD, professor, JSS College of Pharmacy, Ootacamund, Tamil Nadu, India.

Suggested daily intake: Two tablespoons right before or early in the meal. (More is not more effective.)

If you're using vinegar in a salad dressing, the ideal ratio for blood sugar control is two tablespoons of vinegar to one tablespoon of oil. Eat the salad early in the meal so that it disrupts the carb-digesting enzymes before they get a chance to work. Or dip premeal whole-grain bread in a vinaigrette dressing.

SOY FOODS

A recent 10-year study published in *Journal of the American Society of Nephrology* found that the mortality rate for people with diabetes and kidney disease was more than 31%. Statistically, that makes kidney disease the number-one risk factor for death in people with diabetes.

Fortunately, researchers have found that there is a simple way to counter kidney disease in diabetes—eat more soy foods.

Standout scientific research: Dozens of scientific studies show that soy is a nutritional ally for diabetes patients with kidney disease. But the best and most recent of these studies, published in *Diabetes Care*, shows that eating lots of soy can help reverse signs of kidney disease, reduce risk factors for heart disease—and reduce blood sugar, too.

The study involved 41 diabetes patients with kidney disease, divided into two groups. One group ate a diet with protein from 70% animal and 30% vegetable sources. The other group ate a diet with protein from 35% animal sources, 35% textured soy protein and 30% vegetable proteins. After four years, those eating the soy-rich diet had lower levels of several biomarkers for kidney disease. (In another, smaller experiment, the same researchers found that soy improved biomarkers for kidney disease in just seven weeks.) In fact, the health of the participants' kidneys actually improved, a finding that surprised the researchers, since diabetic nephropathy (diabetes-caused kidney disease) is considered to be a progressive, irreversible disease.

Those eating soy also had lower fasting blood sugar, lower LDL cholesterol, lower total cholesterol, lower triglycerides and lower C-reactive protein, a biomarker for chronic inflammation.

How it works: Substituting soy for animal protein may ease stress on the delicate filters of the kidneys. Soy itself also stops the overproduction of cells in the kidney that clog the filters...boosts the production of nitric oxide, which improves blood flow in the kidneys...and normalizes the movement of minerals within the kidneys, thus improving filtration.

Suggested daily intake: The diabetes patients in the study ate 16 grams of soy protein daily.

Examples: Four ounces of tofu provide 13 grams of soy protein...one soy burger, 13 grams...one-quarter cup of soy nuts, 11 grams... one-half cup of shelled edamame (edible soybeans in the pod), 11 grams...one cup of soy milk, 6 grams.

WHAT'S WRONG WITH DIABETES DRUGS?

Doctors typically try to control high blood sugar with a glucose-lowering medication such as *metformin* (Glucophage), a drug most experts consider safe. But other diabetes drugs may not be safe.

Example #1: Recent studies show that *sitagliptin* (Januvia) and *exenatide* (Byetta) double the risk for hospitalization for pancreatitis (inflamed pancreas) and triple the risk for pancreatic cancer.

Example #2: *Pioglitazone* (Actos) can triple the risk for eye problems and vision loss, double the risk for bone fractures in women and double the risk for bladder cancer.

FDA Lifts Restrictions on Diabetes Drug Avandia

Yehuda Handelsman, MD, endocrinologist and incoming president, American College of Endocrinology, Tarzana, California.
Ronald Tamler, MD, clinical director, Mount Sinai Diabetes Center, The Mount Sinai Hospital, New York City.
Bob Eckel, past president, American Heart Association
Steven Nissen, MD, head, cardiology, Cleveland Clinic, Ohio.
U.S. Food and Drug Administration, statement.

The U.S. Food and Drug Administration has lifted the tough safety restrictions it imposed on the diabetes drug Avandia three years ago (based on studies that linked it to heart problems). The decision was finalized in November 2013.

The agency's decision was expected, and followed up on a June 2013 vote by an expert advisory panel to rescind the restrictions, based on new data that suggested the medication may not be as harmful as once thought.

Avandia was taken off drug store shelves in 2011, and its use restricted to patients who first signed a waiver saying they understood the possible risks. Only specially registered pharmacies could dispense Avandia.

But an independent review by Duke University researchers, based on Avandia's original clinical trial, concluded that patients had no elevated risk of heart attack or death compared with those taking standard diabetes drugs.

"Our actions reflect the most current scientific knowledge about the risks and benefits of this drug," Janet Woodcock, MD, director of the FDA's Center for Drug Evaluation and Research, said in a statement. "Given these new results, our level of concern is considerably reduced. Thus, we are requiring the removal of certain prescribing restrictions."

BACKGROUND ON AVANDIA

Steven Nissen, MD, head of cardiology at Cleveland Clinic, first sounded the alarm about Avandia in 2007 with an analysis of 42 studies that showed that the medication caused a 43% increased risk of heart attack.

Following his study, an FDA analysis of more than 50 studies concluded that Avandia was linked to an increased risk of heart problems, and the agency decided to pull the drug from pharmacy shelves.

However, the FDA also asked drug maker GlaxoSmithKline to review key aspects of Avandia's clinical trial related to heart safety. This was the review that led to the FDA's recent reversal.

Dr. Nissen condemned the FDA's latest action.

"This decision is not in the public interest," Dr. Nissen said. "It's really more about the FDA than it is about the drug. It does not make any good regulatory sense, and in fact it's rather bizarre."

EXPERTS VARY ON FINAL CALL

Not everyone agreed with him, however.

Yehuda Handelsman, MD, an endocrinologist in Tarzana, California, and incoming president of the American College of Endocrinology, applauded the FDA for "doing what's right by standing up for the science."

"I thought it was about time. Many of us never thought the information brought against the drug was very scientifically solid or correct," Dr. Handelsman said of the announcement.

Big Breakfasts May Be Better for People With Diabetes

People with type 2 diabetes who ate a large breakfast that included protein and fat for three months had lower blood glucose levels and lower blood pressure than people who ate smaller breakfasts. Nearly one-third of the big-breakfast eaters were able to reduce the amount of diabetes medication they took. And big-breakfast eaters reported themselves less hungry later in the day.

Caution: The calorie, protein and fat contents of the large breakfasts (which were about one-third of the subjects' daily calories) were carefully arranged and monitored. Talk to your doctor before making any changes in your diet.

Study by researchers at Hebrew University of Jerusalem, presented at the annual meeting of the European Association for the Study of Diabetes in Barcelona.

For his part, Bob Eckel, MD, a past president of the American Heart Association, greeted the news with more of a shrug.

"I think they've made the appropriate decision based on the updated evidence," Dr. Eckel said. "It's consistent with the latest evidence."

Both Drs. Nissen and Eckel agreed that widespread use of Avandia is not likely to resume, regardless of the FDA's change of heart, because too many concerns have been raised regarding the drug's safety.

"The good news is physicians are not going to start using this drug again. It's basically an obsolete drug, so this will have no practical implications," Dr. Nissen said. "Who's going to use it? What patient is going to take it and what doctor is going to prescribe it, given everything we know?"

Another expert concurred. "The decision by the FDA is irrelevant in clinical practice," said Ronald Tamler, MD, clinical director of the Mount Sinai Diabetes Center at The Mount Sinai Hospital in New York City. "Patients have been reading about increased risk of cardiovascular events with Avandia since 2007 and will not abandon their concerns overnight, despite the FDA decision. Moreover, a medication with similar properties, *pioglitazone* [Actos], is available as a generic drug at a much lower cost."

But Dr. Handelsman said Avandia—or its generic form—might still have a bright future.

It's entirely possible that Avandia could come back in generic form, and that diabetes doctors might start prescribing it again as a viable option to other medications. "For us, it's not a problem to use," he said.

In its heyday, Avandia was a blockbuster diabetes drug for maker GlaxoSmithKline, with about $3.2 billion in sales posted in 2006.

Under the FDA's decision, the drug's information will be changed to reflect that Avandia may be used along with diet and exercise to improve control of blood sugar in type 2 diabetes patients. Patients will be able to receive the medication through regular and mail-order pharmacies.

A Simple Scoring System Helps Predict Dementia Risk in People With Type 2 Diabetes

The diabetes-specific dementia risk score (DSDRS) is based on factors such as age, education, acute metabolic events, heart disease and depression. The system will make it easier for doctors to monitor patients at the highest risk for dementia.

Study of 29,961 patients by researchers from Kaiser Permanente Northern California Division of Research, Oakland, and University Medical Centre Utrecht, the Netherlands, published in *The Lancet Diabetes & Endocrinology*.

Vaccine May Stop Immune Attack in Type 1 Diabetes, Study Suggests

Lawrence Steinman, MD, professor, pediatrics, neurology and neurological sciences, Stanford University School of Medicine, California.

Richard Insel, MD, chief scientific officer, JDRF, New York City.

Joel Zonszein, MD, director, clinical diabetes center, Montefiore Medical Center, New York City.

Science Translational Medicine

A new type of vaccine may stop the autoimmune attack that occurs in people with type 1 diabetes, researchers report.

Although an initial trial of the vaccine wasn't able to free anyone from their daily insulin injections, it did boost insulin production, which could help prevent some of type 1 diabetes' most devastating complications.

Instead of increasing the immune system's activity like the polio or influenza vaccine does, the new vaccine turns off a portion of the immune response, acting as a reverse vaccine. The researchers were able to isolate a part of the immune response that only seems to be involved with type 1 diabetes, according to the study. That means the vaccine likely wouldn't have the risks that medications that suppress the immune system do.

"We were able to destroy the rogue cells that are attacking the insulin-producing cells without destroying any other part of the immune

Diabetes Medications Affect Cancer Risk Among Women

According to a recent study, women with type 2 diabetes taking insulin sensitizers, including the diabetes medication *metformin* (Glucophage), or thiazolidinediones, such as *pioglitazone* (Actos), had 21% lower risk for cancer than women taking insulin secretagogues. Insulin secretagogues include sulfonylureas, such as *glimepiride* (Amaryl), and meglitinides, such as *nateglinide* (Starlix).

Sangeeta Kashyap, MD, is an endocrinologist and associate professor of medicine at the Cleveland Clinic's Endocrinology & Metabolism Institute. She is lead author of a study published in *Diabetes, Obesity and Metabolism.*

system, and that's truly exciting," said senior study author Lawrence Steinman, MD, a professor of pediatrics and neurology and neurological sciences at Stanford University School of Medicine.

"Once the immune attack is stopped, I believe there's great potential for recovery in the beta cells," Dr. Steinman added.

BACKGROUND ON INSULIN

Beta cells in the pancreas produce the hormone insulin. In people with type 1 diabetes, it's believed that the immune system mistakenly destroys the healthy beta cells, leaving the person with no or too little insulin.

Insulin is a crucial hormone because it's involved in the metabolism of carbohydrates. It allows the glucose (sugar) from carbohydrates to fuel the cells in the body and brain. Without enough insulin, a person will die. That's why people with type 1 diabetes must take multiple daily injections of insulin, or deliver insulin through a catheter inserted under the skin that's attached to an insulin pump.

HOW THE VACCINE WAS DESIGNED

The vaccine was designed by changing a piece of immune-system DNA so that it would shut down the immune system's response to signals in the body that have previously triggered the mistaken destruction of beta cells. These signals come from fragments of a protein (peptides) called *proinsulin,* which is found on the surface of beta cells. Proinsulin is a precursor to insulin.

"We just wanted to throw the off switch for the one cell being attacked," Dr. Steinman explained.

STUDY DETAILS

The researchers recruited 80 volunteers diagnosed with type 1 diabetes during the past five years. They were randomly placed in one of five groups. Four groups received various doses of the vaccine, and the fifth group received placebo injections. Shots were given weekly for 12 weeks.

No one in the study was able to stop using insulin. "That's a possible goal, but it's too early to start saying cure," Dr. Steinman noted.

It's difficult to measure insulin levels, because they can vary rapidly and dramatically. Instead, researchers measured an increase of a substance called C-peptide, a part of proinsulin that stays in the body longer than insulin. C-peptide levels are used as measure of insulin production.

C-peptide levels improved at all doses of the vaccine compared with the placebo, according to the study. And, it's believed that higher levels of C-peptide may be related to a reduction in some of the serious complications associated with type 1 diabetes, such as eye disease, kidney problems and heart disease.

No serious adverse events occurred during the trial.

Dr. Steinman said it's too soon to know how the vaccine might work in the real world. It's not clear how often someone would need to be given the vaccine, and how well the body might recover its ability to produce insulin once the autoimmune attack has stopped. It's also not clear if the vaccine might be more effective in people who've recently developed the disease, or in people who have a high risk of developing type 1 diabetes.

Dr. Steinman said he hopes to have future trials under way soon.

The study appeared online in the journal *Science Translational Medicine.*

EXPERT RESPONSE

Richard Insel, MD, chief scientific officer at JDRF (formerly the Juvenile Diabetes Research Foundation), said, "The encouraging results from this initial trial…in established type 1 diabetes not only demonstrated safety, evidence during the vaccine dosing period showed preservation of beta cell function, a decrease in detectable immune cells [that likely attack the beta cells], and a relationship between the two."

He added that further clinical trials will be needed to figure out the optimal dose for vaccine efficacy and safety.

The study was funded by Bayhill Therapeutics, which helped to develop the vaccine. JDRF provided funding for the trial, as did the Iacocca Family Foundation.

info Learn more about type 1 diabetes from the U.S. National Library of Medicine website at *http://www.ncbi.nlm.nih.gov/pubmedhealth/PMH0001350/*.

People With Type 1 Diabetes May Still Have Insulin-Producing Cells

University of Exeter, news release.

Most people with type 1 diabetes still have active insulin-producing cells in their pancreas, a recent study shows.

The finding suggests it may be possible one day to preserve or replenish these cells.

Type 1 diabetes occurs when the body's immune system destroys insulin-producing beta cells, and it was believed that all these cells were lost within a few years of developing the disease.

But British researchers used new technology that enabled them to detect far lower levels of insulin than was previously possible. They tested 74 people with type 1 diabetes, and found that 73% of them had working beta cells that produced low levels of insulin, regardless of how long they'd had the disease.

The study was published in the journal *Diabetologia*.

"It's extremely interesting that low levels of insulin are produced in most people with type 1 diabetes, even if they've had it for 50 years," study leader Dr. Richard Oram, of the University of Exeter Medical School in the United Kingdom, said in a university news release. "The fact that insulin levels go up after a meal indicates these remaining beta cells can respond to a meal in the normal way—it seems they are either immune to attack or they are regenerating."

Dr. Matthew Hobbs, head of research for Diabetes UK, added: "We know that preserving or restoring even relatively small levels of insulin secretion in type 1 diabetes can prevent hypoglycemia [low glucose levels] and reduce complications, and therefore much research has focused on ways to make new cells that can be transplanted into the body."

"This research shows that some of a person's own beta cells remain, and therefore it may be possible to regenerate these cells in the future," Dr. Hobbs said. "It is also possible that understanding why some people keep insulin production while others lose it may help answer key questions about the biology of type 1 diabetes and help advance us toward a cure for the disease."

info The Nemours Foundation has more about type 1 diabetes at *Nemours.org*.

Bottom Line's
HEALTH
BREAKTHROUGHS 8

Diet, Fitness & Nutrition

Foods That Rev Up Your Metabolism and Help You Drop Those Extra Pounds for Good

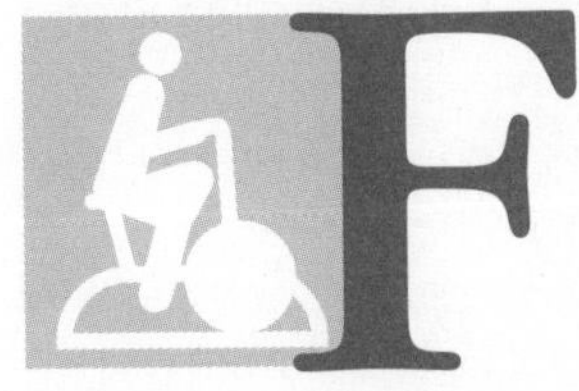

Forget about calories! Most people who are trying to lose weight worry too much about calories and not enough about the actual cause of those extra pounds.

The real culprit: Out-of-balance hormones.

Best approach for controlling weight: A diet that rebalances the body's hormones. Carefully chosen foods and food combinations rebalance levels and/or efficiency of metabolism-regulating hormones, such as ghrelin, leptin and thyroid hormone. You'll burn more calories, and your body will be less likely to store calories as fat. *Here's how...*

TWEAKING THE BEST DIETS

Hands down, the Mediterranean diet is one of the healthiest diets out there. With its emphasis on plant-based foods (such as vegetables, fruits, grains and nuts) and healthful fats (from fatty fish and olive oil), it is good for your heart and helps control blood sugar levels.

But for more efficient weight loss, you need to go a step further. That's where the Protein-Rich Oriental Diet, developed by Korean researchers, enters the picture. With its heavy focus on high-protein foods, this diet has been found to provide twice the weight loss offered by calorie restriction alone.

To achieve and maintain an optimal body weight: The diet I designed includes elements of both these diets—as well as some important additional tweaks such as timing your meals (see page 132) and consuming a mix of

Ridha Arem, MD, an endocrinologist, director of the Texas Thyroid Institute and clinical professor of medicine at Baylor College of Medicine, both in Houston. He is a former chief of endocrinology and metabolism at Houston's Ben Taub General Hospital and is author of *The Thyroid Solution Diet* (Atria). *AremWellness.com* proteins in order to get the full complement of amino acids, which is essential for increasing metabolism and controlling hunger. On my diet, you will eat a combination of at least two proteins, good fats and vegetables at each meal. *For example...*

•**Fish, turkey and chicken** contain all of the essential amino acids that are in red meat, but with fewer calories and less saturated fat. They're particularly rich in arginine, an amino acid that increases the speed at which your body burns calories.

My advice: Aim for six to eight ounces of these foods as the primary protein for dinner. You also can include these foods at breakfast and lunch as one of your protein choices.

•**Reduced-fat cottage cheese, ricotta, yogurt and goat cheese.** Certain forms of dairy are high in branched-chain amino acids, which suppress appetite and increase the ability of mitochondria (the energy-producing components of cells) to burn fat.

My advice: Each day, eat about a half-cup of low-fat or nonfat dairy as a protein.

•**High-protein beans,** lentils and grains, such as black beans, kidney beans, quinoa and brown rice. Eat one of these protein sources (three-fourths cup to one cup) at lunch—usually combined with a small serving of fish or lean meat. In addition to packing plenty of protein and fiber, these foods provide large amounts of amino acids that will help you get fitter and have more energy.

•**Egg whites** contain all of the amino acids that you need for efficient weight loss, and they are my favorite choice as a protein for breakfast. An egg-white omelet with onions, mushrooms and other vegetables can be prepared in just a few minutes. Limit your intake of egg yolks due to their cholesterol.

LOW-GLYCEMIC CARBS

Carbohydrates that are digested quickly—mainly refined and processed foods such as juices, white rice and French fries—increase insulin and fat storage. Carbohydrates with a lower glycemic score are absorbed more slowly and don't cause unhealthy changes in insulin or fat storage.

Good choices: Whole oats, chickpeas and fruit (see below) at breakfast and lunch, and vegetables at each meal.

MORE FIBER

The fiber in such foods as beans and vegetables reduces appetite and slows digestion, important for preventing insulin "spikes." Research shows that people of normal weight tend to eat significantly more fiber than those who are overweight or obese.

For efficient weight loss: Get 35 g of fiber daily.

Fruit is also a good source of fiber. Just be sure that you choose fresh fruit that's low in natural sugar (fructose).

Good choices: Raspberries, strawberries, papayas, apples and cranberries. Avoid fruit at dinner to make it the lowest glycemic meal.

GREEN TEA

Green tea is high in epigallocatechin gallate (EGCG), a substance that can decrease the accumulation of body fat. It also increases insulin sensitivity and improves an obesity-related condition known as metabolic syndrome. Drink a few cups every day. Do not sweeten the tea with honey or other sweeteners—they are among the main causes of high insulin and weight gain.

FISH OIL SUPPLEMENTS

The omega-3 fatty acids in fish increase the rate at which calories are burned. However, even if you eat fish every day, it doesn't contain enough omega-3s for long-term weight control.

Solution: Take a daily supplement with 600 mg of EPA and 400 mg of DHA—the main types of omega-3s. Check first with your doctor if you take blood thinners or diabetes medication, since fish oil may interact with these drugs.

NOT JUST FOR WEIGHT LOSS

A hormone-balancing eating plan can rev up your metabolism even if you don't need to lose weight, giving you more energy and mental focus. If you aren't overweight and you follow this eating plan, you may lose a pound or two, but mostly you'll just feel better.

The Easiest Diet Ever

Marla Heller, RD, a Los Angeles–based registered dietitian who developed plans to bring the DASH diet from the research phase to patients. She is author of *The DASH Diet Action Plan: Proven to Lower Blood Pressure and Cholesterol Without Medication, The DASH Diet Weight Loss Solution* and *The Everyday DASH Diet Cookbook* (all from Grand Central). *www.DashDiet.org*

Following a healthful diet is undoubtedly one of the best things we can do to protect ourselves from chronic disease. So why is it such a struggle?

Unfortunately, many diets just aren't practical over the long haul. Sure, you may be able to white-knuckle it for the first few days or weeks. But what happens when you can no longer withstand the unhealthful temptations at parties, restaurants and just about anywhere else? *The solution...*

A POWERHOUSE DIET

Many people are surprised to learn that one of the most widely studied diets is also perhaps the easiest to follow on a long-term basis because it provides enough food choices to be truly appealing—even enjoyable—to virtually anyone.

Perhaps you've heard of the DASH diet. It is commonly known as the "blood pressure diet." Short for Dietary Approaches to Stop Hypertension, the DASH plan has long been known to effectively lower blood pressure—sometimes in just 14 days, according to research.

Now: After years of scientific scrutiny, this "sleeper" of a diet, with its wide range of foods—vegetables, fruits, low-fat and nonfat dairy, whole grains, lean poultry and fish, and nuts, beans and seeds—is winning more proponents because of its other health benefits.

In addition to being linked to a lower risk for heart disease and stroke, this diet has also been shown to cut risk for kidney stones by 45% and risk for colon cancer by 20%. If that's not enough, the DASH diet also prevents (and sometimes even reverses) diabetes by controlling blood sugar spikes. And it makes you feel younger and lighter, because the low-sodium component helps you to retain less fluid.

The "Best" diet: Because of its many health benefits, nutritional completeness and the ease with which it can be followed, the DASH diet was named "Best Overall Diet" in 2013 by *US News & World Report*, based on analyses by experts in nutrition and various chronic diseases. The DASH eating plan beat other better-known diets, such as the Mediterranean Diet and Weight Watchers.

WHY DASH WORKS

The DASH diet might seem like nothing more than a commonsense eating plan, but very few Americans actually eat according to its basic principles. Not only are most of us sorely lacking in vegetables and fruits, but we take in an average of 3,500 mg of blood pressure–raising sodium per day—far more than the amount that's recommended for healthy adults (up to 2,300 mg daily) or the amount for people with high blood pressure (up to 1,500 mg).

The magic behind DASH lies in its high amounts of potassium, calcium and magnesium. Potassium, found in fruits and vegetables, naturally lowers blood pressure by ridding the body of excess sodium. Calcium from dairy and other sources, including broccoli and fish with bones, such as sardines, works in the same way—plus it relaxes your blood vessels, making it easier for blood to pass through. Magnesium, found in whole grains, nuts and seeds, also promotes healthy blood vessels.

Better Weight-Loss Strategy

If you're trying to lose weight, don't let others pressure you. In a recent study of 1,300 adults ages 20 to 31, more than 40% had used unhealthy diet tactics, including fasting and substituting smoking for eating. Nearly half said a significant other had encouraged them to lose weight. Binge eating was nearly twice as common in this group versus those who weren't pressured to lose weight.

Marla E. Eisenberg, ScD, MPH, associate professor of pediatrics, University of Minnesota Medical School, Minneapolis.

MAKING IT EASY

When first considering the DASH daily eating plan, you may think that you'd never be able to eat such a seemingly large amount and wide variety of food, but that's not true.

The standard 2,000-calorie plan includes…*

- **Fruits**—Four to five servings per day (one serving equals one medium-sized whole fruit or one cup diced raw fruit).
- **Vegetables**—Four to five servings per day (one serving equals one-half cup cooked vegetables or one cup leafy greens).
- **Low-fat/nonfat dairy**—Three daily servings (one serving equals one-half cup fat-free or low-fat cottage cheese or eight ounces skim or low-fat milk or low-fat or fat-free yogurt).
- **Whole grains**—Three daily servings (one serving equals one slice of bread, one-half cup cooked brown rice or one ounce dry cereal).
- **Refined grains**—A few servings a week (one serving equals one-half cup pasta or one cookie as a treat).
- **Healthy fats (such as olive oil and avocado)**—Two to three daily servings (one serving equals one teaspoon olive oil or one-eighth of a small avocado).
- **Lean meat, poultry or fish**—Seven ounces daily.
- **Beans and nuts**—Four to five servings per week (one serving equals one-quarter cup beans or nuts).

Why so much food and so many different choices? The diet delivers all the disease-fighting benefits that can be derived from good nutrition. Plus, the emphasis on low-calorie, high-volume produce and hunger-fighting protein means that you'll feel satisfied and less likely to give in to cravings for unhealthful foods that cause weight gain.

If five daily servings of veggies sounds daunting, think of it this way: A dinner including one cup sautéed broccoli (two servings)…a small side salad (one serving)…and one cup roasted potatoes (two servings) equals five full servings of veggies.

Other ways to meet DASH goals…

Fruits: Try one small banana at breakfast, one plum at lunch, one cup berries as a midafternoon snack, one-half cup sliced Bartlett pears for dessert.

Low-fat/nonfat dairy: Try an eight-ounce serving of nonfat milk on cereal (pour it on, then drink the rest), one ounce light Swiss cheese added to a sandwich for lunch, one cup light yogurt as an afternoon snack.

Whole grains: Try three-quarters cup whole-wheat cereal or oatmeal, two slices thin-sliced whole-wheat bread at lunch, one small whole-wheat dinner roll.

Healthy fats: Try one tablespoon salad dressing and a few avocado slices.

Lean meat, poultry or fish: Try three ounces of turkey slices at lunch and four ounces of salmon at dinner.

Beans and nuts: Try a small handful of nuts for a snack.

If you are eating out, try these DASH-friendly items…

- **A Grande Starbucks Caffé Latte with nonfat milk,** or any 16-ounce coffee drink with eight ounces milk.
- **A slice of thin-crust veggie pizza plus a salad.**
- **A Subway double-meat six-inch roasted chicken sandwich topped with all of your**

Timing Matters!

When you eat is almost as important as what you eat…

- **Plan on eating four or five daily meals**—breakfast between 6 am and 8 am…an optional (and light) late-morning snack…lunch between 11 am and 12:30 pm…a mid-afternoon snack…and supper between 5 pm and 7 pm.
- **Plan your meals so that you get more protein at supper.** It will stimulate the release of growth hormone, which burns fat while you sleep.
- **Avoid all food three hours before bedtime.** Eating late in the evening causes increases in blood sugar and insulin that can lead to weight gain—even if you consume a lower-calorie diet (1,200 to 1,500 calories a day).

*2,000 calories daily is appropriate for men age 51 and older. Women age 51 and older usually need 1,600 calories daily. Younger adults can have more calories. Weight loss requires less calories and fewer servings.

favorite veggies, minus the top half of the bread.

For a tasty DASH snack at home, try celery dipped in hummus.

info For a free copy of the complete DASH diet, go to *www.NHLBI.NIH.gov/health/public/heart/hbp/dash/new_dash.pdf.*

Food-Free Stress Relief

Susan Albers, PsyD, psychologist, Cleveland Clinic, Wooster, Ohio. Dr. Albers specializes in eating issues, weight loss, body image concerns and mindfulness, and is author of many books including *50 Ways to Soothe Yourself Without Food* (New Harbinger) and *Eat Q: Unlock the Weight-Loss Power of Emotional Intelligence* (HarperOne). *EatingMindfully.com*

Guess how much of the overeating people do is triggered by emotions—10%? 25%? Actually, it's about 75%, experts estimate. Considering how stressed out people today tend to feel, it's no wonder so many Americans are overweight!

Fortunately, there are many enjoyable and effective ways to calm down that have nothing to do with eating, said psychologist Susan Albers, PsyD, author of *50 Ways to Soothe Yourself Without Food.* So whenever you feel tempted to eat, first ask yourself whether you are truly physically hungry. If the honest answer is no, try one of these tactics instead.

Do-anywhere techniques for when you're out and about...

•**Adopt a "blanket substitute."** You know Linus from the comic strip Peanuts? He uses his beloved blanket as a source of comfort whenever he feels overwhelmed or anxious. Of course, you're not going to drag a blankie around, but you can carry a small object—a smooth stone, a silk handkerchief—in your pocket or purse. When you feel the urge to eat emotionally, close your eyes for a moment and rub your fingers across the object, finding comfort in its familiar feel.

•**Take a few cleansing breaths.** Inhale slowly and deeply through your nose...hold for a few seconds...then purse your lips and exhale through your mouth in short bursts as you imagine all your toxic thoughts or worries falling into a heap on the floor. This technique has been proven to calm the body and mind, Dr. Albers said.

•**Go for a stroll.** This is not a power walk, and it isn't about burning calories or trying to outpace your cravings. Rather, it's a deliberate opportunity to notice and enjoy the scenery... the people...the sounds...the scents all around you. *At-home tactics that can keep you from raiding the fridge...*

•**Clean house.** It doesn't matter what you clean—the garage, the attic, your office, a closet (though the kitchen would not be your best bet)—because your actual goal is to scrub away stress. Try cleaning for 10 minutes, then see whether the urge to nosh has abated, Dr. Albers suggested...if it hasn't, scrub for another three minutes.

Bonus: When you're done, your well-deserved sense of accomplishment will help keep comfort food cravings at bay.

•**Have a snooze.** Sleep-deprived people tend to eat more, probably in an attempt to increase energy levels. Ask yourself whether what your body really needs is a rejuvenating rest, and if the answer is yes, allow yourself a 30-minute nap. When you get up, chances are good that you'll no longer feel the immediate need to eat.

•**Take up a hobby that uses your hands.** Whittling, knitting, model building, painting and drawing are all good examples. Not only do they keep your hands busy so you can't reach for food, the hand movements themselves relieve tension...and your brain is pleasantly engaged, so you're not thinking about eating.

•**Weed your garden.** Sure, digging in the dirt is good exercise...but more importantly, gardening helps to ease your mind, especially

A Cool Way to Drop Pounds

Shivering stimulates the release of irisin, a hormone that increases metabolism and burns calories. It's the same hormone that's released by muscles during exercise.

Cell Metabolism

when you're stressed or angry. Dr. Albers suggested, "As you pull up each weed, imagine that you're pulling your negative or anxiety-provoking thoughts right out of your mind—and casting them away for good."

Food-Portion Descriptions Affect How Much We Eat

When a portion of spaghetti was labeled regular, people ate more of it than when the same portion was labeled double-size. Portion labels affect willingness to pay for restaurant meals, too—when a portion was labeled half-size, people were willing to pay only half as much for it as when the same portion was labeled regular.

Study by researchers at Dyson School of Applied Economics and Management, Cornell University, Ithaca, New York, published in *Health Economics*.

4 Dangerous Fitness Myths—How Not to Get Injured

Wayne L. Westcott, PhD, an instructor of exercise science at Quincy College in Massachusetts and a strength-training consultant for the American Council on Exercise, the American Senior Fitness Association and the National Youth Sports Safety Foundation. He is author, with Thomas R. Baechle, EdD, of *Strength Training Past 50* (Human Kinetics).

Don't believe everything you hear when you are trying to get in shape or stay in shape. There are plenty of myths and half-truths.

Among the most dangerous fitness myths to avoid…

***Fitness Myth #1:* A little pain means you're getting maximum benefit from your workout.** Despite the popular cliché "no pain, no gain," you should never feel prolonged, stabbing or sharp pain during a workout or continue to exercise when something hurts.

The risk: Pain means damage. It could be a warning sign that you have overstressed or overstretched a muscle, tendon or ligament. It also can indicate joint damage. People who continue to exercise when they hurt risk more serious injuries, such as torn muscles or tendinitis (inflammation of a tendon).

Exception: A little soreness after exercise means that you have had a good workout. When you exercise hard, the muscles develop microscopic tears that lead to rebuilding of tissue and an increase in strength. If you are very sore, however, you have overworked your muscles.

Warning: Don't believe the myth that you can exercise longer and harder if you take an anti-inflammatory pain reliever, such as *ibuprofen* (Motrin), before going to the gym. Taking a preworkout anti-inflammatory may reduce muscle performance and prevent you from feeling an injury while working out.

Important: If you have arthritis or another painful condition that requires daily treatment with aspirin, ibuprofen or another anti-inflammatory medication, ask your doctor if it's safe to take the drug prior to workouts. The combination of exercise and anti-inflammatories might increase the risk for damage to the gastrointestinal lining, according to recent research.

***Fitness Myth #2:* You should stretch before exercising.** Trainers used to advise everyone to stretch before lifting weights, going for a run, etc. Do not do it.

The risk: Tendons and ligaments take longer to warm up than muscles. People who stretch when they're "cold" are more likely to suffer from muscle and tendon strains and other injuries than those who begin their workouts with a progressive warm-up. Static stretches, in which you stretch a muscle to a point of tension and hold the stretch for a certain period of time, can be particularly harmful before a workout.

Recent finding: Recent research also has shown that people who do static stretches before working out can't exercise as long and may have reduced muscle strength.

Exception: You can start a workout with dynamic stretches, slow movements that mimic the exercise patterns you're about to do. Before taking a run, for example, you could do some fast walking and slow jogging. This type of stretching is safe and prepares the muscles for exercise.

Also: Stretch *after* vigorous activity. That's when muscles and tendons have the best blood flow and elasticity, and you're less likely to get injured. *Good postworkout stretches...*

• **Figure Four.** Sit on the floor with both legs out in front of you. Bend your left leg, placing the sole of your left foot against your right inner thigh. With your right hand, reach for your right ankle and hold for 30 seconds. Perform twice on each side to stretch your hamstrings and calves.

• **Letter T.** Lie faceup on the floor with your arms in a T-position. Slowly cross your left leg over your body, allowing your torso to rotate so that your left foot is near your right hand. Keep your leg as straight as possible. Hold for 20 seconds. Perform twice on each side to stretch your hips and lower back.

***Fitness Myth #3:* Do not rest during workouts.** You have probably heard that the best strength-training workouts involve nonstop action, with no rest (or very little rest) between exercises.

The risk: Failing to rest will cause muscle fatigue and poor form, a common cause of injuries. Also, you won't fully train the muscles because they need time to recover.

When you're working the same muscles, you need to rest 30 to 90 seconds between sets.

Example: Do eight to 12 biceps curls...take a 30- to 90-second break...then curl the weight again.

Exception: With circuit training, you move quickly from one exercise to the next. You might do a biceps exercise, then a leg exercise, then return to the biceps. Even though you're constantly moving (and getting a good cardiovascular workout), you're allowing one group of muscles to rest while you work a different part of the body.

***Fitness Myth #4:* High-heat exercise works the muscles more.** Some people believe that high-temperature workouts—including "hot" yoga, spinning and others in which the room temperature may be 90°F or even hotter—make the muscles more limber and improve the body's ability to remove toxins.

I do not recommend it. For the average person, exercising in high temperatures will reduce their performance because the body has to work harder to fend off the heat.

The risk: It forces the heart to do double-duty—not only to bring oxygen to the muscles and remove wastes that accumulate during exercise, but also to pump more blood to the skin to dissipate the extra heat. If you're tempted to try high-heat workouts, ask your doctor first.

A Better Move to Avoid Lower-Back Pain

"Core"-strengthening exercises help prevent low-back pain by strengthening abdominal and back muscles. However, one of the most popular of these workouts, which involves lying on your back and simultaneously raising both legs in the air, causes a pronounced arch in the low back that can trigger—or worsen—low-back pain.

Better: Bicycle maneuver. Lie with your lower back pressed against the floor, your hands clasped behind your head and your knees bent. Simultaneously lift your head and shoulders off the floor. Bring your left knee to your right elbow, while straightening your right leg. Using a bicycle-pedaling motion, alternate sides. Extend your legs as far as you comfortably can without arching your back.

Typical number of reps: 10 to 15 times on each leg with slow and controlled movements.

Rx: Take a Walk and Call Me in the Morning

Jordan D. Metzl, MD, a sports medicine physician at the Hospital for Special Surgery in New York City. The author of *The Exercise Cure: A Doctor's All-Natural, No-Pill Prescription for Better Health & Longer Life* (Rodale), Dr. Metzl maintains practices in New York City and Greenwich, Connecticut, and is a medical columnist for *Triathlete Magazine*. He has run in 31 marathons and finished 11 Ironman competitions.

A recent study made international headlines when it found that exercise was just as effective as—or sometimes even outperformed—drugs when treating such conditions as heart disease and stroke.

The details: After examining about 300 medical trials involving more than 330,000 patients, Harvard researchers found that frequent exercise and powerful drugs, such as beta-blockers and blood thinners, provided very similar results. And in the case of stroke recovery, regular workouts were actually more effective than taking anticoagulant medications.

A troubling fact: Only one-third of clinicians "prescribe" exercise, which could not only boost the health of Americans significantly but also save the average patient thousands of dollars a year in medical costs.

My recommendations for condition-specific routines that contribute to a healthy, disease-free future...*

HEART ATTACK AND STROKE

Drugs such as beta-blockers help treat heart disease, but side effects can include fatigue, dizziness, upset stomach and cold hands. Meanwhile, a single 40-minute session of aerobic exercise has been shown to lower blood pressure for 24 hours in hypertensive patients, and regular workouts can reduce both systolic (top number) and diastolic (bottom number) blood pressure by five to 10 points. Consistent exercise also can improve cholesterol levels.

Why exercise works: The heart is a muscle, and cardiovascular exercise forces it to pump longer and eventually makes it stronger, preventing the buildup of plaques that can rupture and lead to a heart attack or stroke. Many heart attack and stroke survivors are afraid to exercise, but it's crucial that they move past this fear. Those who exercise require less medication...need fewer major surgeries such as bypasses...and are 25% less likely to die from a second heart attack than their couch potato counterparts.

What to do: Five times a week, do 30 to 40 minutes of cardiovascular exercise at a "Zone 2" level of exertion (see page 137). You have lots of choices for this exercise. Options include very fast walking, jogging, swimming, using an elliptical machine or recumbent bike, or taking an aerobics class. Pick an activity you enjoy to help you stay committed. After just six weeks, you'll likely have lower blood pressure, and by three months, your cholesterol levels should be improved.

Note: People with heart failure, a condition in which the heart cannot pump enough blood to the rest of the body, should avoid resistance exercises, such as push-ups and heavy weight lifting, that force muscles to work against an immovable or very heavy object. Such activities can put an excessive burden on the heart and cause further injury to it.

DEPRESSION

Exercise really is nature's antidepressant. Several studies have shown that working out is just as effective, if not more so, than medication when it comes to treating mild-to-moderate depression. Exercise also can help reduce the amount of medication needed to treat severe cases of depression...and even prevent depression in some people.

A Norwegian study that tracked about 39,000 people for two years found that those who reported doing moderate-to-high physical activity, including daily brisk walks for more than 30 minutes, scored significantly lower on depression and anxiety tests compared with nonexercisers.

There are many effective antidepressant drugs, but they are frequently accompanied by bothersome side effects, including sexual dysfunction, nausea, fatigue and weight gain. And while most of these drugs can take a month to work, a single exercise session can trigger an immediate lift in mood, and consistent aerobic exercise will make an even more lasting positive impact.

What to do: The key is to boost your heart rate high enough to trigger the release of endorphins, feel-good chemicals that elicit a state of relaxed calm. Spend 30 to 45 minutes at a "Zone 3" level of exertion (see page 137), three to five days a week, to benefit.

You also may want to try exercising outdoors. A study published in *Environmental Science & Technology* found that outdoor exercise produces stronger feelings of revitalization, a bigger boost

*Be sure to check with your doctor before starting any fitness program. If your condition is severe, he/she may initially want you to use exercise as an adjunct to medication, not as a replacement. Never stop taking a prescribed drug without talking to your doctor. *Caution:* With any of these workouts, seek immediate medical attention if you experience chest pain, shortness of breath, nausea, blurred vision or significant bone or muscle pain while exercising.

Think of Lunch to Eat Less at Dinner

Did you know that thinking about what you had for lunch will help you eat 10% less at dinner? When we focus on what we ate earlier—and the amount of calories we consumed—we make a deliberate effort to eat less at the next meal.

Study by researchers at University of Birmingham, England, reported in *Real Simple*.

of energy and a greater reduction in depression and anger than exercising indoors.

Strength training also is effective in treating depression—lifting weights releases endorphins and builds a sense of empowerment. For a strength-training program, ask your doctor to recommend a physical therapist or personal trainer.

If it's difficult to motivate yourself to exercise when you're depressed, relying on a personal trainer—or a "workout buddy"—can help.

BACK PAIN

Back pain strikes roughly half of Americans. Pain medications are available, but many are addictive and merely mask the symptoms rather than address the underlying problem. Muscle relaxants cause drowsiness...overuse of nonsteroidal anti-inflammatory drugs (NSAIDs), such as *ibuprofen*, can lead to ulcers...and steroid injections, which can be given only a few times per year, can cause infection or nerve damage and long-term side effects such as osteoporosis or high blood pressure.

What to do: There's a very powerful low-tech solution—a foam roller. Widely available at sporting goods stores, these cylindrical rollers have a record of preventing and relieving back pain. With the cylinder on the floor, move various muscles (your hamstrings, quadriceps and lower back) back and forth over the foam roller slowly. Roll each area for one to two minutes. If you hit an especially tender spot, pause and roll slowly or hover in place until you feel a release. The entire routine should take about 10 minutes.

Note: Rolling muscles can feel uncomfortable and even painful at first. But the more painful it is, the more that muscle needs to be rolled. Frequency eases discomfort.

In addition to rolling your muscles, start a back- and core-strengthening program. Avoid using heavy weights, especially within an hour of waking—that's when your muscles are tighter and you're more likely to strain a muscle.

Instead, opt for higher repetitions (three sets of 15) with lighter weights (three to five pounds for women and eight to 10 pounds for men) to build endurance in your back and core, which is more protective than sheer strength.

A good core-strengthening exercise: The plank. In a push-up position, bend your elbows and rest your weight on your forearms (your body should form a straight line from shoulders to ankles). Pull your navel into your spine, and contract your abdominal muscles for 30 seconds, building up to a minute or two at a time. Perform the plank once a day.

THE 3 EXERCISE EXERTION ZONES

There are three main levels of exertion that are based on how easy it is for you to talk...

Zone 1: Talking is easy while moving. An example of Zone 1 exertion might be a moderate-paced walk.

Zone 2: Talking is tough but manageable. In Zone 2, there should be a little huffing and puffing but no gasping for air.

Zone 3: Carrying on a conversation is quite difficult at this level of exertion due to panting.

7 Mistakes That Can Sabotage Your Walking Workout

Robert Sweetgall, president of Creative Walking, a Kirkwood, Missouri, company that designs walking and fitness programs for schools, corporations and other clients. He is the only person to have walked through all 50 states in 365 days. He is coauthor, with Barry Franklin, PhD, of *One Heart, Two Feet: Enhancing Heart Health One Step at a Time* (Creative Walking, Inc.). *www.creativewalking.com*

We all know that walking is very good for us. But what most people don't realize is just how powerful this simple exercise is. Studies have shown that walking promotes heart health, strengthens bones, spurs weight loss, boosts mood and even cuts risk for cancer and Alzheimer's.

Latest development: In recent studies involving patients with peripheral artery disease (PAD), plaque buildup in the arteries that can contribute to heart attack or stroke, walking improved their painful symptoms as much as medication and, in some cases, even more than bypass surgery or balloon angioplasty to treat the affected artery.

What's more, even a small amount of walking goes a long way toward improving health. Recent research has found that walking just a half-mile a day helps prevent diabetes, and another study has shown that walking for just two hours a week reduces breast cancer risk by 18%.

While many people take walking for granted, the majority of walkers could significantly improve the health benefits by tweaking their walking techniques and using the right equipment.

Common walking mistakes—and what to do instead…

Mistake #1: **Tilting forward.** Some walkers tilt their upper bodies forward, as though they're walking into the wind. They think that this position increases speed. It does not—and it greatly increases pressure on the lower back while straining the shins.

Better: Walk with your head high and still, shoulders relaxed and chest slightly out. In this position, you can rotate your eyes downward to survey the path and look ahead to view the scenery around you.

Mistake #2: **Swinging the arms inefficiently.** Many walkers waste energy by swinging their arms side to side or pumping their arms up and down. These exaggerated movements add little to cardiovascular fitness and make walking less efficient because arm energy is directed upward or sideways rather than straight ahead.

Better: For maximum efficiency, pump your arms straight ahead on a horizontal plane, like you're reeling in a string through your midsection. This motion improves balance, posture and walking speed.

Mistake #3: **Using hand and/or ankle weights.** While some people like to walk with weights to boost the intensity of a walking workout, the risk for injury far outweighs the benefits of using weights. The repetitive stress of swinging weights can cause microtears in the soft tissues of the arms and legs.

Better: To increase exertion, walk uphill or on an inclined treadmill.

Another good option: Try Nordic walking for a total-body workout. With this type of walking, you use specially designed walking poles (one in each hand) to help propel your body forward.

Compared with regular walking, Nordic walking can increase your energy expenditure by 20%, according to a study from The Cooper Institute. It works the abdominal, arm and back muscles and reduces stress on the feet, ankles, knees and hips while improving endurance.

Mistake #4: **Not doing a warm-up.** You're inviting muscle soreness and potential injury if you hit your top speed at the start.

Better: Be sure to warm up. Start slowly, accelerating over the first five to 10 minutes…and end slowly, decelerating over the last five minutes. A slow start allows your muscles to warm up and become flexible, while enabling your cardiorespiratory system to get used to higher workloads. A proper cooldown helps eliminate the buildup of lactic acid, which can lead to muscle soreness.

Mistake #5: **Doing the same walk every day.** It's best to alter your routine for maximum health benefits and to maintain motivation.

Better: Do shorter, faster-paced walks some days (cardiovascular conditioning) and longer, moderate-paced walks on other days (calorie burning). Also try walks on steeper terrains and walks that alternate faster intervals with slower intervals.

Oreos Are as Addictive as Cocaine

Cookie addiction is real! If you have trouble putting down the Oreos, take heart. In a recent study, lab animals that ate cookies had brain activity similar to that which ordinarily occurs with drug use.

Connecticut College. *ConnColl.edu*

***Mistake #6:* Not keeping a walking log or journal.** Every day, indicate how far and fast you walked and any other observations you wish to record in a notebook or on your computer. Keeping a journal helps foster a sense of accomplishment and self-esteem and is the single most effective method for ensuring that you'll stick to a walking program.

***Mistake #7:* Choosing cushy shoes.** A study in *The American Journal of Sports Medicine* found that, on average, expensive, high-tech footwear caused twice the injuries as shoes costing half as much.

Some high-priced, cushiony shoes can make you feel as if you're walking on a foam mattress, but they have an inherent "wobble" that can cause your foot to move side to side, leading to potential foot, ankle, knee and hip injuries.

Better: Thin-soled shoes with minimal support. They force the muscles in the legs and feet to work harder, which improves strength and balance and helps prevent injuries.

When transitioning to thinner-soled shoes, make the switch gradually, breaking them in on shorter walks. They can feel awkward at first, so give your feet time to adjust.

Of course the right shoe is a very individual choice, but I like Karhu shoes, which promote forward momentum.

Cost: About $55 to $140, depending on the model. Other people like the so-called "barefoot" shoes, such as Vibram FiveFingers.

Helpful: Avoid cotton socks, which can lose their support and shape after a few washings. Try socks made from blends that include acrylic fibers, Coolmax and/or spandex/elastic. Soft wool socks also can work.

Tip: Powder your feet with cornstarch before a long walk to reduce friction, heat buildup and blisters.

TAKE THE LONGEVITY TEST

The more steps it takes you to walk the same distance each year, the weaker your core muscles are becoming.

Self-test: Each year on your birthday, go to a track and walk one lap, recording the number of steps on your pedometer. Aim to complete the lap in about the same number of steps each year. If it takes you more steps each year, you are regressing toward the "senior shuffle" and compromising your core-muscle strength and overall vitality.

What to do: In addition to walking regularly, start a core-muscle strengthening regimen and a stretching program to tone your hip and leg muscles.

Jump Training...Pros and Cons

Wayne L. Westcott, PhD, professor of exercise science at Quincy College in Massachusetts.

"Plyometric" exercise, also known as jump training or plyo involves rapidly stretching a muscle and then contracting it. It's often done in athletic-conditioning programs, for example, by jumping off a box and immediately jumping back up. Plyo exercise has been shown to significantly increase muscle speed and power.

The risk: In some plyo workouts, participants are instructed to hold dumbbells or wear weighted vests to increase the difficulty of the workout. This can increase the risk for joint or muscle damage. A highly trained athlete can do weighted plyo exercise—the average person shouldn't attempt it.

Tai Chi Gives You More of a Workout Than You Think—And Benefits You'd Never Imagine

Peter M. Wayne, PhD, an assistant professor of medicine at Harvard Medical School and research director of the Osher Center for Integrative Medicine, jointly based at Harvard Medical School and Brigham and Women's Hospital, both in Boston. He has trained in tai chi for more than 35 years and is author, with Mark L. Fuerst, of *The Harvard Medical School Guide to Tai Chi* (Shambhala).

Perhaps you've seen people performing the graceful, seemingly slow-motion movements of tai chi in a nearby park. If you've never tried it before, you may think that this form of exercise is easy to do and provides little more than a mild workout.

The truth: Even though tai chi consists of slow, gentle movements, this exercise is no pushover. Long known for its stress-reducing benefits, it also gives you an aerobic workout that's as intense as walking at a moderate pace...increases muscle strength and flexibility...improves breathing...improves posture and balance (to help prevent falls)...and focuses the mind.

What's new: Tai chi, which was developed centuries ago in China as a means of self-defense, is now linked to a number of new health benefits, including improved cardiovascular health and bone density...and reduced back and neck pain.

Even better: Tai chi is safer than many forms of exercise because of its 70% rule: You never move your joints or exert yourself beyond 70% of your maximum potential.

Recently discovered benefits...

BETTER BREATHING

Many Eastern-based practices, including yoga, meditation and tai chi, emphasize diaphragmatic breathing, in which the muscles of the diaphragm (rather than the chest) are used to take in more oxygen. This style of breathing not only helps the lungs to move with less effort but also allows more oxygen to pass into the bloodstream.

Efficient breathing is more important than you might think. Multiple studies indicate that healthy breathing—as measured by "forced expiratory volume," the amount of air that you can exhale in one second—may help you live longer.

LOWER BLOOD PRESSURE

The stress relief that can come from tai chi, along with improved breathing and other factors, make it an ideal exercise for lowering blood pressure. In fact, research suggests that tai chi is at least as effective for lowering blood pressure as lifestyle changes that are usually recommended, such as losing weight and cutting back on sodium.

A Johns Hopkins study found that light-intensity tai chi improved blood pressure almost as much as moderate-intensity aerobic exercise.

PERIPHERAL NEUROPATHY

Millions of people with diabetes and other conditions have peripheral neuropathy, nerve damage in the hands and/or feet that causes numbness, tingling or pain. The condition is particularly troublesome because reduced sensations in the feet can impair balance and increase the risk of falling.

Research has found that people with peripheral neuropathy who practiced tai chi had improved sensitivity in the soles of the feet. They also had better balance and walking speed.

STRONGER BONES

You don't need to lift weights to increase bone strength and reduce risk for osteoporosis. Researchers in Hong Kong found that women who did tai chi three times per week had increased bone density within 12 months.

IT'S EASY TO GET STARTED

Tai chi classes are commonly offered at health clubs, YMCAs and even some hospitals. Classes are particularly useful because of the feedback given by the instructor and the group support, which helps keep you motivated.

Good goal: Two one-hour tai chi classes a week—plus at-home practice for at least 30 minutes, three times a week.

One Minute at a Time!

Don't have 10- or 30-minute blocks of time for exercise? Researchers may have found just the answer you are looking for. According to a recent study of more than 4,500 adults, short, intense bouts of moderate-to-vigorous exercise such as stair-climbing or brisk walking every day are sufficient to lose or maintain weight.

What to do: If you're short on time, do high-intensity exercise one minute at a time throughout the day.

Jessie X. Fan, PhD, professor of family and consumer studies, The University of Utah, Salt Lake City.

You can find a tai chi expert in your area at *www.AmericanTaiChi.net.*

A TASTE OF TAI CHI

Tai chi consists of dozens of different moves. *Here's one called "Tai Chi Pouring"...*

What to do: Stand with your feet shoulder-width apart. Slightly bend one knee and allow your weight to shift to that side. Briefly pause, and then gently bend your other knee and shift your weight in that direction. Pause again. "Pour" your weight back and forth for a few minutes while breathing deeply and feeling a relaxed flow connecting your whole body.

Supercharge Your Diet!—How to Get a Lot More Nutrients from Your Foods...

Susan Levin, MS, RD, director of nutrition education for the Physicians Committee for Responsible Medicine, a Washington, DC–based nonprofit group that is dedicated to promoting preventive medicine, better nutrition and higher standards in research. *PCRM.org*

If you eat a cup of yogurt and the label says it has 300 mg of calcium, don't assume that's how much of the mineral your body will absorb. You'll actually get just under 100 mg of calcium, on average, from the yogurt.

This kind of disconnect between what foods contain and what they give you comes as a surprise to many people—even those who pride themselves on eating wholesome, fresh foods that are known to be packed with nutrients.

Why it matters: The bioavailability (the amount of nutrients your body actually absorbs) of foods can vary widely depending on which foods you eat and how they are prepared—and even how they're combined with other foods. Absorption of nutrients also can be affected by some health conditions, such as autoimmune diseases and digestive problems, and by certain medications, such as antacids and some antibiotics. *To get more of these nutrients from the foods you eat...*

CALCIUM

You need calcium for healthy blood pressure and to keep your muscles moving and your bones strong. Yet many Americans don't get enough.

Dairy products, such as milk, yogurt and cheese, are widely considered to be our primary sources of calcium. But the truth is, only about 30% of the calcium in most dairy products is absorbed by your body.

To get more calcium: Eat more greens. Some varieties have nearly double the calcium bioavailability of dairy foods.

Examples: You will absorb about 61% of the calcium in broccoli...59% of the calcium in kale...and 54% of the calcium in bok choy. Even though these greens do not contain as much total calcium as dairy products, when you factor in the higher bioavailability of these plant foods, you'll see that they can be excellent sources of the mineral.

Just make sure you get the right greens if you're trying to maximize your calcium absorption. The calcium is poorly absorbed from some greens, such as spinach and Swiss chard, that contain oxalic acid or phytic acid. These chemical compounds bind to calcium and other minerals, reducing their absorption by the body. Spinach and Swiss chard are, however, good sources of iron and folate.

Stop Exercise Heartburn

Prevent heartburn after a workout by avoiding fatty and greasy foods before working out...and waiting a few hours after eating to exercise.

Also: Sip water slowly during and after your workout to avoid filling your stomach with water and air.

If you still get heartburn: Try taking an over-the-counter medicine, such as Pepcid, Zantac or Prilosec, 30 minutes before your workout...or talk to your doctor.

William D. Chey, MD, professor of internal medicine, University of Michigan, Ann Arbor, quoted in *Shape*.

Instant Coffee Has the Same Health Benefits As Brewed

In fact, studies have found that the way instant coffee is produced causes it to contain a higher concentration of healthful antioxidants, such as phenols and flavonoids. Instant coffee also has about the same levels of chlorogenic acid, which may have cardiovascular benefits.

BerkeleyWellness.com

ALLICIN

Allicin, one of the chemical compounds that gives onions and garlic such a powerful smell, has been linked to lower cholesterol, better blood pressure and a reduced risk for heart disease and some cancers.

To get more allicin: Mince fresh garlic and onions. Mincing (rather than slicing or coarse chopping) releases more of an enzyme that interacts with a different compound in onions and garlic to trigger the formation of allicin.

Also helpful: After mincing, leave the onions or garlic on the cutting board for about 10 minutes. This short time-out allows the allicin-producing process to continue.

CAROTENOIDS

Carotenoids are the substances that give tomatoes, carrots and other brightly colored produce their brilliant hues. The most studied carotenoids, such as lycopene and beta-carotene, have been linked to lower rates of cancer, heart disease and eye diseases such as cataracts. Raw produce is rich in carotenoids, but you'll generally absorb even more when the produce is cooked—the heat helps break down the cell walls so that the nutrient can be released.

To get more carotenoids: Instead of eating raw tomatoes, simmer them in a sauce. Also, cook carrots to allow more lycopene to be released. Spinach and kale release more beta-carotene when cooked.

Helpful: Buy processed tomatoes—they actually have more lycopene than fresh. But use tomato paste and tomato sauce in glass jars rather than canned varieties, which can expose you to bisphenol A (BPA), an industrial chemical that's in many metal cans and plastic bottles. It has been linked to cancer, heart disease, diabetes and other health problems.

GLUCOSINOLATES

While cooking tomatoes and carrots coaxes optimal absorption, it's best to eat cruciferous vegetables, such as broccoli and cabbage, raw to get their cancer-fighting benefits. Cruciferous vegetables contain compounds called glucosinolates that help protect against cancer. Boiling these veggies for nine to 15 minutes results in a 20% to 60% decrease in glucosinolates, which are leached into the water. And steaming or microwaving cruciferous vegetables on high may deactivate myrosinase, an enzyme that breaks down glucosinolates into compounds that may eliminate carcinogens.

To get more glucosinolates: Eat cruciferous veggies raw or microwave on low power.

FAT-SOLUBLE NUTRIENTS

All of the fat-soluble nutrients and antioxidants—such as vitamin E, beta-carotene and lycopene—require a little bit of fat in order to be absorbed by the body. The average meal contains plenty of fat to get the job done.

But if you're eating, say, a simple salad and want to ensure that you absorb the most nutrients, a small amount of added fat will help.

Recommended: Have no more than 10% of calories from saturated fat a day.

To get more fat-soluble nutrients: Toss some healthful fat-containing foods into your salad—good choices include cooked grains (such as quinoa), slivered nuts and/or a few olives. You'll also be adding exciting flavors!

The Best "New" Superfoods...These Fermented Foods Are Great Sources of Healthful Probiotics

Delia Quigley, a nutrition educator, natural-foods and macrobiotic chef, and founder of the StillPoint Schoolhouse, a holistic nutritional center based in Blairstown, New Jersey. She is coauthor of six books, including *The Everything Superfoods Book* and *Super Charge with Super Foods* (both from Adams Media). *DeliaQuigley.com*

Ask an American to name a good food source of healthful probiotics, and yogurt, that mainstay of the dairy aisle, is likely to top the list. Lesser-known sources of probiotics include pickles, red wine, dark chocolate and some cheeses.

But in many countries, from Japan to India to Poland, people enjoy a much wider variety of delicious probiotic-packed foods—and you can enjoy them here in the US, too.

Until recently, probiotics were known mostly for their ability to help with digestion—which they are very good at doing.

Now: Researchers are discovering that probiotics also can boost the immune system, reduce allergy symptoms and even improve one's mood. Several probiotic superfoods also rid the body of yeast overgrowth—a powerful one-two punch when it comes to good health.

Here are the best probiotic foods you're probably not eating...*

KIMCHI

A staple in the Korean diet, this fermented side dish consists of vegetables and an assortment of seasonings. A traditional kimchi dish includes Chinese cabbage, red chili pepper flakes, ginger, garlic and green onions. Other vegetables used to make kimchi include white or red radishes, leeks and carrots.

Upon opening a jar of kimchi, you'll see bubbles rise to the surface, a sure sign that this superfood contains lots of good bacteria such as Lactobacillus, Leuconostoc and Weisella. Kimchi is also a good source of vitamins B-1, B-2 and C, niacin, fiber and beta-carotene.

How to use it: Try kimchi on top of a burger...mix it with fried rice...or add it to eggs to give your breakfast an extra kick. Just one-half cup a day will go a long way toward soothing your intestines.

Where to find it: Look for kimchi in the refrigerated section of Asian food stores, in the dairy section of natural-food stores, such as Whole Foods Markets and Trader Joe's, or at Rejuvenative.com, which offers different varieties of kimchi.

DARK MISO

Miso, a paste made from soybeans, salt, grains and a fungus called koji, has been enjoyed in China and Japan for more than 2,500 years. In the US, it's commonly served as the main ingredient in miso soup. The darker the hue of miso, the longer the fermentation process, which means that it's chock-full of good bacteria. Dark varieties, such as barley miso or brown rice miso, taste earthier and saltier than the lighter ones commonly used in miso soup.

Dark miso is a good source of protein, vitamins A and K, minerals like calcium and potassium and Lactobacillus probiotic cultures.

How to use it: You can thin out dark miso with cooking water and then use this as a sauté sauce for vegetables or add dark miso to stews and soups. Use sparingly, as it's powerful stuff and contains a lot of sodium.

Where to find it: Miso is typically sold as a thick paste in small, plastic containers or glass jars. It's carried in major natural-food stores, typically in the dairy section—but these days, you can find it in many supermarkets, too. Good brands include South River Miso Company (SouthRiverMiso.com) and the American Miso Company (Great-Eastern-Sun.com).

COCONUT WATER KEFIR

Kefir is a silky-smooth, probiotic-rich drink popular in northern and eastern Europe. It's made by adding kefir grains to cow, goat or sheep milk. An excellent nondairy version is derived from coconut water—the juice of the

*Fermented foods should be refrigerated to preserve probiotic properties.

young, or green, coconut. Coconut water kefir is packed with several kinds of Lactococcus cultures, along with magnesium, potassium, calcium and B vitamins.

How to use it: Use kefir instead of milk in smoothies and dressings or enjoy it right out of the bottle (it has a mild, sweet taste and will not add the strong taste of coconut).

Where to find it: Kefir is available in most supermarkets and, of course, at most natural-food stores. Coconut water kefir is available at natural-food stores and MyTonix.com.

SAUERKRAUT

You probably know that a mound of sauerkraut on a hot dog gives you a nice helping of probiotics. In fact, cabbage, the key ingredient in sauerkraut, is one of the best probiotic-producing foods, as it stands up well to days of fermentation.

Classic sauerkraut is made from three ingredients—cabbage, salt and vinegar. But it contains lots of good stuff, including vitamin C, vitamin K, potassium, fiber, folate, iron and the Leuconostoc, Pediococcus and Lactobacillus strains of probiotics.

How to use it: You may not have much experience using sauerkraut creatively. But in fact, it goes great with lots of meats besides hot dogs, including corned beef and pot roast, and in stews and soups, such as potato leek soup.

For a tangy guacamole dip: Chop sauerkraut and mix with avocados, garlic and a dash of lemon juice.

Where to find it: Buy sauerkraut labeled "raw" and "unpasteurized."

Good choices: Deep Root Organic, available at Whole Foods, and Ultimate Kraut at Rejuvenative.com.

GET YOUR PROBIOTIC KICK

When cooking with probiotic foods, add them at the very end of the heating process—for example, just a minute before you serve stew—to preserve the live cultures. Also, be sure to choose brands that are unpasteurized for the same reason.

And remember: Kimchi and sauerkraut are easy and economical to prepare at home. For recipes, go to AllRecipes.com or EdenFoods.com.

THE VINEGAR TRICK

So, if a probiotic is a healthful type of bacteria that stays viable in the gut after eating, what is a prebiotic? A prebiotic acts as food for a probiotic. In other words, it's the fuel in your body that probiotics need to thrive.

An excellent example of a prebiotic is raw, organic, unrefined apple cider vinegar, which contains strandlike chains of protein enzyme molecules rich in nutrients. Apple cider vinegar—be sure it's the unrefined kind!—is nirvana for probiotics. Sprinkle it on vegetables or use in salad dressings to help your good bacteria help you!

This Snack Food Helps You Live Longer

David Grotto, RD, founder and president of Nutrition Housecall, LLC, a Chicago-based consulting firm that provides nutrition communications, lecturing and consulting services along with personalized, at-home dietary services. He is author of *The Best Things You Can Eat* (Da Capo Lifelong). *DavidGrotto.com*

Want a simple way to live longer? Eating nuts may be the answer.

A recent study published in *The New England Journal of Medicine* followed 119,000 men and women for 30 years. The researchers found that those who ate walnuts, peanuts, almonds and/or other nuts seven or more times a week were 20% less likely to die from any cause during the study period than those who didn't eat nuts.

Overall, nut eaters tend to be slimmer and have better cholesterol levels, less arterial inflammation and better blood sugar levels than people who don't eat nuts.

Here, the health benefits of specific nuts. Aim to consume one ounce of nuts a day, choosing a variety of kinds.

Raw, Roasted, Shelled or Spread?

Are salted, roasted nuts bad for you? Not really. Assuming that you limit yourself to one ounce of nuts a day, you will get only 110 milligrams (mg) of extra sodium by eating salted varieties. The extra oil that comes with oil-roasted nuts is not an issue—that adds up to only about one gram per serving.

Those supersweet nut spreads are another story.

Example: Nutella, a popular brand using hazelnuts, is high in saturated fat and loaded with sugar—5.5 teaspoons of sugar in two tablespoons. It is more like frosting than like a true nut butter.

Also, the "crunch" from whole nuts seems to trigger satiety, the feeling of fullness that causes you to stop eating. This doesn't occur when you eat nut butters—even the crunchy kind—so to control calories, go easy on nut butters.

Although nuts are good for you, they are highly caloric. So if you must watch your weight, buy nuts in the shell and, as you eat them, pile up the shells where you can see them. According to a recent study, people who ate shelled pistachios consumed 211 calories at a sitting but those who removed the nut from the shell ate only 86 calories.

ALMONDS

If you are one of the millions of Americans who takes medication to reduce cholesterol, you might want to add almonds to the mix.

One three-month study tested 27 men and women with high cholesterol. People who ate about a handful of almonds a day lowered their "bad" LDL cholesterol by an average of 4.4%. Those who ate two handfuls lowered it by 9.4%.

BRAZIL NUTS

These are higher in selenium than just about any other food. Selenium is an antioxidant that reduces cholesterol and decreases the risk for blood clots and heart attacks.

Important for men: The body needs selenium to produce testosterone, the hormone that helps maintain a man's bone density, muscle strength and sex drive.

Brazil nuts are higher in fat than many other nuts, but they aren't the "fat bombs" most people imagine. When you eat Brazil nuts, filberts or other hard nuts, the cell walls aren't completely broken down during digestion. You will absorb less fat than you would with softer nuts, such as macadamias (see below).

CASHEWS

Despite their velvety texture, cashews are one of the lowest fat nuts at 13 grams (g) of fat per ounce—with the majority of fats, including phytosterols and tocopherols, being good for the heart. Cashews also are good for your weight. When you eat a handful of cashews, the body releases *cholecystokinin*, a hormone that increases feelings of fullness. As long as you eat the nuts slowly enough to allow the hormone to kick in, you will find that you say "enough" before you've overdone it.

MACADAMIA NUTS

These are delicious—and high in fat. But more than 82% of the fat in macadamias is monounsaturated. Olive oil, another "good" fat that has been linked to cardiovascular health, is between 55% and 83% monounsaturated.

Macadamia nuts also are a good source of fiber, with 2.3 g per one-ounce serving. A *Journal of Nutrition* study found that people who got most of their fiber from macadamia nuts had a greater reduction in LDL and total cholesterol than those who ate a similar diet without the nuts.

PEANUTS

Peanuts technically are a legume, but they act like nuts. They reduce the risk of dying from cancer, heart disease and other conditions.

Peanuts are rich in *resveratrol*, a potent antioxidant that reduces inflammation. The large, multidecade Harvard Nurses' Health Study found that people who regularly ate peanut butter, peanuts or other nuts were less likely to develop diabetes.

PECANS

It may be carrots that have a reputation for improving eye health, but you also might want to take a 20/20 look at pecans.

Reason: Cataracts, macular degeneration and other serious eye diseases are caused in part by free radicals. The antioxidants in nuts and other plant foods help prevent free radicals from damaging eye tissues. One study found that antioxidants—including the vitamin E in pecans and other nuts—helped slow the progression of macular degeneration by about 25%.

When USDA researchers measured the antioxidant capacity of more than 100 foods, they found that pecans were at the top of the nut pack.

PISTACHIO NUTS

This is another nut that men should love. In one study, men with erectile dysfunction were given 100 g (a little more than three ounces) of pistachios daily for three weeks. They showed an increase in IIEF scores (a measure of the ability to get erections) and improvements in blood flow. They also had an increase in HDL, which helps prevent cholesterol from clogging arteries in the penis.

Pistachios are particularly high in arginine, an amino acid used by the body to produce nitric oxide, a gas that causes blood vessels to dilate. It is important not just for sexual health but for overall cardiovascular health as well.

WALNUTS

Walnuts are rich in alpha-linolenic acid (ALA), a plant-based form of the omega-3 fatty acids that are found in fish. A one-ounce serving of walnuts has 2.5 g of ALA, compared with about 0.5 g in pecans and none in other nuts. The ALA in walnuts appears to rival the health benefits of the longer-chain omega-3s in fish. One study, published in *Diabetes Care*, found that people who ate walnuts had an increase in beneficial HDL cholesterol and a drop in harmful LDL. The fatty acids in walnuts may slow the progression of arterial plaques that produce clots, the cause of most heart attacks.

Bonus: A recent study found that eating walnuts with meals decreased the inflammation that occurs immediately after eating a steak or other foods high in saturated fat. Inflammation is linked to cardiovascular disease, cancer, Alzheimer's and other diseases.

Wait to Refrigerate

Recent research shows that nonrefrigerated produce may have a nutritional edge over its refrigerated counterparts.

Possible reason: Harvested fruits and vegetables continue to produce healthful phytochemicals when they are exposed to daily cycles of light and dark.

Current Biology

The Truth About Sugar and Artificial Sweetners

Karen Collins, RDN, a registered dietitian nutritionist, speaker and consultant, and nutrition adviser to the Washington, DC–based American Institute for Cancer Research, *AICR.org*. She is author of the weekly syndicated newspaper column "AICR HealthTalk" and blogs at *KarenCollins Nutrition.com/smartbytes*. She has taught patients how to cut down on sugar for more than 25 years.

We all know that getting too much added sugar carries a slew of health risks—from weight gain and heart disease to diabetes and obesity-linked cancers.

In fact, research shows that most Americans are getting so much sugar in their daily diets that they are increasing their heart attack risk by 20%. But with so many natural and artificial sweeteners to choose from—and new studies coming out all the time that raise questions about their safety—it's tough to know which claims are valid and which are not.

Facts you need to choose the best sweeteners for you…*

TRADITIONAL SWEETENERS

If you're not cutting calories and eat a healthful diet, it's OK to have up to two to three teaspoons of these sugars daily. But if your diet includes high-sugar snacks, cereals, drinks or

*People with diabetes can use any type of sweetener in their diets but must include it in their total daily carbohydrate limit recommended by their doctors or registered dietitians. Artificial sweeteners themselves have no carbohydrates, but the foods containing them usually do. To cook or bake with artificial sweeteners, check the labels for instructions.

other processed foods, limit these sugars to a few times a week.

•Brown and white sugars. You may think of brown sugar as a more wholesome choice than white sugar. But the fact is, they're both processed—white sugar is derived from sugarcane or sugar beets, while brown sugar is a combination of white sugar and molasses. These sugars also have roughly the same number of calories—16 calories per teaspoon for white sugar...and 17 for brown sugar.

How safe? When consumed in modest amounts, brown and white sugars are safe for most individuals. Brown sugar is really no more healthful than white sugar, but it does make baked goods moister and adds a hint of caramel flavor. Follow your taste preference.

•Honey. Even though honey contains trace amounts of minerals (mainly potassium, calcium and phosphorus), its nutritional value is not significantly different from that of white or brown sugar. Honey is about 25% to 50% sweeter by weight than sugar, so you can use less and still get a nice sweet taste.

How safe? Honey is safe for most adults when consumed in modest amounts. However, honey should never be given to babies under one year of age—it could contain bacterial spores that produce a toxin that causes infant botulism, a serious form of food poisoning. Honey's stickiness also may contribute to cavities in everyone else.

Better Milk for Heart Health

When the nutritional content of 384 samples of organic and conventional whole milk from around the country was analyzed, the organic milk had 62% more healthful omega-3 fatty acids and 25% less harmful omega-6s than conventional milk.

Reason: Organic-fed dairy cows spend more time grazing on pasture grasses that contain omega-3s than do cows used to produce conventional milk. A balance of omega-3s and omega-6s is essential for heart health.

Charles Benbrook, PhD, research professor, Center for Sustaining Agriculture and Natural Resources, Washington State University, Puyallup.

•Agave (ah-GAH-vay) nectar. Made from the juice of the agave plant, this sweetener reminds some people of a sweeter, thinner version of honey. Agave and honey have about the same number of calories (21 calories per teaspoon).

How safe? Overall, agave is no more healthful than other types of added sugar. Compared with the same amount of white sugar, agave causes smaller increases in blood sugar, triggering fewer of the metabolic changes that can lead to diabetes and heart disease. However, agave is higher in fructose than other natural sugars, which may not be healthy in large amounts.

•Molasses. This syrupy liquid is created from the juice of sugarcane and beet sugar during the refining process. The type of molasses is determined by the degree of boiling that occurs—light molasses comes from the first boiling...dark molasses, which is darker and thicker than the light variety, comes from the second boiling...and blackstrap molasses, which is quite thick and dark, comes from the third boiling.

How safe? Molasses is safe for most people. Dark and blackstrap molasses provide health-protective polyphenol compounds. Blackstrap molasses is also a good source of iron. All types of molasses contain about 20 calories per teaspoon.

LOW- OR NO-CALORIE SWEETENERS

Many people believe almost as a matter of principle that all artificial sweeteners are harmful and should be avoided. But that view is simplistic. Here is what the science shows about artificial sweetener safety...

•Aspartame. Sold in a light blue packet as NutraSweet or Equal, this artificial sweetener has no calories and is about 200 times sweeter by weight than white or brown sugar. Aspartame is used in soft drinks, chewing gum, pudding and gelatins and hundreds of other products.

How safe? Some individuals get headaches and/or feel dizzy when they ingest too much aspartame. Despite animal studies that have linked aspartame to cancer, no such association has been found in humans. However, a recent study linked consumption of diet soft drinks containing aspartame to an increased risk for non-Hodgkin's lymphoma and multiple myeloma in men. The watchdog group Center for Science in the Public Interest (CSPI) advises against using aspartame. In addition, people with phenylketonuria should avoid aspartame completely—this genetic disorder makes it difficult to metabolize phenylalanine, one of the protein building blocks used to make the sweetener.

•**Saccharin.** Found in a pink packet and sold as Sweet'N Low, it is 300 to 500 times sweeter than sugar. Saccharin has less than four calories per packet.

How safe? Despite concerns about saccharin causing bladder cancer in male rats, many human studies have shown no link to cancer risk. Even so, CSPI believes the research is inconsistent and recommends against its use. There's some evidence that saccharin can cross the placenta, so some experts advise women to limit it during pregnancy.

•**Stevia.** A highly purified extract made from the leaves of a South American shrub, stevia (sold as stevia, rebiana and under the brand names PureVia and Truvia) has zero calories and is about 250 times sweeter than sugar.

How safe? No health risks have been uncovered in a wide range of studies on stevia, but research is ongoing. Stevia may cause an allergic reaction in people who are allergic to ragweed and could interact with diabetes and blood pressure drugs.

•**Sucralose.** Known as Splenda and sold in a yellow packet, it has four calories per packet and tastes about 600 times sweeter than white or brown sugar. Sucralose is a processed sweetener derived from a molecule of sucrose (table sugar).

How safe? There's no evidence that sucralose harms humans when consumed in small amounts. One recent study suggested that it increases diabetes risk, but this was a small study of obese people looking at how sucralose affected their ability to metabolize a very large sugar load—about 19 teaspoons consumed all at once. More research is needed on how sucralose may affect metabolism with a more typical diet.

PROCESSED FOOD SWEETENERS

•**High fructose corn syrup (HFCS).** Derived from cornstarch, HFCS is found in a vast and sometimes surprising array of processed foods, ranging from many breads and yogurts to certain brands of applesauce and even macaroni and cheese. Beverages that contain HFCS include a wide variety of soft drinks, sports drinks and even tonic water.

How safe? Most experts have long insisted that there's no research showing that HFCS is any worse than other sweeteners—and, in fact, most HFCS contains only a little more fructose than regular table sugar. However, some studies have now linked HFCS-containing beverages (one or more servings a day) to greater risk for heart disease, diabetes, weight gain and obesity. But these associations may be due to increased calorie consumption from foods that contain HFCS, such as soda, rather than the HFCS itself.

Best: Avoid these beverages and limit processed foods to substantially cut consumption of HFCS and calories.

•**Sugar alcohols.** Sorbitol, mannitol and erythritol are processed sweeteners that do not actually contain alcohol or sugar. They're about half as sweet as white sugar, with fewer calories. Sugar alcohols are slowly absorbed, so they don't raise blood sugar quickly. A serving of food with less than 5 g of these sweeteners generally will not affect blood sugar. Consuming

Some Canned and Frozen Foods Are Healthier Than Their Fresh Counterparts

Tomatoes: The heat used in canning raises their antioxidant level and content of lycopene, which protects against heart disease and some cancers.

Corn and spinach: Compared with fresh versions, canned and frozen corn and spinach—which are processed with heat—have higher levels of lutein, which protects against macular degeneration. **Canned peaches** have significantly more vitamin C, antioxidants and folate than fresh ones. **Boiled peanuts** have four times the antioxidants of raw or roasted peanuts or peanut butter.

Roundup of experts in the nutritional content of produce, reported in *Environmental Nutrition*. *Environmental Nutrition.com* more than 20 g at once can lead to gas, bloating and diarrhea.

Are You Overdosing on Calcium?

Susan Levin, MS, RD, director of nutrition education for the Physicians Committee for Responsible Medicine, a Washington, DC–based nonprofit group dedicated to promoting preventive medicine and higher standards in research. *PCRM.org*

Getting a little older...and worried about your bones? Pop a calcium supplement. That's long been the message that American women and men have received from their doctors.

What's changed: A spate of recent studies suggests that calcium supplements, which now are used by nearly half of US adults, might not be as innocuous as once thought.

Troubling research finding: A report that appeared in the *British Medical Journal* concluded that women who took calcium supplements had about a 30% increased risk for a heart attack. Other studies have also linked calcium supplementation to cardiovascular disease in men and women.

What most people don't realize: While some medical experts dispute these findings, a recommendation issued earlier this year by the US Preventive Services Task Force (USPSTF)—that postmenopausal women should not take calcium supplements to prevent bone fractures—signals a possible shift in medical consensus.

This recommendation, made by an expert panel that reviewed more than 100 scientific studies, also concluded that there was not enough evidence to prove that calcium supplements prevented bone fractures in healthy premenopausal women and men. In addition, the panel concluded that there was insufficient evidence to support the use of vitamin D-3 to help promote calcium absorption. (The recommendations do not apply to women or men with osteoporosis or vitamin D deficiency—for whom supplements presumably do offer more benefit than risk.)

KEY QUESTIONS TO ASK

The research has raised important questions. How much calcium is too much? Is supplemental calcium riskier than calcium in foods? So far, there are no clear answers.

A daily calcium intake that doesn't exceed the recommended amounts (see next page) has long been presumed to be safe. In fact, most studies have found that calcium is either neutral (no good or bad effects) or slightly beneficial because it promotes bone health—and heart health by increasing HDL "good" cholesterol levels and lowering blood pressure. But researchers are now investigating whether the equation changes when some or most of the calcium comes from supplements. Some experts suspect that a "flood" of calcium created by taking a supplement leads to vascular calcification, deposits of calcium on the inside of arteries that increase atherosclerosis and the risk for clots and heart attacks.

Putting the issue in context: This wouldn't be the first time that a substance that's healthy when consumed from foods becomes harmful when it's taken as a supplement. A now-famous study found that smokers or former smokers who took beta-carotene supplements were more likely to get lung cancer than those who got beta-carotene only from food sources.

And what about calcium in food? When you eat calcium-rich foods, you're getting a mixture of nutrients that includes a variety of vitamins, minerals and other substances. Some experts now theorize that our bodies are not biologi-

Nondairy Source of Calcium

One cup of stinging nettle tea provides about 500 milligrams (mg) of calcium, compared with 300 mg in a cup of milk. Put one ounce of dried nettles in 32 ounces of water, and let it steep for four to 10 hours. Stinging nettle is available at health-food stores.

Jennifer Adler MS, CN, certified nutritionist and natural foods chef, writing in *Speed Healing* (Bottom Line Books).

cally programmed to process certain single-substance supplements, such as calcium.

HOW MUCH CALCIUM FOR YOU?

Calcium is necessary not only for strong bones but also for muscle contractions, a healthy heartbeat and many other functions. For adults, the recommended daily amount of calcium from food and supplements (if necessary) ranges from 1,000 mg to 1,200 mg. (The exact amount varies with age and sex.)*

An ongoing problem: Many Americans do not eat enough calcium-rich foods and take a daily supplement "for insurance." However, it is easy to exceed the recommended daily amount because many people don't track their calcium intakes—or they mistakenly assume that more must be better.

Best: Until there is definitive research, play it safe and get as much of your calcium as possible from your diet. Discuss the use of supplements with your doctor, and be sure to also do weight-bearing exercise (such as walking and/or running) and strength-training (including the use of hand weights and resistance machines) to keep your bones strong.

If you have osteoporosis or significant risk factors, such as a vitamin D deficiency, or your doctor OKs a calcium supplement for some other reason, take no more than 500 mg at one time—the body can't absorb more than that, especially if you're over age 50, take acid blockers or have an absorption disorder. Calcium citrate is the best choice for absorption.

*Recommended daily amount set by the Institute of Medicine is 1,000 mg for women ages 19 to 50 and men ages 19 to 70...and 1,200 mg for women ages 51 and older and men ages 71 and older.

Best Calcium-Rich Foods

Susan Levin, MS, RD, director of nutrition education for the Physicians Committee for Responsible Medicine, a Washington, DC–based nonprofit group dedicated to promoting preventive medicine and higher standards in research. *PCRM.org*

For now, no one is sure if calcium supplements really pose health risks, or how big (or small) the risks may be. Most experts agree, however, that getting calcium from one's diet is the best approach. The standard advice to eat a nutritious, balanced diet isn't sexy, but it works. Calcium is one of the easiest nutrients to get enough of. *For example...*

- **One cup of cooked curly-leaf Scotch kale** has 172 mg of calcium. Other green, leafy vegetables (including beet greens, spinach, watercress and collard greens) also are good sources of calcium.
- **Yogurt is another high-calcium food.** You'll get 338 mg in a six-ounce container of plain, skim-milk yogurt—much more than plain, nonfat Greek yogurt, which provides 187 mg per six-ounce container.
- **Fish** is among the healthiest ways to get more calcium because it also provides heart-healthy omega-3 fatty acids. For example, a 3.75-ounce can of sardines (with bones) has 351 mg of calcium...a three-ounce can of pink salmon (with bones), 181 mg.
- **Almonds** contain 76 mg of calcium per ounce (about 23 nuts). Other good choices are Brazil nuts and hazelnuts.

Better Than Meat—Other Proteins You Should Be Eating

Dawn Jackson Blatner, RD, a registered dietitian in private practice in Chicago. She is author of *The Flexitarian Diet: The Mostly Vegetarian Way to Lose Weight, Be Healthier, Prevent Disease, and Add Years to Your Life* (McGraw-Hill) and the nutrition consultant for the Chicago Cubs. As a flexitarian expert, she gets most of her protein from plants. *DawnJacksonBlatner.com*

When it comes to getting enough muscle-building protein, most people do just fine by having a juicy steak, a generous chicken breast or a tasty fish fillet a few times a week.

The problem is, most Americans need to get more protein from other foods and a little less from animals, since research suggests a more plant-based diet decreases risk for chronic health problems, such as heart disease, diabetes, cancer and obesity. Balancing animal protein (from meat, for example) with protein from plants and other foods is one of the simplest ways to improve your diet. Of course, you don't have to be a vegetarian or vegan to enjoy meat-free protein foods.* *My favorite options...*

FOR BREAKFAST

If you want protein in the morning, you may reach for some eggs and sausage. But not so fast! *Here are some other great ideas...*

•**Quinoa.** Often used as a dinner side dish, quinoa also can be eaten as a great nutty-tasting grain for breakfast. Technically a seed, quinoa wins points for being a high-protein whole grain with 8 g per cooked cup. It's also naturally gluten-free—a bonus for those who can't safely eat most oatmeal, since oats may be contaminated in the field or through processing with gluten-containing foods.

For a great protein-packed breakfast: Have a bowl of quinoa with chopped fruit and nuts...or top it with sautéed spinach and a poached egg. To make things easier, there's nothing wrong with buying precooked, frozen quinoa—it is now sold at lots of markets.

•**Cottage cheese.** It is not a plant-based food, but it's an excellent source of protein. In fact, you may be surprised to find out that a half cup of 1% milkfat cottage cheese contains more than twice as much protein (14 g) as an egg.

Caution: Most cottage cheese is high in sodium, so be sure to stick to the low-sodium variety if you are on a low-sodium diet.

Not a fan of curds? Puree it. Make "whipped cottage cheese" in your blender and flavor it with cinnamon for a delicious spread to smear on apple slices or add chives and basil for a veggie dip.

FOR LUNCH OR DINNER

Want a quick and easy protein for lunch or dinner? Tofu or beans are excellent choices, but you may want to try something new. *Here's what I suggest...*

*Adults over age 19 should consume 0.37 g of protein per pound of body weight, according to the Institute of Medicine (IOM). *Example*: If you weigh 150 pounds, you need about 55 g of protein daily.

•**Split peas.** A bowl of delicious split pea soup will add some variety. Dried peas have four times more protein than brown rice—and four times more fiber. If you don't want to cook your own split pea soup, certain prepared varieties are worth trying.

Good choices: Fantastic Foods Split Pea Soup Mix and Tabatchnick Split Pea Soup.

•**Spinach.** Most people don't realize that cooked spinach—at 4 g per half cup—offers more protein than most other vegetables. Not only that, spinach is incredibly nutrient-dense—it contains antioxidant vitamins A, C and E and is a rich plant source of iron and calcium.

To get a lot of spinach, buy it frozen. Since frozen spinach is precooked, it's easier to eat more—toss it into soups, pasta sauce, bean burritos or lasagna—than if you are downing it raw in, say, a salad. Frozen spinach is picked at peak season before freezing, so it retains its nutrients for months. And it's a great value!

FOR SNACKS

You already know that nuts are excellent protein-rich snacks. *Some other options you may want to try...*

•**Edamame.** These young green soybeans are a versatile protein source. One-half cup of frozen edamame contains 6 g of protein...and a quarter cup of roasted soybeans has an impressive 15 g (roasting concentrates the protein by removing the water). Soy foods contain

Have a Beer for Your Health!

Good news for brewski lovers: Researchers are finding that beer, like wine, is an excellent source of health-promoting flavonoids. Beer also provides a good amount of B vitamins and bone-strengthening silicon—and may even reduce risk for kidney stones by a whopping 41%!

Just go easy: No more than one (12-ounce) glass for women per day and two for men. The darker the beer, the more flavonoids you get!

Sandra Woodruff, MS, RD, LDN, registered dietitian and nutrition consultant based in Tallahassee, Florida. *EatSmartToday.com*

Healthful Food Facts

Chicken Thighs Are More Nutritious Than Chicken Breasts

Thighs have twice as much iron and nearly three times as much zinc—which boosts the immune system. Skinless thighs contain only one more gram of fat per serving than skinless breasts—and are less likely to dry out during cooking. Thighs cost less, too.

Prevention. Prevention.com

Lamb Is a Highly Nutritious Red Meat

It is a good source of omega-3 fatty acids, which may protect against heart disease and stroke...and is rich in iron, which can boost energy and help prevent anemia. Choose lean cuts of lamb from the leg, loin and shank.

Reader's Digest. *ReadersDigest.com*

Surprising Source of Vitamin D

In a 12-week study of 30 adults, consuming white button mushroom powder provided almost as much vitamin D as the same amount in a vitamin D supplement.

To boost your vitamin D levels: Add mushrooms to your diet. All varieties contain vitamin D—read package labels to find out how much per serving.

Michael Holick, MD, PhD, professor of medicine, Boston University School of Medicine.

phytochemicals that may help slow or protect against certain cancers.

•**Hummus.** Here's a great way to spice up the hefty protein kick you get from beans.

What to do: Blend two 15.5-ounce cans of rinsed, drained garbanzo beans with one-quarter cup each tahini, lemon juice and water. Add one tablespoon each of olive oil and Frank's RedHot Cayenne Pepper Sauce (or any brand of pepper sauce you like). Cayenne pepper contains pain-relieving capsaicin. Then finish it off with one clove of minced garlic and one-half teaspoon of sea salt. Use it as a hearty dip with whole-grain pita bread or veggies...and maybe some tabouli. It's scrumptious!

Digestive Disorders

Digestive Enzymes to the Rescue

If you watch the TV ads, you might think that a good probiotic is the answer for all your digestive problems. Don't believe it.

While it is true that probiotic supplements can help relieve gas and diarrhea—and boost your immunity—when your intestinal bacteria are out of whack, that's not always the issue.

Perhaps your gut has plenty of "friendly" bacteria, but you are still plagued by gut-related problems such as flatulence, heartburn, lactose intolerance, diarrhea or abdominal pain. What then?

It is time to think about taking digestive enzymes.* These supplements not only help relieve the digestive problems described above, they can also have powerful healing effects for other ailments, such as arthritis and sinusitis, that have nothing to do with the digestive system.

When to consider taking a digestive enzyme—most are available at drugstores or health-food stores...

TIME FOR DIGESTIVE ENZYMES

•**Flatulence.** Most people have heard of the over-the-counter flatulence preventive known as Beano, but they do not necessarily know how it works.

This product is actually a digestive enzyme called *alpha-galactosidase.* Taken just before consuming gassy foods, such as cabbage, beans, cauliflower and broccoli, it breaks down some of the complex carbohydrates into easily digestible sugars, thus preventing intestinal gas.

•**Heartburn.** I have seen some great responses in patients with frequent heartburn who take digestive enzymes along with—or

*Digestive enzymes are generally safe, but check first with your doctor if you have a chronic condition or regularly take any medication or supplement.

Leo Galland, MD, director of the Foundation for Integrated Medicine in New York City. He is author of *The Heartburn and Indigestion Solution* (Renaissance Workshops).

instead of—over-the-counter remedies such as Tums with calcium, which tightens the valve between the stomach and esophagus. It is not clear how these enzymes help. It is possible that they deactivate some of the body's *pepsin*, a stomach enzyme that plays a crucial role in digestion but that surges upward from the stomach in some patients, damaging tissue in the esophagus. This is what causes the "burn" in heartburn.

What to try: A blend that includes different enzymes, such as *lipase*, *protease* and *amylase*. Some good products include AbsorbAid powder, Botanic Choice Digestive Enzyme Complex and Twinlab Super Enzyme Caps.

How to use it: Take the supplement with or just after meals.

•**Dairy sensitivity.** It's estimated that up to 50 million Americans have symptoms of lactose intolerance, a sensitivity to dairy foods that can cause bloating, gas, cramps and other digestive problems.

Humans are born with high levels of lactase, the enzyme that is required to digest a sugar (lactose) in dairy foods. But the levels drop in the first years after birth, so by adulthood, many people don't have enough lactase to comfortably digest dairy.

What to try: Supplemental lactase will replace the enzyme that's missing from the intestine. People who take lactase supplements can usually enjoy dairy foods without discomfort.

How to take it: Chew or swallow a tablet just before eating dairy...for milk and other liquidlike dairy, you can use lactase drops if you prefer.

Yet another option: Lactaid Milk, which comes with added lactase.

It's Not What You Eat—It's How You Eat

If your gut acts up during or after a meal, you may want to change how you eat before trying a digestive enzyme.

What to do...

•**Eat slowly and chew your food well.** This gives the enzymes in your saliva a better chance to start breaking down your food before it reaches your stomach.

•**Enjoy your food and relax.** People who are stressed have an increase in dopamine and adrenaline, hormones that inhibit normal digestion.

Be aware of any tension you feel in your body...relax your shoulders and jaw...and breathe slowly (your abdomen should expand and your chest should not rise when you breathe in).

•**Take a walk after eating.** It increases metabolism and helps you digest more efficiently. It also stimulates motility, the intestinal movements that move food (and wastes) through your system. Walk for at least five minutes—a leisurely pace is fine to promote digestion.

•**Gluten intolerance.** If you are one of the millions of Americans who is sensitive to gluten, a protein that is contained in wheat, barley and rye, you already know that a simple slice of bread or a bowl of wheat cereal can lead to hours of digestive problems, such as diarrhea, stomach cramps and flatulence.

Important: Many people who think that they're gluten-intolerant actually have fructose malabsorption, which occurs when the small intestine can't absorb fructose, a plant sugar. Get checked by a doctor before assuming that gluten is the problem. Fructose malabsorption is typically diagnosed with a hydrogen breath test—after ingesting a fructose solution, the amount of hydrogen in your breath is measured. An increase in hydrogen means that the fructose has not been properly digested.

What to try: If you are sensitive to gluten, you can try taking a supplement such as GlutenEase, which contains a blend of protease enzymes. You might be able to eat small amounts of wheat and other gluten-containing foods without discomfort.

How to use it: Take one capsule with meals. Double the dose if one capsule isn't effective.

If your gluten sensitivity is caused by celiac disease: Don't depend on any supplement. Patients with celiac disease must avoid even trace amounts of gluten, and supplements are unlikely to help.

RELIEF FOR OTHER PROBLEMS

•**Arthritis.** A study published in *Clinical Rheumatology* found that a European product known as Phlogenzym, a blend of the enzymes bromelain and trypsin and rutosid (a flavonoid), was as effective at treating osteoarthritis of the knee as a commonly prescribed anti-inflammatory drug. Researchers believe that this particular mix of enzymes may help with all forms of osteoarthritis.

What to try: Consider buying Phlogenzym online from a European pharmacy. Take two capsules three times daily, on an empty stomach.

Phlogenzym's major ingredients—bromelain, trypsin and rutosid—also can be found in US health-food stores. Follow dosage instructions on the product label.

Caution: If you take these enzymes for arthritis relief, be sure to do so only under the supervision of a physician. In some individuals, the protein-digesting components can damage the lining of the stomach.

• **Sinusitis.** Bacterial sinusitis usually responds to antibiotics, but some people can have chronic sinusitis that lasts 12 weeks or more—even when they are taking medication.

What to try: Bromelain or other protease enzymes (with protease or trypsin on the label). They are not a replacement for antibiotics if you have a stubborn bacterial infection, but they can help to reduce inflammation and discomfort while the infection is active and even while you are taking an antibiotic.

How to take it: Follow the directions on the product label. The dosing directions will depend on the specific enzymes, concentrations, etc.

WHAT ARE DIGESTIVE ENZYMES?

Digestive enzymes are present in saliva, the stomach and the small intestine. Their job is to break down the food you eat into smaller components.

After about age 50, the pancreas produces only about half the amount of digestive enzymes that it did when you were younger. Some individuals find that they have less gas, bloating or fullness when they take an enzyme supplement during or after meals.

Dangers of a "Slow Stomach"

Gerard Mullin, MD, an associate professor of medicine at The Johns Hopkins University School of Medicine and director of the Celiac Disease Clinic, Integrative GI Nutrition Services and the Capsule Endoscopy Program at Johns Hopkins Hospital, all in Baltimore. He is author of *The Inside Tract* (Rodale).

When you eat a meal, you probably don't think about the amount of time it takes your body to digest the food. But for many people, this is the key to uncovering a host of digestive ills—and even some seemingly unrelated concerns such as chronic fatigue.

WHEN FOOD MOVES TOO SLOWLY

In healthy adults, digestion time varies, but it generally takes about four hours for a meal to leave the stomach before passing on to the small intestine and colon.

What happens: When food enters the stomach, signals from hormones and nerve cells trigger stomach acid, digestive enzymes and wavelike peristaltic contractions of the muscles in the stomach wall. Together, they break down the meal into a soupy mixture called *chyme*, which peristalsis then pushes into the small intestine.

This process is known as gastric motility. And when gastric motility is impeded—when stomach emptying slows to a crawl, even though nothing is blocking the stomach outlet—it's called gastroparesis.

Surprising fact: An estimated one out of every 55 Americans suffers from gastroparesis—but the condition is diagnosed in only one out of every 90 people who have it.

When gastroparesis goes undetected: The symptoms of gastroparesis often are obvious—for example, nausea, vomiting, feeling full right after starting to eat a meal, bloating and abdominal pain. But the condition can cause other health problems such as unwanted weight loss and even malnutrition. It also can interfere with the absorption of medications and wear you down physically (one study found that 93% of people with gastroparesis were fatigued).

GETTING THE RIGHT DIAGNOSIS

If you're experiencing the symptoms of gastroparesis, see your primary care physician. He/she may refer you to a gastroenterologist. It's likely the specialist will order the "gold standard" for diagnosing gastroparesis, a test called gastric emptying scintigraphy.

Next step: At the test, you'll eat a meal that contains radioactive isotopes. (Radiolabeled Egg Beaters with jam, toast and water are typical.) A scan is taken at one, two and four hours after the meal with a scintigraph, or gamma camera. A one-hour scan after drinking liquid also is recommended. If images from any of the scans show that your stomach isn't emptying normally, you are diagnosed with gastroparesis.

Another approach: When I perform an endoscopy on a patient with gastroparesis-like symptoms (a thin, flexible tube with a light and camera on the end is inserted down the esophagus and into the stomach), if I see a significant amount of retained fluids or food despite an overnight fast, I make the diagnosis then and there, saving time and money.

Tips for Digestion

Many dietary and lifestyle habits can improve stomach motility...

- **Eat smaller, more frequent meals.** Eat smaller amounts of food every two, three or four hours.
- **Reduce dietary fiber and fat.** Both slow stomach emptying.
- **Chew food thoroughly.**
- **Chew sugarless gum.** Do so for about one hour after eating to stimulate peristalsis.
- **Take a leisurely five- or 10-minute (or longer) walk** after every meal.

FINDING THE CAUSE

Experts haven't discovered the exact mechanisms underlying gastroparesis. In fact, an estimated 40% of cases are idiopathic—the cause is unknown. Gastroparesis is a complication for about 30% of people with type 1 or type 2 diabetes.

What happens: Diabetes can damage the vagus nerve, which runs from the cranium to the abdomen and plays a key role in digestion.

Medication also can cause gastroparesis.

Examples: Narcotic pain relievers, such as *oxycodone* (OxyContin), and anticholinergics, a class of drugs that includes certain antihistamines and overactive bladder medications.

Small intestine bacterial overgrowth, in which abnormally large numbers of bacteria grow in the small intestine, also can lead to gastroparesis.

GETTING THE BEST MEDICAL CARE

I have found that an integrative approach that combines conventional and alternative medicine is the best way to control gastroparesis.

Conventional treatment typically includes medications that either speed stomach emptying or help control the symptoms of gastroparesis such as nausea and vomiting. *For example...*

- ***Metoclopramide*** **(Reglan).** This is currently the only FDA-approved medication for gastroparesis. Reglan works by blocking receptors of the neurotransmitter dopamine, which accelerates gastric motility.

Problem: The FDA has approved Reglan for no more than 12 weeks of use because long-term intake can cause *tardive dyskinesia*—involuntary, repetitive body movements, such as grimacing. Because of this risk, I rarely prescribe metoclopramide for my patients.

Another medication option: The drug *domperidone* has the same dopamine-suppressing action in the digestive tract as Reglan, but it does not cross the blood–brain barrier and, therefore, is much less likely to cause tardive dyskinesia. Risks include breast tenderness and worsening of the heart condition Long QT Syndrome.

However, according to clinical guidelines for the management of gastroparesis published in *The American Journal of Gastroenterology*, domperidone "is generally as effective" as metoclopramide with "lower risk of adverse effects."

Domperidone is readily available in most countries, where it is a standard treatment for heartburn, but not in the US. However, your doctor can obtain it under the FDA's Investigational New Drug program.

- **Antinausea drugs.** *Prochlorperazine* (Compazine) and *ondansetron* (Zofran) are commonly prescribed for gastroparesis.

New Blood Test for IBS

Among 221 adults who had acute gastroenteritis and were screened with a new blood test, those with irritable bowel syndrome (IBS) were identified by a biomarker (antibodies to a protein called *vinculin*).

Implication: The test will help distinguish between IBS and inflammatory bowel disease (IBD), two conditions that have similar symptoms but very different treatments. IBS is now diagnosed by frequency of symptoms. The blood test should be available late 2014.

Mark Pimentel, MD, director, GI Motility Program, Cedars-Sinai Medical Center, Los Angeles.

- **Botox.** Injections of botulinum toxin into the pylorus (the opening from the stomach into the small intestine) can help some patients for four to six months, after which the injection must be repeated.

New approaches: Physicians at Johns Hopkins are now using a new and effective procedure called through-the-scope transpyloric stent placement. With this procedure, an endoscope is used to place a stent (tube) that helps transfer stomach contents into the small intestine.

Another new approach, pioneered by John Clarke, MD, of Johns Hopkins, involves placing a stent across the pylorus to drain the stomach.

ALTERNATIVE THERAPIES

Certain alternative therapies may also help with stomach motility and/or with nausea and vomiting...*

- **Peppermint oil.** This can help gastroparesis, but it also can worsen heartburn in people with gastroesophageal reflux disease (GERD). If you have gastroparesis but not GERD, an enteric-coated softgel of peppermint oil may help you.

Recommended dose: 90 mg once a day.

- **Iberogast.** This pharmaceutical-grade, multi-herbal tincture can help with gastroparesis, studies have shown.

Recommended dose: 20 drops, two to three times a day, before meals. (Iberogast does contain alcohol.)

***Be sure to check with our doctor before trying these therapies, which are available online and at most health-food stores.**

- **Ginger.** Gingerroot may help with nausea and improve gastric motility.

Recommended dose: 1,200 mg daily.

- **Acupuncture.** This treatment can help control the symptoms of gastroparesis. Acupuncture has been shown to be effective for nausea and vomiting and abdominal pain and bloating.

Chronic Heartburn May Raise Odds for Throat Cancer

Scott Langevin, PhD, postdoctoral research fellow, Brown University, Providence, Rhode Island.
Cancer Epidemiology, Biomarkers & Prevention

People who suffer from frequent heartburn may be at increased risk for cancers of the throat and vocal cords even if they don't smoke or drink alcohol, a recent study says.

Interestingly, common over-the-counter antacids seemed to protect against these cancers while prescription medications such as Prilosec, Nexium and Prevacid didn't, the researchers said.

"There has been a controversy about whether heartburn contributes to cancers of the larynx or pharynx," said lead researcher Scott Langevin, PhD, a postdoctoral research fellow at Brown University in Providence, Rhode Island.

"And we found out that it does elevate the risk of these cancers. There is about a 78% increase in the risk for cancer in people who experience heavy heartburn," he said. "This is important in figuring out who to monitor more closely."

The other finding, which Dr. Langevin called "surprising," was the protective effect of common antacids in reducing the risk of cancer.

"We didn't see that protective effect with prescription medications. But it should be noted that people who take them are those who get the worst heartburn, so we shouldn't read too much into that," he said.

Dr. Langevin added that it's hard to explain that medication finding, and other studies will be needed to see if it's really the case. "It's possible that these drugs didn't have that protective effect because these were the worst cases of heartburn," he said.

STUDY DETAILS

Dr. Langevin's research group compared more than 600 patients with throat or vocal cord cancer with more than 1,300 people without a history of cancer. All the patients answered questions about their history of heartburn, smoking and drinking habits, and family history of cancer.

In addition, since some head and neck cancers are caused by the human papillomavirus (HPV), the researchers tested all the participants for antigens to the virus.

The researchers found that among those who weren't heavy smokers or drinkers, frequent heartburn increased the risk for cancers of the throat and vocal cords by 78%.

The researchers also found that taking antacids—but not prescription medications or home remedies—reduced the risk for these cancers by 41%. The protective effect of antacids was independent of smoking, drinking or infection with HPV, they said.

The report was published in the journal *Cancer Epidemiology, Biomarkers & Prevention*. And while it uncovered an association between heartburn and cancer of the throat and vocal cords, it didn't prove a cause-and-effect relationship.

info For more information on throat cancer, visit the American Cancer Society at *http://www.cancer.org/cancer/laryngealandhypopharyngealcancer/overviewguide/*.

Finally...a Way to Prevent IBD

Jenifer Fenton, PhD, MPH, assistant professor, department of food science and human nutrition, College of Osteopathic Medicine, Michigan State University, East Lansing. Her study was published in *The Journal of Nutrition*.

Life can be a waiting game—an anxious and decidedly unfun game—for people whose family history puts them at high risk for inflammatory bowel disease (IBD).

An umbrella term for a group of digestive disorders, IBD includes ulcerative colitis, which usually is confined to the colon and rectum... and Crohn's disease, which can appear anywhere along the lining of the digestive tract.

Symptoms can be really terrible, including diarrhea, constipation, abdominal pain, gas, bloating, bloody stools, malnutrition and more.

Do you know if IBD has affected anyone in your family?

You should—because you no longer have to just wait for it to hit you. *Now, there is news about something you can do to lower your risk of getting it...*

FEEDING THE GOOD

Before discussing this exciting research, here's a little background on your gut...In your intestines are trillions of bacteria, with the specific types varying from person to person based on factors such as diet and environment. One theory about IBD suggests that it is caused by an overactive immune response to some "bad" bacteria in the intestines.

The "good versus bad bacteria" idea is nothing new—in fact, it's one reason why you want that "live, active cultures" label on your yogurt. Those live, active cultures are probiotics, beneficial bacteria that you can ingest directly. A prebiotic is different—it is food for bacteria, so you can use it to support certain types of beneficial bacteria that are already in your gut.

TESTING, TESTING

For this study, the researchers wanted to use a prebiotic supplement (basically a type of fiber) to feed and thus increase a specific population of beneficial bacteria before IBD developed. The goal was to see whether the prebiotic might help prevent the development of the disease or make it less severe if it did develop.

Researchers performed the study on mice that did not have symptoms of the disease but were genetically predisposed to develop colitis after infection with "bad" bacteria. One group of mice received a prebiotic supplement of galacto-oligosaccharides (GOS) daily for six weeks...a second group did not get GOS. After the first two weeks, the researchers purposely infected all the mice with a pathogen to trigger the onset of colitis.

Results: Compared with mice that did not get GOS, those that were fed the prebiotic developed significantly less severe colitis...and their lab tests showed much less inflammation and dysplasia (abnormal tissue development) in their digestive tracts.

Researchers hypothesize that the prebiotic helps by increasing the number of protective bacteria in the gut, which in turn enhances immune function, reduces intestinal inflammation and/or reduces colonizing of harmful pathogens.

IS IT RIGHT FOR YOU?

We spoke with lead researcher Jenifer Fenton, PhD, MPH, an assistant professor in the department of food science and human nutrition at Michigan State University in East Lansing. She emphasized that because this study was conducted in mice, the results—though encouraging—cannot be directly translated to people. So human studies definitely are needed. In the meantime, however...

Patients who already have IBD should consult the physician treating their IBD before deciding whether to take GOS. "The problem with having a chronic disease such as IBD for years is that it leads to a dramatic change in the intestinal tissue. A supplement could theoretically make it worse," she explained. What's more, because GOS is a type of fiber, it may not be well-tolerated by IBD patients, who often cannot eat a high-fiber diet.

So who is most likely to benefit from GOS? People with a family history of IBD (meaning that their parent, sibling or child has or had the disease)...and perhaps those who are at risk for exposure to pathogenic gut bacteria (for instance, because they are traveling to a new country).

To determine whether GOS is appropriate for you, consult a doctor with expertise in nutrition. You may be given a test called a comprehensive digestive stool analysis. As for dosage, follow your doctor's guidelines. (By way of comparison, Dr. Fenton mentioned one human study published in *American Journal of Clinical Nutrition* in which participants took daily doses of up to five grams of GOS.) GOS generally is safe, though it may cause an increase in flatulence and/or mild gastrointestinal discomfort, particularly in people who are not accustomed to consuming much fiber.

You may face a challenge in getting hold of GOS because the supplement isn't easy to find in the US. One available option is ProBiota Immune from Seeking Health (available at *SeekingHealth.com*). On the label, the suggested serving size is about one to two teaspoons per day. Several GOS-containing products also are available from Europe, such as Bimuno IBAID (*Bimuno.com/buy-now*).

Better Care for Irritable Bowel

In a recent study of 45 adults who had irritable bowel syndrome with diarrhea (IBS-D)—but not celiac disease—those who ate a gluten-free diet for a month had significantly fewer bowel movements per day than those whose diets included gluten (a protein found in wheat, barley and rye).

Possible explanation: Gluten can irritate the lining of the small intestine, even in people who do not have celiac disease.

Michael Camilleri, MD, professor of medicine, pharmacology and physiology, Mayo Clinic, Rochester, Minnesota.

Extra Vitamin D May Ease Crohn's Symptoms, Study Finds

Tara Raftery, research dietitian and PhD candidate, Trinity College, Dublin, Ireland.

John White, PhD, professor, physiology, McGill University, Montreal, Canada.

Neera Gupta, MD, co-chair, Crohn's & Colitis Foundation of America, pediatric affairs committee, and assistant professor, pediatrics, New York-Presbyterian Morgan Stanley Children's Hospital/Columbia University Medical Center, New York City.

Vitamin D supplements may help those with Crohn's disease overcome the fatigue and decreased muscle strength associated with the inflammatory bowel disease, according to recent research.

Extra vitamin D "was associated with significantly less physical, emotional and general fatigue, greater quality of life and the ability to perform activities of daily living," said Tara Raftery, a research dietitian and doctoral candidate at Trinity College Dublin.

BACKGROUND

Besides boosting bone growth and remodeling, vitamin D is thought to improve neuromuscular and immune function, reduce inflammation and help with other bodily tasks. Children and adults aged one year to 70 are advised to get 600 IUs a day; older adults, 800, according to the U.S. National Institutes of Health (NIH).

Vitamin D is found in fatty fish such as salmon, in smaller amounts in cheese, egg yolks and beef liver, and in fortified foods such as milk.

Sometimes called the sunshine vitamin, vitamin D is also produced when the sun's rays strike the skin.

Crohn's can affect any part of the gastrointestinal tract, but most commonly affects the end of the small bowel and the beginning of the colon. Symptoms vary, but may include persistent diarrhea, rectal bleeding, abdominal cramps, and pain and constipation. About 700,000 Americans are affected, according to the Crohn's & Colitis Foundation of America.

Its cause is not well understood, but Crohn's is thought to involve heredity and environmental factors. Experts believe that in those with Crohn's, the immune system attacks harmless intestinal bacteria, triggering chronic inflammation and, eventually, the disease symptoms.

STUDY DETAILS

Raftery and her colleagues evaluated 27 patients who had Crohn's in remission. (Even in remission, fatigue and quality of life can be problematic.) The patients were assigned to take either 2,000 IUs (international units) of vitamin D a day or a dummy vitamin for three months.

Before and after the study, the researchers measured hand-grip strength, fatigue, quality of life and blood levels of vitamin D.

"Hand-grip strength is a proxy measure of muscle function," Raftery said. "Muscle function has been known to be reduced in Crohn's disease."

The daily vitamin D supplement benefitted participants in many ways, Raftery found. "When levels of vitamin D peaked at 30 ng/mL (75 nmol/L) or more [a level considered healthy], muscle function in both the dominant and nondominant hands were significantly higher than in those who had levels less than 30 ng/mL," she said.

Quality of life improved more for the D-supplement group, too. Using a standard measure to evaluate quality of life, the researchers found those who achieved a healthy blood level of the vitamin scored 24 points higher than those not on supplements. A 20-point difference is considered meaningful from a "real-world" perspective, Raftery said.

ADDITIONAL STUDIES

The study results echo those of other researchers, including John White, PhD, professor of physiology at McGill University, Montreal. He said the research findings "show collectively that vitamin D acts in the intestine to stimulate the innate immune system to defend against pathogenic bacteria, and to enhance the barrier function of the intestinal epithelium [the lining of the intestine]."

Other researchers, including Raftery, have also shown vitamin D can help improve muscle strength, he said.

EXPERT RESPONSE...AND A CAUTION

Vitamin D is getting a lot of attention in inflammatory bowel disease treatments, said Neera Gupta, MD, co-chair of the Crohn's & Colitis Foundation of America's pediatric affairs committee.

More study is needed to determine the benefits of maintaining vitamin D levels higher than currently recommended, she said.

Dr. Gupta cautioned those with Crohn's not to self-dose with vitamin D. "Discuss your vitamin D status with your primary gastroenterologist to determine whether or not vitamin D supplementation is indicated in your particular situation," she said.

Dr. White said supplements are inexpensive and safer than too much sun exposure. A daily intake of 2,000 IUs is considered safe, he said.

The safe upper limit for adults is 4,000 IUs, according to the NIH.

The data and conclusions of research presented at medical meetings should be viewed as preliminary until published in a peer-reviewed journal.

info To learn more about vitamin D, visit the U.S. National Institutes of Health website at *http://ods.od.nih.gov/factsheets/VitaminD-QuickFacts/.*

What Your Kidneys May Be Telling You—Don't Miss These Subtle Warnings...

Rajiv Saran, MD, professor of medicine and associate director of the University of Michigan's Kidney Epidemiology and Cost Center in Ann Arbor. He's also a principal investigator on a national chronic kidney disease surveillance system (*CDC.gov/ckd*), a project funded by the Centers for Disease Control and Prevention (CDC) and in partnership with the University of California, San Francisco.

Are your kidneys working normally? If you're like most people, you probably don't really know.

About one in every nine American adults suffers from chronic kidney disease (CKD). But many of these people have no idea that they're affected until they develop cardiovascular disease due to kidney disease...or have kidney failure or even end-stage renal disease, necessitating dialysis treatments or a kidney transplant.

What's new: With up to 44 million people in the US potentially affected by CKD—a startling number that rivals the diabetes epidemic—scientists now are developing new ways to detect and fight this problem. *What you need to know...*

WHO'S AT RISK

If you have early-stage kidney disease, chances are you won't experience any pain and may, in fact, feel fine. Any signs that do appear are likely to be vague (for example, a slight increase in frequency of urination or becoming fatigued more easily) and even may resemble those triggered by other conditions, such as prostate enlargement or anemia.

Anyone can develop kidney disease, but it's long been known that people who are over age 60 and/or those who have high blood pressure, diabetes or heart disease are at increased risk. People who have a family history of kidney disease, especially in a parent or sibling, are also at increased risk for CKD.

But certain other risk factors are often overlooked. These include obesity, a history of kidney stones and rheumatologic conditions such as lupus. Acute kidney injury, caused by such conditions as dehydration, infection or trauma, also may lead to CKD.

BEYOND THE USUAL RED FLAGS

The classic red flags for CKD may include slight changes in typical urine output (either more or less) and swelling of the ankles, feet or eye area due to fluid retention.

Surprising signs: Foamy urine that resembles foam on the surface of eggs as they are beaten can indicate an abundance of protein in the urine, a sign of kidney damage.

Other unusual symptoms that may, for unknown reasons, signal CKD include nonspecific muscle pains (especially at night) or dry, itchy skin (anywhere on the body) without obvious skin disease.

GETTING THE RIGHT TESTS

If you have any of the risk factors for CKD or symptoms, as described above, you should have certain screening tests at least once a year.

Don't overlook this test: A urinalysis, sometimes dubbed the "dipstick" test, checks more than a dozen components in urine, such as pH level, protein, glucose, nitrites and ketones. The presence of urine protein, in particular, offers an immediate clue that kidney damage may have occurred. If your doctor doesn't ask you for a urine sample to perform a urinalysis during your yearly checkup, talk to him/her about getting the test. *Routine tests to screen for kidney disease...*

- **Serum creatinine and estimated glomerular filtration rate (eGFR).** The latter test estimates how well your kidneys are filtering blood. As kidney disease worsens, your level of creatinine goes up and your eGFR goes down. An eGFR of less than 60 (for three months or longer) indicates CKD.

• **Urinary albumin-to-creatinine ratio (UACR).** Albumin, a protein in the blood that passes through the kidneys' microscopic filtering cells, signals kidney damage. The lower the number the better, with a normal UACR being less than 30.

Important: Exercising strenuously or eating a lot of meat before a test could raise creatinine levels, erroneously signaling a problem. Herbal supplements containing creatinine also can falsely elevate levels. This naturally occurring substance, which helps muscles make energy, often is taken by weight lifters.

AVOIDING CKD

High blood pressure and diabetes cause more than two-thirds of CKD cases in the US. Modifying those risk factors through lifestyle changes, such as limiting sodium and sugar intake, losing weight and taking prescribed medications, is crucial.

The hidden dangers: Daily use of over-the-counter nonsteroidal anti-inflammatory drugs (NSAIDs), such as *ibuprofen* (Advil) or *naproxen* (Aleve), can increase one's risk for CKD over time by constricting the blood vessels in the kidneys. For this reason, people who have CKD should avoid NSAIDs. Many herbal supplements contain compounds that can be toxic to the kidneys. Be sure to discuss these products with your doctor before using them, especially if you have CKD. For more on this, go to *Kidney.org* and search "Herbs."

If you need an imaging test that requires the use of dyes that contain iodine—these are used as contrast agents for computed tomography (CT) and other imaging scans—discuss your CKD risk with your doctor.

If your kidney function is normal, the dyes typically won't harm you. But these contrast agents can be toxic to the kidneys, causing acute injury to the organs if kidney function is already compromised. If this type of scan is needed by a person with advanced CKD, serum creatinine levels should be monitored before and after the scan. These patients also need to stay well-hydrated, and their kidney function must be closely followed to minimize the risks of contrast agents.

Best and Worst Drinks for Preventing Kidney Stones

Pietro Manuel Ferraro, MD, physician, department of internal medicine and medical specialties, Catholic University of the Sacred Heart, Rome, Italy. His study was published in *Clinical Journal of the American Society of Nephrology.*

Mention kidney stones and everyone within earshot winces—because we've all heard how painful these stones can be. So if you want to be stone-free, you're probably following the common advice to drink lots of liquids. But instead of focusing on how much you drink, the crucial question is what you drink, a recent study reveals. Certain beverages—including some very surprising ones, such as beer!—are particularly helpful in protecting against stones, while other drinks do more harm than good.

Unfortunately, kidney stones are common, plaguing 19% of men and 9% of women in the US at least once in their lifetimes—and recurrences are quite common. Drinking plenty of water helps prevent stones from forming...but actually, there are other fluids that can be even more effective.

DRINK THIS, NOT THAT

Using data from three large studies, researchers followed 194,095 people, none of whom had a history of kidney stones, for more than eight years. Participants periodically completed questionnaires about their diet and overall health. During the course of the study, there were 4,462 cases of kidney stones.

Researchers adjusted for health factors (age, body mass index, diabetes, medications, blood pressure) as well as various dietary factors (including intake of meat, calcium and potassium) known to affect kidney stone risk. Then they calculated the stone risk associated with various types of beverages.

How the comparison was done: For each analysis, the effects of drinking an average of one or more servings per day were compared with drinking less than one serving per week. Because data from three different studies were used, serving sizes were not necessarily alike across the board. But in general, a serving was considered to be 12 ounces of soda or beer...eight ounces of coffee, tea, milk or fruit punch...five ounces of wine...and four to six ounces of juice. The researchers' findings were eye-opening.

- **Kidney stone risk boosters...**
  - Sugar-sweetened noncola sodas increased kidney stone risk by 33%.
  - Sugar-sweetened colas increased risk by 23%.
  - Fruit punch increased risk by 18%.
  - Diet noncola sodas (but, surprisingly, not diet colas) increased risk by 17%.
- **Kidney stone risk reducers...**
  - Beer reduced kidney stone risk by 41%.
  - White wine reduced risk by 33%.
  - Red wine reduced risk by 31%.
  - Caffeinated coffee reduced kidney stone risk by 26%.
  - Decaf coffee reduced risk by 16%.
  - Orange juice reduced risk by 12%.
  - Tea reduced risk by 11%.

Consumption of milk and juices other than orange juice did not significantly affect the likelihood of developing kidney stones.

Theories behind the findings: Because sugar-sweetened sodas and fruit punch are associated with higher risk, researchers suspect that their high fructose concentration may increase the amount of calcium, oxalate and uric acid in the urine—and those substances contribute to kidney stone formation. So how to explain the beneficial effects of orange juice, which is also high in fructose? Perhaps orange juice's high concentration of potassium citrate offsets the fructose and favorably changes the composition of urine.

Regarding the beneficial effects of coffee and tea, it could be that their caffeine acts as a diuretic that promotes urine production and thus helps prevent stones. Tea and coffee, including decaf, also contain antioxidants that may help combat stone formation. Alcohol, too, is a diuretic, and wine and beer contain antioxidants as well—though of course, with any type of alcoholic beverage, moderation is important.

Vitamin C Supplement Raises Risk for Kidney Stones

Men who took supplements of 1,000 milligrams (mg) or more per day were twice as likely to develop kidney stones as those who did not take supplements. Multivitamins—which usually contain about 60 mg of vitamin C—were not associated with increased risk, nor were foods rich in vitamin C.

Agneta Åkesson, PhD, associate professor, IMM Institute of Environmental Medicine, Karolinska Institute, Stockholm, and leader of a study published in *JAMA Internal Medicine.*

Light Exercise Might Reduce Risk of Kidney Stones

American Society of Nephrology, news release.

Just a little exercise each week—jogging for an hour or walking for about three hours—can reduce the risk of developing kidney stones by up to 31%, according to a recent study.

Researchers looking at data on more than 84,000 postmenopausal women found that engaging in any type of light physical activity can help prevent the formation of these pebbles in the kidneys. Even light gardening might curb their development, according to the study, which was published recently in the *Journal of the American Society of Nephrology.*

"Even small amounts of exercise may decrease the risk of kidney stones," said study author Mathew Sorensen, MD, of the University of Washington School of Medicine. "It does not need to be marathons, as the intensity of the exercise does not seem to matter."

BACKGROUND

Kidney stones, which usually affect men more often than women, are becoming more prevalent among women. Each year in the United States, more than 300,000 people go to emergency rooms for kidney stone problems. Larger stones can get stuck in the urinary tract and block the flow of urine, causing severe pain or bleeding.

During the past 15 years, research has shown that kidney stones might actually be a systemic problem, involving more than just the kidneys. Recent research has linked the stones to obesity, diabetes, metabolic syndrome and heart disease.

NEW STUDY

In conducting the study, the researchers analyzed information compiled since the 1990s on the women's eating habits and level of physical activity.

After taking into account the women's body-mass index (a measurement of body fat based on a ratio of height and weight), the researchers found that obesity was a risk factor for the development of kidney stones. Eating more than 2,200 calories a day could increase the risk for kidney stones by up to 42%, they found.

IMPLICATION

"Being aware of calorie intake, watching their weight and making efforts to exercise are important factors for improving the health of our patients overall, and as it relates to kidney stones," Dr. Sorensen said.

EXPERT COMMENTARY

John Lieske, MD, of the Mayo Clinic in Rochester, Minnesota, said the study, which included only postmenopausal women, must be replicated in a larger, more diverse population. Women who engage in regular physical activity also likely have other healthy habits that help lower their risk for kidney stones, he added.

"Nevertheless, conservative counseling for patients with stones often centers almost exclusively on diet, stressing increased fluid intake, normal dietary calcium, lower sodium, moderate protein and reduced dietary oxalate," Dr. Lieske wrote in a journal editorial accompanying the study.

The results of this study suggest that a recommendation for moderate physical activity might reasonably be added to the mix, he said. The study did not, however, prove a cause-and-effect link between exercise and decreased risk for kidney stones. It showed only an association between the two in a small portion of the population.

info For more information on kidney stones, visit the website of the National Kidney and Urologic Diseases Information Clearinghouse, *http://kidney.niddk.nih.gov/kudiseases/pubs/stones_ez/*.

Poo in a Pill to Treat Gut Infection

Thomas Louie, MD, professor, medicine, University of Calgary, Alberta.

Thomas Moore, MD, clinical professor, medicine, University of Kansas.

IDWeek conference, San Francisco, presentation.

Researchers report they have found a more palatable way to deliver a decidedly unappealing treatment that can cure a potentially deadly intestinal infection.

Until now, the transplantation of healthy fecal bacteria into a patient's gut to tackle Clostridium difficile infections could only be done one of three ways: With an enema; a colonoscopy (placing a tube in the colon); or via a tube snaked through the nose and down the throat. But Canadian scientists have created capsules containing a concentrate of fecal bacteria that can simply be swallowed by the patient.

"It's much more palatable for patients," said Tom Moore, MD, a clinical professor of medicine at the University of Kansas, who was not involved with the study. "It takes a lot of the 'ick factor' out."

Even better, the capsules stopped recurring bouts of C. difficile, the Canadian researchers discovered. They reported their findings at IDWeek 2013, the infectious diseases society conference in San Francisco.

BACKGROUND ON C. DIFFICILE

A reliable cure for C. difficile is in high demand. The U.S. Centers for Disease Control and Prevention (CDC) recently named the harmful bacteria one of the three most urgent health threats caused by the rise of antibiotic-resistant microbes.

C. difficile itself is not antibiotic-resistant, but it gains a foothold in the gut when healthy intestinal flora are decimated by strong antibiotics used to overcome the resistance of other bacteria.

Once active, C. difficile causes severe diarrhea in already weakened patients. About 250,000 people in the United States suffer from C. difficile infections every year and about 14,000 die, according to the CDC.

HOW TO MAKE FECAL PILLS

Doctors crafted the capsules by running healthy stool through a sieve, and then using a centrifuge to separate out the fecal bacteria and "discard everything but the bug," said study author Thomas Louie, MD, a professor of medicine at the University of Calgary, in Alberta.

The remaining fecal bacteria resembles off-white river clay, Dr. Louie said. It is scooped into a gelatin capsule, which is then placed inside two other layers of gelatin capsule to ensure that the bacteria will make it through the stomach to reach the colon.

RESEARCH DETAILS

The researchers provided the pills to 27 patients with C. difficile and reported a 100% success rate. None of the patients had a recurrence of the infection, even though all of them previously had had repeat bouts with the germ. Patients ingested between 24 and 34 capsules containing fecal bacteria, often donated by family members.

AN EXPERT ELABORATES

Dr. Moore compared fighting C. difficile with fecal bacteria to restoring a lawn that has become infested with weeds.

C. difficile can be destroyed using antibiotics, much like using herbicides to get rid of the weeds, but that does nothing to restore the "lawn" within the gut to proper balance.

Alternatively, one can choose to reseed the lawn with fresh grass seed and hope the new grass crowds out the weeds. In the case of C. difficile, probiotics can sometimes boost healthy intestinal flora that crowd out the bad bug, Dr. Moore explained.

Fecal transplantation is more akin to planting fresh sod across the entire lawn, he suggested.

"This study confirms what has been suspected for quite some time, that fecal transplants are the most effective and most efficient way to restore gut health in patients with recurrent C. diff," Dr. Moore said.

Further, he believes using capsules will make the process much easier for people.

Dr. Moore said he sees no reason why doctors can't begin using handmade fecal bacteria capsules to treat C. difficile, particularly since the U.S. Food and Drug Administration has lifted a moratorium it had placed on the practice.

info For more information on C. difficile, visit the website of the U.S. Centers for Disease Control and Prevention at *http://www.cdc.gov/HAI/organisms/cdiff/Cdiff_infect.html.*

Emotional Well-Being

The Color That Prevents Mistakes—and Other Surprising Forces That Shape Your Thinking

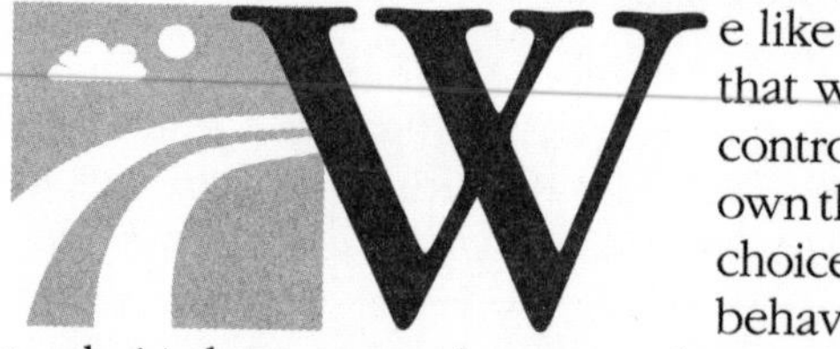

We like to think that we are in control of our own thoughts, choices and behavior. The truth is that external cues and triggers shape many of our decisions and actions.

We can avoid potential problems and improve our success and well-being by recognizing how we are influenced by these forces—and how we can compensate for them.

Here, some of the ways subtle cues shape us...

• **Color affects creativity.** Brain scans show that seeing the color red activates a part of the brain associated with avoiding failure. This avoidant mind-set promotes caution and vigilance but works against creativity and insight, which require openness to new experiences.

It doesn't take a lot of color to have this effect. In one study, students proofreading text against a red background were far more vigilant and accurate than when the text had a blue background. On tasks that required creativity, the presence of red was associated with poorer performance.

The explanation may be a combination of culture and biology. We associate red with danger—stop signs, fires and blood—while blue is associated with calming images such as a cloudless sky. Red signals that something is amiss, leading us to focus on preventing something bad. Blue makes us feel safe, suggesting that it's OK to relax our focus and explore the unknown.

How to use this information: Don't paint the walls of your work area red or blue—you

Adam Alter, PhD, assistant professor of marketing at the Stern School of Business, New York University, New York City. He has been featured on PBS, BBC and other media and is author of *Drunk Tank Pink—and Other Unexpected Forces That Shape How We Think, Feel, and Behave* (Penguin).

need to shift between creativity and vigilance to be effective. Keep a red book or a piece of red paper visible when you need to do detail-oriented work, such as checking numbers or proofreading. Put the red away, and keep a blue surface visible when you want to think more creatively.

•**Eyes make you more ethical.** People behave more honestly when they know someone is watching, but they also are more honest when all they see is an image that reminds them of being observed. Researchers at Newcastle University in England found that cash contributions to the office coffee "honor box" increased dramatically when a picture of a pair of eyes was posted over the box. Other studies have found that people are less likely to cheat on a task, and more likely to treat companions fairly, when they can see themselves in a mirror.

The sense that someone is looking at us—or that we're looking at ourselves—seems to create social pressure that makes us think twice about acting on unethical impulses.

How to use this information: Reduce minor infractions at work by placing a mirror or a picture of eyes at the site of the problem.

Example: Attach a picture of eyes or a mirror to the front of an office-supply cabinet to discourage people from taking supplies home for personal use.

You also can use a mirror to encourage yourself to live up to your own commitments.

Example: If you are dieting and trying to cut back on snacks, put a mirror on the refrigerator door.

•**A little nature makes a big difference.** We all know that nature can be restorative, but even a little exposure has a powerful effect on stress and physical health. Dutch researchers found that people who had just viewed a gruesome, upsetting video, followed by a seven-minute video depicting a walk through a forest, were happier and more relaxed than people whose second video showed an urban stroll. The forest-video group also performed better on a challenging mental task.

In a Pennsylvania study, patients who had gallbladder surgery recovered more quickly and experienced less pain if their hospital rooms faced a small stand of trees rather than a brick wall.

New Treatment for Alcoholism

The drug *gabapentin*, which has been approved for treating seizures and neuropathic pain, may help alcoholics cut down or quit drinking. It is not metabolized by the liver—which often is damaged by alcohol abuse—and has no evidence of abuse potential. Ask your doctor for details on when its use might be appropriate.

Barbara J. Mason, PhD, is codirector of Pearson Center for Alcoholism and Addiction Research, The Scripps Research Institute, La Jolla, California. She led a study published online in *JAMA Internal Medicine*.

Why does the sight of nature—even in a video or through a window—reduce stress, improve concentration and speed physical recovery? One plausible theory—called attention restoration theory—holds that urban environments drain us by aggressively directing our attention to demanding tasks, such as dodging pedestrians and traffic. Natural landscapes also capture our attention but in an undemanding way. We can enjoy sights such as a bird alighting on a tree without feeling compelled to do anything about them. This undirected attention is deeply replenishing.

How to use this information: Spend time in greenery every day. If you live in a city, bring natural elements into your home, such as potted plants or a small fountain. Although pictures of nature are pleasant to look at, they are less effective than actual plants or water. The random changes in natural objects, such as movement of water or leaves, is part of what captures the restorative, undemanding type of attention.

•**A hard-to-pronounce name can hinder your success.** When two colleagues and I analyzed names of lawyers at American law firms, we found that lawyers with easy-to-pronounce names became partners more quickly than people with complex names. Having a simple name may help others feel familiar and comfortable with you, building trust more quickly. It also is likely that when a name is hard to pronounce, people say it somewhat less often, leading to fewer recommendations and introductions that could pave the way to advancement.

How to use this information: If your name is unusual, help others become comfortable with it quickly by saying, "It rhymes with..." or comparing it to something familiar.

Example: "Zajonc sounds like science, but starts with a Z."

Also, look for opportunities to repeat your name more often than you naturally would so that people get used to hearing it. Repetition will make the name seem simpler and encourage others to use it.

• **Having an audience improves your performance...**but only on certain tasks. Many competitive cyclists and runners perform faster in front of a crowd. In a study of pool players, experienced players made more shots when a group of people watched. However, novice pool players did worse in front of others...and people learning a maze struggled more in front of an audience than people learning the maze alone.

Having an audience seems to exaggerate a person's dominant instinctive response, so an experienced runner will run faster in the presence of an audience. But if your dominant response to a situation is uncertainty or anxiety, or if you need to draw on mental resources, thinking about the audience can overload you, depleting those resources and draining motivation.

How to use this information: Think about your confidence in performing a task and about the type of resources needed. Then determine when the presence of others would be helpful.

Example: In brainstorming, contrary to popular opinion, people don't come up with their best ideas in a group. The pressure of being around others and potentially being judged by them uses up mental energy and constrains thinking. Have people generate ideas on their own at first, then get the group together to build on those ideas. At that point, the stimulation of being in a group will help new ideas grow from existing ones.

Feel-Good Strategies for Life's Disappointments

Guy Winch, PhD, a clinical psychologist in private practice in New York City. He is author of *Emotional First Aid: Practical Strategies for Treating Failure, Rejection, Guilt, and Other Everday Psychological Injuries* (Hudson Street). *GuyWinch.com*

We try to shrug off the little things that make us feel bad. We tell ourselves it doesn't matter that we were snubbed by a neighbor. We reason that it's no big deal that our plan to get new customers failed. We reassure ourselves that our feelings of loneliness after retirement will pass. But recent research suggests that minor emotional challenges such as these can lead to major mental-health issues when left unaddressed.

Example: A study published last year in *Psychological Science* found that the more minor daily emotional stresses participants reported, the more likely they were to suffer from other serious psychological disorders such as depression 10 years later.

Minor emotional challenges are the psychological equivalent of cuts and scrapes. They don't require surgery, but a little basic first aid will reduce the odds that they will become infected.

Effective first-aid strategies for three common emotional challenges...

REJECTION

Even minor rejections can wound us far deeper than logic suggests they should.

Example: A study published in *Annual Review of Psychology* found that people feel significant emotional pain when a pair of strangers who are throwing a ball back and forth fail to include them in the game, a rejection of seemingly no consequence. Remarkably, this emotional pain persists even after study subjects are told that the rejection is not real—the ballplayers were instructed to leave them out of the game as part of the experiment.

The hurt we feel when we're rejected is very real—the brain pathways that react to rejection are the same ones that react to physical pain. In fact, pain and rejection seem so similar to our brains that taking Tylenol temporarily eases the sting of rejection. The reason rejection affects us so deeply is probably evolutionary—early humans could not survive if they were rejected by their social group. *To recover from rejection, here's a three-step plan...*

1. Assume it's them. When people end romantic relationships, they sometimes say, "It's not you, it's me." This may be a cliché—but it's also an important distinction. When you feel rejected, go ahead and tell yourself that it really is the person doing the rejecting who has mishandled the situation, not you. That won't eliminate the sting of the rejection, but it should reduce the odds that you will fall into a downward spiral of self-criticism.

2. Focus on aspects of yourself that you deeply value. Take some time to think about this, and pay special attention to talents and attributes related to the aspect of your life where the rejection occurred—your key professional skills if the rejection was career-related, for example.

Once you've identified several characteristics, choose one and write a brief essay on why it's important to you. We are more convinced by things we write than by things we think, because writing activates additional parts of the brain.

3. Spend time around people who understand your worth. Being around people who value us can effectively counter the sting of rejection.

Example: If you have a falling-out with a friend, have lunch with another friend who cares about you.

LONELINESS

Surveys suggest that 40% of us will feel lonely at some point in our adult lives. Loneliness is particularly common when we leave our parents' home as young adults and when we retire and no longer have workplace relationships.

Loneliness can become a downward spiral. Lonely people often come off as desperate or defensive, reducing the odds that the people they meet will want to spend time with them. *A three-step plan for coping with loneliness...*

1. Figure out what you're doing that's keeping other people away from you (or keeping you away from other people). Lonely people tend to become defensive when it's suggested that they are partially to blame for their loneliness. But if they accept this as true, they usually can identify and correct some aspect of their behavior that's limiting their ability to form relationships.

Example: Lonely people often convince themselves that they cannot join existing conversations at social functions, even though doing so usually is perfectly acceptable. Just say, "Excuse me, I don't know anyone here. Is it OK if I join your group?" You will almost always be welcomed in. Outright social rejections at social gatherings occur among teens, but they're very rare among adults.

2. Replace "it's not worth going" pessimism with "any connection is a good thing" optimism. Lonely people often conclude that it's not worth going out to meet people because previous attempts to make new friends have failed. But while the odds are low that on any particular outing you will meet a lifelong friend or future spouse, there's a good chance that you could make a connection or have a conversation—and a single conversation will make a big difference to your emotional state if you have been feeling lonely.

3. Deepen existing relationships. The best cure for loneliness isn't more relationships, it's deeper relationships. Even very lonely people usually have some social connections—perhaps a distant relative or an old friend they have barely spoken with in years. Search your address book for people such as these, then make an effort to stay in closer contact with them.

Helpful: The best way to deepen relationships is to make a conscious effort to see things from the other person's perspective and empathize with him/her.

FAILURE

It isn't just the big, life-altering failures that affect us. If we're not careful, small failures can undermine our confidence and optimism, too. *A three-part strategy for overcoming the pain of minor failures...*

1. Blame your goal-setting strategy, not your abilities. People often take on big projects and set themselves tight deadlines—then blame their skills when they fall short. Instead, set a series of smaller, incremental, achievable goals. You're likely to reach at least some of these incremental targets, easing any feelings of failure if others are missed.

Example: Rather than try to lose 30 pounds in three months, try to lose one pound a week for 30 weeks.

2. Focus on factors within your control. Failing can make you feel helpless, as though you have tried your best and don't know what else you can do. Such feelings can damage your motivation when making future efforts or make you give up entirely. The best thing to do is to focus on factors within your control.

Example: You exhausted your contacts, you're out of leads, and you still haven't found a new job. Focus on the interim goal of expanding your contacts and professional network. Send a quick message to your Facebook friends and other social-media contacts asking if they know people in your field...and/or join relevant LinkedIn groups.

3. Learn the simple trick that could keep you from choking next time. Let's say a bowler makes nine strikes in a row, then rolls a gutter ball on the tenth. What happened? He choked—he became so anxious that he overthought something that didn't require much thought at all. Everyone chokes on occasion. Trouble is, once we've choked, we might start to worry that we'll do so again, undermining our confidence.

There's a simple way to reduce the odds of choking—whistle. This works best when playing sports but can come in handy at other times, too. Whistling requires just enough brainpower to distract the part of our mind that might otherwise overthink things. If you're bowling, start humming or whistling a tune (softly) as you pick up the bowling ball, and continue whistling until the ball is rolling toward the pins.

Love Your Way to Better Health

Barbara L. Fredrickson, PhD, professor of psychology and director of the Positive Emotions and Psychophysiology Laboratory at the University of North Carolina, Chapel Hill. She is author of *Love 2.0: How Our Supreme Emotion Affects Everything We Feel, Think, Do, and Become* (Plume).

Ask people how they stay healthy, and you are likely to hear a lot about eating well... exercising...getting enough sleep...etc.

But loving more? This isn't likely to appear high on the list for even the most health-conscious people.

A shocking risk to your health: Your doctor probably won't bring it up at your next checkup, but not having enough love in your life—and we don't mean sex, but any kind of love—can be as hazardous to your health as well-known risk factors such as smoking, obesity and a sedentary lifestyle, according to a recent analysis of more than 300,000 people.

Anyone can bring more love into his/her life. I'll tell you how. *But first, here's how love can improve your health...*

GOOD FOR YOUR BODY

While love has long been known to promote emotional well-being, researchers have begun to uncover some of the actual physiological effects that can result in improved physical health. *For example...*

•**Heart health improves.** The expression and/or receipt of love has been linked to increased activity of the vagus nerve, which runs from the brain, through the face and neck to the

Check Your Night-Light If You're Feeling Blue

Animals exposed to blue light at night are more likely to have depression-like symptoms than those exposed to red light—and both fare worse than those exposed to no light.

The Journal of Neuroscience

chest and abdomen. This nerve calms the heart and steadies its rhythm as you breathe.

Recent scientific evidence: When people habitually practice an exercise to increase the number of "loving moments" in their lives, their vagus nerves function at a higher level, and their cardiovascular health improves. Improved vagal tone also promotes better regulation of glucose and immunity.

•**Antistress hormones rise.** Each person's levels of oxytocin, the hormone linked to trust and attachment, tend to go up.

A NEW WAY OF LOVING

Your capacity for love is like a muscle—whether it grows or shrinks depends on how much exercise it gets. However, most people are too restrictive in the way they think about love. It's reserved primarily for, say, a romantic partner, a parent, child or longtime friend.

The fact is, however, the same elements of love that bring about positive physiological changes (so-called "micromoments of connection") can be present with a casual acquaintance, a coworker or a barista at your favorite coffee shop. During these moments, it's typical for your eyes to meet as you exchange pleasantries, you each may smile, your gestures are likely to mirror one another's and you may even echo each other's words.

While it's true that the connections you have with acquaintances are not as deep as those you may have with family members, research shows that the frequency of these encounters has more effect on one's well-being than the intensity.

LEARNING TO LOVE

Fortunately, you can have a loving moment in just about any reasonably relaxed, safe setting where feelings can be freely exchanged. While eye contact isn't absolutely necessary—tone of voice, even over the phone, can convey a lot of feeling—face-to-face encounters are the most likely triggers.

The potentially bad news is that real-time conversation, especially in person, is going out of style—texting, e-mails and social media make such moments of real connection increasingly rare.

Green Tea May Fight Depression

People who drank two to three cups of green tea daily were about 40% less likely to report feeling depressed than those who drank one cup a day or less.

Possible reason: Antioxidants in green tea may help reduce levels of cortisol, a stress hormone associated with depression. Fresh-brewed green tea delivers more antioxidants than bottled tea.

Studies of green tea by researchers at Tohoku University, Sendai, Japan, published in *The American Journal of Clinical Nutrition*, and Rutgers University, New Brunswick, New Jersey, published in Cancer *Epidemiology, Biomarkers & Prevention.*

To reap the benefits of more love, you will have to pay less attention to your cell phone—Love Enemy No. 1—and more to the person you are riding with on the elevator!

Getting started: Just becoming aware of the possibility of connection is a major step forward.

Try this: Each night for several weeks, set aside a few minutes to review your day and consider encounters and interactions you had with others.

Focus on the three longest and ask yourself: Did I feel "in tune" with the other person? Did I feel a closeness to him/her? Rate these statements from 1 (not true at all) to 7 (very true). Record your self-ratings in a notebook or computer file.

Researchers were surprised to discover that when study participants simply kept track of these encounters, without trying to change how they behaved or felt, their positive emotions and feelings of connection with others significantly increased and their vagal tone also improved. The nightly exercise may have served as a reminder during the day so that people were more open to the possibility of positive, loving connections with others.

Going a step further: For a more active approach, make it your intention to connect more fully with three people in the course of each day. You can't force such moments to happen, but you can slow down, forget your to-do list momentarily, pay attention to those you meet and look for opportunities to share positive feelings.

In any situation where it seems natural, smile, make eye contact and really listen to the other person. Try to think of his good qualities and offer a favor if appropriate.

Even better: Meditation, which provides its own health benefits, prepares you for such loving encounters (see below).

HOW TO MEDITATE FOR LOVE

A type of meditation known as "loving-kindness" strengthens your capacity for positive connections with others...

What to do: Sit comfortably in an upright, relaxed position that allows you to breathe deeply. Bring your attention to the region of your heart. Think of someone for whom you already have warm and compassionate feelings—your spouse, a child, a parent or a beloved friend. Visualize that individual's face, bringing his/her best qualities to mind.

Take a few minutes to slowly repeat to yourself phrases of goodwill...

- **May (this person) feel safe.**
- **May (he/she) be happy.**
- **May (he/she) feel healthy.**
- **May (he/she) live with ease.**

Sit for a moment with these warm feelings. Then imagine someone else in your circle of friends, and go through the same process. When you feel ready, extend the practice to other people with whom you share a connection—no matter how slight. End your meditation by reminding yourself that you can generate such feelings anytime, anywhere.

Research has shown that just 60 minutes of this practice a week can provide the health benefits described above as well as more happiness in daily life. While you're likely to get the most benefit from daily meditation, doing so for 15 to 20 minutes three to five times a week will also be extremely helpful.

Do You Really Need an Antidepressant?—Don't Bury Important Emotions

Michael D. Banov, MD, medical director of Northwest Behavioral Medicine and Northwest Behavioral Research Center, both in Atlanta. He is author of *Taking Antidepressants: Your Comprehensive Guide to Starting, Staying On, and Safely Quitting* (Sunrise River).

The statistics are truly shocking—more than one out of every 10 Americans takes an antidepressant. That includes nearly 4% of all adolescents (ages 12 to 17) and more than 20% of women ages 40 to 59.

Use of antidepressants is controversial. Some people believe that they're extremely dangerous...some think they are little more than overused "happy pills"...and others insist that these medications are literally lifesaving for people who suffer from depression.

WHAT'S THE TRUTH?

How does one decide whether to take an antidepressant? Whether or not to take an antidepressant is a personal decision. There are many forms of depression and no diagnostic test to tell when an antidepressant is "absolutely necessary."

But there are a number of basic clues. How well are you functioning? Perhaps you've lost your job or someone close to you has died, and you're very sad about it. But if you still get up each morning, go to work (or look for work), see friends, do what needs to be done, you may not benefit from an antidepressant. In fact, medication may have a negative effect, masking normal emotions and the grieving process. Mild-to-moderate depression, such as this, often responds well to psychotherapy alone—without the use of medication. But even in these cases, you may want to try an antidepressant if you and your doctor believe that you could benefit.

With more severe depression—for example, you are not eating or sleeping...you're not getting out of bed—it's usually more clear-cut that you need medication. Also, if you have a family history of depression...have been depressed a number of times before...or if depression first started when you were an adolescent or younger, this indicates that your depression is biochemical in nature—that is, there may be a shortage of certain mood-regulating neurotransmitters or a dysfunction in how neurons respond to them. With biochemical depression, medication is typically an important part of treatment.

BEST ALTERNATIVES TO DRUGS

Some people prefer to avoid medication if at all possible. What are the best alternatives to antidepressants? Psychotherapy helps. Just be sure to choose one of the types shown to work for depression, such as cognitive behavioral therapy (which addresses self-destructive thinking and behavior) or interpersonal psychotherapy (which focuses on patterns in relationships that promote depression). This may also be a good first step with children and adolescents because the evidence that antidepressants work isn't as strong for them, and the possible side effects, such as increased risk for suicide, are greater.

Some people also have found natural remedies such as the herb St. John's wort, omega-3 fatty acids or SAMe to be helpful. *L-methylfolate* (Deplin), a prescription compound related to the B-vitamin folic acid, is the newest addition to the "natural antidepressant" roster. Some people are unable to convert folic acid, which is found in food and dietary supplements, to methylfolate, which appears to help regulate mood.

If you try any of these treatments, just be sure to do it under the supervision of a psychiatrist who is knowledgeable about natural medicine and mental health. Above all, do not let depression go untreated, and be ready to reconsider antidepressants if other methods don't work or your symptoms worsen within four to six weeks.

Moderate Drinking Guards Against Depression

People who drank two to seven small glasses of wine each week were 30% less likely to develop depression than nondrinkers.

Possible reason: A compound found in grapes helps protect parts of the brain from inflammation that is linked to depression.

Study of more than 5,500 people ages 55 to 80 led by researchers at University of Navarra, Pamplona, Spain, published online in *BMC Medicine*.

ANTIDEPRESSANTS ARE NOT MAGIC BULLETS

Even if an antidepressant corrects biochemistry, lifestyle adjustments and sometimes psychotherapy are critical for recovery. Lifestyle changes help alleviate symptoms as they do for other medical conditions such as heart disease.

Regular exercise is also important. It can be as effective as antidepressants for some people with mild depression. In addition, take time for activities you enjoy, reach out to friends, get enough sleep, control stress, eat properly and if you drink alcohol, do so only in moderation.

Does a family doctor have the expertise to prescribe an antidepressant effectively, or should a depressed individual see a psychiatrist or other mental-health professional? Most antidepressant prescriptions are written by primary care physicians (such as a family doctor, internist, pediatrician or ob-gyn), and there's nothing wrong with this if he/she has stayed up-to-date on the use of these medications through reading medical literature and/or taking classes.

But not all doctors, competent as they may be in other areas, are expert in diagnosing depression and knowing when to prescribe an antidepressant, how to deal with side effects, and when to adjust the dose, switch or add drugs. Far too often, nonspecialists are familiar with only three or four antidepressants, among the roughly 50 that are available, making it hard to get the best one for you.

Besides psychiatrists, certain clinical nurse specialists or nurse practitioners have advanced training in psychiatry and are proficient in prescribing antidepressants. Check with your mental-health insurance provider to find a referral.

CAN ANTIDEPRESSANTS DAMAGE YOUR BRAIN?

There's been no evidence of long-term detrimental effects on the brain. But, of course, there are no guarantees...issues with some medications have come to light only after years of use.

On the other hand, we do know that untreated depression can damage the brain. Imaging studies show that areas such as the hippocampus

Midlife Stress Linked to Late-Life Dementia

Among 800 women tracked for nearly 40 years, those who experienced significant stress (divorce, widowhood, loss of a child or mental illness in a loved one) were 21% more likely to develop Alzheimer's disease.

Why: Stress may cause structural and functional changes in the brain, which may linger for years after a stressful event.

If you're facing midlife stress: Try psychotherapy, meditation and/or yoga.

Lena Johansson, PhD, researcher, University of Gothenburg, Mölndal, Sweden.

actually shrink, which can cause severe memory and thinking problems. The more severe your depression and the longer it goes untreated, the worse and more lasting these deleterious changes are likely to be. So the goal should be to take an antidepressant as long as necessary—but no longer.

WHEN AND HOW TO STOP TAKING ANTIDEPRESSANTS

How do you know whether it's time to stop taking an antidepressant? Generally, six to 12 months of medication are sufficient for a first episode of depression. If this is your second episode, longer may be better. And after three or more episodes, research shows that it may be advisable to stay on an antidepressant indefinitely.

In any case, you should not stop until you are no longer depressed (the more residual symptoms you have, the more likely it is that depression will come back)...your physical health is good (or any chronic medical condition is being controlled)...and you're maintaining a healthy lifestyle. If you are under unusual stress at work or at home, have recently dealt with a loss, like a death in the family, or you are drinking more than moderately, consider waiting.

Some people have trouble stopping antidepressants. "Discontinuation syndrome" bothers about 20% of people when they stop antidepressants, probably due to a drop in the neurotransmitter *serotonin* or *norepinephrine*. It's not true withdrawal, because your body isn't dependent on these medications as it might be with narcotics and other drugs that can be abused.

Discontinuation problems include flulike symptoms, fatigue, unusual sensations (like pins and needles in hands or feet) or anxiety. In most people, they are relatively mild and go away within a week, but they may last up to a month or two.

To minimize discontinuation problems, taper the dose slowly under the guidance of your doctor. If you are particularly sensitive, the process may take up to six weeks.

Sometimes it helps to switch from a drug that leaves the body very quickly, such as *paroxetine* (Paxil) or *venlafaxine* (Effexor), to one that is naturally eliminated slowly, like *fluoxetine* (Prozac). Or switch to a liquid formulation (if one is available for your drug) or have the druggist compound very small doses—both approaches allow you to slow the tapering process. Antidepressants available in liquid form include Prozac, Lexapro, Celexa, Zoloft and Paxil.

If a Loved One Has Vision Loss, Be on the Lookout for Depression

Xinzhi Zhang, MD, PhD, senior epidemiologist, National Institute on Minority Health and Health Disparities, National Institutes of Health, Bethesda, Maryland.

Among 10,500 adults (average age 47), the rate of clinical depression among those with vision loss was 11.3%, compared with 4.8% for those with good eyesight. Depression was significantly higher in those with chronic conditions, such as macular degeneration, glaucoma and cataracts, and whose poor vision kept them from everyday activities, such as reading the newspaper, watching television and driving.

If your loved one has vision loss: Encourage him/her to be screened for depression if symptoms develop.

What You Eat and Drink Can Negatively Affect Your Mood

Mind, Mood & Memory

Trans fats, alcohol and too much sugar can make you sad and anxious. Replace sugary beverages with water or unsweetened drinks...processed foods with natural foods such as fruits, vegetables, nuts and fish...and simple carbohydrates (such as table sugar and white bread) with complex carbohydrates, such as whole-grain breads, pastas and cereals. Drink no more than two caffeinated drinks a day. Increase your healthy fat intake with olive, canola and vegetable oils, fish, avocado, flaxseeds and nuts.

Risk of Depression May Rise With Too Much or Too Little Sleep

Sleep, news release
Nathaniel Watson, MD, associate professor of neurology and codirector of the University of Washington Medicine Sleep Center, Seattle.
Robert Roberts, PhD, professor of behavioral sciences, School of Public Health, University of Texas Health Science Center, Houston.
M. Safwan Badr, MD, president of the American Academy of Sleep Medicine, Darien, Illinois.

Too much or too little sleep can increase the risk of depression, according to two recent studies.

Inappropriate amounts of sleep may activate depression-related genes, researchers report in the journal *Sleep*.

STUDY #1

One study included more than 1,700 adult twins. Among those who got normal amounts of sleep (seven to nearly nine hours a night), the genetic influence on symptoms of depression was 27% versus 53% for those who slept only five hours a night, and 49% among those who slept 10 hours a night.

"Both short and excessively long sleep durations appear to activate genes related to depressive symptoms," said lead investigator Nathaniel Watson, MD, an associate professor of neurology and codirector of the University of Washington Medicine Sleep Center in Seattle.

Ensuring that patients get optimum levels of sleep may be one way to boost the effectiveness of treatments for depression, he added.

STUDY #2

The second study included more than 4,100 youngsters aged 11 to 17. It found that sleeping six hours or less per night increased their risk for major depression, which in turn increased their risk for too little sleep.

"These results are important because they suggest that sleep deprivation may be a precursor for major depression in adolescents, occurring before other symptoms of major depression and additional mood disorders," said principal investigator Robert Roberts, PhD, professor of behavioral sciences in the School of Public Health at the University of Texas Health Science Center in Houston.

"Questions on sleep disturbance and hours of sleep should be part of the medical history of adolescents to ascertain risk," he added.

EXPERT COMMENTARY

"Healthy sleep is a necessity for physical, mental and emotional well-being," according to M. Safwan Badr, MD, president of the American Academy of Sleep Medicine, based in Darien, Illinois. "This new research emphasizes that we can make an investment in our health by prioritizing sleep."

info For more information about sleep, visit the website of the U.S. National Institute of Neurological Disorders and Stroke, *www.ninds.nih.gov*, and search "Understanding sleep."

Don't Suffer with OCD—This Unique Treatment Can Help

James Greenblatt, MD, an integrative psychiatrist board-certified in child and adult psychiatry. He is founder and medical director of Comprehensive Psychiatric Resources in Waltham, Massachusetts, and a clinical faculty member in the department of psychiatry at Tufts University School of Medicine in Boston. *IntegrativePsychMD.com*

You wash your hands so often that they're red and raw. Perhaps you repeatedly rearrange the food in your kitchen cabinets so that all items are facing a certain way.

Or you may check over and over again to make sure that your front door is locked. Perhaps you hoard newspapers and other everyday objects until your house is filled with junk—or count to yourself whenever you drive through a stoplight.

If you or someone you know experiences these or similar symptoms, it could be a red flag for obsessive-compulsive disorder (OCD).

WHAT IS OCD?

Obsessive-compulsive disorder (OCD) is a psychiatric illness that affects more than two million Americans.

The condition is characterized by repetitive, upsetting thoughts (obsessions) and an overwhelming urge to perform behaviors or rituals (compulsions) to help alleviate related anxiety. The cause is unknown, but genetics may play a role.

Inside the mind of an OCD sufferer: People with this disorder have disturbing, unwanted thoughts, such as the belief that they are contaminated by germs or are about to be in a horrible car crash. These obsessive thoughts cause intense anxiety that the sufferer attempts to ease with compulsive behaviors (or rituals) such as repeated hand-washing or counting in unusual patterns.

Suffering in silence: For people who have never experienced OCD, the symptoms seem entirely irrational. The irony is, even those who have the disorder know that their thoughts and behaviors are irrational but, for unknown reasons, they just can't stop them. As a result, people with OCD are usually ashamed of their symptoms and often go to great lengths to hide them from their friends, family or doctor. Unfortunately, more than half of Americans with this disorder never receive treatment.

Even when a person with OCD sees a doctor for it, the condition is very difficult to treat. The conventional approach—usually, an antidepressant and psychological counseling called cognitive behavioral therapy—reduces the severity of symptoms by about 50%, according to research, but achieves complete recovery in only 20% of cases.

New approach: A technique called integrative psychiatry—using conventional treatments and natural therapies such as nutritional supplements—is likely to produce far better results than conventional treatment alone. *Best approaches...*

SEROTONIN BOOSTERS

Serotonin is a neurotransmitter (brain chemical) that plays a key role in regulating mood, appetite and sleep. Low levels of serotonin are believed to be a contributing cause of OCD. Many factors can reduce serotonin. For example, it's thought that serotonin levels can be lowered by a diet high in processed foods, sugar and fat...stress...and chronic inflammation.

Selective serotonin reuptake inhibitor (SSRI) antidepressants help OCD by blocking the absorption of serotonin in the brain, which keeps levels in the body higher. Medication is quite helpful for some OCD patients, while others find that it increases their obsessive thinking.

Best Bedtime Snack for Better Sleep...

Peanut butter on toast...or a small serving of fruit and yogurt.

Reason: The protein in these snacks contains the amino acid tryptophan. The carbohydrates make tryptophan more available to your brain, where the relaxation neurotransmitter serotonin is produced.

Tasneem Bhatia, MD, medical director and founder, Atlanta Center for Holistic & Integrative Medicine, writing in *Prevention*.

The integrative approach: Several nutritional supplements boost serotonin and thereby help reduce or eliminate OCD symptoms.

Work with your doctor to determine which of the following supplements (one or more may be recommended) would be the most useful for you. To find an integrative doctor near you, go to *www.IntegrativeMedicineforMentalHealth.com.*

HELPFUL SUPPLEMENTS...*

•Vitamin B-12. A deficiency of this serotonin-boosting B vitamin is common in people with OCD. If you have this disorder, your doctor should test your blood levels of vitamin B-12.

My advice: Most conventional doctors consider blood levels of 200 pg/mL to 1,100 pg/mL to be "normal," but I treat any patient with a level below 500 pg/mL with weekly B-12 injections until his/her blood level reaches 900 pg/mL. B-12 is also available in sublingual and liquid forms. Some patients have a dramatic decrease in OCD symptoms with this treatment alone.

•Folate. This B vitamin is also crucial for serotonin production and can boost the effectiveness of antidepressants. However, some OCD patients can't absorb folate properly due to a genetic abnormality.

My advice: For patients with OCD, I typically recommend having an MTHFR test (methylenetetrahydrofolate reductase mutations) to check for the enzymes that are necessary to process folate. If the test is positive, you may need to take 7.5 mg to 15 mg daily of a medication called *L-methylfolate* (Deplin) that supplies a high dose of the nutrient.

•Omega-3s. The brain is nearly 60% fat. To work optimally, it needs healthful fats such as the omega-3 fatty acids EPA and DHA found in fish oil. Omega-3s can be obtained by eating fatty fish two or three times a week, but I have found that OCD patients often have an aversion to fish.

My advice: Try a daily supplement containing 3 g of omega-3 fatty acids with an EPA to DHA ratio of 2:1.

*Check with your doctor before trying these or any other nutritional supplements. Some may interact with prescription medications or affect medical conditions.

Try This "Psychobiotic"

Probiotic foods containing healthy gut bacteria, such as yogurt, were recently found in a meta-analysis to help alleviate chronic fatigue, depression and other mood disorders.

Theory: "Good" bacteria help produce serotonin and other beneficial brain chemicals. Researchers are still studying exactly how much yogurt you need to get these benefits.

Ted Dinan, MD, PhD, professor of psychiatry, University College Cork, Ireland.

•5-HTP (5-hydroxytryptophan) is a compound that boosts serotonin levels.

My advice: I typically recommend a daily dose of 100 mg to 300 mg of 5-HTP for OCD sufferers.

Important: Serotonin syndrome is a potentially dangerous condition (with agitation, rapid heart rate, blood pressure fluctuations and hot flashes) that can develop when patients take 5-HTP in addition to some painkillers and cough medicines. 5-HTP should not be used with an antidepressant unless the patient is under the guidance of a medical professional.

•Inositol. In some OCD patients, supplementing with inositol (a vitamin-like compound that plays a role in serotonin receptors on cells) improves symptoms of the condition dramatically.

My advice: I typically have OCD patients start with 1 g to 3 g a day and increase slowly to 10 g to 12 g daily. The dose should be divided so it's taken two to three times a day. (Taking too much inositol too quickly can cause digestive trouble.)

SLOW DOWN THE INFLAMMATION

Inflammation anywhere in the body disrupts serotonin metabolism—and people with OCD are often in a state of chronic, low-grade inflammation.

To reduce chronic inflammation...

•Get enough vitamin D. Ask your doctor to test you for vitamin D deficiency (which I define as a blood level below 30 ng/mL). If you're deficient, take 2,000 international units (IU) to

4,000 IU of vitamin D daily to reach the level recommended by your doctor.

•**Take magnesium.** This mineral is also thought to reduce inflammation. In addition, it's required to balance levels of the stress hormone cortisol. If you have OCD, ask your doctor if you should take a magnesium citrate or magnesium glycinate supplement.

Important: Don't take magnesium supplements if you have kidney disease, since you may not be able to excrete excess magnesium.

•**Get better sleep.** Treat insomnia with the basics—for example, go to bed at the same time every night and get up at the same time every morning, giving yourself at least seven hours in bed.

•**Reduce stress.** Stress not only causes inflammation but also worsens the symptoms of OCD. Reduce stress with mindfulness-based stress-reduction techniques, such as meditation, yoga, playing a musical instrument and/or exercise.

PROBIOTICS FOR OCD

The toxic gut bacteria Clostridia can generate HPHPA, a compound that disrupts normal brain function. High levels of HPHPA are a feature of many psychiatric diseases, including OCD. If OCD symptoms increase after use of an antifungal or antibiotic (both of which may allow HPHPA growth), ask your doctor about testing for HPHPA.

Your doctor can order a urine test for HPHPA from a lab that specializes in digestive disorders, such as the Great Plains Laboratory, *www.GreatPlainsLaboratory.com*, or Genova Diagnostics, *www.GDX.net*. If HPHPA is detected, consider trying high-dose probiotics that supply 50 billion to 300 billion CFUs (colony-forming units) daily. Consult your doctor for any additional treatment you may need.

Natural Remedy for Anxiety

The light, soothing fragrance of lavender oil has long been used in aromatherapy to ease anxiety and insomnia. You also can try a lavender oil supplement. For example, Calm Aid by Nature's Way contains Silexan, a type of lavender oil shown in clinical studies to ease anxiety as effectively as the benzodiazepine drug *lorazepam* (Ativan). Those who took the supplement also reported better sleep quality. I recommend taking one 80-mg softgel in the morning with a glass of water. Side effects are rare but can include nausea, constipation and headache. Check with your doctor before trying.

Holly Lucille, ND, RN, naturopathic doctor based in West Hollywood, California. *DrHollyLucille.com*

Tricks to Get Yourself to Meditate Daily

Sharon Salzberg, cofounder of the Insight Meditation Society in Barre, Massachusetts, and author of numerous books, including *Real Happiness: The Power of Meditation* and most recently *Real Happiness at Work* (both from Workman). *SharonSalzberg.com*

Can you count to 10? Of course you can, and that means you also can meditate. This is just one trick (see below) that can make meditation easier.

Studies show that daily meditation helps relieve high blood pressure, pain, insomnia, depression and more.

Latest research: When participants did a simple 20-minute meditation for eight weeks, beneficial genes, such as those involved in insulin function, were activated, while genes related to inflammation and cancer were suppressed.

But many of us just can't seem to make meditation part of our everyday routine—it seems so difficult to set aside the time...sit still...or quiet our minds. *Here are three easy ways to work meditation into your life now...*

•**5-minute meditation.**

What to do: Find the place where you feel the breath most clearly—nostrils, chest or abdomen—and bring your attention there. Take a normal breath without trying to change it. Repeat in sets of 10 (counting to yourself) for five minutes. If you take only three breaths before you start thinking about something else, bring your focus back to your breath. You don't need

Exercise May Prevent Job Burnout

According to a recent study, men who did better on a cycling fitness test were less likely to report feeling burned out by work than men with lower fitness scores.

Possible reason: Exercise can help refresh you mentally and—if done with other people—expand your social circle. Both effects may help protect against burnout.

Best: 30 minutes a day of moderate-to-intense activity.

Study by researchers in the department of psychology at University of Basel Institute for Sport and Sport Sciences, Switzerland, published in *BMC Research Notes.*

absolute quiet. You can do this in your doctor's waiting room or while walking the dog.

- **Single-task meditation.** Choose a simple activity you do often, like drinking a cup of tea, and pay close attention to the sensations that occur while doing it. Feel the heat of the mug in your hands, the warmth and aroma of the steam, and the taste of the liquid in your mouth. When your mind wanders, draw your attention back to the experience.

Other activities to try this with: Cooking, mowing the lawn or exercising.

- **"On cue" meditation.** With this type of meditation, you use cues in your environment to prompt you to focus and breathe. Let your phone ring three times before answering it. Use the sound of the phone as a reminder to be in the moment and take a few deep, relaxing breaths.

Other cues: Stopping at a red light or sitting down at your desk.

Do You Have Misophonia?

Michelle R. Berman, MD, editor of the medical information website *CelebrityDiagnosis.com.*

Extreme reactions to everyday noises could indicate a neurological disorder known as misophonia, literally "hatred of sound." Hearing a sound produces a fight-or-flight response resulting in extreme anger or high levels of anxiety. Misophonia usually begins at ages 10 to 12, and most often involves sounds connected with eating and breathing. The closer the person with misophonia is emotionally to the person producing the sound, the more he/she tends to react to the noise. Misophonia cannot be cured, but treatments are available—including habituation therapy, hypnosis, cognitive behavioral therapy and antianxiety medication.

Video Glasses May Ease the Anxiety of Minor Surgery

David Waldman, MD, PhD, chair, department of imaging sciences, University of Rochester Medical Center, Rochester, New York.

Society of Interventional Radiology, news release.

Wearing special video glasses while undergoing certain types of outpatient procedures may help reduce patients' anxiety, a recent study suggests.

"Whether they were watching a children's movie or a nature show, patients wearing video glasses were successful at tuning out their surroundings," said lead author David Waldman, MD, PhD, chair of the department of imaging sciences at the University of Rochester Medical Center in Rochester, New York.

"It's an effective distraction technique that helps focus the individual's attention away from the treatment," he added.

STUDY FINDINGS

The study included 33 men and 16 women, ages 18 to 87. They either underwent a biopsy —removal of tissue for examination—or placement of a catheter in the arm or chest to receive medication to treat cancer or infection.

About half of the patients wore video glasses and watched TV shows or movies during their procedure.

The patients who used the video glasses were 18% less anxious after the procedure than they were before. Those who did not have video glasses were only about 8% less anxious after the procedure, the findings showed.

The video glasses didn't bother the doctors or the patients, and had no significant effect on blood pressure, heart rate, respiratory rate, pain, procedure time, or amount of sedation or pain medication, the researchers found.

The study was presented at the Society of Interventional Radiology's annual meeting in San Diego.

VIDEO GLASSES MORE EFFECTIVE THAN OTHER STRATEGIES

Other drug-free methods of reducing patients' anxiety—such as listening to music or hypnosis—have been assessed but provided slight benefits at best, according to the researchers.

"Patients told us the video glasses really helped calm them down and took their mind off the treatment, and we now offer video glasses to help distract patients from medical treatments going on mere inches away," said Dr. Waldman. "It is really comforting for patients, especially the ones who tend to be more nervous," he explained.

Addiction Can Be Hard to Spot in Loved Ones

What to look for—dramatic shifts in energy throughout the day...inconsistent sex drive... abnormal weight gain or loss in a short time... missing valuables or depleted supplies of alcohol and/or prescription drugs...new and/or unfamiliar friends or social events, which may indicate a lifestyle change.

Adi Jaffe, PhD, executive director of Alternatives Behavioral Health, Los Angeles, and author of the blog All About Addiction, writing in *Psychology Today.*

Drug Duo Might Help Smokers Quit Better Than Single Med

Jon Ebbert, MD, professor of medicine, Mayo Clinic, Rochester, Minnesota.

Sidney Braman, MD, senior faculty, pulmonary, critical care and sleep medicine, Mount Sinai Hospital, New York City.

Len Horovitz, MD, pulmonary specialist, Lenox Hill Hospital, New York City.

Journal of the American Medical Association

Two drugs in combination might be better than one when it comes to helping hardcore smokers quit, at least in the short term, a recent study suggests.

Smoking accounts for 62% of deaths among women smokers and 60% of deaths among men who smoke, the researchers said.

The drugs—*varenicline* (sold under the brand name Chantix) and *bupropion* (Wellbutrin)—taken together increase the rates of quitting over 12 weeks compared with Chantix alone, the researchers found. After a year, however, relapse rates were similar using both approaches.

"We believe this evidence strongly supports the idea that varenicline helps everybody quit," said lead researcher Jon Ebbert, MD, a professor of medicine at the Mayo Clinic in Rochester, Minnesota. "But for heavier smokers and more dependent smokers, combination therapy with varenicline plus bupropion will increase quit rates more than varenicline alone."

"This is how we are going to treat patients," he said.

HOW THE DRUG COMBINATION WORKS

Combination therapy works better than a single medication because the two drugs act in different ways, Dr. Ebbert said.

"With any addiction there are multiple parts of the brain involved," he said. "These drugs have different effects on the brain. Perhaps one of the keys to treatment of any addiction may be to target different parts of the brain to increase success."

STUDY DETAILS

For the study, 315 smokers were randomly selected to take Chantix and Wellbutrin or Chantix and a placebo for 12 weeks.

Dr. Ebbert's team found that 53% of those taking both drugs had quit smoking after 12 weeks, compared with about 43% of those taking Chantix alone.

After about six months, 37% of people in the two-drug group remained smoke-free, compared with 28% of those who took Chantix alone.

After a year, however, the difference narrowed, with about 31% in the combination group and about 25% of those taking Chantix alone still not smoking, the researchers found.

SIDE EFFECTS

More patients using the combination treatment reported anxiety and depression than those taking only Chantix. "Those are important symptoms to monitor, but we don't feel it's more than would occur with normal treatment," Dr. Ebbert said.

DEALING WITH RELAPSE

The study, published in the *Journal of the American Medical Association*, found that although many quitters relapsed, a significant number who had combination therapy didn't take up the habit again.

"You're looking at a 30% quit rate [with combination therapy] versus a 24% quit rate [with one drug]," Dr. Ebbert said.

It's not surprising that many people eventually reached for cigarettes again, he said.

"Relapse is part of the addiction process," Dr. Ebbert said. "The important part of long-term treatment of these patients is to re-engage them in the quitting process and use different types of medication in combination with each other to increase quit rates."

Len Horovitz, MD, a pulmonary specialist at Lenox Hill Hospital in New York City, said breaking an entrenched smoking habit likely will take more than drug therapy.

"Behavioral therapies clearly need to be considered," Dr. Horovitz said.

Dr. Ebbert agreed, and said counseling to help patients overcome some behavioral aspects of tobacco addiction was offered to all of the study participants.

Sidney Braman, MD, a senior faculty member in pulmonary, critical care and sleep medicine at Mount Sinai Hospital in New York City, said most smokers who eventually quit have tried an average of six times to break the habit.

"Most trials of smoking cessation have shown that the long-term success rate is a tough nut to crack," he said.

Dr. Braman said he anticipates that significant advances in understanding—and therefore treating—addiction will be made in the near future.

Until then, Dr. Braman said, "You have to try again and again and again."

info For more information on quitting smoking, visit the American Cancer Society's website, *www.cancer.org*, and search "quitting smoking."

Four-Part Plan Helps People Quit Smoking

The program includes counseling by a nurse…brochures on smoking cessation…referral to a quit-smoking phone hotline…and a six-week supply of nicotine patches at no charge. Patients using the program were four times more likely to quit before surgery than patients who were advised to quit but did not use the program. Thirty days after surgery, 29% of patients in the quit-smoking program said that they had not started smoking again, compared with 11% of those not in the program.

Study of 168 smokers due for elective surgery by researchers at University of Western Ontario, London, Canada, published in *Anesthesia & Analgesia*.

Doctors Aren't Doing Enough to Discourage Problem Drinking

Thomas Frieden, MD, MPH, director, U.S. Centers for Disease Control and Prevention.

Doctors aren't talking often enough with their patients about the harmful effects of alcohol, even if those patients are binge drinkers, US health officials recently reported.

Only one in six adults says a doctor or health professional has ever discussed alcohol use with them, even though drinking too much can be harmful to health, according to a U.S. Centers for Disease Control and Prevention report.

That lack of dialogue holds true even for binge drinkers. Only one in four binge drinkers reported discussing their drinking with a health professional. And among drinkers who binge 10 or more times a month, only one in three has had a serious talk with their doctor regarding alcohol use, the report said.

Only 17% of pregnant women said their doctor discussed alcohol use with them, even though drinking can harm the developing fetus, the CDC researchers added.

Such counseling can provide significant help to people who are problem drinkers, CDC director Thomas Frieden, MD, MPH, said.

"Counseling for no more than 15 minutes can result in a substantial reduction in problem drinking," Dr. Frieden said. "It should be a part of routine patient care. In the same way we screen for high blood pressure and high cholesterol, we should be screening for excess alcohol use and treating patients appropriately."

HOW MUCH IS TOO MUCH

At least 38 million American adults drink too much, even though most aren't alcoholics, Dr. Frieden said.

"For every one person who is [an] alcoholic, there are six who are problem drinkers," he said. *Dr. Frieden said problem drinking can involve...*

- **Binge drinking, or drinking too much on one occasion.** Binge drinking is defined as five or more drinks within a few hours for a man, and four or more drinks for a woman.

- **Excessive average weekly drinking.** For men, that's 15 or more drinks, on average, a week, and eight or more drinks a week for women.

- **Any drinking by pregnant women or people under age 21.**

A drink is defined as 5 ounces of wine, 12 ounces of beer, or 1.5 ounces of 80-proof distilled spirits or liquor.

HEAVY ALCOHOL CONSUMPTION A MAJOR HEALTH ISSUE

Problem drinking causes an estimated 88,000 deaths in the United States each year. It contributes to health problems such as heart disease, breast cancer, high blood pressure and sudden infant death syndrome. It also increases rates of motor vehicle crashes, violence, suicide and sexually transmitted diseases, according to the CDC.

"We are not saying people should not drink at all," Dr. Frieden said. "What we're saying is for people who drink heavily there are serious health problems."

The CDC used patient survey data from 44 states and the District of Columbia to assess whether doctors are talking at all with those under their care about problem drinking.

The researchers found that despite increased understanding of the health risks of problem drinking, doctors are talking with patients about alcohol use about as often as they did back in 1997, the last time the CDC looked at this problem.

"The health-care system is not doing a good enough job," Dr. Frieden said.

RESOURCES FOR DOCTOR-PATIENT DIALOGUE

These days, doctors and health professionals have access to screening forms that can provide patients with a quick idea of whether they're drinking too much, Dr. Frieden noted.

Such screening is also provided free of charge to patients under the Affordable Care Act as a preventive health service, he added.

Such frank talk with a doctor could reduce the amount of alcohol consumed by 25% among people who drink too much, the CDC suggests.

"Alcohol screening and brief counseling can help people set realistic goals for themselves and achieve those goals," Dr. Frieden said. "Health-care workers can provide this service to more patients and involve communities to help people avoid dangerous levels of drinking."

info For more on problem drinking, visit the U.S. National Institutes of Health website at *http://rethinkingdrinking.niaaa.nih.gov/WhatCountsDrink/HowMuchIsTooMuch.asp.*

The Mental Illness Trap

Charles B. Inlander, a consumer advocate and health-care consultant based in Fogelsville, Pennsylvania. He was the founding president of the nonprofit People's Medical Society, a consumer advocacy organization, and is author or coauthor of more than 20 consumer-health books.

Anyone who has a mental illness, such as major depression, bipolar disease or schizophrenia, is likely to have a hard enough time keeping that condition under control. But over the past several years, a plethora of studies have found that these individuals have an added burden—they often receive poor medical care for conditions that are unrelated to their mental health.

And now, recent studies have found that the problem has worsened. The most startling recent research suggests that people with serious mental health problems die 25 years earlier, on average, than the general population. And 60% of those deaths are not from mental illness but from conditions such as cardiovascular, pulmonary and infectious diseases—often triggered by the medications prescribed for the individual's mental condition.

Unfortunately, many doctors presume that a health problem affecting someone with mental illness is due to the mental condition when, in fact, it often is not. *To protect yourself or a loved one or friend with a mental issue...*

• **Don't give up on going to the doctor.** Studies show that many patients with mental health problems simply stop going to their primary care or other non–mental health practitioners (such as cardiologists and pulmonologists) out of sheer frustration when their physical complaints are not taken seriously. Sadly, these people are more likely to commit suicide or to die from another condition (such as diabetes or breast cancer)—mainly because they avoid doctors and don't get screened for such diseases—than people without mental illness.

Insider tip: If you or a loved one has trouble convincing a doctor that an ailment may not be caused by mental illness, seek out another practitioner. Contact your local Mental Health Association or your county mental health office for referrals to primary care doctors and specialists who have experience treating physical ailments in people with mental illness.

• **Never go alone!** During a doctor's appointment, a friend or family member can quickly point out that the symptom, pain or problem seems to be unrelated to a mental problem. The advocate can also, if necessary, help the patient communicate better with the practitioner. This is especially important for patients who have dementia (technically considered a mental illness).

Insider tip: If you are working with a psychiatrist or other mental health professional, ask him/her to regularly communicate with your doctors.

• **Keep a close eye on mental health medications.** As beneficial as some may be, drugs that are used to treat depression, schizophrenia, anxiety and dementia often have severe side effects, such as significant weight gain (which can lead to diabetes and/or cardiovascular conditions) and dizziness (which can lead to falls). For any drug you are prescribed, ask your doctor or pharmacist for a detailed list of possible side effects.

Insider tip: Make sure that your doctor monitors you for illnesses that can develop from the medications being taken (check the side effect disclosure section of the guide that comes with your prescription). And insist that all symptoms be checked out.

Pets Can Get Depressed, Too

They may lose their appetite and become reclusive or lethargic. If you notice these symptoms, go to your veterinarian—depression can indicate arthritis, cancer or other conditions. Comforting your animal can help—so can extra playtime, a set routine and serving food at the same times each day. Try dietary changes—avoid food high in additives and artificial preservatives. Consider acupuncture or acupressure—find a vet who knows these techniques through the International Veterinary Acupuncture Society, IVAS.org.

Natural Health. NaturalHealthMag.com

11 Bottom Line's HEALTH BREAKTHROUGHS

Family Matters

Hiring an In-Home Caregiver—What You Must Know

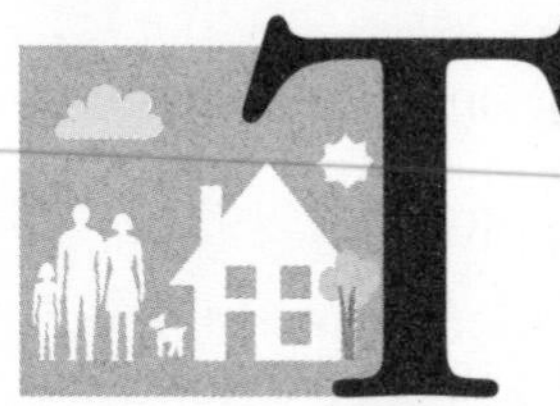

The vast majority of Americans would rather remain in their homes than move to an assisted-living facility, according to recent surveys by AARP. Hiring an in-home caregiver could make it possible to remain at home even after you no longer can live fully independently—but it's a trade-off in challenges compared with a nursing home–type facility. The experience can be pretty horrible, in fact, if you don't take the right steps.

Here's how to select and manage an in-home caregiver...

ASSESSING YOUR NEEDS

As a first step, it is very worthwhile to have a professional geriatric care manager assess the senior's needs. For example, does the senior mainly need companionship during the day? Housekeeping? Meals prepared and served? Medication doled out? Does he/she need help with activities of daily living, such as toileting, bathing and dressing? Are there health issues that require trained assistance, such as giving injections to a person with diabetes or assistance with physical therapy exercises? Do you need an aide who can drive—on outings, errands and to doctor appointments...and will you provide a car or will you require the use of the aide's car? (The care manager also can recommend caregiver agencies and/or caregivers.)

This assessment usually takes about two hours at $100 to $150 an hour. The National Association of Geriatric Care Managers* (CareManager.org) can help you find a care manager in your area. Or ask local senior centers, Area Agency

* Jullie Gray is past-president of this organization.

Jullie Gray, LICSW, CMC, principal of Aging Wisdom, a geriatric-care-management company based in Bellevue, Washington. She is a certified care manager and licensed independent clinical social worker with three decades of experience working with older adults. *AgingWisdom.com* on Aging offices or the senior's doctor if he/she can recommend agencies or care providers.

HIRE THROUGH AN AGENCY

In-home caregivers can be hired directly or through an agency, but agencies are the safer and simpler option.

Hiring in-home help directly might save you a few dollars an hour, but in general, the savings are significant only for people who hire an undocumented immigrant and/or don't pay the required taxes. Doing either of these things could lead to legal problems for both of you. (If you hire someone directly, that person will be your employee, creating insurance and tax obligations—you are required to pay payroll taxes, obtain the worker's liability insurance and file employer tax forms with the state and federal governments.)

Hiring directly also means that you will have to conduct a background check on this person yourself and find a replacement on short notice if he/she is sick, needs time off, quits or is fired. Hiring an undocumented immigrant also makes it virtually impossible to run a full background check on the caregiver. That's a big risk when you consider that this person essentially will be unsupervised in the senior's home.

A reputable agency should handle all of these issues for you.

When you speak with an agency, ask the following...

Are you licensed by the state? Some, though not all, states require licensing—your local Area Agency on Aging office should know if yours does.

Are you a member of the American Association for Homecare? Belonging to this professional association suggests a commitment to professionalism (AAHomeCare.org).

Also ask about the process for requesting a new caregiver if the first one assigned doesn't work out or is sick. You should be able to do this relatively quickly and easily.

Make sure the senior meets any potential caregivers during the interview process so that he will be more welcoming when you actually make a hire.

MAKING THE CAREGIVING RELATIONSHIP WORK

•**Be very clear with the caregiver about your expectations.** Explain precisely what you want him/her to do. Are there specific household or personal tasks that should be prioritized? Is social interaction for the senior a priority?

Lack of communication about needs and expectations is a common cause of problems. If you want something done, ask. If you don't like how something is being done, give instructive feedback.

•**Lock up all valuables,** or move the valuables to the home of a trusted relative before allowing a caregiver to work in the home. Secure any checkbooks, credit cards and documents containing Social Security numbers or other personal data, too, and keep a close eye on accounts and credit reports for any signs of identity theft. These measures are important even if you eventually come to know and trust a caregiver.

•**Plan ahead for backup.** It is best to hire multiple caregivers on a rotating schedule—possibly one for weekdays and one for weekends—if your caregiving needs are truly full-time. Even if you hire a live-in, no one can work 24/7. And even if the caregiver tells you that he wants to work every day to make more money, everyone needs days off for vacation, sick days and doctor visits. It will be easiest on your senior, both physically and emotionally, if his care is consistently provided by caregivers he knows and who are adequately trained in his needs.

•**Visit randomly.** Close friends and relatives of the senior should drop in without warning occasionally when the caregiver is working to make sure that he is doing his job and that the senior is happy and safe in his care.

WHAT WILL THIS COST?

Extensive in-home support is expensive. In-home care costs an average of $18 an hour—around $19 if "personal care" such as help bathing, dressing and/or using the bathroom is required. These hourly rates vary by region and can easily reach $25 or more per hour in high cost-of-living areas. Agencies typically have four-hour minimums per day. Round-the-clock

Better Life Combo for Seniors

Planned multigenerational communities give special attention to residents 55 and older but are not age-restricted—so parents can live near adult children or so aging baby boomers, who are notorious for keeping a youthful perspective on life, can be close to younger people.

Example: One planned community in Seattle includes an independent and assisted-living facility that shares a courtyard and amenities with non-age-restricted apartments. Developments of this type are likely to increase as baby boomers continue to age.

Roundup of experts in housing, reported at *MarketWatch.com*.

live-in assistance averages around $350 a day, nearly three times the price of the typical assisted-living facility. There might be additional onetime costs associated with remaining in the home as well, such as modifying the house to allow wheelchair access, installing an easy-access bathtub and grab bars throughout the home or adding a bedroom for a live-in caregiver.

Finally...There's a Way to Connect with a Loved One Who Has Dementia

Gerontologist Tom Brenner, MA, cofounder, with his wife, Karen Brenner, MA, of Brenner Pathways, a consulting and educational company in Chicago that specializes in the Montessori Method for Positive Dementia Care, *BrennerPathways.org*. He and his wife are also coauthors of *You Say Goodbye and We Say Hello: The Montessori Method for Positive Dementia Care* (Brenner Pathways). A researcher for the State of Illinois Department on Aging, Brenner trains caregivers and case managers through the Illinois Community Care Program.

Henry had been diagnosed with early-onset Alzheimer's and was quiet and withdrawn. When he was younger, he had collected vintage cars, so his caregiver gave him some old hubcaps and polish. After 30 minutes of polishing, Henry began talking with a great deal of emotion about his time as a soldier. Perhaps the process of polishing the hubcaps reminded him of polishing his boots, and an important memory was triggered. This activity enabled Henry and his caregiver to connect, even if only for a short time.

One of the most heartbreaking and frustrating aspects of caring for a loved one with dementia is the loss of meaningful interaction.

But there's good news on this front: The Montessori Method for Positive Dementia Care, a nondrug approach (often used in combination with medication), is now being used by some caregivers in home-care settings and nursing homes with dramatic results.

Through basic Montessori principles (see below), this method offers ways to be in the moment with a dementia patient and possibly have a deep connection. Patients become more secure, confident and calm. And caregivers are less likely to get frustrated and burn out.

Recent research: In a study involving nine residential facilities in Melbourne, Australia, dementia patients were two times more actively engaged when participating in Montessori-based activities than when they were not doing these activities.

Background: Developed more than 100 years ago as a method of teaching "unreachable" children with learning disabilities, the Montessori approach encourages the use of all five senses to stimulate different areas of the brain and the use of "muscle memory"* to develop small-muscle coordination and promote confidence. The Montessori method also advocates an environment that meets the specific physical and emotional needs of those using it.

Montessori classrooms for children are uncluttered but homey and filled with natural light and materials to promote use of the senses. Students are free to move about and engage in activities that appeal most to them. This sets the stage for focused and calm activity. Research has shown that Montessori pupils learn to excel at problem solving, adapting to change and social skills—all areas that are difficult for adults with dementia.

*Sometimes called procedural memory, this involves physical movements fixed into memory through repetition (think of riding a bike or playing a musical instrument).

Key Montessori tenets and how they can help dementia patients…

•Emphasis on environment. The surroundings of the dementia patient should be familiar and comforting and designed to foster as much independence as possible. For example, the layout of a facility, or your home if a loved one is living with you, should be uncomplicated so there is less potential for confusion. Visual cues, such as large-print labeling indicating what can be found in drawers, are also very helpful. Clutter should be minimized, but the use of natural elements—such as plants, pictures of nature, natural lighting, etc.—can induce a feeling of calm.

•Muscle memory stimulation. While the mind of a dementia patient might be faltering, the muscles often "remember" how to do an activity that was done repetitively and enjoyably in the past. The key is to discover a patient's unique strengths, passions and interests—not only tapping muscle memory but strong emotions as well. Focusing on a physical task and having success helps dementia patients feel more secure and confident and less angry and agitated.

A caregiver might take a former golfer to the driving range to jump-start his/her muscle memory. Or a long-retired handyman might be given a toolbox with a tape measure, paintbrushes and a level so that he can tinker.

These activities also build muscle coordination and can simply make life more pleasant and enriching for a dementia patient.

•Sharing stories. This is one of the most effective tools for helping dementia sufferers stay connected. Moments when patients share their stories, even if the time is fleeting, can enable the patient and caregiver to feel a deep connection, boosting the patient's sense of security.

To encourage a patient to share a story: A caregiver might give him a meaningful object to hold—something important from the patient's life or an object from nature. This simple act can help spark a memory and get the patient talking.

•Art therapy. Painting, singing and playing an instrument can provide patients new avenues of self-expression and strengthen their spirits. These activities also can give patients the opportunity to engage their senses.

Good activity: Flower arranging. Patients are encouraged to feel and smell the flowers, cut stems and pour water. This exercise calls on small motor skills, essential for independence and range of motion. Key areas of the brain are also exercised when deciding how to arrange the flowers.

•The Knobbed Cylinder. This classic Montessori tool—a long wooden block with 10 different-sized holes in which the user places matching cylinders—builds focus and small-muscle coordination. Dementia patients might be asked to fill only two holes—the point is for the patient to feel success and build confidence through this activity.

•Finish a phrase. Old sayings may never leave our minds. With this technique, the caregiver holds up the first half of a statement on a piece of paper ("The whole nine…") and asks the patient to finish the saying ("…yards"). It's astonishing to see dementia sufferers suddenly become very vocal and involved.

Benefits for the caregivers: The Montessori method gives the caregiver more tools to care for a dementia patient. It encourages the caregiver to use his imagination and allows him to act more like a guide than a director. Plus, patients are less agitated and aggressive, so they

How to Talk to Someone With Hearing Loss

Don't shout. Instead, speak in a normal voice. Do not lean into the person's ear—many people with hearing loss read lips, so they need to see what you are saying. Try to eliminate background noise that can interfere with hearing, such as a TV program or an air conditioner. In a group meeting, try to have one general conversation rather than several overlapping ones. If someone does not hear what you say after you try two or three times, rephrase your comment and try again. Do not say, "Never mind. It doesn't matter." It matters to the person who can't hear.

Katherine Bouton, author of *Shouting Won't Help: Why I—and 50 Million Other Americans—Can't Hear You* (Picador).

are easier to be with. All this helps minimize caregiver burnout and frustration.

Try out a few of these exercises with your loved one. To find a facility that offers this specific approach, you'll need to ask the director of the center you are considering.

Thanks, Sis!

Grown children from large families are less likely to get divorced than those who had no siblings.

Theory: Living with multiple siblings improves interaction and communication skills.

The Ohio State University

Mistakes Parents Make That Push Adult Children Away

Jeffrey Jensen Arnett, PhD, a research professor in the department of psychology at Clark University, Worcester, Massachusetts. He is coauthor, with Elizabeth Fishel, of *When Will My Grown-Up Kid Grow Up?* (Workman). *JeffreyArnett.com*

Our children will always be our children, but once they turn 18 or leave home, they also are adults with lives increasingly separate from our own. It's a challenge for parents to step back while also staying connected to their grown-up kids.

Much of the angst between parents and adult children stems from the tug-of-war over whose life it is. There often is a disconnect between parents who still want to shape their grown-up kids' future course and the kids who are determined to live their lives their own way.

For loving parents, their grown children's trials and errors, including failed projects and teary breakups, can be anguishing. It can be wrenching to let go of the old parental omnipotence and not be able to fix everything. But when grown kids cope with these ups and downs, they develop into resilient, self-sufficient people with the confidence that comes from standing on their own feet.

Seven "don'ts" to keep in mind when dealing with grown children...

MONEY AND CAREER

It takes a long time these days for grown kids to achieve financial independence, and my research shows that money issues are the number-one topic of conflict between parents and kids 18 to 29 years old.

•**Don't use your financial support to control your adult kids.** If you're supplying money to your adult child, you certainly can set ground rules about how that money is used—but you should not threaten to withdraw your support if the adult child doesn't make life changes unrelated to finances.

Example: It's reasonable to tell your adult child that money you're providing cannot be spent on a vacation—but don't tell him that it can't be spent on a vacation unless he leaves the girlfriend you don't like.

•**Don't push your kids to take a job in a field that pays well but that they don't like.** Not only might they hold their unhappiness with the hated job against you, their lack of passion for the field could inhibit their career growth.

Also: Don't make snide comments about the job prospects of your college-age child's field of study or the earnings potential of his line of work. It is reasonable to discuss career and earnings outlooks with your kids before they choose a college major, field of graduate study or first job. But trying to control the big decision of what field your adult child will choose is sure to stir up resentment. Keep in mind that although college majors do vary in their future earnings, getting a college degree, in any area, is the most important goal for enhancing lifelong career prospects.

•**Don't insist that your kids find their own way after college rather than return home.** These days, many adult children live at home for a short time. Almost always, their return home is temporary because they prefer to live independently as soon as they can afford to do so.

Helpful: Agree on a division of household responsibilities. The adult child is now an adult member of the household and should do an adult share of the housework, laundry and cooking.

COMMUNICATION

Most adult children like talking to their parents and enjoy having a more adultlike relationship than they did in their teens. *But...*

•Don't ask probing questions about your children's lives. If they want to share something personal, they will. Adult children vary a lot in how much they want their parents to know about their lives and how much they want to confide in them.

Take special care not to raise subjects that your adult child has historically been disinclined to discuss. Resist the urge to ask follow-up questions on the rare occasions when your child does raise one of these subjects.

Example: Many adult children prefer not to discuss their love lives with their parents.

•Don't overdo it. Today's technology makes it cheap and easy to stay in contact with loved ones, and many adult children and their parents are in contact with one another nearly every day. However, for some grown kids, that's a bit too much togetherness at a time when they are striving to become self-sufficient. In general, it's best to follow your adult children's lead on communications. If they contact you weekly via text message, then contact them weekly via text message, too. Text messaging might not be your preferred communication method, but it's a great way to touch base with today's young

How to Give Advice to an Adult Child

Many young adults spend their 20s acting in ways that seem irresponsible to their parents. They might change jobs or romantic partners frequently or rely on their parents for financial support or housing.

This is all perfectly normal and does not mean that the young adult is destined to act this way forever.

And while adult children might seem to be in desperate need of advice, there's a good chance that they will react poorly if their parents offer it. Such guidance makes them feel as if their parents still see them as children. This puts parents in a difficult position—they want to help their grown-up kids avoid missteps, but any wisdom they offer is likely to be poorly received.

Usually parents' best option is to bite their tongues and not offer their adult children advice when it hasn't been requested. Such advice might harm the relationship, and there is a good chance it won't be heeded anyway. *But speaking up could be wise if...*

•You believe your adult child's safety is at risk. It's worth putting the relationship at risk when safety is at stake.

Examples: Don't offer unsolicited advice if you think your adult child is staying out too late—but do if you suspect he's driving home drunk. Don't tell your daughter you don't like her new boyfriend—but do speak your mind if your daughter has a black eye and you suspect that the boyfriend is responsible.

•The topic is money-related and you're providing financial support. If your money is on the line, it's perfectly reasonable to voice concerns about the adult child's questionable financial decisions or even set ground rules for spending. But it will help the relationship if after voicing these concerns or setting these rules, you add something such as, "The final decision is yours, and I will continue to support you emotionally whatever you decide. I just can't continue to support you financially if you make this decision."

Example: You're paying your child's rent while he searches for a job, but you notice that he hasn't been looking for work lately.

•You obtain permission to provide advice. The odds of a negative reaction decline greatly if you ask the child if he would like your input before you offer it.

Warning: Respect the child's answer. If he says he prefers to work through the problem on his own, keep your advice to yourself.

When you feel you must provide advice, also ask the adult child for his advice on a different topic about which he is knowledgeable. This can keep the relationship balanced.

adults without seeming pushy. You can always slip in a phone call now and then.

Helpful: Don't feel offended if kids go a few days without answering your text message or voice mail. It doesn't mean that they don't care. It could just mean that they are busy—or that they're not that eager to discuss that particular topic.

ROMANCE

An adult child's romantic relationships can be a minefield for parents...

•**Don't confide that you "never liked" an ex-boyfriend or ex-girlfriend or provide reasons why your adult child is better off without this former mate.** Keep in mind that ex-boyfriends and ex-girlfriends sometimes re-enter the picture. That could create awkwardness if you've previously expressed a dislike.

•**Don't overlook your adult child's romantic partners at family get-togethers.** If your adult child has been seeing someone for a while, be sure to include the partner in family gatherings, then do your best to make him/her feel welcome and comfortable. The more comfortable your grown child's partner is with you, the more you are likely to see of your child.

Family Conflicts Can Impair Child's Brain Development

Nicholas Walsh, PhD, a lecturer in developmental psychology at the University of East Anglia, England.
University of East Anglia, news release.

Exposure to common family problems early in life can impair a child's brain development, according to recent research.

Tension between parents, arguments and lack of affection or communication between family members can affect growth of the cerebellum, a brain area involved in skill learning, stress regulation and sensory-motor control, the researchers found. This might lead to mental health problems for children later in life, the researchers said.

"These findings are important because exposure to adversities in childhood and adolescence is the biggest risk factor for later psychiatric disease," said study leader Nicholas Walsh, PhD, a lecturer in developmental psychology at the University of East Anglia, England.

Previous studies have focused on the effects of severe abuse and neglect, but this study found common and ongoing family problems can also cause psychiatric ills in young people.

STUDY DETAILS

Using brain-imaging technology, the researchers examined the brains of 58 teenagers between the ages of 17 and 19. The teens' parents were asked to report any negative events their children had experienced between birth and age 11. Nearly half of the children—27—were classified as having been exposed to childhood family problems. When the teens were 14 and 17, they were also asked about any troubles they, their friends or their family faced over the course of the past year.

The study, published in *NeuroImage: Clinical*, found the teens who faced mild to moderate family troubles from the time they were born until age 11 had a smaller cerebellum.

The study's authors pointed out that a smaller cerebellum is found in just about all cases of mental illness.

The researchers noted the teens who faced family problems early in life were more likely to have a diagnosed mental illness, have a parent with a mental health disorder and have negative views of their family life.

IMPLICATIONS

"We show that exposure in childhood and early adolescence to even mild to moderate family difficulties, not just severe forms of abuse, neglect and maltreatment, may affect the developing adolescent brain," noted Dr. Walsh.

"We also argue that a smaller cerebellum may be an indicator of mental health issues later on," Dr. Walsh added. Reducing exposure to adverse social environments during early life may enhance typical brain development and reduce subsequent mental health risks, she said.

"This study helps us understand the mechanisms in the brain by which exposure to

Vaccinating Provides Protection for the Whole Family

Vaccinating babies against rotavirus, which causes stomach illness, prevents older children and adults from developing the potentially fatal infectious disease. The Centers for Disease Control and Prevention (CDC) recommends that all children be vaccinated against the disease starting at two months. Adults generally do not need to be vaccinated against the rotavirus.

Study by researchers at the division of viral diseases, CDC, Atlanta, published in *The Journal of the American Medical Association.*

problems in early-life leads to later psychiatric issues," added Dr. Walsh. "It not only advances our understanding of how the general psychosocial environment affects brain development, but also suggests links between specific regions of the brain and individual psychosocial factors."

info The U.S. Department of Health and Human Services has more information on the environment and brain development at *www.childwelfare.gov.* Search "environment and brain development."

Keep Out of Reach of Children

Study by Safe Kids Worldwide, Washington, DC. *Safe Kids.org*

Accidental ingestion of medicine sent more than 64,000 children to emergency rooms in 2012 (latest data available).

In three out of four of these cases, the medicine belonged to a parent or grandparent. One in eight grandparents now provide care on a regular basis for a grandchild. And 74% of grandparents say they take prescription medication every day. Among those who use easy-open containers, 42% keep medicine on a bathroom or kitchen sink, counter, table or shelf.

Self-defense: If you are concerned that you might forget to take pills you cannot easily see, use a cell-phone alarm or other reminder to alert you when it is time for your medication.

High Praise Might Backfire on Kids With Low Self-Esteem

Association for Psychological Science.

Eddie Brummelman, visiting scholar, Ohio State University, Columbus and doctoral candidate in psychology at Utrecht University, the Netherlands.

Brad Bushman, PhD, professor of communication and psychology at Ohio State University, Columbus.

Although children who feel good about themselves might thrive on praise from their parents or other adults, exaggerated compliments could have the opposite effect on kids with low self-esteem, researchers have found.

Adults might sometimes try to boost children's confidence with high praise. But this type of inflated encouragement might put too much pressure on kids with low self-esteem, causing them to shy away from challenges, a recent study suggests.

"Inflated praise can backfire with those kids who seem to need it the most—kids with low self-esteem," said study lead author Eddie Brummelman, PhD candidate, and a visiting scholar at Ohio State University.

STUDY #1

In conducting the study, which was published in the journal *Psychological Science*, the researchers defined inflated praise as a compliment that included an additional adverb or adjective. For example, rather than a simple compliment (e.g. "You are good at this"), inflated praise would include an extra word ("You are incredibly good at this").

Adults naturally shower kids with low self-esteem with twice as much inflated praise, the researchers found. Too much praise however, might actually discourage children from taking on greater challenges, said Brummelman and his colleagues.

STUDY #2

In a second experiment conducted in participants' homes, 114 parents gave their kids 12 timed math tests. Several days before the tests, the kids completed an assessment that measured their self-esteem.

After the math tests, the parents scored their child's work. The researchers were not present in the room, but videotaped the testing sessions. Following the tests, they counted the number of times the parents praised their child. They divided the compliments into two groups—inflated praise and non-inflated praise.

The study showed that parents praised their children about six times throughout the testing session. The most common non-inflated compliments included "Well done!" and "You're good at this!"

The researchers pointed out, however, that 25% of the praise was inflated. The inflated compliments most often used were "You answered very fast!" and "Super good!"

Parents gave more inflated praise to children with low self-esteem than kids with a lot of confidence, said study co-author Brad Bushman, PhD, professor of communication and psychology at Ohio State.

"Parents seemed to think the children with low self-esteem needed to get extra praise to make them feel better," Dr. Bushman said. "It's understandable why adults would do that, but we found in another experiment that this inflated praise can backfire in these children."

STUDY #3

In a third experiment, 240 children drew Wild Roses, a famous Vincent van Gogh painting. These kids received a note with either an inflated compliment or a non-inflated compliment from someone identified as a professional painter, or no praise at all.

After they received their note, the kids were told to copy another picture. This time, however, they could draw anything they wanted. The kids were told that if they chose an easy picture, they wouldn't learn much. They also were told that they might make mistakes if they chose a difficult picture, but that they would learn a lot.

The study showed that kids with low self-esteem were more likely to select an easier picture if they received inflated praise. Meanwhile, kids with high self-esteem who were given inflated praise were more likely to select a difficult picture.

CONCLUSIONS

"If you tell a child with low self-esteem that they did incredibly well, they may think they always need to do incredibly well," said Brummelman, who is also a doctoral student in psychology at Utrecht University in the Netherlands. "They may worry about meeting those high standards and decide not to take on any new challenges."

"It goes against what many people may believe would be most helpful," Brummelman said. "But it really isn't helpful to give inflated praise to children who already feel bad about themselves."

info The American Academy of Pediatrics has more information on helping children develop a healthy sense of self-esteem at *www.healthychildren.org*. Search "self-esteem."

Let Them Eat Fat

Restricting infants' and toddlers' fat intake may increase their chances of being overweight. Researchers who examined 73 children in the first two years of their lives and then as adults found that those who had higher fat intakes as children were less likely to be overweight. Restriction of dietary fat in early life may activate adaptive mechanisms that increase the susceptibility to being overweight later in life.

The results substantiate current recommendations that fat intake should not be restricted in young children.

Study led by researchers at University of Paris, France, published in International *Journal of Obesity*.

Combination Treatment Best for Recurrent Ear Infections

Thijs van Dongen, MD, physician and doctoral candidate, department of epidemiology, Julius Center for Health Sciences and Primary Care, Utrecht, the Netherlands.

Ruby Roy, MD, assistant professor, pediatrics, University of Chicago, and chronic disease physician, La Rabida Children's Hospital, Chicago.

New England Journal of Medicine

An eardrop that combines antibiotics and steroids might be the best ear infection treatment for children who already have ear tubes because of recurrent infections, a recent study finds.

New research compared the eardrop treatment to oral antibiotics and to a wait-and-see approach. After two weeks, just 5% of children receiving the eardrops had continuing discharge from their ears. But 44% of those given oral antibiotics still had signs of infection, as did 55% of those managed with observation, according to the study.

"Children treated with eardrops had a shorter duration of the initial episode, and a lower total number of days of ear discharge, and a lower number of recurrences during six months of follow-up than children treated with oral antibiotics or initial observation," said the study's lead author, Thijs van Dongen, MD, a physician at the Julius Center for Health Sciences and Primary Care in Utrecht, the Netherlands.

ABOUT EAR TUBES

Most children experience at least one ear infection during childhood, according to the American Academy of Otolaryngology—Head and Neck Surgery. But for some children ear infections are a near-constant problem.

For these kids, small tubes—known as tympanostomy tubes—inserted into the eardrum help preserve or restore a child's hearing. The tubes help fluid drain and allow air in the middle ear so that it can function properly.

Each year, more than a half million children in the United States have surgery to place ear tubes, according to the academy.

A condition called acute tympanostomy tube otorrhea is a common complication after the procedure. It means fluid is draining from the tube, and it may be accompanied by a foul odor, pain and fever.

STUDY DETAILS

The best treatment option for acute otorrhea hasn't been well-studied, and those studies that have been done were small. For this study, published in the *New England Journal of Medicine*, the researchers randomly assigned 230 children between the ages of one and 10 years old who had ear tubes to one of three treatments.

Seventy-six children were put into the antibiotic/steroid eardrop group, while another 77 children were assigned to receive oral antibiotics. The final 77 children were assigned to the observation group. After two weeks, the children's ears were examined again.

The combination eardrops were significantly more effective than the other two practices, the investigators found.

"Next to being the most effective in treating acute ear discharge in children with tympanostomy tubes, we also found that the increase in quality-of-life scores was largest in children treated with eardrops," said Dr. van Dongen.

Children May Be Allergic to Dustless Chalk

Children with milk allergies may also be allergic to dustless chalk, which contains the milk protein casein. Many teachers opt for dustless chalk to keep hands and classrooms clean, but chalk particles still get in the air. When the particles are inhaled by children with a milk allergy, symptoms can include coughing, sneezing, wheezing, shortness of breath, nasal congestion and a runny nose.

If your child is allergic to milk: Ask that he/she be seated as far from the chalkboard as possible. Inform teachers, coaches and the school nurse about your child's allergies.

Study by researchers at the American College of Allergy, Asthma and Immunology, published in *Annals of Allergy, Asthma Immunology*.

Side effects were mild and no complications of middle-ear infections were reported, Dr. van Dongen added.

SWIMMER'S EAR STUDY

A second study published in the journal *Otolaryngology—Head and Neck Surgery* found that eardrops worked better than oral antibiotics for the painful condition known as swimmer's ear. This infection of the outer ear canal is often caused by water that remains in the ear after swimming, which aids bacterial growth.

However, one expert cautioned that the current study's findings are not applicable to most children with ear infections.

"This study showed—in this very select group of kids—that eardrops were much better than oral antibiotics and much better than observation," said Ruby Roy, MD, a pediatrician and assistant professor of pediatrics at the University of Chicago.

Because the children in the study have ear tubes, it allows the eardrops to travel right to the source of the infection, Dr. Roy said. In kids without ear tubes, this isn't the case, she added.

"Not using systemic antibiotics when you don't need to means that you've protected this small group of kids from side effects like stomach irritation and diarrhea," noted Dr. Roy.

It's also known that antibiotic pills help promote resistant bacteria.

RECOMMENDATION ON DROPS

Dr. Van Dongen said he disagrees with doctors who advise parents to wait until ear drainage has gone on for a week before contacting their child's doctor.

"We would recommend parents to contact a physician when otorrhea occurs . . . so that children can be treated with eardrops shortly after the onset of ear discharge, and improve more quickly and have fewer recurrences in following months," said Dr. van Dongen.

info To learn more about ear tubes, visit the website of the American Academy of Otolaryngology—Head and Neck Surgery at *www.entnet.org/HealthInformation/Ear-Tubes.cfm.*

When Moms Get Active, Kids Follow

Esther van Sluijs, PhD, group leader, MRC Epidemiology Unit and Centre for Diet and Activity Research, School of Clinical Medicine, University of Cambridge, England.

Bernard Fuemmeler, PhD, MPH, associate professor and codirector of mHealth@Duke, Duke University Medical Center, Durham, North Carolina.

Leann Birch, PhD, professor, department of foods and nutrition, University of Georgia, Athens.

Pediatrics

Want to keep your little kids active? A new study suggests that mothers may be the key—Preschool children with more active moms appear more likely to be active themselves.

The research doesn't confirm that physical activity in mothers directly affects how much their kids walk or run around. And the findings don't say anything about the role of fathers.

Still, the study provides evidence that mothers should be encouraged to move around, said lead author Esther van Sluijs, PhD, group leader with the MRC Epidemiology Unit and the Center for Diet and Activity Research, at the University of Cambridge School of Clinical Medicine, in England.

"If activity in mothers and children can be encouraged or incorporated into daily activities so that more time is spent moving, activity levels are likely to increase in both," she said. "In

One-Fifth of Children Outgrow Asthma

According to a recent finding, among children who had asthma at age seven or eight, 21% had had no wheezing for three years by age 19. About 26% of boys and 14% of girls seemed to outgrow asthma. Remission was less common in children with severe asthma and those sensitive to furry animals, such as dogs or cats.

Study of 248 children by Swedish researchers of Obstructive Lung Disease in Northern Sweden studies, Norrbotten Council in Lulea, Sweden, published in *Pediatrics*.

return, this is likely to have long-term health benefits for both."

BACKGROUND

The researchers launched their study to build on other research into how the physical activity of mothers and their kids are connected, Dr. van Sluijs said.

According to the researcher, parents seem to affect their kids' physical activities in three ways—by acting as role models, by helping kids be active (by taking them to the park, for instance), and by being active with them. "All three aspects are thought to be important," Dr. van Sluijs said, "but it has generally been unclear how directly mother and child's physical activity are related."

STUDY DETAILS

In the study, the researchers used devices called accelerometers to track 554 children, all four years old, and their mothers for as many as seven days. "The more activity a mother did, the more active her child," Dr. van Sluijs noted.

Specifically, for every single minute of moderate-to-vigorous activity that the mother did, her child was more likely to do 10% more of a similar level of activity. Those extra minutes add up over time, the researchers pointed out.

Does that mean active mothers make their kids more active or the other way around? Or could another factor such as genetics or the places where families live affect the level of physical activity in both mother and child? It's not clear.

However, "it is likely that activity in one of the pair influences activity in the other," Dr. van Sluijs said.

The study was published in the journal *Pediatrics*.

EXPERT COMMENTARY

The research matters because "better understanding activity patterns in preschool-age children can inform the ways we approach prevention and intervention," said Bernard Fuemmeler, PhD, MPH, an associate professor and codirector of Duke University Medical Center's mHealth@Duke, which explores the use of technology to improve health. Dr. Fuemmeler was not involved with the study.

Another expert focused on the issue of fathers and what role they might play.

Age Limit for Cold Medicine

Do not give cough and cold medicine to kids under age four—even if the products are labeled as being for children. More than 40% of parents say that they give their children under age four cough medicine or multisymptom cough and cold medicine. But these medicines do not reduce the time an infection lasts—and they can cause serious side effects in young children, including uneven heart rate, sleep problems, confusion, hallucinations, nausea and constipation. Products marketed as being for children have been labeled since 2008 as not for kids under age four—but the information usually is in small print and is easy to miss.

C.S. Mott Children's Hospital National Poll on Children's Health at University of Michigan, Ann Arbor.

"This is a big question not addressed here," said Leann Birch, PhD, a professor at the University of Georgia's department of foods and nutrition who studies children and obesity. But, she said, research on parenting suggests that fathers tend to engage in more rough-and-tumble and high-action play with kids than mothers.

Also, she said, "some of our own work showed that reported activity by dads was more important than by moms in predicting the activity of daughters, especially in organized sports during later childhood."

FUTURE STUDIES
TO TRACK CHILDREN
AS THEY AGE

As for future studies, lead author Dr. van Sluijs said researchers hope to investigate whether the link between physical activity in mothers and children will change as kids grow older. They also want to study "ways to engage the family and help parents to effectively change their own and their children's health behaviors," she said.

info For more about children's fitness, visit the website of the American Academy of Pediatrics, *www.healthychildren.org*, and search "fitness."

HPV Shot Doesn't Encourage Sexual Activity in Young Girls

Jessica Kahn, MD, professor, department of pediatrics, University of Cincinnati College of Medicine and Cincinnati Children's Hospital Medical Center.
Ginny Ryan, MD, obstetrician-gynecologist, University of Iowa, Iowa City.
Pediatrics, online

A recent study finds no evidence that getting the cervical cancer vaccine will encourage young girls to engage in sexual activity or give them a false sense of security about sex.

The study found that what a girl believes about the human papillomavirus (HPV) vaccine has no bearing on her decision to become sexually active or engage in risky sexual behavior.

Experts hope the research will reassure parents who fear that the vaccine might encourage sexual activity.

"Parental concerns have, in part, driven the relatively low acceptance rates of HPV vaccines compared to other adolescent vaccines and present a barrier to clinicians," said study author Jessica Kahn, MD, who practices adolescent medicine at Cincinnati Children's Hospital Medical Center.

ABOUT THE HPV VACCINE

Despite the fact that HPV vaccines protect against viruses that cause about 70% of all cervical cancers, and about half of all cancers of the mouth, throat and esophagus, they've been a tough sell.

Pace the Gum Chewing

Gum-chewing teens may be giving themselves migraines by stressing the TMJ joint, a common cause of headaches.

Recent study: Headaches disappeared entirely in 19 of 30 teens who gave up chewing gum for a month.

Tel Aviv University

Only one-third of teenage girls got all three recommended doses of the vaccine in 2012, and only half got a single dose, according to data from the U.S. Centers for Disease Control and Prevention.

RECENT STUDY

For the study, Dr. Kahn and her colleagues surveyed more than 300 girls who were between the ages of 13 and 21 when they got their first dose of the vaccine.

She asked about their sexual experience, and about the need to practice safe sex. She also asked them how worried they felt about getting sexually transmitted infections other than HPV after their shots.

Dr. Kahn asked the same questions two and six months later to see if anything had changed. She also wanted to know if how the young women felt about the protection they were getting from the shots might be linked to subsequent sexual behavior.

She found nothing to suggest the shots were influencing the girls' sexual activity.

Overall, 58% of girls reported that they had been sexually active with a man or woman, while 42% said they were sexually inexperienced at the start of the study. Whether or not a girl was sexually experienced largely depended upon her age. Older girls were more likely to be sexually active than younger ones.

Out of 99 girls who were sexually inexperienced at the start of the study, 20 had become sexually active six months after they got the vaccine.

Among girls who were already sexually active when they started the vaccine, most said they were using condoms with intercourse two and six months later. And a minority, 34%, reported having more than two male partners during that time.

"We didn't find anything concerning," Dr. Kahn said.

The study was published in the journal *Pediatrics*.

STUDY WITH SIMILAR FINDINGS

The finding echoes the conclusions of a smaller study published in the *Journal of Pediatric and Adolescent Gynecology*. That study, which surveyed 153 young women who'd been vaccinated against HPV and compared them with 70 who'd not had the shots, found no significant differences in the age girls started having sex or in their numbers of sexual partners. There were also no differences in high-risk sexual behaviors or attitudes about safe sex between the two groups.

"By far, the weight of evidence would dispel that myth of disinhibition for teen girls," said Ginny Ryan, MD, an obstetrician-gynecologist at the University of Iowa, in Iowa City.

Dr. Ryan has studied the HPV vaccine and sexual behavior in young women, but she was not involved in the current research.

She said her study, and others, have found that most girls come away from the vaccination a bit savvier about their sexual health.

"Not only do these studies generally prove that they're not participating in any earlier or riskier sexual behavior, but they also might get a little education out of the whole process of being vaccinated. So they tend to be a little more knowledgeable about the virus and other sexually transmitted infections," Dr. Ryan said.

info For more information about the HPV vaccine, visit the website of the National Cancer Institute, *www.cancer.gov*, and search "Human Papillomavirus Vaccines."

FDA OKs Sale of "Morning-After" Pill Without Age Limit

Planned Parenthood Federation of America, statement. Associated Press.

The so-called morning-after pill is now over-the-counter, with the U.S. Food and Drug Administration (FDA) announcing that it has approved unrestricted sales of Plan B One-Step.

The move follows a decision earlier in 2013 by the Obama administration to drop its effort to fight a court order that would make the emergency contraceptive pill available over-the-counter to all women and girls of child-bearing age.

Plan B prevents implantation of a fertilized egg in a woman's uterus through the use of *levonorgestrel*, a synthetic form of the hormone progesterone used for decades in birth control pills. Plan B contains 1.5 milligrams of levonorgestrel, more than the birth control pill contains. It is considered a form of birth control, not abortion. The drug prevents pregnancy if taken within 72 hours of sexual intercourse. Effectiveness rate is stated as "seven out of every eight women who would have gotten pregnant will not become pregnant," according to the Plan B website.

EMERGENCY BIRTH CONTROL BATTLE

After fighting for an age threshold on the nonprescription use of the Plan B One-Step pill for months, the FDA said June 2013 that it would heed the ruling of Judge Edward Korman, of the United States District Court for the Eastern District of New York.

Korman first issued his order in April 2013, igniting a battle over whether young girls should be allowed access to emergency contraception without a prescription. A day later, on May 1, the Obama administration stepped in to appeal the Korman decision.

FDA CITES RESEARCH TO SUPPORT DECISION

At the time of the FDA's move to remove the age limit, agency Commissioner Margaret Hamburg, MD, said that "research has shown that access to emergency contraceptive products has

Common Scoliosis Treatment Gets a Thumbs-up

For more than 50 years, doctors have advised adolescents with scoliosis to wear a back brace, but until recently, studies of its effectiveness had produced mixed results.

Recent finding: 72% of children who wore a brace were successfully treated. If the brace was worn for more than 13 hours a day, the treatment was 90% successful.

Study of 242 adolescents by researchers in the department of orthopedics and rehabilitation, University of Iowa, Iowa City, published in *The New England Journal of Medicine*.

the potential to further decrease the rate of unintended pregnancies in the United States."

The Associated Press reported that the FDA's recent decision only applied to Plan B One-Step. Other brands of emergency contraception include Next Choice and Ella.

Planned Parenthood has long pushed for wider access to emergency contraception. But conservative groups have objected to such a move.

info For more information about emergency contraception, visit the website of the World Health Organization at *http://www.who.int/mediacentre/factsheets/fs244/en/*.

Best Remedy for Lice

Pesticide shampoos do not get rid of all head lice and nits. Neither do organic substances such as lavender, rosemary, tea-tree oil, olive oil or mayonnaise.

What does work: Manual removal. The LiceMeister comb, developed by the National Pediculosis Association, uses highly polished, precision-spaced tines to comb out lice and nits from hair.

Cost: About $13 at SchoolHealth.com. Other, similar combs also are available, but older-style plastic cradle-cap or stamped-aluminum combs are not as effective.

Deborah Altschuler, president and cofounder, National Pediculosis Association, Newton, Massachusetts.

How to Tell the Kids That You Have a Serious Health Problem

Hollye Jacobs, RN, MS, MSW, a palliative-care nurse and social worker based in Santa Barbara, California. She is a breast cancer survivor, mother of four and author of *The Silver Lining: A Supportive and Insightful Guide to Breast Cancer* (Atria). *TheSilverPen.com*

When a serious medical diagnosis comes into a family, children deserve to know. Silence is not golden. Discussing illness candidly and openly, in developmentally appropriate ways, teaches children that parents are trustworthy and that honesty is a family priority.

Parents diagnosed with serious health issues often put off sharing the news with their children because they think that keeping their kids in the dark will protect them. However, children will almost certainly figure out on their own that something is very wrong. In truth, this tends to increase their fear and anxiety.

When children are not told what's happening, they are left alone with their fear and confusion. When this happens, children often imagine that things are far worse than reality or that they are somehow responsible.

Sharing news of a medical diagnosis is emotionally difficult. Despite the fact that I am a nurse, social worker and child development specialist, talking with our children was the hardest part of my cancer experience. But it needs to be done, and it can be done.

Here's how to tackle this very difficult conversation, plus specific tips for helping children of different ages through this challenging time...

11 TIPS FOR TELLING THE KIDS

- **Bring notes.** Prior to the conversation, jot down the key points you want to mention. Depending on the child's age, these points might include the specific type of illness you have and the treatment you will be pursuing. Without notes, you might forget something important or give your child the impression that things are worse than they really are. This conversation could become emotional, and that's OK.

- **Choose a time for the conversation that makes sense for your child.** This timing needs to be when children are most awake and alert. Weekends are optimal because they give the child some time to process the news before going back to school.

- **Have the conversation at the child's eye level, literally.** This encourages conversation and engagement. It also is respectful. With a young child, it might mean sitting the child on your lap.

- **Open with a "warning shot."** This introductory sentence prepares the listener for the gravity of the conversation ahead.

Example: "I have some important news to tell you..."

•Speak clearly, calmly and confidently. Our kids hear our mood as much as our words. If you are calm and confident during this conversation, it will help your kids feel calm and confident, too. Pause a few seconds between sentences to let important information sink in.

•Be honest if the child asks if you're going to die. If your illness is very treatable, you might respond by saying, "I don't think so, and my doctors and I will do everything we can to prevent that from happening." If the diagnosis is potentially life-threatening, you might respond with, "I don't know, but my doctors and I will do everything we can to prevent that."

•Do not promise that you won't die. That sows doubt in the child's mind about whether he/she is being told the whole truth and robs the child of his chance to come to terms with the possibility of your death.

•Share your emotions with the child. If you're sad, worried or angry, say so—it encourages your kids to be open about their feelings, too. Reassure your children that the family will get through this challenge together and that they will be kept informed.

•Maintain a consistent schedule and normal discipline with your kids. Kids draw a sense of security and normalcy from consistency.

•Head off kids' common misunderstandings and fears. If your kids are younger than age 12, stress that they did not do anything to cause your illness and that there always will be family members to take care of them no matter what. Repeat these points during future conversations.

•Encourage questions. Tell your child that he can ask questions or express his feelings about your illness at any time.

TAILORING THE TALK TO THE CHILD'S AGE

•Toddlers (ages one to two)—Toddlers cannot fully understand what it means to have a serious illness, but they are able to sense when something is wrong and deeply fear being separated from their parents.

What to do: Maintain a consistent environment with predictable caregivers. Provide comfort through touch, rocking and routine.

•Preschool and kindergarten (ages three to six)—Preschoolers can understand the seriousness of an illness, but they often engage in magical thinking and associative logic. They can imagine that waving a toy wand will cure their parent or that the disease was caused by something that they did or thought.

What to do: Use simple terms to explain that you are sick, but provide more detail than you would with a toddler. These details might include the specific name of the illness and where it is in your body. Stress that the illness is not a result of anything he did, nor is it a punishment for anything he might have done wrong. Ask the child to explain back to you the important points to make sure that he understands. Continue to maintain a consistent schedule with predictable caregivers.

•Middle childhood (ages seven to 12)—These children have the capacity for a deeper understanding of your illness, but they still might become confused by big words and complicated topics. They also might not admit when they don't fully understand something you have told them.

What to do: The advice for ages three to six still applies, but add even more specifics—kids this age derive security from concrete facts. Provide details about your illness and treatments. Carefully explain all difficult words and concepts.

Write out schedules for upcoming days and weeks so that the child knows what to expect. You even might want to ask the child if he would like to meet your doctor, assuming that is OK with the doctor.

•Adolescents (ages 13 to 18)—Teenagers can understand the biological and psychological implications of a serious illness. They often are self-centered and might voice concerns or complaints about how the parent's illness affects them rather than about the parent's welfare. This could result in the teenager feeling guilty.

What to do: Provide the basics about your diagnosis and treatment, then ask the teen what he already knows about your illness and what he would like to know. Don't force the conversation if the teen resists. Let him know that you are available to talk whenever he likes, but don't be surprised if he prefers to talk with another adult, such as a trusted coach, teacher or relative.

If your teen wants to learn more about your disease, encourage him to do the research with you. There tends to be a great deal of inaccurate information on the Internet, and even accurate information might not apply to your specific situation. It is very important that your teen has accurate information.

TALKING TO ADULT KIDS ABOUT ILLNESS

The news that a parent has a serious illness is likely to come as a huge emotional blow even to adult children. The adult child might want to drop everything and rush to the parent's side—and might feel helpless or guilty if this is not feasible.

What to do: Consider waiting until you have details about your diagnosis, treatment plan and prognosis before sharing the news. That way, you can give the adult child a more complete picture of the situation, minimizing his fears as much as possible.

If an adult child who lives far away offers to drop everything to come help you, consider suggesting that he postpone such drastic action (unless your prognosis is extremely dire). Better that he save his vacation days and travel budget for times when you might need his help more, such as immediately following surgery.

If the child insists on helping, suggest specific forms of support that can be provided from afar, such as calling or Skyping you often or researching doctors or caregivers on your behalf.

Fast Music and Safe Driving Don't Mix

Teen risk for traffic violations increases when they listen to fast music. When teenagers were allowed to drive while listening to music with fast-paced vocals, about 98% of them made driving errors, such as speeding. When they listened to a softer, easy-listening background, driver errors declined by 20%.

Study of 85 teens by researchers at Ben-Gurion University of the Negev, Beer-Sheva, Israel, published in *Accident Analysis & Prevention.*

The 6 Things to Do If Your Spouse Is Sick

Dan Shapiro, PhD, a psychologist and professor of medical humanism and chair of the department of humanities at Penn State College of Medicine in Hershey. He is author of *And in Health: A Guide for Couples Facing Cancer Together* (Trumpeter-Shambhala). *DanShapiro.org*

If your spouse were diagnosed with cancer or some other life-threatening illness, would you feel fully prepared to deal with the challenge? Virtually no one is.

Someone who knows what works—and what doesn't—is Dan Shapiro, PhD, a psychologist who has battled cancer twice himself—and helped his wife recover from breast cancer. Here's his advice...*

YES, YOU CAN!

When you find out your spouse is seriously ill, it's natural to feel overwhelmed by fear and confusion.

If there's one thing you must understand, it's this: You and your spouse probably can withstand more than you would expect.

Professionals who work with seriously ill patients see this all the time—the vast majority of patients and families do manage to cope, even those who were scared out of their minds at first.

What's most helpful: Remind yourself that you don't have to cope with everything all at once. Instead of worrying about the big picture, focus on what you have to contend with right now—the potentially painful procedure your spouse has scheduled for this morning or the bandage change you help with every afternoon.

*This article does not address the complexities of dealing with a spouse who has dementia or some other cognitive illness.

DON'T OVERDO OPTIMISM

Some people are naturally optimistic, while others have a darker outlook often described as "realistic." When couples are out of sync in this regard, friction can result.

What makes things worse is a belief that even a peek at negative possibilities can lead to relapse, complications and worse. The fact is, there's no hard evidence that optimism makes a real difference in mortality from cancer—and except for some mental-health conditions, it probably doesn't have a significant effect on other diseases.

Not helpful: Uncalibrated optimism from the well spouse—such as "I'm sure it's nothing," while waiting for test results...or "This new treatment is sure to work," when the last one failed. If the patient's fears turn out to be justified, it may be hard to forget your too-casual attitude.

What's most helpful: "Survivor optimism"—a basic belief that "whatever results come back, whatever we have to do, wherever we have to go to get the best treatment, we'll get through it, and we'll make the best of it."

YOU'RE IN IT TOGETHER

When someone you love is scared or in pain, the natural response often is to try to "fix" it. But while this may make you feel better, your spouse may find it much more supportive if you simply show that you understand what he/she is going through.

Example: Your spouse may say, "My surgery scar really hurts!" Rather than responding with, "Let's take you to the emergency room," try, "That sounds so uncomfortable...You've been so brave!"

And if you're scared yourself, you may try to keep up a brave front so your spouse won't worry about you. But if carried too far, this can give the impression that you don't care, which can be deeply injuring.

What's most helpful: A balanced approach where you are honest with yourself about your feelings and share them with your spouse—at least some of the time. Don't overdo gloom and doom, but be open enough about your fears and concerns to convey that we're in this together.

DEALING WITH THE DOCTOR

In many couples, it's common for one person to be highly suspicious of doctors, while the other person tends to trust them and give them the benefit of the doubt.

If this sounds like you and your spouse, consider it a strength rather than a point of contention. By combining your beliefs, you can avoid extreme biases that may prevent your loved one from receiving the best medical care. (And the truth is, sometimes doctors are right, and sometimes they are not!)

What's most helpful: Plan your doctor visits together in advance. Decide what each of you wants to know, who will ask which questions and who will write things down. You may need to assertively ask the doctor to stay long enough to answer follow-up questions from you and your spouse. When treatment choices must be made, you can help your spouse gather information and weigh pros and cons.

But remember: It's the person who is sick who should ultimately make the decision.

SET ASIDE TIME

It's easy for a serious illness to dominate your life together.

What's most helpful: Compartmentalize. Consider setting aside some time every week (it might be 10 minutes or could be an hour or more, depending on what you need to discuss) to focus on the "business" of your lives and how illness has impacted it.

This may include getting household chores done despite crowded therapy schedules or discussing financial issues. This will allow you to still enjoy your life together.

Even better: Also plan regular "date nights" or "date days" when discussion of illness is off-limits. Go out to a restaurant or a movie if you're able.

A WORD ABOUT SEX

Serious illness and its treatment can have a powerful impact on sexual function, but they needn't put an end to intimacy.

What's most helpful: Many couples rarely, if ever, talk about their sex lives when they are both healthy—let alone when one of them is ill. What will really help now is having the gumption to simply be candid with each other. Discuss how things have changed and how you can make the best of it.

Intercourse isn't always necessary for satisfaction, and intimacy in all its forms can express your love and show your spouse you find him/her attractive regardless of change and limitation. Aim for a healthy dose of enthusiasm for new ways of relating to each other.

Movies Save Marriages

Newlyweds who watch five relationship movies are half as likely to divorce or separate within three years as ones who do not, reports Ronald D. Rogge, PhD. Watching five movies from the more than 100 listed at Couples-Research.com and then discussing them using the site's interactive tools help couples actively set aside time to prioritize and focus on their relationship, thus strengthening bonds.

Ronald D. Rogge, PhD, associate professor in the department of clinical and social sciences in psychology, University of Rochester, Rochester, New York, and leader of a study published in *Journal of Consulting* and *Clinical Psychology.*

Should You Have Sex Just to Please Your Partner?

Amy Muise, PhD, a postdoctoral fellow in psychology at the University of Toronto Mississauga in Ontario, Canada. She has authored or collaborated on dozens of scientific papers on sexuality and relationships, and writes the blog "The Passion Paradox" for *Psychology Today.*

What happens when your partner wants to have sex, but you're just not in the mood? Should you do it anyway to please him or her? Or is no sex better than sex for the "wrong reasons"? Recent studies led by Amy Muise, PhD, a researcher who specializes in human sexuality, offer helpful insights. *Below, she answers some questions on her latest research...*

You study sexual motivation. What role does motivation play in a couple's sex life? It's well-known that couples who have more and better sex are happier. But our research shows that what motivates couples to have sex—the reasons they have it—also has a major impact on relationship satisfaction.

In one study, we gave 108 dating couples questionnaires to fill out every night for several weeks, and in another study, we gave the questionnaires to 44 couples who were married or living together. In both groups, participants rated themselves more sexually satisfied and happier in their relationships when they had sex for what we term "approach goals" than when they had sex for so-called "avoidance goals."

Approach goals include having sex to pursue a positive outcome, such as pleasure or greater closeness, for yourself and/or your partner. Avoidance goals include avoiding a negative outcome for yourself, such as feeling guilty about saying no to sex...or avoiding conflict or disappointing your partner.

What's more, we found that a person's reason for having sex affected his or her partner's feelings, too. When an individual's motivation was positive, the partner felt more desire and relationship satisfaction than when it was negative.

Why does one partner's motivation influence the other partner's feelings? If a person is having sex for positive reasons, desire and satisfaction will be evident and can carry over to the partner. Conversely, if the reason for sex is negative, the person enjoys it less, and the partner will probably pick up on this fact through body language, perhaps, and respond accordingly.

Does motivation really make a difference in the overall health of a couple's sexual relationship? There's good reason to think so. We contacted the married and cohabiting couples four months after they did the original questionnaires and found that the more often individuals reported sex for positive reasons when first surveyed, the more sexual desire they felt at this later time. Individuals reporting sex for negative reasons when first surveyed had lower sexual satisfaction after four months, and their partners reported less sexual satisfaction and less commitment.

It sounds like the conclusion is, if one partner doesn't want sex, it's better for him or her to say "no." That's not necessarily true. We found, as others have, that couples generally feel closer after having sex for whatever reason. If some nights you're doing it mostly to avoid upsetting your partner, there's probably no harm in that and even some benefit. But if this is a chronic pattern, it's likely to be undermining your relationship.

What can a person who chronically doesn't want to have sex do to change that feeling? We know from research into other social interactions that motivation can be changed. In the case of sex, feelings generally aren't 100% positive or negative, but a mix. The first step is to take some time to think about how you feel about having sex with your partner.

Once you're aware of how you feel, you might try shifting your thoughts toward the positive—what you've enjoyed about sex in the past, how this is an opportunity to express love for your partner, and how it will bring you closer. It could enhance the experience and even alter your motivation.

Despite this advice, there will inevitably be times when sex isn't mutually agreeable—due to life circumstances, medical conditions, etc. Honest talk promotes compromise—maybe you can find something that's pleasurable for you both at the time. You might provide affection, attention and the expression of love in ways other than sex. Perhaps you don't want to cuddle when you're not in the mood for sex, fearing it will be interpreted as a gateway to sex, but this gesture could make both of you happy.

Can a certain kind of motivation keep desire alive in long-term relationships? It certainly seems so. In our group of married and cohabiting couples, we asked participants how strongly they were motivated when having sex to please their partners and meet their partners' needs. We also questioned participants on how much they focused on their own pleasure.

We found that individuals who made their partners' sexual needs a priority reported stronger feelings of desire. Additionally, this generous approach seemed to prolong desire—four months later, desire was just as strong, while in those who cared less about pleasing their partners, it had declined.

Aren't there risks involved in putting your partner's needs before your own? Most people think that giving is good for the self and for relationships. We would all agree that giving a partner a back rub or going to a work function just to make him or her happy is fine. But when it comes to sex, doing something solely to please a partner somehow raises a red flag.

We didn't look at this in the study, but in general, if one person adopts a partner-pleasing mentality, the other one will, too...and there needs to be some give and take, or the relationship simply won't last. Just remember to keep your own desires and limits in mind, even as you try to make your partner happy.

What's the single best piece of advice you can give to help people make their partners happier sexually? Many people find it hard to talk about sex openly, but it's vital. In fact, a recent study found that partners are particularly likely to be satisfied if they give feedback and communicate what they're feeling while in bed, rather than before or after.

A Happy Husband Is Key for a Happy Marriage

James Iveniuk, PhD candidate, department of sociology, University of Chicago.
Jamila Bookwala, PhD, professor of psychology, Lafayette College, Easton, PA.
Journal of Marriage and Family

Long-term unions tend to stay happy if the husband has an agreeable personality and is in good health, according to a recent study.

Whether a wife is agreeable and in good health, however, doesn't play as big a role in predicting marital harmony, the researchers found.

"It's the husband's health more than the wife's that is associated with conflict in marriage," said James Iveniuk, lead study author and a PhD candidate at the University of Chicago.

BACKGROUND

While previous studies have looked at the quality of a marriage or long-term partnership and its effect on health, Iveniuk and his team wanted to understand how the reverse direction might work.

So, they looked at how health and personality characteristics affect late-life marital conflict.

STUDY DETAILS

For the study, Iveniuk used data from a national survey that analyzed 953 heterosexual couples, married or cohabitating. The men and women were aged 63 to 90 and their relationships, on average, had lasted 39 years.

The study was published in the *Journal of Marriage and Family.*

The researchers analyzed information about each partner's health and other characteristics, such as their tendency to be agreeable and a measure the authors describe as "positivity" —how important it was for the partner to be viewed in a positive light.

Personality traits, such as extroversion, were also considered. Extroversion describes not only how outgoing a person is, Iveniuk said, but also how energized that person is by socializing, how impulsive and their degree of self-control.

To gauge marital conflict, the researchers took into account how much one partner tended to criticize the other, make too many demands or get on the other's nerves.

"If the husband's health is bad, the wife is more likely to report high levels of conflict," Iveniuk said.

But the opposite was not true. The husband's health may have a greater impact on the wife, Iveniuk noted, because wives are more likely to be asked to provide nurturing and caretaking. If the wife is ill, the husband may get another family member to step in and help, he suggested.

If the husband had high levels of positivity, there was also less conflict, Iveniuk found. The opposite was not true—the amount of positivity the wives displayed had no effect on the husbands' reports of conflict.

However, if men were easily stressed out or were very extroverted, the wives tended to complain more about the marriage, Iveniuk found. The stressed-out person tends to be a difficult person to live with, he said, and wives may bear the brunt of that more than husbands with stressed-out wives.

Wives married to husbands who score high on extroversion may find it difficult to "tame them," Iveniuk said, and find it hard to deal with their high energy level and impulsivity.

EXPERT COMMENTARY

An expert who was not involved with the study said its findings may also reflect women's tendency to take things personally.

Traditionally, "women are far more responsive to the feelings of others, the behavior of others. We're reared to be more sensitive to how others relate to us," said Jamila Bookwala, PhD, a professor of psychology at Lafayette College, in Easton, Pennsylvania, who also studies marital quality.

If a husband is more positive, the wife is likely to feel her marriage is much better. "If she's a grouch, he is less affected by it," she said. Men may simply be better at shrugging off perceived slights and criticisms, she suggested.

Other research has found, in general, that older men rate marriage quality higher than do older women, Dr. Bookwala said.

RELATIONSHIP ADVICE

Couples in long-term unions might take a step back and think about whether they could do things differently to preserve or increase harmony, Dr. Bookwala and Iveniuk agreed.

"Take a look at your reaction [to conflict]," Iveniuk said. If a man's inclination is to withdraw at the first sign of trouble and leave the discussion, maybe he could stay and talk it out.

Women might realize that they tend to be more relationship focused, and also be aware that this can actually make them more vulnerable to criticism, Dr. Bookwala said.

info To learn more about keeping relationships healthy, visit the website of the American Psychological Association at *www.apa.org/helpcenter/healthy-relationships.aspx.*

Heart & Stroke

How Does the Weather Affect Your Heart?

The arctic blast that brought tundralike temperatures to much of the country during the winter of 2013-2014 left behind more than frozen pipes and frost-nipped noses. During a typical winter, there are up to 36% more circulatory-related deaths than during warmer months.

And it's not just cold weather that puts you at risk. Researchers have identified other types of weather—throughout the year—that trigger spikes in hospitalizations and death.

For details on the effects that weather can have on your heart, we spoke to Barry A. Franklin, PhD, a leading expert in cardiac rehabilitation.

We hear a lot about cold weather being hard on the heart. At what temperature does this really become an issue?

When it's cold enough to wear a winter jacket, it is cold enough to think about the health of your heart. In fact, research that was recently presented at the European Society of Cardiology Congress shows that the risk of having a heart attack increases by 7% for every 18°F drop below 73°F.

Why exactly is cold weather so dangerous?

Cold temperatures cause blood vessels throughout the body to temporarily constrict, raising blood pressure. Since the arteries that supply the heart are only about the thickness of cooked spaghetti, even a slight narrowing can cause reduced blood flow.

Winter temperatures aren't generally a problem if you are young and active. But risk rises as you hit middle age and beyond. The risk is highest for adults who are ages 65 and older, particularly those with underlying health problems, such as diabetes, obesity or preexist-

Barry A. Franklin, PhD, director of preventive cardiology and rehabilitation at William Beaumont Hospital in Royal Oak, Michigan. Dr. Franklin is coauthor of *109 Things You Can Do to Prevent, Halt & Reverse Heart Disease* (Workman).

ing heart disease. For people in these groups, spending even a few minutes in below-freezing temperatures can trigger a 20- to 50-point rise in blood pressure.

That's why I advise older adults, in particular, to stay indoors on the coldest days if possible. When you do go outdoors, don't depend on a light jacket—you should really bundle up by wearing a hat and gloves and dressing in multiple loose layers under your coat. Each layer traps air that's been heated by the body and serves as insulation.

And what about hot weather—does it harm the heart?

Actually, heat kills more people every year than any other type of weather.

High temperatures, generally above 80°F, but especially greater than 90°F, can cause heat syncope (sudden dizziness and/or fainting)...heat edema (swelling in the feet/ankles)...and heat stroke, in which the body's core temperature can rise above 104°F. People with atrial fibrillation or dementia are at a 6% to 8% increased risk of dying on hot days. Dementia affects the brain's ability to regulate the body's heat response.

Why is strenuous exertion so dangerous for many people during weather extremes?

Snow shoveling provides a good example. This activity creates a "perfect storm" of demands on the heart. With snow shoveling, the real danger—particularly for those who are older and/or sedentary—is the exertion itself.

Moving snow is hard work. Each shovelful weighs about 16 pounds (including the weight of the shovel). If you lift the shovel once every five seconds and continue for 10 minutes, you'll have moved nearly one ton of snow. This exertion can have adverse effects on the heart.

Here's why: Snow shoveling involves isometric exercise and unaccustomed muscle tension, which increases heart rate and blood pressure. Your legs may stay "planted" when you shovel, which allows blood to pool and reduces circulation to the heart.

Also, people tend to hold their breath (this is known as a Valsalva maneuver, and it often occurs when people are straining to lift heavy loads) when they are wielding a shovel, which causes a further rise in heart rate and blood pressure. That's why every year, we read or hear about people who dropped dead while shoveling snow.

Is there any way to reduce the risk associated with snow shoveling?

If you have or suspect you have heart disease, I suggest that you don't shovel your own snow. Hire someone to do it for you.

If you are in good shape and want to shovel your own snow, it may be safer in the afternoon. In general, most heart attacks occur between 6 am and 10 am, when heart rate and blood pressure tend to be higher. You're also more likely to form blood clots early in the day.

Then be sure to shovel slowly...work for only a few minutes at a time...and keep your legs moving to circulate blood. And remember, it's best to push snow rather than lift it. This helps keep your legs moving and takes less exertion than lifting. There are snow shovels designed for pushing snow.

What types of exertion are especially dangerous during hot weather?

Racket sports, water skiing, marathon running and certain highly competitive sports seem to be associated with a greater incidence of cardiac events in hot, humid weather. Why? Heart rates are disproportionately increased. Electrolytes,

Skipping Breakfast May Hurt the Heart

In a study of nearly 27,000 men over age 45, those who reported regularly skipping breakfast were 27% more likely to suffer heart attacks or die from coronary disease than those who didn't miss the meal.

Why: Skipping breakfast may contribute to other coronary risk factors, such as obesity, diabetes, high blood pressure and high cholesterol.

Good way to start the day: A breakfast of chopped fruit and nuts on a bowl of whole-grain cereal or steel-cut oats, topped with milk or yogurt.

Leah Cahill, PhD, research fellow, Harvard School of Public Health, Boston.

The Flu Shot Protects Your Heart

The flu vaccine offers surprising benefits, we hear from Jacob A. Udell, MD, MPH. A review of six studies of more than 6,700 adults found that the flu vaccine lowered risk for heart attack, stroke, heart failure or death from any cardiac cause by 36%.

Theory: The vaccine may reduce flu-related inflammation that can make plaque in the arteries unstable and trigger a heart attack or other cardiac event. Violent coughing, elevated heart rate, pneumonia and other flu symptoms also may stress the heart.

Jacob A. Udell, MD, MPH, cardiologist, Women's College Hospital, University of Toronto, Canada.

such as sodium and potassium, also are lost, which can lead to dangerous heart rhythms.

What steps should people take to protect themselves in hot weather?

Everyone knows to drink water when it's hot. But even people who are consciously trying to stay hydrated often do not drink enough. Drink plenty of cool liquids before, during and after heat exposure. If you're sweating a lot, you might want to drink an electrolyte-rich sports drink such as Gatorade or Powerade. And be sure to wear lightweight, loose-fitting clothing when you go outdoors.

In addition, think about any medications you may be taking. Many common drugs, including certain antihistamines and antidepressants, have anticholinergic effects—they inhibit your body's ability to cool off.

To help your body adapt to heat and humidity: As the weather grows hotter, gradually increase your daily exposure to the heat. The body's circulation and cooling efficiency increases, generally in eight to 14 days. Afterward, the body is better able to cope with extremes in heat and humidity.

Do You Have a Heart Attack Gene?

Bradley F. Bale, MD, cofounder of the Heart Attack & Stroke Prevention Center, Nashville, and medical director of the Grace Clinic Heart Health Center, Lubbock, Texas. He is coauthor, with Amy Doneen, ARNP, and Lisa Collier Cool, of *Beat the Heart Attack Gene: The Revolutionary Plan to Prevent Heart Disease, Stroke, and Diabetes* (Turner).

Even if you do everything right—you don't smoke, you're not overweight and you manage your cholesterol and blood pressure—your odds of having a heart attack might be higher than you think.

An eye-opening case: One of our patients, a 44-year-old executive whom we nicknamed "Superman," looked very healthy. His Framingham Risk Score—a standard measure of heart disease risk predicted that he had only a 1% risk of having a heart attack over the next 10 years. That should have been good news—except that other tests we did, which most doctors do not routinely give, showed that his real risk was about 40 times higher.

THE TESTS YOU NEED

Many of the tests that are used to detect heart disease are decades old. Some look for risk factors (such as arterial narrowing) that have less to do with the actual risk of having a heart attack than most people think. Many of the tests that can make a difference still aren't used by most doctors.

Most cardiologists routinely recommend angiography, an imaging test that looks for large blockages in the coronary arteries. If a blockage of 70% or more is found, a patient might be advised to receive a stent or undergo a bypass, surgical procedures that don't always help and can have a high rate of complications.

Severely blocked arteries can be a problem, but a more common, and typically overlooked, threat is from small deposits inside artery walls. A patient might have dozens or even hundreds of deposits that are too small to be detected with angiography.

The risk: When these "hidden" deposits are exposed to inflammation—triggered by insulin resistance, smoking, a poor diet or stress, for example—they can rupture, tear the blood vessel lining and trigger a clot, the cause of most heart attacks.

New approaches: Doctors can now predict the risk for a heart attack with far more accuracy than in the past—if you know which tests to ask for. Tests I recommend…

• **Carotid intima-media thickness (CIMT).** This is an effective way to measure atherosclerosis inside an artery wall (between the intima and media layers). The FDA-approved test uses an ultrasound wand to look for the thickening of the carotid arteries that occurs when plaque between the two layers accumulates and pushes outward.

An isolated area of thickness measuring 1.3 mm or greater indicates plaque—and an increased risk for a heart attack or stroke.

Most patients who have excessive arterial thickening will be advised to exercise more, eat a healthier diet and take a daily baby aspirin to reduce the risk for clots. A cholesterol-lowering statin drug also may be prescribed.

• **Genetic tests.** More than half of all Americans have one or more gene variations that increase the risk for a heart attack and a stroke. According to research published in *Circulation*, up to 70% of patients who are given the genetic tests described below will be reclassified as having a higher heart attack risk than their doctors originally thought. The cost of testing has dropped to about $100 per gene. Your insurance may cover the cost. *Important gene tests…*

• **9P21.** If you inherit two copies of this "heart attack gene" (one from each parent), your risk of developing heart disease or having a heart attack at an early age (in men, under age 45…in women, under age 55) is 102% higher than that of someone without the gene. And increased risk continues if you are already past these ages.

You'll also have a 74% increased risk for an abdominal aortic aneurysm, a dangerous weakening in the heart's largest blood vessel. If you test positive, your doctor will advise earlier and more frequent abdominal aortic scans. If you smoke, stop now. Most aortic aneurysms occur in smokers.

You should also exercise for at least 22 minutes daily (the amount found in research to be protective) and maintain healthy cholesterol and blood pressure levels.

Important: Patients with the 9P21 gene often are advised to have an ankle-brachial index test, which involves measuring blood pressure in the arms and ankles. It's used to diagnose peripheral artery disease (PAD), plaque buildups in the legs that quadruple or even quintuple the risk for a heart attack or stroke.

• **Apo E.** This gene affects how your body metabolizes nutrients. There are different types of Apo E. The 3/3 genotype—64% of Americans have it—increases cardiovascular disease, but not as much as the 3/4 or 4/4 types. Those with 3/4 or 4/4 need to eat a very low-fat diet (with no more than 20% of calories from fat). Those with the 3/3 genotype are advised to eat a Mediterranean-style diet—focusing mainly on plant foods…fish…and olive oil.

• **KIF6.** Patients with the so-called arginine gene variant have up to a 55% increased risk for cardiovascular disease. There are no particular lifestyle changes known to be especially helpful for these patients. It's also useful to know if you're a noncarrier of KIF6—as such, you won't receive significant risk reduction if you are prescribed either *atorvastatin* (Lipitor) or *pravastatin* (Pravachol), two of the most popular statin drugs. Instead, you'll need a different statin, such as *lovastatin* (Mevacor).

ANOTHER CRUCIAL TEST

An oral glucose tolerance test can detect insulin resistance years or even decades before it progresses to diabetes. But many doctors still use the simpler A1C test. It's more convenient—it doesn't require fasting—but it often fails to detect insulin resistance, one of the main causes of heart attacks and strokes. Insulin resistance leads to inflammation that can trigger plaques to rupture and form clots.

With an oral glucose tolerance test, your blood sugar is measured. Then you drink a sweet solution, and your blood sugar is measured again two hours later. A level of 100 mg/dL to 139 mg/dL could indicate insulin resistance. Higher levels may indicate prediabetes—or, if they're high enough, full-blown diabetes.

Next steps: Regular exercise is critical if you have insulin resistance or diabetes.

Also helpful: Weight loss, if needed, reduced intake of sugary beverages and foods, and a diet rich in fruits, vegetables and grains.

Taking Aspirin Before Bed May Lower Heart Attack Risk

People taking low-dose aspirin because they are at high risk for a heart attack should consider taking it at night rather than in the morning. Nighttime aspirin consumption significantly reduces blood platelet activity in the morning. Platelet activity is associated with heart attacks and strokes, which occur most often in the morning.

Study of 290 people by researchers at Leiden University Medical Center, the Netherlands, presented at the American Heart Association's Scientific Sessions in Dallas.

Gardening, Housework Help Boost Your Heart Health

Elin Ekblom-Bak, doctoral student, Swedish School of Sport and Health Sciences, and Karolinska Institute, Stockholm.
Gregg Fonarow, MD, professor, cardiology, University of California, Los Angeles.
Samantha Heller, RD, senior clinical nutritionist, exercise physiologist, NYU Langone Medical Center, New York City.
British Journal of Sports Medicine

Activities, such as gardening, do-it-yourself projects and housework, may be as good as formal exercise when it comes to reducing the risk for heart attack and stroke, Swedish researchers say.

For people age 60 and older, just keeping busy with daily activities can reduce the risk of cardiovascular problems by nearly 30% and even prolong life, they added.

Being on your feet and active cuts the time spent sitting around, pointed out lead researcher Elin Ekblom-Bak, a doctoral student at the Swedish School of Sport and Health Sciences and the Karolinska Institute, in Stockholm.

"Sitting is mainly replacing time you spend in daily activity and vice versa," Ekblom-Bak said. A recent study found long periods of sitting actually increased the risk for diabetes, cardiovascular disease and death, she noted.

STUDY DETAILS

For the recent study, researchers collected data on more than 3,800 men and women in Sweden who were born in 1937 and 1938. Participants were asked about their lifestyle, which included information on their diet, whether they smoked or drank alcohol, and how physically active they were.

The participants were also asked how often they took part in activities, such as gardening, do-it-yourself projects, car maintenance and blackberry picking over the past year. They were also asked about any exercise they did.

To see how heart-healthy they were, the researchers examined the participants and took blood samples to assess levels of fat and sugar. They also checked for high levels of blood-clotting factor, which is linked to a raised heart attack and stroke risk.

During more than 12 years of follow-up, 476 of the participants died from or experienced a first heart attack or stroke, and 383 died from other various causes.

People whose daily activities kept them moving reduced their risk of a heart attack or stroke by 27% and the risk of dying from any cause by 30%, compared with people who spent the least amount of time on their feet.

The report was published in the *British Journal of Sports Medicine.*

IMPLICATIONS

"The results of this study showed that activities of daily life are as important as regular intentional exercise for older adults for cardiovascular health and longevity," she said.

But that doesn't mean formal exercise isn't important. "We saw that those who exercised regularly and that also had a daily physically active life had the lowest risk of all," Ekblom-Bak explained.

The time people spend exercising, however, is only a small part of the day, which leaves a lot of time for daily activities or sitting, she added.

"Promoting daily life activities is as important as recommending regular exercise for older adults for cardiovascular health and longevity," Ekblom-Bak said.

"This is particularly important for older adults as they tend to spend a greater portion of their active day performing non-exercise physical activity, as they often find it difficult to achieve recommended exercise intensity levels," she said.

STRATEGIES TO INCREASE PHYSICAL ACTIVITY

Traditional notions of retirement often don't support continued physical activity at this stage of life. "It is almost expected that as we age, we move less," said Samantha Heller, RD, a senior clinical nutritionist and exercise physiologist at NYU Langone Medical Center, in New York City.

"Retirement, a patient told me, is for sitting around, resting and watching TV," she said. "Unfortunately, sedentary lifestyles now range across all ages with the same unhealthy results—increased risk for diseases such as cardiovascular disease, metabolic syndrome and certain cancers."

The human body is designed to be moving a good portion of the day, Heller said. "The less one physically moves, the less they are able to move," she said.

Regular physical activities such as house cleaning, gardening, lawn care and climbing stairs help keep the body mobile and strong, Heller said.

"You can burn up to six times as much energy per minute when house cleaning as you do when you are sitting still. People of all ages need to be encouraged to get up off the couch and turn off the computer and TV and move," she said.

Heller said there are simple ways to add more physical activity into the day, such as the following...

- **Stand up when talking on the phone.**
- **March in place when watching TV—at least during the commercials.**
- **Get up from your desk every hour** and do jumping jacks, knee lifts or knee bends for three to five minutes.
- **Climb a flight of stairs every few hours.**
- **Vacuum the house.**
- **Mop the floor.**

MORE REASONS TO MOVE

Gregg Fonarow, MD, a professor of cardiology at the University of California, Los Angeles, said sitting for too long may have adverse effects including burning fewer calories, and increasing insulin resistance and fats in the blood.

"Greater time spent in non-exercise physical activities can potentially counter these effects," Dr. Fonarow said. "These findings further emphasize the importance of decreasing sedentary time and encouraging everyday regular non-exercise physical activity to improve cardiovascular health."

info For exercise advice, visit the American Heart Association website, *www.heart.org*, and search "physical activity in adults."

Reduce Risk for Dangerous Aneurysms

People who eat more than two servings of fruit daily are 25% less likely to develop abdominal aortic aneurysms (AAAs) than people who eat little or no fruit—and they are 43% less likely to have aneurysms that rupture. If an AAA ruptures, life-threatening bleeding may occur.

Otto Stackelberg, MD, a PhD student at Institute of Environmental Medicine, Karolinska Institute, Stockholm, and lead author of a study of 80,426 people, published in *Circulation*.

New Way to Predict Heart Problems

Gregory Marcus, MD, director of clinical research, division of cardiology, University of California, San Francisco.

Left anterior fascicular block (LAFB) is an indicator of possible heart scarring that's long been viewed as a benign condition.

New thinking: LAFB, which shows up in a standard electrocardiogram (EKG), may signal an increased risk for several serious heart conditions. A 16-year analysis of the EKGs of 1,664 healthy people over age 65 found that those with LAFB had an 89% greater risk for atrial fibrillation...a 243% greater risk for heart failure...and a 57% increased risk for death from any cause.

At your next EKG: Ask your doctor if the test shows LAFB. If so, discuss how to lower your risk for the conditions mentioned above.

Vegetarians Have 32% Lower Risk for Heart Attack Than Meat Eaters

Vegetarians also have lower blood pressure and better cholesterol levels than nonvegetarians. Avoiding meat reduces the likelihood of plaque buildup and artery blockages that can lead to heart attack.

Study of about 45,000 adults by researchers at University of Oxford, UK, published in *The American Journal of Clinical Nutrition*.

Can You Survive When Your Heart Just Stops?

Norman S. Abramson, MD, chair of the board of directors of the Sudden Cardiac Arrest Foundation, SCA-Aware.org, based in Pittsburgh, and a former professor of emergency medicine at the University of Pittsburgh. His research focuses on improving neurological outcomes among survivors of cardiac arrest.

Sudden chest pain isn't something you're likely to ignore. This symptom—along with breathlessness, cold sweats and other classic heart attack symptoms—is a clear sign that you need to call 911.

While a possible heart attack is scary enough, the reality actually could be even worse. With sudden cardiac arrest (SCA), brain damage is almost certain unless you are treated within just a few minutes. And unlike a heart attack, which many people survive, SCA is almost always fatal. But what if that grim picture could be improved?

A chance of survival: Recent research suggests that paying close attention to early signs that may precede SCA—as well as being prepared in your home, where this killer condition most often strikes—could mean the difference between life and death.

What you need to know...

WHEN THE HEART JUST STOPS

A heart attack occurs when a blood clot interrupts blood flow to a section of the heart. In contrast, with SCA, an electrical malfunction in the heart triggers a dangerous abnormality in the heart rhythm (arrhythmia) that disrupts blood flow to the brain and other organs.

Only about 10% of people who suffer SCA live long enough to get to a hospital. Most—such as newsman Tim Russert who succumbed to SCA in 2008—collapse and then die within minutes.

ARE YOU AT RISK?

More than 400,000 Americans (not including hospitalized patients) suffer SCA each year. If your doctor has warned you about elevated cholesterol, high blood pressure or other cardiovascular risk factors, you know that you could be setting yourself up for a heart attack. But the same conditions also mean that you're at risk for SCA.

For certain other people, SCA is truly a stealth killer. It sometimes occurs in those who have "silent" (often congenital) cardiovascular disease. Abusing drugs or alcohol also increases risk for SCA.

KNOW THE SIGNS

When someone suffers cardiac arrest, the only symptoms that occur simultaneously tend to be sudden collapse and a loss of consciousness. The victim also will have stopped breathing and won't have a detectable pulse.

What's new: Many individuals do have advance warning of SCA—even if they choose to ignore it.

In fact, when researchers recently looked into this, they found that 53% of SCA patients had prior symptoms, including chest pain, shortness of breath, heart palpitations and/or fainting. The symptoms—identical to those that often accompany heart attacks—occurred anywhere from one hour to four weeks before the SCA. Since SCA is so closely tied to heart disease, it makes sense that many victims will have heart disease symptoms before they suffer from SCA. If you have any of these symptoms, consult a doctor!

PROTECT YOURSELF

Most of the same approaches that will protect you from a heart attack—such as maintaining a healthy weight and not smoking—will help you avoid SCA. *Also useful for people concerned about SCA...*

- **Consider buying an automated external defibrillator (AED).** It can triple the likelihood of survival when used within the first minute or two of SCA. An AED is about the size of a laptop computer. The cost ranges from $1,200 to $2,500 but might be covered by insurance or Medicare if you have a high-risk arrhythmia or another heart condition. The device is easy to operate. Once it's turned on, a voice and screen explain where to attach the electrodes and when to push the buttons.

Be sure to act quickly: If someone collapses, use the device immediately. It won't prompt you to deliver a shock unless the person is experiencing SCA. For each one-minute delay, the chance of survival from SCA drops about 10%.

Important: I advise everyone who has heart disease or heart disease risk factors to talk to his/her doctor about owning one of these devices (or sharing one with close neighbors)—and to watch an online video or take an in-person class on how to use it. AEDs are available online.

- **Chest compressions.** Even if an AED is available, give chest compressions until it is ready to be placed on the victim's chest. If the heartbeat hasn't started after following AED voice prompts, do chest compressions for two minutes and use the AED again. Or if there's no AED, do chest compressions alone. Don't waste time checking for a pulse or giving mouth-to-mouth breathing—it's the chest compressions that are needed to restart the victim's heart. If someone collapses and is unresponsive and you suspect it's SCA, call 911 first. Then give the compressions, and don't stop (it's hard work, so you may need help from a bystander) until the emergency medical service arrives.

How to do compressions: Put the heel of one hand on the center of the chest (between the nipples)...place the heel of your other hand on top of the first hand for strength...position your body over your hands...and press hard about two inches into the chest. Try to give at least 100 compressions per minute (almost two per second).

For a hands-only CPR video: Go to *Heart.org/HandsOnlyCPR.* For more detailed instruction, sign up for in-person training at your local hospital or fire department.

HOSPITAL CARE

If you suffer SCA in the hospital (or if you get to an ER in time), you'll be given treatments to restart the heart and re-establish heart, brain and lung functions.

Induced hypothermia, a promising therapy to reduce the damage from SCA, is available at many hospitals. This therapy involves rapid cooling of the body to about 89°F for about 24 hours. Cooling the body as soon as the heart has been restarted lowers the metabolic requirements of the brain and reduces the risk for long-term neurological problems, such as coma.

People who survive SCA may need additional treatments to prevent a second cardiac arrest.

Examples: Some are given an implantable cardioverter defibrillator (ICD), a surgically implanted device that analyzes the heartbeat and administers shocks to treat ventricular fibrillation. Another approach, radio-frequency ablation, uses radio-frequency energy to destroy abnormal heart cells that can cause irregular rhythms.

Better Surgery Prep for Heart Patients

According to a recent study, among adults with severe heart disease who underwent noncardiac surgery, those given beta-blocker drugs beforehand were 40% less likely to have a stroke or heart attack or die during the 30 days following surgery than those who did not take these drugs.

Possible reason: Beta-blockers lower blood pressure and slow heart rate, which can help ease stress on the heart during and after surgery.

If you have heart disease and need noncardiac surgery: Ask your doctor if you should take a beta-blocker.

Charlotte Andersson, MD, PhD, cardiology researcher, Gentofte Hospital, Hellerup, Denmark.

Could You Work the Device That Restarts Hearts?

U.S. Food and Drug Administration, news release.

Potentially life-saving devices called automated external defibrillators are common in public places across the United States and can help rescue people suffering a sudden cardiac arrest, government health officials say.

Sudden cardiac arrest—a leading cause of death in the nation—results from a malfunction in the heart's electrical system. Automated external defibrillators deliver an electrical shock to restore the heart's normal rhythm. The devices are found in many shopping malls, grocery stores, airports, schools and offices.

Each year, emergency medical responders treat about 383,000 Americans with sudden cardiac arrest. Less than 12% of those patients survive. For every minute that a person in sudden cardiac arrest has an abnormal heart rhythm, the chances of survival fall by 7% to 10%, according to Oscar Tovar-Calderon, MD, a medical officer at the FDA. "Defibrillation is a time-sensitive issue," he said.

WHAT TO DO

Someone who suddenly collapses and is unresponsive and not breathing normally may have suffered sudden cardiac arrest. Bystanders need to call 911, start CPR and then look for an automated external defibrillator. If the automated external defibrillator fails to deliver an electric shock, bystanders should continue CPR until an emergency responder arrives, says Dr. Tovar-Calderon.

Automated external defibrillators are not difficult to use and provide voice prompts to guide users, but the FDA highly recommends that people get trained in their use. Training is frequently offered, along with CPR instruction, by groups, such as the American Red Cross, the American Heart Association and private companies.

People who have a heart condition and are most at risk for sudden cardiac arrest may want to talk to their doctor about having an automated external defibrillator at home, Dr. Tovar-Calderon said.

info For more on automated external defibrillators, visit the website of the U.S. National Heart, Lung, and Blood Institute at *www.nhlbi.nih.gov/health/health-topics/topics/aed/.*

You Can Be Healthy But Still Need a Pacemaker

Jeffrey L. Williams, MD, medical director of electrophysiology at The Good Samaritan Hospital, with a private practice in cardiology and heart-rhythm disorders at Lebanon Cardiology Associates, both in Lebanon, Pennsylvania. He directs the Heart Rhythm Center, HeartRhythm-Center.com, an online forum on pacemakers and related equipment/procedures, and is author of *What Is a Pacemaker? A Cardiologist's Guide for Patients and Care Providers* (CreateSpace).

You might think that you'd never be a candidate for a pacemaker. Perhaps your doctor has told you that your cholesterol levels are good. Maybe your blood pressure readings are normal, too. But these facts don't mean that the electrical components of your heart, which control the speed and rhythm of your heartbeats, are firing on all cylinders.

Common misconceptions: Many people assume that pacemakers are needed only by individuals who have serious cardiovascular disease or are approaching the end of their lives. Neither assumption is true.

It can be common for someone who needs a pacemaker to be otherwise healthy—in these cases, the heart just needs help to generate the signals that make it pump efficiently. And even though people who get pacemakers usually are over age 60, a person of any age may need the device, which is about the size of two poker chips stacked on top of one another. Those with cardiovascular disease also are more likely to need a pacemaker.

WHAT CAN GO WRONG

The heart normally beats 60 to 100 times a minute. The rate and rhythm of the heart are set by a natural pacemaker—a cluster of cells known as the sinoatrial, or SA, node.

What can go wrong: Electrical signals that are delayed or interrupted, due to conditions such as those described later in this article, cause the heart to beat too slowly (a condition known as bradycardia)...or to pump insufficient amounts of blood (a condition known as heart failure).

These problems can lead to unexplained symptoms, such as dizziness, shortness of breath, fatigue and/or episodes of syncope (a sudden loss of consciousness). More subtle symptoms include chest pain, swelling, coughing, difficulty walking and weight gain.

When such symptoms occur, doctors routinely recommend an EKG and/or use of a Holter monitor, a device that's worn at home to record the heart's electrical activity over 24 to 48 hours. An echocardiogram (an ultrasound test that shows how well the heart is working) and/or an intracardiac electrophysiology study (to pinpoint where the heart's electrical system is damaged) also may be needed.

Note: Many heart failure patients need defibrillators, which are different from pacemakers. If a potentially fatal arrhythmia is detected by the device, it can give the patient a lifesaving shock. Pacemakers do not have this ability.

WHEN THE HEART NEEDS HELP

After certain problems are ruled out, you may be advised to get a pacemaker for these conditions...*

• **SA-node dysfunction.** It's common for these electricity-producing cells to slow with age. The heart might beat as little as 30 to 40 times a minute—not allowing the heart to circulate enough of the blood the body needs, particularly during exercise. A pacemaker can help the heart beat more quickly and prevent patients from suffering such symptoms as dizziness and fatigue.

What doctors check before suggesting a pacemaker: Patients with angina (chest pain caused by reduced blood flow to the heart) may be advised to take a beta-blocker drug, such as *atenolol* (Tenormin), to reduce the heart's demand for oxygen. But this type of medication may slow the heart too much and cause bradycardia. Calcium channel blockers, such as

*Doctors should follow the American College of Cardiology's evidence-based guidelines when deciding whether a patient needs a pacemaker. To read these guidelines, go to CardioSource.org (under "Science & Quality," click on "Guidelines & Quality Standards" and search for "Pacemaker").

Better Treatment for Atrial Fibrillation

Recent study: An analysis of health data from 4,060 atrial fibrillation (AF) patients found that those taking the heart drug digoxin were 35% more likely to suffer a cardiovascular-related death and 61% more likely to die due to an arrhythmia (irregular heartbeat) than AF patients not taking the drug.

If you have AF and take digoxin: You may want to discuss medication alternatives with your doctor (such as beta-blockers or calcium channel blockers) to control fast heart rates. If your doctor concludes that digoxin is the best drug for you, talk to him/her about using the lowest possible dose and ask that you be closely monitored.

Samy Claude Elayi, MD, associate professor of medicine, Gill Heart Institute, University of Kentucky, Lexington.

> **Help for Aging Hearts**
>
> *Rapamycin*, a drug used to keep the body from rejecting an organ transplant, has been found to improve age-related heart problems. It extended the lifespans of laboratory animals by 14%. Research on humans is under way.
>
> *Aging Cell*

diltiazem (Cardizem), or other anti-arrhythmics, such as *amiodarone* (Pacerone), also can slow heart rates.

What to try first: If a drug you're taking is causing bradycardia, it's possible that changing the drug and/or dose will help. Be sure to discuss this option with your doctor. If a different drug and/or dose doesn't help within several weeks, you may need a pacemaker.

•Acquired AV (atrioventricular) block. The AV node is an area of heart tissue that conducts electrical impulses from the upper heart chambers, atria, to the lower chambers, ventricles. AV block occurs when there's an electrical conduction delay between the heart's upper and lower chambers—or, in more serious cases, when there's a complete electrical block. The heart still beats but in a disorganized fashion.

What doctors check before suggesting a pacemaker: In some cases, an AV block is temporary—for example, due to Lyme disease or a potassium deficiency.

What to try first: If your doctor says that you are experiencing an AV block, ask about blood tests to check your electrolytes (including potassium) and to ensure that you don't have Lyme disease, which can lead to forms of AV block that usually resolve on their own when the underlying condition is treated.

A "third-degree" AV block is potentially the most serious. It can occur with aging and may even follow a heart attack because the interruption in circulation from a blood clot can damage the AV node.

Important: The AV node usually recovers on its own within a day or two after a heart attack is treated. If the node recovers, you won't need a pacemaker...if symptoms continue, a pacemaker is almost always needed.

•Atrial fibrillation (AF). This common rhythm disturbance causes the atria to beat very fast and send a signal to the ventricles to beat very fast. Most AF patients need medication to control the fast heartbeat (tachycardia), which can lead to bradycardia when normal rhythm returns. This is called tachycardia-bradycardia syndrome, and these patients may benefit from a pacemaker.

Other conditions that can cause a slow and irregular heartbeat that may require a pacemaker include congestive heart failure, neuromuscular diseases (such as Parkinson's disease) and carotid sinus hypersensitivity.

A SPECIAL TRAVEL PRECAUTION

If you have a pacemaker, it's safe to pass through freestanding security systems at airports. But ask security officers to avoid holding a metal-detecting wand near the pacemaker area for more than a second or two because the magnet inside the wand may affect the operation of the pacemaker. Always carry your pacemaker ID card.

Better Heart Attack Care

James J. DiNicolantonio, PharmD, medication therapy management specialist, Wegmans Pharmacy, Ithaca, New York.

In a review of 13 studies of 3,629 patients who had suffered heart attacks up to 24 years earlier, those who took the amino acid L-carnitine experienced significantly improved cardiac health—deaths from all causes were reduced by 27%, ventricular arrhythmias by 65% and angina by 40%—compared with those who took a placebo.

Theory: During a heart attack, blood levels of L-carnitine are depleted.

If you've had a heart attack: Talk to your cardiologist about starting on 2 g daily of L-carnitine and increasing the dose as needed.

Caution: It may interact with thyroid medication and increase risk for seizure in people with a history of seizures.

Tragedies Do Cause Broken Hearts, Study Suggests

American College of Cardiology, news release.
Sadip Pant, MD, internist, University of Arkansas for Medical Sciences, Little Rock.

The stress of natural disasters can break people's hearts, according to a recent study.

Researchers found dramatic rises in "broken heart syndrome" in Vermont after a huge storm ravaged the state and in Missouri after a massive tornado.

BACKGROUND

People with broken heart syndrome—formally called Takotsubo cardiomyopathy—suffer a temporary enlargement and weakening of the heart. The condition is often triggered by extreme emotional or physical stress, such as losing a loved one or being in an automobile accident.

"Despite the seemingly increasing number of natural disasters we have, there is limited data about how it might affect the heart," said lead investigator Sadip Pant, MD, an internist at the University of Arkansas for Medical Sciences.

"Our findings suggest two disasters—one in Vermont and one in Missouri—might have been possible triggers for the clustering of Takotsubo cardiomyopathy cases in these regions," Dr. Pant said.

STUDY DETAILS

For the study, a university team looked at data from nearly 22,000 people in the United States who were diagnosed with broken heart syndrome in 2011. They mapped the cases state by state and found that Missouri and Vermont had the highest rate of cases—169 and 380 per one million residents, respectively.

Most states had fewer than 150 cases per million people. In 2011, Tropical Storm Irene devastated Vermont, and an enormous tornado tore through Joplin, Missouri, and killed at least 158 people.

New Heart-Valve Treatment

Mitral valve regurgitation is a condition in which a heart valve doesn't close all the way—it can cause fatigue, difficulty breathing and heart damage. Until now, the only treatment was open-heart surgery. Now the MitraClip—recently approved by the FDA—can be used to fasten together the loose flaps of the valve. The device is implanted through a catheter, a minimally invasive procedure. It currently is available at the 52 medical centers that participated in the clinical trials. Other hospitals will use the therapy soon.

Ted Feldman, MD, director of the Cardiac Catheterization Laboratory at NorthShore University HealthSystem in Evanston, Illinois.

The study was presented at the American College of Cardiology annual meeting, in Washington, DC.

SYMPTOMS AND TREATMENT

Broken heart syndrome is "a perfect example of our brain-heart connection," Dr. Pant said. "The emotional stress we have in our brain can lead to responses in the heart, and not much is known about this condition."

Symptoms of broken heart syndrome include chest pain and shortness of breath. The condition typically resolves within one or two months, but can lead to serious complications, such as heart failure, heart rhythm disorders and stroke in some cases.

"By and large, it is a very reversible form of cardiomyopathy, but in the acute phase these patients need to be monitored closely to be sure they are stable and to prevent and manage problems," said Dr. Pant.

"It's also something that emergency doctors and medical personnel need to be aware of as they are often on the frontlines seeing patients after disaster strikes," he said.

info For more information about broken heart syndrome, visit the Johns Hopkins University website, *www.hopkinsmedicine.org*, and search "broken heart syndrome."

Better Pump for Heart Failure

Edward K. Kasper, MD, director of clinical cardiology, The Johns Hopkins Hospital, Baltimore.

The FDA recently approved a new pump, which is implanted in the patient's chest near the heart, to treat heart failure. In clinical trials of the device, called the HeartWare Ventricular Assist System, 91% of 140 advanced heart-failure patients were alive six months after the new pump was implanted—these survival rates are comparable to those for patients using the currently available left ventricular assist device (LVAD). This older device, however, must be placed in the abdomen, which is not suitable for some heart-failure patients.

No Need to Screen All Adults for Clogged Neck Arteries

Peter Faries, MD, chief, vascular surgery, Mount Sinai Hospital, New York City.
Jessica Herzstein, MD, MPH, a board certified specialist in preventive and internal medicine and member of the U.S. Preventive Services Task Force.
Michael LeFevre, MD, vice chair, department of family and community medicine, University of Missouri School of Medicine in Columbia and co-vice chair of the U.S. Preventive Services Task Force.
U.S. Preventive Services Task Force, news release.

Adults in the general population should not be screened for narrowing of the neck arteries, according to a draft recommendation from the influential U.S. Preventive Services Task Force (USPSTF).

ABOUT CAROTID ARTERY STENOSIS

Narrowing of the neck arteries, formally called "carotid artery stenosis," reduces blood flow to the brain and is a risk factor for stroke.

"The carotid artery is the blood vessel that brings blood to the brain," explained Peter Faries, MD, chief of vascular surgery at Mount Sinai Hospital in New York City. "It starts in the chest and travels through the neck until it enters the skull."

Dr. Faries, who was not involved in drafting the new recommendations, explained that a buildup of fatty deposits in the carotid artery can lead to "narrowing or blockage of the blood flow to the brain. These carotid narrowings, or stenosis, can lead to a stroke in the patients that have them."

He said, "Often times, the first indication that a stenosis is present in the carotid artery is when the patient suffers a stroke."

SCREENING RECOMMENDATIONS

Doctors have long wondered then if routinely screening adults for narrowed neck arteries might be a good idea. But the USPSTF panel said that their review of the available evidence does not favor widespread screening.

The recommendation does not apply to adults with any history of stroke, mini-stroke, or signs and symptoms of stroke, however.

Carotid artery narrowing "is uncommon in the general adult population, so screening everyone would lead to many false positive results," explained Jessica Herzstein, MD, MPH, a board certified specialist in preventive and internal medicine and member of the USPSTF panel. "This can lead to follow-up tests and surgery that carry risk of serious harms, including stroke, heart attack, and death."

Sign of Heart-Valve Disorder

Visibly distended neck veins may be a sign of a common heart-valve disorder. People with tricuspid valve disease may have destruction of the valve caused by a bacterial infection in the heart. In addition to distended neck veins, people with tricuspid valve disease may have shortness of breath, a distended abdomen and swelling in the legs. If you have any of these symptoms, talk to your doctor.

Juan Crestanello, MD, a surgeon in the division of cardiac surgery at The Ohio State University Wexner Medical Center, Columbus.

A false positive result occurs when a test indicates that a person has a condition that's not actually there.

"Screening for carotid stenosis can be performed using ultrasound," Dr. Faries added. "The carotid screening ultrasound test is safe, simple, quick, effective, completely non-invasive, does not require any exposure to radiation, and inexpensive."

Dr. Faries agreed with the USPSTF panel that screening is important for patients at risk for the development of carotid artery blockage and stroke. That includes people over the age of 65 who are at high risk for "hardening of the arteries," with conditions such as high cholesterol, heart disease, a family history of stroke or a history of smoking.

In such cases, "screening can be an effective method of identifying blockages in the carotid artery, allowing them to be treated and thereby preventing a stroke from occurring," Dr. Faries explained.

REDUCING YOUR RISK FOR STROKE

All the experts agreed that preventing vessels from narrowing in the first place is the best option of all.

"The good news is that we have ways to reduce the risk of a stroke—control blood pressure and cholesterol, don't smoke, be physically active, and eat a healthful diet," said task force co-vice chair Michael LeFevre, MD.

Dr. Faries, who is vice chair in the department of family and community medicine at the University of Missouri School of Medicine in Columbia, echoed that notion. "Preventing a stroke before it occurs is obviously preferable to treating the blockage after a patient has suffered a stroke," he said.

The draft recommendation is posted on the task force's website at *www.uspreventiveservicestaskforce.org/uspstf13/cas/casdraftrec.htm.* The task force is an independent advisory group of health experts.

info The U.S. National Library of Medicine has more information about carotid artery stenosis at *www.nlm.nih.gov/medlineplus.* Search "carotid artery disease."

The New Way to Prevent Stroke

Louis R. Caplan, MD, senior neurologist at Beth Israel Deaconess Medical Center and a professor of neurology at Harvard Medical School, both in Boston. He has written or edited more than 40 books, including *Stroke (What Do I Do Now?)* and *Navigating the Complexities of Stroke* (both from Oxford University).

What if there were more to preventing a stroke than keeping your blood pressure under control...getting regular exercise...watching your body weight...and not smoking? Researchers are now discovering that there is.

New thinking: While most stroke sufferers say that "it just came out of the blue," an increasing body of evidence shows that these potentially devastating "brain attacks" can be caused by conditions that you might ordinarily think are completely unrelated.

Once you're aware of these "hidden" risk factors—and take the necessary steps to prevent or control them—you can improve your odds of never having a stroke. *Recently discovered stroke risk factors...*

INFLAMMATORY BOWEL DISEASE

Both Crohn's disease and ulcerative colitis can severely damage the large or small intestine. But that is not the only risk. Among patients who have either one of these conditions, known as inflammatory bowel disease (IBD), stroke is the third most common cause of death, according to some estimates.

During flare-ups, patients with IBD have elevated blood levels of substances that trigger clots—the cause of most strokes. A Harvard study, for example, found that many IBD patients have high levels of C-reactive protein (CRP), an inflammatory marker that has been linked to atherosclerotic lesions, damaged areas in blood vessels that can lead to stroke-causing clots in the brain.

If you have IBD: Ask your doctor what you can do to reduce your risk for blood clots and inflammation. Some patients with IBD can't take aspirin or other anticlotting drugs because these medications frequently cause intestinal bleeding. Instead of aspirin, you might be advised to take an autoimmune medication such as *azathioprine* (Azasan, Imuran), which suppresses the immune system and reduces inflammation. During flare-ups, some patients are given steroids to further reduce inflammation.

Side effects, including nausea and vomiting with azathioprine use and weight gain and increased blood pressure with steroid use, usually can be minimized by taking the lowest possible dose.

Some physicians recommend omega-3 fish oil supplements for IBD, which are less likely to cause side effects. Ask your doctor whether these supplements (and what dose) are right for you.

Important: Strokes tend to occur in IBD patients when inflammation is most severe. To check inflammatory markers, CRP levels and erythrocyte sedimentation rate (ESR) can be measured. Tests for clotting include fibrinogen and d-dimer. The results of these tests will help determine the course of the patient's IBD treatment.

MIGRAINES

Migraine headaches accompanied by auras (characterized by the appearance of flashing lights or other visual disturbances) are actually a greater risk factor for stroke than obesity, smoking or diabetes (see below), according to a startling study presented at the American Academy of Neurology's annual meeting in 2013.

When researchers use MRIs to examine blood vessels in the brain, they find more tiny areas of arterial damage in patients who have migraines with auras than in those who don't get migraines. (Research shows that there is no link between stroke and migraines that aren't accompanied by auras.)

If you have migraines with auras: Reduce your risk by controlling other stroke risk factors—don't smoke...lose weight if you're overweight...and control cholesterol levels.

Also: Women under age 50 who have migraines (with or without auras) may be advised to not use combined-hormone forms of birth control pills—they slightly increase risk for stroke. In addition, patients who have migraines with auras should not take beta-blockers, such as *propranolol* (Inderal), or the triptan drugs, such as *sumatriptan* (Imitrex), commonly used for migraine headaches. These drugs can also increase stroke risk. For frequent migraines with auras, I often prescribe the blood pressure drug *verapamil* (Calan) and a daily 325-mg aspirin. Ask your doctor for advice.

Garbled Texts Could Signal Stroke

Neurologists report that a patient who appeared normal wrote text messages that were completely garbled. This condition could be the only symptom of stroke-related language problems.

Henry Ford Hospital

RHEUMATOID ARTHRITIS

Rheumatoid arthritis, unlike the common "wear-and-tear" variety (osteoarthritis), is an autoimmune disease that not only causes inflammation in the joints but may also trigger it in the heart, blood vessels and other parts of the body.

Arterial inflammation increases the risk for blood clots, heart attack and stroke. In fact, patients with severe rheumatoid arthritis were almost twice as likely to have a stroke as those without the disease, according to a study published in *Arthritis Care & Research*.

If you have rheumatoid arthritis: Work with your rheumatologist to manage flare-ups and reduce systemic inflammation. Your doctor will probably recommend that you take one or more anti-inflammatory painkillers, such as *ibuprofen* (Motrin). In addition, he/she might prescribe a disease-modifying antirheumatic drug (DMARD), such as *methotrexate* (Trexall), to slow the progression of the disease—and the increased risk for stroke. Fish oil also may be prescribed to reduce joint tenderness.

Strokes tend to occur in rheumatoid arthritis patients when inflammation is peaking. Ask your doctor if you should have the inflammation tests (CRP and ESR) mentioned in the IBD section.

DIABETES

If you have diabetes or diabetes risk factors—such as obesity, a sedentary lifestyle or a family history of diabetes—protect yourself. People with diabetes are up to four times more likely to have a stroke than those without it.

High blood sugar in people with diabetes damages blood vessels throughout the body, including in the brain. The damage can lead to both ischemic (clot-related) and hemorrhagic (bleeding) strokes.

If you have diabetes: Work closely with your doctor. Patients who achieve good glucose control with oral medications and/or insulin are much less likely to suffer from vascular damage.

Also important: Lose weight if you need to. Weight loss combined with exercise helps your body metabolize blood sugar more efficiently. In those with mild diabetes, weight loss combined with exercise may restore normal blood sugar levels...and can reduce complications and the need for medications in those with more serious diabetes.

CLOTTING DISORDERS

Any condition that affects the blood's normal clotting functions can increase risk for stroke.

Examples: Thrombocytosis (excessive platelets in the blood)...an elevated hematocrit (higher-than-normal percentage of red blood cells)...or Factor V Leiden (an inherited tendency to form blood clots). Clotting tests (fibrinogen and d-dimer) are recommended for these disorders.

If you have a clotting disorder: Ask your doctor what you can do to protect yourself from stroke.

Example: If you have an elevated hematocrit, your doctor might advise you to drink more fluids.

This is particularly important for older adults, who tend to drink less later in the day because they don't want to get up at night to urinate. I recommend that these patients drink approximately 80 ounces of noncaffeine-containing fluids during the day, stopping by 7 pm. People who don't take in enough fluids can develop "thick" blood that impedes circulation—and increases the risk for clots.

Work Fast When Stroke Symptoms Occur

When adults who had mild or moderate strokes got the clot-busting drug tissue plasminogen activator (tPA) within 90 minutes of having symptoms (rather than within 4.5 hours, as is generally recommended), they were much more likely to have little or no disability at a three-month follow-up than those who were given tPA later.

Takeaway: Call 911 if you have any sign of stroke—sudden numbness or weakness on one side of the body, facial drooping, speech difficulties, inability to walk or loss of vision—even if it lasts for only a few minutes.

Daniel Strbian, MD, PhD, associate professor of neurology, Helsinki University Central Hospital, Finland.

Ambulance Is Best for Stroke Patients

Jeffrey L. Saver, MD, director, UCLA Comprehensive Stroke Center, Los Angeles.

Even though an ambulance is the fastest way for someone suffering symptoms of a stroke to get to a hospital—a crucial factor in stroke survival and recovery—the records of 204,591 stroke patients show that more than one in three were driven by someone else or they drove themselves. Among the ambulance patients, 67.3% received a clot-busting drug within three hours (an important cutoff period for this stroke treatment), compared with 44.1% of the others.

Bonus: Ambulance personnel can contact the hospital in advance so staff is ready when the stroke patient arrives.

Dry Brushing for Stroke

Mao Shing Ni, DOM, PhD, LAc, Oriental medicine practitioner at Tao of Wellness, Santa Monica, California.

Strokes often injure the motor fibers connected to movement, causing immobility.

Immobility affects blood circulation and impairs the delivery of nutrients to cells and the elimination of toxins and waste products—both essential for good health. Dry brushing, massage and reflexology will help stimulate circulation.

Dry brushing, a rubdown of the body with natural-bristle brushes, can activate circulation of the lymphatic system, which is necessary for warding off infections.

Massage also can help to activate circulation and eliminate waste products, such as lactic acid, that cause muscle stiffness and pain. Reflexology (pressure to trigger points on hands, bottoms of the feet and other areas) and acupuncture may also be effective.

New Stroke Fighter: Red Peppers

Eating red peppers and other vitamin C–rich fruits and veggies may reduce your risk for intracerebral hemorrhagic stroke (a blood vessel rupture in the brain). And what's so great about red peppers? At 190 mg per cup, they contain three times more vitamin C than an orange. Other good sources of vitamin C—broccoli and strawberries. Researchers believe that this vitamin may reduce stroke risk by regulating blood pressure and strengthening collagen, which promotes healthy blood vessels.

Stéphane Vannier, MD, neurologist, Pontchaillou University Hospital, Rennes, France, from research being presented at the annual meeting of the American Academy of Neurology.

New Guidelines Aim to Lower Stroke Risk in Women

Cheryl Bushnell, MD, MHS, associate professor, neurology, and director, Stroke Center, Wake Forest Baptist Medical Center, Winston-Salem, NC.

Andrew Russman, DO, neurologist, Cerebrovascular Center, Cleveland Clinic, Ohio.

Suzanne Steinbaum, MD, director, Women's Heart Health, Heart and Vascular Institute, Lenox Hill Hospital, New York City.

Stroke

For the first time, guidelines have been created to help prevent stroke in women.

The author of the new guidelines, published in the journal *Stroke*, said women share a lot of stroke risk factors with men—namely high blood pressure, high cholesterol, diabetes, smoking and obesity—but they also have a set of unique concerns that need to be addressed.

Pregnancy, childbirth and hormones play a role in stroke risk for women, explained Cheryl Bushnell, MD, MHS, director of the Stroke Center at Wake Forest Baptist Medical Center, in Winston-Salem, North Carolina.

"The basic message is that women live longer, and so they actually have a higher lifetime risk of stroke," Dr. Bushnell said. "They also tend to do worse after they have had a stroke. They're more likely to end up in long-term nursing care and have a worse quality of life. For those reasons, we thought it was important to emphasize prevention and to start those strategies early in the childbearing years for women."

BACKGROUND ON STROKE

A stroke happens when a blood vessel that carries oxygen and nutrients to the brain is either blocked by a clot or it bursts, keeping oxygen from reaching the brain, and killing brain cells, according to the American Stroke Association.

Each year, about 55,000 more women than men experience a stroke, and non-Hispanic black women are most at risk, the American Heart Association reports.

NEW STROKE PREVENTION GUIDELINES

Dr. Bushnell said she and colleagues scoured the existing scientific literature to develop the new guidelines, which include recommendations for women of all ages.

"There's risk across a woman's lifespan," said Dr. Bushnell. "Without a doubt, the highest risk is as women get older, especially as they accumulate other risk factors," such as high blood pressure.

But, she added, while complications from stroke are rare during pregnancy, that's when the first signs of vascular disease can appear. She said women who have eclampsia and preeclampsia during pregnancy (a dangerous condition marked by high blood pressure), for example, are at twice the risk for stroke later in life and four times the risk for high blood pressure later.

Dr. Bushnell added that taking birth control pills can raise a woman's risk for stroke, especially in middle age. And women who get migraines with aura are also at higher risk, so they need to consider preventive strategies earlier in life.

Some recommendations in the new guidelines include...

- **Women with a history of high blood pressure before pregnancy** should be considered for low-dose aspirin therapy or calcium supplementation while pregnant.
- **Pregnant women with elevated blood pressure (150-159 mm Hg/100-109 mm Hg)** should talk with their doctor about possible blood pressure medication.
- **Pregnant women with severe high blood pressure** (160/110 mm Hg or above) should take medication.
- **Women should be screened for high blood pressure** before taking birth control pills.
- **Women who suffer from migraines with aura should quit smoking.**
- **Women over age 75 should be screened for atrial fibrillation (irregular heartbeat) risks.**

"There isn't a specific prevention strategy for women because we haven't studied it enough to find one," Dr. Bushnell said. "But all of the healthy lifestyle recommendations apply equally to men and women."

EXPERT COMMENTARY

According to Andrew Russman, DO, a neurologist at the Cleveland Clinic's Cerebrovascular Center, "They did a good job putting the guidelines on paper. I think it's terribly important that there's now a set of guidelines that help women understand some of their unique stroke risks, which change throughout life—from pregnancy, through menopause and later in life."

Suzanne Steinbaum, MD, director of Women's Heart Health at the Heart and Vascular Institute at Lenox Hill Hospital in New York City, said she hopes the new guidelines will help women be more aware of stroke risk and cardiovascular health.

"Whenever I give a talk, I ask what people think is the greatest risk to women's health and they say breast cancer," Dr. Steinbaum said. "I don't think stroke is on the same level of consciousness. Awareness is the first step," she noted.

"The first step is, if you have any risks for cardiovascular disease, heart disease or stroke, it's important to visit your doctor," Dr. Steinbaum said. "Then, know your numbers—your blood pressure, your cholesterol, your blood sugar, your BMI [which is a score based on height and weight]. Knowing your family history is also very important. To prevent stroke it comes down to the basics, lifestyle changes. These are critical issues to address in order to reduce cardiovascular disease and prevent stroke."

To recognize the warning signs of stroke and learn about the acronym FAST, visit the American Stroke Association website, *www.strokeassociation.org*, and search "Stroke warning signs and symptoms."

Brain-Training Device May Ease Stroke Paralysis

Vivek Prabhakaran, MD, PhD, director, functional neuroimaging in radiology, University of Wisconsin-Madison.

Rafael Ortiz, MD, director, neuro-endovascular surgery and stroke, Lenox Hill Hospital, New York City.

Radiological Society of North America annual meeting, presentation.

Scientists are testing a new thought-controlled device that may one day help people move limbs again after they've been paralyzed by a stroke.

Strokes occur when blood flow to the brain stops. This happens because a blood clot blocks a blood vessel in the brain or a blood vessel breaks in the brain. Strokes often cause problems with movement and language.

The device combines a high-tech brain-computer interface with electrical stimulation of the damaged muscles to help patients relearn how to move frozen limbs.

Several patients who had lost movement in one hand have been through several weeks of therapy with the device. They reported improvements in their ability to complete daily tasks—"Things like combing their hair and buttoning their shirt," explained study author Vivek Prabhakaran, MD, director of functional neuroimaging in radiology at the University of Wisconsin-Madison.

"These are patients who are months and years out from their strokes," Dr. Prabhakaran said. "Early studies suggested that there was no real room for change for these patients, that they had plateaued in the recovery. We're showing there is still room for change. There is plasticity we can harness."

HOW THE TOOL HELPS PARALYSED LIMBS

To use the new tool, patients wear a cap of electrodes that picks up brain signals. Those signals are decoded by a computer. The computer, in turn, sends tiny jolts of electricity through wires to sticky pads placed on the muscles of a patient's paralyzed arm. The jolts act like nerve impulses, telling the muscles to move.

A simple video game on the computer screen prompts patients to try to hit a target by moving a ball with their affected arm. Patients practice with the game for about two hours at a time, every other day.

Researchers also scanned the patients' brains before, during and a month after they finished 15 sessions with the device.

The more patients practiced, the more they were able to train their brains, the researchers found.

The brain has two sides, or hemispheres. Researchers say that what seems to be happening is that the side of the brain that wasn't damaged by the stroke learns to take over many of the functions lost on the affected side.

And the more patients are able to recruit the unaffected side, the better their progress, Dr. Prabhakaran said.

Some, but not all, of the positive brain changes remained even a month after patients had finished therapy. Researchers think maintenance sessions may be necessary to help people keep their gains.

Patients with mild to moderate damage seem to get the most help from the device, he added. Patients with milder impairments were able to increase their speed on a task that required them to move pegs on a board. Patients with moderate damage were able to recover movement and strength.

The findings were presented at the annual meeting of the Radiological Society of North America, in Chicago.

EXPERT COMMENT

Though it's an early look at evidence supporting the therapy, one expert who was not involved with the research said the results looked promising.

"Stroke is the largest cause of disability in the country," said Rafael Ortiz, MD, director of neuro-endovascular surgery and stroke at Lenox Hill Hospital in New York City. "Fifty percent of stroke patients end up with severe disability,

Life Changes Work Better Than Stents

Aggressive nonsurgical treatment prevents stroke recurrence more effectively than stents, reports Colin P. Derdeyn, MD.

Recent finding: People at high risk for a second stroke who received anticlotting medications and intense management of cardiovascular risks (blood pressure and cholesterol) and who strictly adhered to a lifestyle-modification program (diet and exercise) had fewer incidences of stroke recurrence than patients who received this treatment in addition to receiving a stent.

Colin P. Derdeyn, MD, professor of radiology, neurology and neurological surgery at Washington University School of Medicine in St. Louis and lead author of a study published in *The Lancet*.

FDA Rules on Naproxen Warning

Naproxen (Aleve), once thought to be safer than other popular over-the-counter (OTC) pain relievers, has about the same risk for cardiovascular blood clots as *ibuprofen* (Advil) and aspirin, an FDA advisory panel has ruled. Labels on Aleve and other OTC nonsteroidal anti-inflammatory drugs (NSAIDs) must continue to carry a warning that long-term use may increase risk for heart attack or stroke.

Takeaway: If you regularly take naproxen, ask your doctor whether you should continue doing so.

Harris McIlwain, MD, rheumatologist in private practice, Tampa.

and that's out of 800,000 strokes that happen a year," he said. Better kinds of rehabilitation for stroke patients are desperately needed, he added.

"Using therapies like this, we can offer hope to patients, even six or 12 months after their stroke," he said.

The study is still in its early stages. Researchers said they won't know for sure how well it works or how useful it may be for long-term recovery until they've tested it on more patients.

info For more information on stroke rehabilitation, visit the website of the National Institute of Neurologic Disorders and Stroke at *http://www.ninds.nih.gov/disorders/stroke/poststrokerehab.htm.*

Infectious Diseases

Hot Spots for Bacteria—Our Bodies Are Breeding Grounds for Germs...

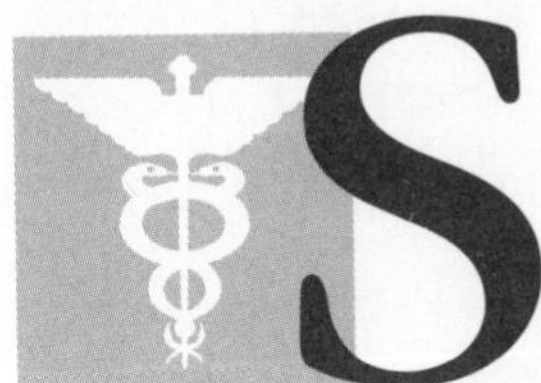

Stinky underarms aren't unusual, but when one man's stubbornly smelly armpits lasted for four years, doctors knew something was, uh, fishy.

According to a report appearing in a recent issue of *The New England Journal of Medicine*, the 40-year-old's underarm hairs were infected with bacteria known as Corynebacterium tenuis. The hair shafts were covered with—beware: what follows is pretty gross!—a creamy, yellow substance that emitted an irrepressible odor.

This man's case is a stark reminder that our skin is crawling, usually unbeknownst to us, with hundreds of types of bacteria. And some of these stealthy germs can lead to serious illnesses such as sepsis (a potentially deadly inflammatory response throughout the body) and pneumonia.

WHERE BACTERIA LIVE

The good news is, most skin bacteria, which outnumber our body's own cells, are harmless and even protect skin cells from more dangerous microorganisms.

For example, harmless Staphylococcus epidermidis takes up space on our skin that the insidious Staphylococcus aureus—usually called "staph"—would otherwise colonize. Scientific research is increasingly indicating that the vast majority of skin bacteria inhibit disease-causing agents or even "educate" the immune system to help us fend off illness.

Harmful bacteria, however, tend to congregate at certain skin sites that are either moist or oily. *Here are four of the most common "hot spots" for harmful bacteria—and the red flags that mean you should get to a doctor...*

Cindy Owen, MD, an assistant professor of dermatology and the residency program director in dermatology at the University of Louisville School of Medicine in Louisville, Kentucky. Dr. Owen's scientific research on skin conditions has been widely published in medical journals.

To Banish a Boil

A nasty collection of pus under the skin, known as a boil, is an infection typically resulting from *Staphylococcus aureus*, more commonly referred to as "staph."

Recurrent boils, however, can signal infection with MRSA, a drug-resistant form of staph that can cause pneumonia or severe infections of the blood, bones, heart valves or lungs. Boils can occur anywhere on the body but are more common in the armpits, groin and the area between the genitals and anus.

Important: Seek medical attention for boils larger than one-half inch in diameter, which should be professionally drained.

The same goes for boils with red streaks around them, which can be a sign of dangerous blood vessel involvement…boils that continue to enlarge…if a fever develops or lymph nodes enlarge…or if the boil is near the anus.

Also, see a doctor about any boil on the spine or face. Boils on the spine can lead to a spinal cord infection, and those in the triangular area between the eyes, cheeks and lip can trigger a dangerous brain infection. Most other boils are small and can be treated at home.

What to do…

- **Apply a compress soaked in warm salt water three times per day for 20 minutes.** Use a fresh washcloth each time.

What not to do…

- **Never squeeze or pop a boil,** which can spread the infection.
- **Do not stick a needle or other object into a boil**—this can cause dangerous bleeding or spread the infection.

•**Hot Spot #1: Tip of the nose.** The anterior nares (the ends of the nostrils) are the most common site for colonized methicillin-resistant Staphylococcus aureus, or MRSA, highly dangerous bacteria that can cause sepsis and even death. MRSA also can colonize in areas inside the nose.

About 2% of people carry MRSA (often harmlessly) on their skin—it also can congregate in adults in the armpits and groin area.

What to look for: Constant irritation at the tip of the nose, which may include tiny skin cracks called fissures, can clue you in to MRSA's presence. Another tip-off is the development of numerous or recurrent boils anywhere on the body. If you develop one of these signs, see a doctor.

•**Hot Spot #2: Between the toes.** The webby region between the toes and the cuticle areas on toes and fingers can harbor Pseudomonas aeruginosa bacteria, which can cause an infection of the toes and feet, especially in people who sweat a lot or are active and wear closed-toe shoes. The infection may cause pain and difficulty walking and can result in cellulitis (an infection just below the skin surface) or sepsis in people with weak immunity.

What to look for: A discharge that may stain socks a green color and a sweet, grape-like odor.

•**Hot Spot #3: Armpits.** The Corynebacteria causing the 40-year-old man's long-term odor have a fondness for armpits and the groin area, coating the hair shafts with a "cheesy" yellow paste. The infection, called trichomycosis axillaris, is most common in tropical or other warm climates. Similar bacteria can cause infections of the feet.

What to look for: A noticeable smell, and if the feet are infected, small, "punched out" pitting of the soles.

•**Hot Spot #4: Scalp/hairy areas.** While the scalp is the most reliably hair-covered spot on our bodies (or so we hope), hair follicles cover almost our entire bodies. In men, of course, the hair tends to be more visibly abundant—for example, on the chest, back and face.

Densely packed areas of hair follicles can be the target of Propionibacterium acnes, which plays a role in the development of inflammatory acne that's typically far worse than a blackhead or two.

What to look for: Pustules and/or large, painful bumps grouped on the face, chest or back.

HOW THE MYSTERY ENDED

And what about the man with the smelly armpit infection? After the hair was shaved, he received an antibiotic for the infection and topical aluminum chloride to curb his armpit sweating, which had created the ideal home for the bacteria.

Remember: Most bacteria are beneficial. Still, it's wise to inspect your skin regularly for the red flags of infection described in this article. Avoid antibacterial soaps unless directed by your doctor. These soaps disrupt the normal skin barriers that protect us from invading bacteria and other pathogens. Plain soap and water are usually the best way to wash.

Recover Fast from Stomach Flu

Jamison Starbuck, ND, a naturopathic physician in family practice and a guest lecturer at the University of Montana, both in Missoula. She is past president of the American Association of Naturopathic Physicians and a contributing editor to *The Alternative Advisor: The Complete Guide to Natural Therapies and Alternative Treatments* (Time Life).

"We've ALL got the stomach flu," my weary patient announced. Exhausted from caretaking and still not feeling well himself, he was at his wit's end. I was happy to assure him that the illness, which is highly contagious, usually passes within a few days, but with the natural remedies below, he could likely speed up their recoveries by at least a day.

Though commonly known as the "stomach flu," this short-lived gastrointestinal (GI) bug is technically gastroenteritis, a medical term meaning inflammation of the stomach and intestines. It can be caused by bacteria, parasites or a virus—which are spread by human contact as well as contaminated food or water. One of its most common causes, norovirus, is often spread when you use a doorknob, for example, that has been touched by someone with the virus on his/her hands, and you then put your fingers (or food you touch) in your mouth. The symptoms of gastroenteritis are well known—nausea, diarrhea, loss of appetite, sometimes vomiting and a mild (99-degree) fever. *How to reduce the severity and duration of your misery...**

- **Stick to clear fluids.** At the first sign of gastroenteritis (typically diarrhea), have only chicken, beef or vegetable broth, herbal tea, diluted fruit juice, ginger ale, club soda and water. Consume these liquids cold, hot or at room temperature—whatever feels most soothing. Avoiding solid foods will reduce both diarrhea and nausea and give your GI tract time to recuperate. When nausea and diarrhea are gone, ease back into eating solid foods with rice, steamed veggies and/or three ounces of chicken or fish.

- **Take a good probiotic.** I recommend a powdered formula containing 3 billion colony forming units (CFUs) of Lactobacillus acidophilus and Bifidobacterium, taken three times a day. If your probiotic comes in a capsule, open it and dissolve the powder it contains directly in your mouth or in only two ounces of water to avoid the vomiting that can accompany gastroenteritis.

- **Consider chamomile.** Lots of herbal teas—such as cinnamon, ginger, chamomile, lemon balm, peppermint and spearmint—soothe nausea and diarrhea. However, I prefer chamomile because it also kills microorganisms, decreases inflammation and reduces intestinal gas. For gastroenteritis, I suggest drinking 32 to 48 ounces of chamomile tea daily. People who are allergic to plants in the daisy family—daisy, ragweed, marigold, chrysanthemum—should avoid chamomile.

- **Use natural antiseptics.** Two natural antiseptics can speed your body's process of shedding an unwanted stomach bug. Oregon graperoot is an antimicrobial, and activated

*If you are frail, elderly or have a compromised immune system...or if vomiting or diarrhea lasts more than 48 hours, see your physician.

charcoal binds to microorganisms so they can be eliminated via the stool. Use these medicines separately, or the charcoal will also sweep the Oregon graperoot out of your body.

My advice: Take one-eighth teaspoon of Oregon graperoot tincture in four ounces water, followed two hours later by two charcoal capsules, opened and mixed with four ounces of water. Do this until you get four doses of each medicine in 24 hours. Consult a pediatrician before giving Oregon graperoot and/or activated charcoal to children.

How Not to Get Sick on a Cruise

James Windeck, MD, a retired physician who formerly worked as a cruise ship doctor for the Royal Caribbean cruise line. He also is a frequent cruise passenger and author of *Cruise Ship Doctor* (Amazon Digital Services).

Norovirus outbreaks on cruise ships inevitably receive media attention, but passengers' odds of contracting this unpleasant gastrointestinal ailment actually are very low. Only a few thousand of the roughly 10 million cruise passengers who depart from US ports each year catch it, according to data compiled by the Centers for Disease Control's Vessel Sanitation Program. In fact, we're no more likely to catch norovirus on a cruise ship than in any other crowded location—we just hear about cruise ship outbreaks most often because cruise lines are required to report them.

With all the attention paid to the norovirus, other more serious and more common cruise health issues often are ignored. *To stay healthy on a cruise...*

•Bring copies of key medical records. Large cruise ships generally have high-quality doctors and well-equipped medical facilities. What they might not have is fast access to your medical records in an emergency (although the ability of cruise ship doctors to obtain digital copies of medical records from sea is improving).

Self-defense: Bring copies of key medical records with you onto the ship. This includes copies of prescriptions for medications that you currently are taking, paperwork related to recent or ongoing medical conditions, your doctor's contact information and—if you've had heart problems—a copy of your most recent electrocardiogram (EKG). Be sure a travel companion knows where this information is.

Also, be sure to bring sufficient quantities of any prescription and over-the-counter medications you currently use—more than you think you'll need. The ship's pharmacy might have these in stock, but it probably won't accept Medicare or health insurance in payment, and its prices likely will be several times what you would pay onshore.

•Control your eating and drinking. Overconsumption of food and alcohol is extremely common on cruises, and it can lead to gastrointestinal distress or worse—binge eating and drinking have been linked to increased risk for heart attack.

•Choose a large ship if you're prone to seasickness (or if you're not certain whether you're prone to seasickness). Ships with passenger capacities of roughly 3,000 or more are so massive that you would barely feel them moving even in a big storm, greatly reducing the risk for seasickness. Larger ships also tend to have more extensive medical facilities.

•Purchase travel health insurance that includes emergency evacuation if your cruise leaves US waters. This is particularly important if your ship calls at ports in parts of the world where the medical care is not as good as in the US. websites SquareMouth.com and InsureMyTrip.com can help you find and compare these policies.

RISKS ON SHORE

Significant portions of the typical cruise vacation take place off the ship—and that's where many cruise health risks can be found...

•Don't rent a motor scooter unless you have extensive experience riding them. Scooter rentals are common in many cruise ship ports, but scooters are dangerous for novices, particularly in parts of the world where road conditions are poor and traffic rules lax.

•**Be picky about restaurants.** When cruise ship passengers get food poisoning, it's usually because of something they ate onshore, not aboard ship. Many restaurants and roadside food stands in common cruise destinations such as the Caribbean pay insufficient attention to cleanliness and food safety.

Lean toward restaurants where you can walk into the kitchen to confirm that the staff is wearing gloves—even better if you see them washing their hands—an indication that the restaurant takes food safety seriously. Drink only bottled or canned beverages, and make sure that the cap still is on the bottle when it arrives at your table.

•**If you're flying to the cruise departure point, be sure to move around the plane.** Remaining in one's seat for the duration of a long airline flight significantly increases the risk for blood clots. Such clots can be fatal if they reach the lungs—particularly if this happens aboard a cruise ship, where medical care is less extensive than in a hospital. Simply strolling around the aircraft's cabin every few hours greatly reduces this risk.

"Cruise Ship Virus" Vaccine a First-Class Idea?

David Bernstein, MD professor, pediatrics, Cincinnati Children's Hospital Medical Center, University of Cincinnati.

Jesse Reeves-Garcia, MD, chief, division of gastroenterology, Miami Children's Hospital.

The dreaded "cruise ship virus" could sink into history some day, if a promising vaccine trial pans out.

Researchers report that an early test of an experimental vaccine for norovirus—the cause of a stomach sickness that fells scores of cruise ship passengers and nursing home residents, among others—reduced symptoms of vomiting and diarrhea by 52%.

Every year, norovirus sickens 19 million to 21 million Americans—or one in 15—and kills as many as 800, according to the U.S. Centers for Disease Control and Prevention.

Pneumonia Warning

Among more than 1,400 adults (age 50 and older) who had been hospitalized, those with pneumonia were twice as likely to suffer cognitive decline and depression as those who had been hospitalized for other reasons.

If you're over age 50: Ask your doctor if a pneumonia vaccination is appropriate for you.

Dimitry Davydow, MD, MPH, assistant professor of psychiatry, University of Washington School of Medicine, Seattle.

"Early results of testing an experimental vaccine for norovirus appear positive, providing optimism that a vaccine can be developed for this common cause of gastroenteritis," said lead researcher David Bernstein, MD, a professor of pediatrics at Cincinnati Children's Hospital Medical Center and the University of Cincinnati.

STUDY DETAILS

For the latest study, Dr. Bernstein's team randomly assigned 98 people, who agreed to drink water laced with the virus, to an injection of the vaccine or placebo.

Among those given the vaccine, 26 were infected as were 29 in the placebo group. Ten people in the vaccinated group had mild, moderate or severe vomiting and/or diarrhea compared with 20 in the non-vaccinated group—a 52% reduction in symptoms.

The vaccine disarms two genotypes of norovirus, one of them the leading cause of U.S. outbreaks, the study authors say.

The results of the study were presented at ID Week 2013, the infectious diseases society conference in San Francisco. Data and conclusions presented at meetings are typically considered preliminary until published in a peer-reviewed medical journal.

"More testing will be necessary to ensure the vaccine is safe and effective," Dr. Bernstein said. "If this can be duplicated in larger trials, it could lead to the availability of a new vaccine for a very common illness."

BACKGROUND ON NOROVIRUS

Currently, there is no treatment or cure for the highly contagious virus, the most common cause of viral gastroenteritis in children and adults. It can spread through infected food or water, contaminated surfaces and even through the air.

Outbreaks occur in close quarters, such as health care facilities, child care centers, schools and military bases in addition to cruise ships, the researchers said.

Not everyone exposed to norovirus gets infected, and of those who are infected not all get sick, Dr. Bernstein said. But it is very common and can be serious, particularly for young children and older adults, he added.

A recent study found the overall cost of the disease in the United States is $5.5 billion a year, the researchers noted.

The vaccine might be useful for people in any of those settings, Dr. Bernstein said. Ocean-going travelers, for instance, could add the vaccine to their to-do list before departure.

But first, Dr. Bernstein hopes to test the vaccine in a larger "real-world" trial.

EXPERT RESPONSE

Jesse Reeves-Garcia, MD, chief of the division of gastroenterology at Miami Children's Hospital, said the idea of a vaccine for norovirus is "fascinating."

"Norovirus ruins people's lives," he said. "They take a vacation, they take a cruise and spend three of four days in the toilet puking or pooping or both."

A vaccine that's effective, safe and reasonably priced would be "great," Dr. Reeves-Garcia continued. "It would be another sickness that I wouldn't see anymore."

info For more information on norovirus, visit the U.S. Centers for Disease Control and Prevention website at *http://www.cdc.gov/norovirus/*.

The Killer Lurking in the Water...and Two Other Dangerous Diseases on the Rise

John Galgiani, MD, professor of medicine at University of Arizona College of Medicine, Phoenix, and director of the Valley Fever Center for Excellence, Tucson, Arizona.

Richard S. Ostfeld, PhD, a senior scientist and disease ecologist at Cary Institute of Ecosystem Studies in Millbrook, New York. He is author of *Lyme Disease: The Ecology of a Complex System* (Oxford University).

Jonathan S. Yoder, MSW, MPH, team leader for the Domestic Water, Sanitation, and Hygiene Epidemiology Team in the National Center for Emerging Zoonotic and Infectious Diseases at the Centers for Disease Control and Prevention, Atlanta. *CDC.gov/naegleria*

The earth is getting warmer, on average—and that is leading to more cases of certain infectious diseases.

Here, three experts explain what you need to know now about three dangerous diseases on the rise...

VALLEY FEVER: GROWING DANGER IN THE DUST

More than half of people who live in or travel to the dry areas of the country—parts of Arizona, California, Nevada, New Mexico, Texas and Utah—run the risk of being infected with Coccidioides, a fungus that lives in the soil.

Coccidioidomycosis, also known as valley fever, causes no symptoms in 60% of people who get it—the immune system eliminates the infection, and no harm is done. But 35% will develop pneumonia, and 5% will become extremely ill when the fungus travels to the brain, bones or other parts of the body. The disease kills more than 150 people a year.

You literally can catch valley fever from the wind. Summer winds that create dust storms scoop up fungal spores from the soil and shoot them downwind. A rainy winter promotes fungal growth and can increase infections the following summer and fall. The number of infections decreases during the wet seasons, then spikes upward in the hot months. You cannot catch the disease from someone who is sick with it.

Between 1998 and 2011, the total number of reported infections increased tenfold. Though valley fever is common in parts of California and the Southwest, infections in the last dozen years have been reported to the CDC from 28 states and the District of Columbia.

Self-defense…

•**See a doctor if you have flulike symptoms**—such as fever, a cough, chest pain, headache and fatigue—that don't start to improve in about a week. Some patients will have painful red bumps on their chest, arms, back or lower legs. Symptoms usually start about one to three weeks after you have been exposed to the fungus.

•**Tell your doctor about recent travels.** Even in areas where valley fever is common, only about 25% of patients get an accurate diagnosis, partly because the infection has symptoms common to other illnesses. The misdiagnosis rate is higher in areas where doctors don't think to test for it.

Antifungal medications, such as *fluconazole* (Diflucan), will control the infection. You might need to take medications for about six months. More serious infections may require *amphotericin B*, an intravenous antifungal medication.

TICKS ON THE MOVE

People who live in the northeastern states are accustomed to checking their skin (and their pets) for ticks. It's a routine that's going to become more common in other states. The blacklegged tick that transmits Lyme disease is taking advantage of warmer temperatures. It has been reported in many parts of the US and is moving into areas where it wasn't seen before, including the colder parts of Maine, Vermont and even Canada.

Other ticks are thriving, too. The American dog tick, for example, which transmits Rocky Mountain spotted fever, is found in every state. The Lone Star tick, found in the eastern and southeastern states, carries ehrlichiosis and tularemia.

The extreme weather that has been linked to climate change is a boon for ticks. The long summer droughts that are natural to some areas served to reduce tick populations. In recent years, some of the same areas have had shorter dry seasons or heavier-than-expected rains, which may have caused an uptick in ticks.

In some parts of the country, tick season appears to be starting earlier and ending later. It's not merely that summers are getting warmer. Winters, on average, are less cold than they used to be. Warmer winters are known to allow tick populations to expand northward and to higher elevations.

Self-defense…

•**Check for ticks.** Check yourself, your children and your pets after spending time outdoors. To reduce risk on hikes, stay on trails. If you plan to leave the path, wear light-colored clothing to make ticks easier to spot. Wear long sleeves, and tuck long pants into your socks.

Also, use insect repellent containing DEET on exposed skin.

•**Know the symptoms.** Tick-related illnesses often are accompanied by flulike symptoms such as fever, fatigue, and aches and pains. Lyme and other tick diseases also can cause distinctive rashes. See your doctor if you develop any of these symptoms, particularly if you develop flulike symptoms when it's not flu season.

Most victims of tick-borne illnesses can be cured with antibiotics, particularly when the infection is detected and treated early. (For more information about Lyme Disease, see page 239.)

RARE BUT DEADLY AMOEBA

This single-cell organism Naegleria fowleri is found in freshwater lakes, rivers, streams and hot springs. It is not found in the ocean or other bodies of saltwater. It rarely causes infection—but when it does, the infection is deadly.

This amoeba thrives in warm, untreated water and can survive in temperatures up to 115°F. It has been identified most often in southern states in the US.

But in 2010, a young girl was infected while swimming in a lake near her home in Minnesota—an area that's typically too cold for the amoeba to survive. Cases also have been reported in Indiana and Kansas. Scientists aren't sure if the warming of the planet has extended the amoeba's range, but it is one possibility.

The infection is rare. Only 31 cases were reported in the US between 2003 and 2012.

Two Chicken Pox Vaccinations Are Better Than One

The rate of chicken pox infection dropped by as much as 76% in children who received a second dose of the vaccine between ages four and six. (The first vaccination was given between 12 months and 15 months.) Infections even declined among adults and infants—who do not usually get the vaccination—because there was less chicken pox virus within the community.

Rachel Civen, MD, medical epidemiologist, Los Angeles County Department of Public Health, and leader of a study published in *Pediatrics*.

What happens: The amoeba enters the body through the nose, usually when people are swimming or diving in contaminated water. It then travels to the brain, where it literally consumes brain tissue.

Symptoms start one to seven days after exposure. The disease progresses rapidly, and there are no effective treatments. The fatality rate is more than 99%.

The organism can cause infection only when it enters the nasal cavities. There is no risk from drinking a glass of water or from typical showering.

Self-defense...

•**When swimming in warm fresh-water lakes, rivers, ponds or streams, wear nose plugs or keep your head above water.** Hold your nose shut, or use nose plugs when jumping or diving into the water.

•**If you use a Neti pot or a bulb syringe to flush congestion from your nose,** always use boiled, properly filtered or sterilized water. Officials recently found Naegleria in a municipal water system in Louisiana, where it caused two deaths—in both cases, the patients had performed nasal flushing.

U.S. Drinking Water Sanitation Still a Concern: CDC

U.S. Environmental Protection Agency.
U.S. Centers for Disease Control and Prevention, *Morbidity and Mortality Weekly Report.*

While US water sanitation has improved, bacteria-laden drinking water continues to cause disease outbreaks, according to a report recently released by federal health officials.

Legionella-tainted plumbing systems, untreated groundwater, and problems with distribution systems were the three main culprits identified in the 33 outbreaks reported to the U.S. Centers for Disease Control and Prevention from 2009 to 2010.

In all, unsanitary drinking water was responsible for 1,040 illnesses, 85 hospitalizations and nine deaths in 17 states during that time.

Legionella in community water systems was behind more than half of the outbreaks, while Campylobacter was the second most common outbreak cause, according to the report published in the CDC's *Morbidity and Mortality Weekly Report.*

Although Legionella, which causes a type of pneumonia known as Legionnaires' disease, led to a greater number of outbreaks, other types of bacteria resulted in more illnesses, including acute gastrointestinal illness, according to the report.

States that reported drinking water-related outbreaks were California, Florida, Georgia, Idaho, Illinois, Maine, Maryland, Minnesota, Missouri, Montana, Nevada, New York, Ohio, Pennsylvania, South Carolina, Utah and Vermont.

WHAT THIS MEANS FOR CONSUMERS

The findings don't mean that consumers should change their source of drinking water.

"Bottled water is not necessarily safer than your tap water," according to the U.S. Environmental Protection Agency. "EPA sets standards for tap water provided by public water systems; the Food and Drug Administration sets bottled water standards. Bottled water and tap water are both safe to drink if they meet these standards."

Local water suppliers must notify customers immediately if a public health threat exists from drinking-water contamination, the EPA website notes.

Identifying and correcting problems with water-distribution systems and untreated groundwater systems could prevent many outbreaks and illnesses, while more research is needed to learn how to better control Legionella, the CDC report concludes.

info The U.S. Environmental Protection Agency has more about groundwater and drinking water at its website, *http://water.epa.gov/drink/index.cfm.*

CDC Sounds Alarm on Antibiotic-Resistant Bacteria

Steve Solomon, MD, director, Office of Antimicrobial Resistance, U.S. Centers for Disease Control and Prevention.

Georges Benjamin, MD, executive director, American Public Health Association.

U.S. Centers for Disease Control and Prevention, Antibiotic Resistance Threats in the United States, 2013.

More than two million people come down with infections from antibiotic-resistant bacteria every year in the US, leading to at least 23,000 deaths, according to a recent report by federal health officials.

The report marks the first time that the U.S. Centers for Disease Control and Prevention (CDC) has performed a comprehensive analysis of the impact on society from antibiotic-resistant bacteria, said Steve Solomon, MD, director of the agency's Office of Antimicrobial Resistance.

"This is scary stuff, and we want people to know about it," he said.

The report outlines how antibiotic resistance occurs in patients and spreads through the community. It also lists medical procedures that have become more dangerous because of these bacteria. Those procedures include dialysis, chemotherapy, complex surgery and organ transplants.

Antibiotic overuse is the single most important factor leading to antibiotic resistance, according to the report. Antibiotics are among the most commonly prescribed drugs, but as many as half of those prescriptions are either not needed or not the best course of treatment for the patient, the report said. (For information on how to avoid antibiotic overuse and alternative treatments, see page 290.)

"Patients need to understand that antibiotics are not the solution for every illness," Dr. Solomon said. "It's important that people not take antibiotics when they aren't necessary. It contributes to resistance, and it also has consequences to the patient in the form of side effects."

The CDC also faulted the use of antibiotics in food animals to prevent, control and treat disease, and to promote their growth. "The use of antibiotics for promoting growth is not necessary, and the practice should be phased out," the report stated.

The centerpiece of the CDC report is a threat-level assessment for 18 bacteria- and antibiotic-related illnesses, broken down into three categories—urgent, serious and concerning.

Three antibiotic-related illnesses are ranked as urgent threats demanding immediate attention...

Having Shingles Can Increase Risk for Heart Attack and Stroke Later in Life

People who had shingles after age 40 had a 10% higher risk for heart attack and a 15% higher risk for mini-stroke, or transient ischemic attack. People who had shingles prior to age 40 were at much greater risk—they had a 50% higher risk for heart attack...were 2.4 times more likely to have a mini-stroke...and had a 74% higher risk for stroke.

If you have had shingles: Get a cardiovascular checkup, and be screened for risk factors, such as high cholesterol and high blood pressure.

Judith Breuer, MD, professor of virology at University College London, and lead author of a study published in *Neurology.*

•**Carbapenem-resistant Enterobacteriaceae,** or CRE, are a family of bacteria that have developed remarkable drug resistance in recent years. Half the people who get bloodstream infections from CRE die. About 9,300 hospital infections of CRE occur each year. "A lot of those bacteria are becoming resistant to every antibiotic we have," Dr. Solomon said of CRE. "We are very concerned about significant spread over the next few years."

•**Neisseria gonorrhoeae**—the bacteria that causes gonorrhea—are showing signs of resistance to the cephalosporin family of antibiotics. The CDC estimated that about one-third of the 820,000 annual gonorrhea infections involve strains that have become antibiotic-resistant. "The cephalosporins are really the last line of defense we have against gonorrhea," Dr. Solomon said. "It has shown its ability to become resistant to every antibiotic we throw at it. If we lost those—if this cephalosporin-resistant gonorrhea spreads—that disease is going to be untreatable."

•**Clostridium difficile** is bacteria that, although not antibiotic resistant, poses an urgent threat because it causes diarrhea linked to at least 250,000 hospitalizations and 14,000 American deaths each year. C. difficile infections occur because of antibiotic use that destroys the good bacteria in people's bodies that protect against illness. "Because there has not been as much success in addressing the problem of antibiotic overuse, we are flagging that as an urgent problem because it has to be brought under control," Dr. Solomon said.

Twelve infections from antibiotic-resistant bacteria are listed as serious, and three as concerning. For each bacteria threat, the CDC offers guidance for what healthcare industry officials, medical professionals and the general public can do to limit its spread.

Infections by antibiotic-resistant bacteria add as much as $20 billion in excess direct healthcare costs, with additional costs for lost productivity as high as $35 billion a year, according to the report.

In its report, the CDC outlined a four-pronged strategy for combating antibiotic-resistant bacteria…

HPV Linked to Poor Dental Health

Among 3,439 adults, those who reported poor oral health were 56% more likely to have oral human papillomavirus (HPV) infection, which can cause oral cancer.

Theory: HPV, which can infect the mouth during oral sex, may enter the body through tiny wounds that may occur with gum disease.

Self-defense: Be sure to practice good dental hygiene and have regular dental checkups.

Christine Markham, PhD, associate professor, The University of Texas School of Public Health, Houston.

•**Preventing infections and preventing the spread of resistance.**

•**Tracking resistant bacteria.**

•**Improving the use of existing antibiotics.**

•**Promoting the development of new antibiotics and new diagnostic tests for resistant bacteria.**

"As different as these problems are, the same strategies to address them are shared in common," Dr. Solomon said. "By helping people understand that those four core strategies are shared among the ways we address all of these antibiotic-resistant bacteria, we put it all in context and provide a glimpse of the big picture."

Georges Benjamin, MD, executive director of the American Public Health Association, said he appreciates the report's frank, down-to-earth manner.

"[The report] gives us a handle. Something we can use to talk with the public," he said. "Obviously, there is an enormous risk to the health of the public by antibiotic resistance, and it's going to take a multiple-sector response to resolving it."

info For more information on antibiotic-resistant bacteria, visit the U.S. Centers for Disease Control and Prevention at its website, *http://www.cdc.gov/drugresistance/index.html.*

Gene Testing Helps Sort Out Bacterial, Viral Infections

Duke University Medical Center, news release.

A new genetic test that distinguishes between viral and bacterial infections could help fight antibiotic resistance and quickly detect new diseases, according to a recent study.

The immune system responds differently when battling a viral or bacterial infection, and these differences are evident at the genetic level.

This new blood test detects a specific genetic signature that a person's immune system expresses in response to viruses, the Duke University Medical Center researchers said.

They assessed the test in 102 people and found that it was more than 90% accurate in distinguishing between viral and bacterial infections in people with respiratory illnesses, according to the study, which was published in the journal *Science Translational Medicine.*

The findings move the test closer to clinical use, where it could help patients get quicker diagnoses and treatments, while reducing the unnecessary use of antibiotics that don't work on viral infections, the researchers said.

"In instances such as pandemic flu or the corona virus that has erupted in the Middle East, it's extremely important to diagnose a viral illness far more accurately and speedier than can be done using traditional diagnostics," study co-senior author Dr. Geoffrey Ginsburg, director of genomic medicine and a professor of medicine, said in a Duke news release.

Current tests rely on evidence of the microbe in a patient's blood and require knowledge of that particular bug to detect it. The new test doesn't have those limitations and could be used to detect new diseases, including potential bioterrorism threats, according to the news release.

"This is important not only in viral pandemics where infection may be caused by unknown viruses but also in routine care where the decision to treat or not with antibiotics is paramount," study lead author Dr. Aimee Zaas, associate professor of infectious diseases and international health, said in the news release.

The researchers plan more, larger studies and say they're trying to reduce the amount of time it takes to get test results. The test currently takes 12 hours.

Better Sore Throat Screening

More than 600 adults with severe sore throats were screened with a new diagnostic tool called the FeverPAIN score, which evaluates patients for inflamed tonsils, cough, fever and other symptoms.

Result: When doctors based treatment on high FeverPAIN scores, antibiotic use decreased by nearly 30%, and symptoms were controlled.

Benefit: The score can help avoid unnecessary antibiotic use.

If you visit your doctor for a severe sore throat: Ask about the FeverPAIN score. *ctu1.phc.ox.ac.uk/feverpain/index.php.*

Paul Little, MD, professor of primary care research, University of Southampton, UK.

Hand Washing and Zinc Top the List for Warding Off Colds

Michael Allan, MD, associate professor and director, evidence-based medicine in family medicine, University of Alberta, Edmonton, Canada.

Aaron Glatt, MD, spokesman, Infectious Diseases Society of America and executive vice president, Mercy Medical Center, Rockville Centre, New York.

CMAJ (Canadian Medical Association Journal)

When the cold season hits, it seems as if everyone swears by their own methods for avoiding infection or treating themselves should they get sick.

Now, a recent review finds that some methods seem to work better than others, namely hand washing and zinc supplements for prevention of a cold, and decongestants and pain relievers for treatment.

STUDY DETAILS

For the study, the team reviewed hundreds of published studies looking at the best ways to prevent and treat colds. The review is published in *CMAJ* (*Canadian Medical Association Journal*).

Some evidence also suggests that probiotics—the "good bacteria" found in some yogurts and elsewhere—helped prevent colds. However, the studies included various combinations of probiotics, so making comparisons about which is best was difficult, said study leader Michael Allan, MD, director of evidence-based medicine in family medicine at the University of Alberta, in Canada.

For the prevention of colds, the evidence wasn't clear for gargling with water (and no benefit was found from gargling with an iodine solution), ginseng, exercise, garlic, homeopathy, echinacea or vitamins C or D.

BEST WAYS TO PREVENT A COLD

For preventing colds, frequent hand washing came out on top, said Dr. Allan.

Besides hand washing, daily zinc supplements appeared to help kids avoid colds, some research found, and Dr. Allan said it would probably work for adults. The evidence was not strong, however.

"It wouldn't be something I'd recommend on a regular basis," he said. Zinc use can lead to nausea and has an unpleasant taste, he noted.

BEST WAYS TO TREAT A COLD

For the treatment of colds, antihistamines by themselves didn't help. But they did help somewhat when used in combination with decongestants, pain relievers or both—but only in children over age five and adults. For fever in kids, he said, parents can use *acetaminophen* or *ibuprofen*, "but ibuprofen is superior to acetaminophen; it's a more potent fever reducer."

Nasal sprays with *ipratropium* (Atrovent)—prescribed for allergies and other conditions—may help runny noses but don't seem to help congestion, Dr. Allan found.

For the cough associated with cold, children over the age of one who get a single dose of honey at bedtime had reduced cough, Dr. Allan said. Honey should not be given to children younger than one due to risk of botulism poisoning.

WHAT TO AVOID

Many other old favorite treatments fell short, Dr. Allan found. Vapor rub was linked with burning of skin, eyes and nose. No clear benefit was found for nasal irrigation, humidified air, echinacea, Chinese medicinal herbs, ginseng or vitamin C. Intranasal zinc spray should not be used, Dr. Allan said. It has no clear benefit and could lead to loss of smell.

EXPERT COMMENTARY

The finding that hand washing is the best preventive rings true, said Aaron Glatt, MD, a spokesman for the Infectious Diseases Society of America and executive vice president of Mercy Medical Center, in Rockville Centre, New York.

Most treatments for the common cold, Dr. Glatt agreed, have minimal benefits.

Whatever cold remedy is chosen…"If you have an underlying disease, see a doctor to be sure there are no complications," said Dr. Glatt.

For example, anyone with heart or lung disease should be aware a cold may impact them more strongly than others. "Those types of patients should check in with their doctor," Dr. Glatt said.

DO WHAT (SAFELY) WORKS FOR YOU

Even without evidence of benefit, Dr. Allan said many of his patients swear by the remedies that have helped them in the past. As long as they present no harms, he tells them to go ahead.

"People have individual reactions to medicines that are not predictable," he said. "There is also, of course, the placebo effect—you think it's going to work [and you feel better]."

info Visit the American Academy of Pediatrics website at *http://www.healthychildren.org/English/health-issues/conditions/ear-nose-throat/pages/Children-and-Colds.aspx* for more on colds in kids.

Flu-Fighting Facts That May Surprise You

William Schaffner, MD, a professor of preventive medicine and infectious diseases at Vanderbilt University Medical Center in Nashville. Dr. Schaffner is the immediate past-president of the National Foundation for Infectious Diseases and has authored or coauthored more than 400 published studies, reviews and book chapters on infectious diseases.

The flu is an illness that you hear so much about year after year that it's easy to assume you know all there is to know about it. That's a mistake. Widely held assumptions about the flu often are wrong—and dangerous. By learning the facts, you can help yourself and loved ones from being among the estimated 36,000 Americans who will die this year due to pneumonia and other flu-related complications. *Common misconceptions...*

Misconception #1: **People who have the flu are contagious only when they have symptoms.** Actually, most people with the flu are able to spread the illness beginning about a day before showing any symptoms and up to seven days after symptoms begin.

And you don't even have to be in very close proximity. The influenza virus can spread to a person six feet away—mainly when the sick person sneezes, coughs or even talks. Of course, you can also become contaminated if you touch your eyes, nose or mouth after coming in contact with an object, such as an elevator button, handrail or doorknob, that harbors a flu virus. These viruses can live up to eight hours on such objects.

Helpful: Wash your hands or use hand sanitizer several times a day—and always after you've been out in public or in contact with someone who has the flu.

Also: If you get the flu and have a fever, stay home until your fever has been gone for at least 24 hours without the use of fever-reducing medication.

Misconception #2: **If you're not running a fever, you don't have the flu.** Flu symptoms aren't always predictable. A fever is common with the illness, but it doesn't occur in everyone. Typical flu symptoms include body aches, extreme fatigue and a dry cough. However, some flu patients may also experience sneezing, a stuffy nose and sore throat—symptoms that usually occur with the common cold. In rare cases, flu patients even suffer vomiting and diarrhea. Although flu symptoms vary, a hallmark of the illness is that it comes on quickly and makes you feel quite sick.

Misconception #3: **If you think you have the flu, you should go right to bed until you feel better.** Getting plenty of rest is important for flu recovery, but if you suspect that you have the flu and are in the high-risk category for flu complications (for example, you are over age 65, pregnant or have a chronic health condition such as asthma or heart disease), you should also alert your doctor right away.*

He/she may recommend a rapid flu test (using a nose or throat swab) that can diagnose the flu in about 30 minutes. If the result is positive, you may be prescribed the antiviral medication *oseltamivir* (Tamiflu).

Key: This drug works best when started within 48 hours of getting sick.

Important: Adults produce much less of the flu virus

Too Healthy to Get the Flu? Think Again!

Many people believe that if they're basically healthy, they won't benefit from flu vaccination and that only high-risk individuals need the vaccine. That's absolutely false. Perhaps you've dodged this bullet in past flu seasons, but that doesn't mean you will this year or in any future year. While it's true that people in high-risk groups are more likely to develop potentially deadly complications (such as pneumonia, dehydration and even heart attacks) from the flu, many perfectly healthy people contract the flu each year, and some of those cases turn out to be devastating. Even people without symptoms can spread the flu: Younger adults (in their 20s and 30s) can get the flu but have no symptoms and pass it on to others, including those in high-risk categories. If younger adults get vaccinated, it helps cut down on the spread of the virus.

*For the entire list of CDC flu recommendations, go to *CDC.gov/flu.*

and for a shorter time than children. If the rapid flu test is negative, it doesn't necessarily mean that you don't have the flu, and your doctor may want to treat you anyway.

If you're generally healthy and get a mild case of the flu, you may simply want to get a lot of rest and drink plenty of fluids. To control symptoms, you can use over-the-counter drugs—cough medicine or *acetaminophen* (Tylenol) or a nonsteroidal anti-inflammatory drug such as *naproxen* (Aleve) for fever, if necessary.

Misconception #4: **The flu vaccine must be given early in the season to be effective.** You will certainly have protection for a greater part of the flu season if you get vaccinated early on, but it's still worth getting the vaccine even as late as January if the flu is still circulating. But don't wait! It takes about two weeks for the vaccine to trigger the development of antibodies and confer maximum protection.

Misconception #5: **All flu vaccines offer the same level of protection.** Again, not true. Traditional flu vaccines, known as trivalent vaccines, protect against three types of viruses-—two strains of Type A (which cause the most severe illness) and one Type B strain.

New option introduced in 2013: Manufacturers have introduced quadrivalent vaccines, which add a second type of B strain to the mix. It is more likely than older vaccines to protect against the variety of virus strains that circulate each year.

Ask your doctor—or the pharmacist where you get your shot—if the new version is available. The extra protection is worth it. The "quad" vaccine will probably become standard in the next few years. In 2013, however, it was in short supply because manufacturers hadn't fully changed their operations.

Important: If the quad vaccine is not available in your area, don't skip your vaccination.

Misconception #6: **People who are allergic to eggs can't get a flu vaccination.** A new vaccine, Flublok, doesn't use eggs in production—as do traditional vaccines that culture flu viruses in eggs. Instead, it's made with recombinant DNA technology in which insect viruses are used to produce a protein found in flu viruses. The vaccine is FDA-approved for adults ages 18 to 49 (the ages of people in a study that was performed). It is just as effective as egg-based vaccines.

Flu Patients Can Emit Germs as Far as Six Feet

This is a much greater distance than previously thought.

Also: People suffering from the worst flu symptoms give off the greatest levels of flu particles into the air.

Study of 94 flu patients by researchers at Wake Forest School of Medicine, Winston-Salem, North Carolina, published in *The Journal of Infectious Diseases*.

Misconception #7: **The flu vaccine doesn't work very well.** In 2012, the CDC reported that the flu vaccine was about 56% effective at overall prevention and about 27% effective in adults age 65 or older.

The immune system gets less robust with age. It produces fewer antibodies in response to vaccines. To help older adults, manufacturers have recently introduced a higher-dose vaccine that research has shown to be about 24% more effective than older vaccines.

Important: These percentages may seem low but represent complete prevention in people who respond to the vaccine. Even though the flu vaccine isn't effective for everyone, it's better than no protection. The vaccine also makes the flu milder in people who do get it and reduces deadly complications such as pneumonia.

If you are age 65 or older, your doctor or pharmacist will probably recommend the Fluzone High-Dose vaccine.

Note: A small percentage of people will have arm soreness and/or a headache.

Misconception #8: **All flu shots contain mercury.** Questionable research that once claimed that the mercury-containing preservative thimerosal caused autism in children has been completely debunked. Even though there's no credible evidence of harm caused by thimerosal, some people refuse to get a flu shot because they are still concerned about the preservative and assume that all flu shots contain it. If you would rather avoid thimerosal, ask your doctor for a single-dose flu vaccine (the preservative is used only in multi-dose vials that provide vaccine for multiple injections). The FluMist nasal spray also doesn't contain thimerosal.

Saliva May Improve With Age for Flu Protection

Journal of Proteome Research, news release

Certain proteins in saliva help protect seniors from influenza, according to a recent study from China.

The findings improve understanding of why older people are better able to fight off the new strains of bird and swine flu than younger people, said researcher Zheng Li and colleagues.

As well as beginning the process of digesting foods, saliva also contains germ-fighting proteins that form a first-line defense against infections. It was already known that a person's age affects their saliva's levels of certain glycoproteins, which are proteins with a sugar coating that combat disease-causing germs.

In this study, investigators sought to learn more about how age-related differences in these saliva proteins affect people's susceptibility to influenza.

The researchers analyzed saliva samples from 180 men and women of various ages and found that glycoproteins in the saliva of people aged 65 and older were more efficient in binding to influenza viruses than those in children and young adults.

The study was published recently in the *Journal of Proteome Research.*

The researchers said their findings suggest that saliva testing may help improve understanding, prevention and diagnosis of some age-related diseases.

info The U.S. Office of Disease Prevention and Health Promotion explains how to protect yourself from seasonal flu at its website, *http://www.healthfinder.gov/HealthTopics/Category/doctor-visits/shotsvaccines/protect-yourself-from-seasonal-flu.*

Almost All Teens and Adults Should Be Screened for HIV

The US Preventive Services Task Force updated its guidelines because of the effectiveness of newer treatments when started early on. All people ages 15 to 65 should be screened for HIV. These recommendations now are similar to those from the US Centers for Disease Control and Prevention, the American College of Physicians and the American Academy of Pediatrics.

Guidelines from US Preventive Services Task Force, Rockville, Maryland.

5 Top Myths About Lyme Disease

Richard I. Horowitz, MD, an internist, integrative medicine practitioner and medical director of the Hudson Valley Healing Arts Center in Hyde Park, New York. He is author of *Why Can't I Get Better? Solving the Mystery of Lyme & Chronic Disease* (St. Martin's). *CanGetBetter.com*

Your risk of getting Lyme disease is higher than you might think. Until recently, it was estimated that about 30,000 new cases occurred in the US each year. A recent report, released by the Centers for Disease Control and Prevention (CDC) in 2013, stated that the number of Lyme cases is roughly 10 times higher—about 300,000 per year.

If you assume that you're safe from Lyme, consider this: Although many people think that this disease occurs in isolated pockets around the country, it's actually now been reported in most parts of the US.

"The great imitator": Lyme, the most common disease that's spread by ticks, causes dozens of symptoms that can easily be mistaken for other conditions, such as chronic fatigue syndrome, fibromyalgia and autoimmune diseases including multiple sclerosis. Many patients with Lyme suffer unnecessarily because they never even know that they have the disease—and those who are diagnosed often are not given the best treatments.

Leading misconceptions about Lyme—and the facts...

***MYTH #1:* Lyme always causes a bull's-eye rash.** People who live in areas where Lyme disease is common are taught to look for a red, expanding rash called erythema migrans. It resembles a bull's-eye and generally appears about seven days after a bite from an infected tick.

Fact: About half of Lyme patients develop a rash. But even when the rash is present, it resembles a bull's-eye in only about half of those cases. It's just as likely to appear as a "simple" rash that's easily mistaken for a spider bite or skin infection.

***MYTH #2:* Joint pain is the telltale symptom of Lyme.** Many Lyme patients will develop Lyme arthritis, severe joint pain and swelling that usually affects the knees or other large joints. But not every Lyme patient develops this symptom—so you can't assume that the absence of joint pain and swelling means that you don't have Lyme.

Fact: Most Lyme patients have at least a dozen different symptoms, but there is no one symptom that everyone with Lyme has. Among the most common symptoms are fatigue, migratory joint and muscle pain, tingling, numbness and burning sensations, a stiff neck, headache, memory and concentration problems and sleep disorders. These symptoms can range from mild to severe. The constellation of symptoms and ruling out other disorders point to Lyme.

***MYTH #3:* Lyme is fairly easy to diagnose with a blood test.** If you have Lyme symptoms, your doctor will probably recommend two-tiered blood testing—the ELISA test, which measures the total amount of antibodies produced by the body in response to the Lyme bacterium (Borrelia burgdorferi)...and if that test is positive, the Western blot, which looks for specific protein patterns that are characteristic of Lyme.

Fact: The tests are not very accurate. One study, conducted by the New York State Department of Health, looked at more than 1,500 patients who had been diagnosed with Lyme disease. Two-tiered testing missed 81% of the cases. If tests are done early in the course of the disease or if the patient has received an antibiotic, test results may indicate a false-negative.

Important: I recommend getting both the ELISA and Western blot tests. If your Western blot shows a 23, 31, 34, 39 and/or 83-93 band, this indicates Lyme. Other tests, such as a DNA test called polymerase chain reaction (PCR) and antibody titers, to check for other common tick-borne infections, such as Babesia (a malaria-like parasite) and Bartonella (which causes cat scratch fever), also can be helpful in diagnosing resistant symptoms.

***MYTH #4: Doxycycline* always cures Lyme quickly.** When Lyme is diagnosed and treated within two to four weeks of the tick bite that transmitted the disease, about 75% of patients will be cured with tetracycline antibiotics such as doxycycline or other antibiotics such as penicillin or cephalosporin.

But about one-quarter of these patients—and a higher percentage of those who don't get quick treatment—will develop a chronic infection that doesn't respond to simple antibiotic therapy. Although some doctors don't think Lyme bacteria survive after 30 days of antibiotic treatment, many studies have shown that they can.

***MYTH #5:* Medication is the only treatment.** Antibiotic therapy is the mainstay of Lyme treatment. But it's usually not enough.

Fact: Many Lyme symptoms—such as fatigue, muscle and joint pain, and memory loss—that persist despite antibiotics may be caused by more than one organism. Chinese herbs such

New Faster Treatment for Hepatitis C

The new drugs *sofosbuvir* and *simeprevir* are specifically designed to stop the hepatitis C virus from replicating. Studies show high cure rates for both drugs. In many patients, including some who previously had been unresponsive to treatment, the infection was gone within 12 to 24 weeks. Hepatitis C is an infectious disease that can scar the liver and lead to liver cirrhosis and/or liver cancer.

Robert Gish, MD, clinical professor of medicine at University of Nevada, and senior medical director of Robert G. Gish Consultants, San Diego, a consulting firm that promotes liver health.

Dogs May Be Able to Sniff Out Deadly Infections

A beagle has been trained to detect the intestinal bacterium C. difficile in stool samples. If other dogs can be trained to detect such bacteria, this may lead to faster detection and better treatment. C. difficile spreads rapidly in hospitals and long-term-care centers. The CDC reports that the bacterium causes 14,000 deaths in the US each year.

Marije K. Bomers, MD, infectious disease specialist, VU University Medical Center, Amsterdam, the Netherlands, and leader of a study published in *BMJ*.

as coptis, artemesia and cat's claw may help treat Lyme and these co-infections.

I often advise patients also to take low-dose *naltrexone*, a medication that helps reduce inflammation. A combination of naltrexone, curcumin (an anti-inflammatory compound found in the spice turmeric) and antioxidants like glutathione have helped relieve fatigue, pain and cognitive difficulty in my patients.

Also helpful: Diet is important. Some people feel better avoiding gluten, and for others, an alkaline diet with lots of fruits and vegetables counteracts the acidity and inflammation caused by infection.

BETTER TICK PROTECTION

People can prevent some cases of Lyme by carefully checking their skin and removing ticks with tweezers after spending time outdoors—but don't count on it.

Fact: The black-legged tick that causes Lyme is about the size of a sesame seed. Most people never see the ticks that bite them.

My advice: Whenever possible, wear long pants and high socks when you go outdoors during tick season. Spraying your clothing with a product that contains permethrin, a flower-based insect repellent, can help repel ticks. If it's just too hot and you prefer shorts or other summer clothes, you can apply the stronger insect repellent known as DEET to your skin, but wash it off as soon as you are out of the tick-infested area to reduce exposure to the chemical.

Lessons Learned from Cantaloupe-Listeria Outbreak

Benjamin Silk, PhD, MPH, epidemiologist, division of foodborne, waterborne, and environmental diseases, U.S. Centers for Disease Control and Prevention.

Marc Siegel, MD, associate professor, medicine, NYU Langone Medical Center, New York City.

New England Journal of Medicine

Of all the dangerous bacteria lurking in foods, perhaps the most deadly is listeria, and the lesson from a 2011 outbreak is to always handle food safely, US health officials say.

In the summer and fall of 2011, cantaloupes contaminated with listeria sickened 147 people in 28 states, killing 33 of them. That listeria outbreak—the deadliest in a decade—was unusual because listeria is rarely associated with fresh produce, according to a recent report from the U.S. Centers for Disease Control and Prevention (CDC).

Although rare, listeria is an important public-health issue because of its severity, said report coauthor Benjamin Silk, PhD, MD, a CDC epidemiologist in the division of foodborne, waterborne and environmental diseases. "Nearly all people who have listeria infections diagnosed are hospitalized, and about one in five die," Dr. Silk said.

The report, published in the *New England Journal of Medicine*, highlights lessons learned from an investigation into the 2011 outbreak.

The authors found that for the 145 people for whom complete records were available, all but two were hospitalized and nearly one-quarter died.

WHO GETS SICK

Most of those sickened were in their 60s or older and suffered from other illnesses. But there also were seven pregnancy-associated infections among four women and three infants. One of the four women miscarried because of the infection.

Overall, this is typical of the general consequences of a listeria outbreak, one expert said.

"Listeria is only a problem for immuno-compromised folks and pregnant women, but in those cases people can and do get quite ill and almost all are hospitalized," said Marc Siegel, MD, associate professor of medicine at the NYU Langone Medical Center in New York City.

"In this case, pregnant women were a small percentage, though they are usually more," he said. "Outbreaks are limited as healthy people don't generally get ill."

HOW CONTAMINATION OCCURS

The contaminated cantaloupes were traced to a Colorado grower, and while the exact cause of the contamination isn't known, unsanitary conditions were likely the culprit, according to the report.

"The problem is that listeria bacteria grows on produce—in this case cantaloupes—and occurs especially when proper precautions aren't taken at the farm or processing facility," Dr. Siegel said.

One possible contributor to the outbreak is inadequate facility and equipment design, which hampered thorough cleaning of surfaces the melons could touch, according to the report. Another possible route to contamination is a truck kept next to the processing line that went to and from a cattle operation.

In addition, the Colorado farm did not cool its cantaloupes before placing them in cold storage, which may have caused condensation that promoted the growth of listeria.

"This outbreak confirms the viability of raw produce, including cantaloupe, as a vehicle for listeriosis and highlights the importance of preventing produce contamination within farm and processing environments," the report noted.

Listeria is associated with about 1,600 infections in the United States annually, Dr. Silk said. A partnership between the CDC and state health departments, known as the Listeria Initiative, enabled the agency quickly to identify the source of the 2011 outbreak, he said.

The CDC continues to monitor and follow up on all listeria cases, Dr. Silk said. In addition, the FDA has stepped up inspections of cantaloupe farms and has issued guidelines to cantaloupe growers.

Popular Meat Substitute May Contain Salmonella

Tempeh, made from fermented soybeans and often used in place of meat, has been linked to a salmonella outbreak among 100 people in five states in 2013. The tempeh had been unpasteurized and made with tainted ingredients imported from Indonesia.

Self-defense: Tempeh should be treated like a meat and thoroughly cooked. Knives and hands should always be thoroughly washed after touching tempeh.

Study by researchers at North Carolina Division of Public Health, Raleigh, published in *Emerging Infectious Diseases.*

SAFETY TIPS FOR HANDLING FOOD

The best way to avoid listeria is to follow common-sense food-safety procedures, Dr. Silk said.

To help prevent infection, the CDC recommends you do the following...

- **Rinse fruits and vegetables thoroughly under running water** before eating, cutting or cooking them.
- **Scrub farm produce,** such as melons and cucumbers, with a clean produce brush.
- **Dry produce with a clean cloth or paper towel.**
- **Separate uncooked meats and poultry** from vegetables, cooked foods and ready-to-eat foods.
- **Wash hands, knives, countertops and cutting boards** after handling and preparing uncooked foods.
- **Because listeria can grow in foods in the refrigerator,** keep the temperature of your refrigerator at 40 degrees or lower and the freezer at 0 degrees or lower.
- **Clean up all spills in the refrigerator,** especially juices from hot dogs, lunch meat, raw meat and raw poultry.
- **Clean the inside walls and shelves of the refrigerator** with hot water and liquid soap, and then rinse.
- **Thoroughly cook beef, pork or poultry.**

info For more information on listeria, visit the U.S. Centers for Disease Control and Prevention website at *http://www.cdc.gov/listeria/.*

First Effective Malaria Vaccine May Be Near, Experts Say

PATH Malaria Vaccine Initiative, news release.

Promising results from a large-scale clinical trial mean that the world's first malaria vaccine may be on the market by year-end 2015 and could potentially save hundreds of thousands of lives a year.

The phase III clinical trial of more than 15,000 infants and young children in Africa found that the vaccine—called RTS,S—continued to protect the youngsters from malaria for up to 18 months after vaccination. The ongoing trial of the RTS,S vaccine is being conducted by 11 research centers in seven African countries, together with the PATH Malaria Vaccine Initiative and drug maker GlaxoSmithKline.

"It appears that the RTS,S candidate vaccine has the potential to have a significant public health impact," Halidou Tinto, lead investigator from the Nanoro, Burkina Faso trial site in West Africa, said in a PATH news release.

"Preventing substantial numbers of malaria cases in a community would mean fewer hospital beds filled with sick children," said Tinto, who is chair of the Clinical Trials Partnership Committee, which oversees the RTS,S phase III program. "Families would lose less time and money caring for these children and have more time for work or other activities. And of course the children themselves would reap the benefits of better health."

During the 18-month follow-up period, there was a 46% reduction in the number of malaria cases in children aged five months to 17 months at first vaccination, working out to 941 fewer cases of malaria for every 1,000 children. (A child can contract more than one case of malaria, the experts noted.) Cases of severe malaria were reduced by 36% and malaria hospitalizations were reduced by 42%.

Among infants who were six to 12 weeks old at first vaccination, there was a 27% reduction in the number of malaria cases during the 18-month follow-up, which works out to 444 fewer cases of malaria for every 1,000 infants. There was also a 15% reduction in cases of severe malaria and 17% fewer hospitalizations for malaria, the investigators found.

The latest findings from the trial were presented at the Multilateral Initiative on Malaria Pan African Conference in South Africa. Based on the data, vaccine maker GlaxoSmithKline plans to apply in 2014 to have the vaccine approved by the European Medicines Agency. If the agency approves the vaccine, the World Health Organization said it could issue a recommendation for the vaccine as early as 2015.

"In Africa we experience nearly 600,000 deaths annually from malaria, mainly children under five years of age," Tinto said.

"Many millions of malaria cases fill the wards of our hospitals. Progress is being made with bed nets and other measures, but we need more tools to battle this terrible disease," Tinto explained.

David Kaslow, MD, vice president of product development at PATH, commented on the importance of the results. "Given the huge disease burden of malaria among African children, we cannot ignore what these latest results tell us about the potential for RTS,S to have a measurable and significant impact on the health of millions of young children in Africa," he said in the news release.

"While we want to be careful about not getting ahead of the data, this trial continues to show that a malaria vaccine could potentially bring an important additional benefit beyond that provided by the tools already in use," Dr. Kaslow added.

info The U.S. Centers for Disease Control and Prevention has more about malaria at its website *http://www.cdc.gov/malaria/about/faqs.html.*

14 Bottom Line's HEALTH BREAKTHROUGHS

Longevity & Optimum Aging

Give Yourself a Natural Face-Lift

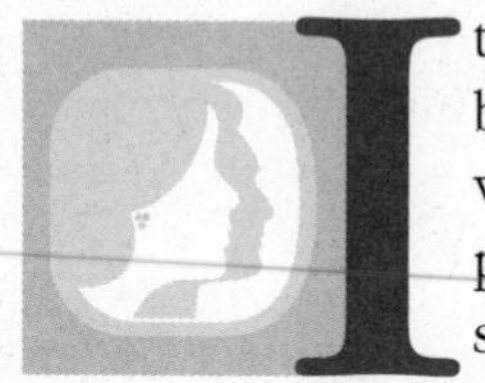

It's a fact of life that our skin becomes more wrinkled as we age. But you may be surprised to learn that our skin starts changing as early as age 30 for both women and men.

What happens: The cells that make up the skin divide more slowly with age, so the top layer of skin gets about 10% thinner every decade. The result? You guessed it—more wrinkles as well as more bruises...uneven skin tone...and sagging skin. Of course, you can "refresh" your appearance with Botox and skin fillers, but even "inexpensive" cosmetic procedures cost hundreds of dollars.

A better option: Natural skin care. Used properly, natural approaches can take years off your appearance.

STEP 1: TWEAK YOUR DIET

While you might think that skin-care products are the logical choice to smooth wrinkled skin, it's wise to first work from the "inside out" to give your skin the nutrients it needs to look its best.

Increasing laboratory evidence and positive reports from patients suggest that the following foods promote younger-looking skin...

- **High-sulfur foods.** Sulfur is known to be one of the "building blocks" of collagen, a protein that strengthens skin and gives it elasticity. Fortunately, sulfur is found in a number of foods.

My advice: At least once a day, eat sulfur-rich foods.

Good choices: Eggs, chives, legumes (such as black, white or kidney beans) and fish that is high in omega-3 fatty acids (such as salmon and sardines).

Eudene Harry, MD, medical director of Oasis Wellness & Rejuvenation Center in Orlando, Florida. She is author of *Live Younger in 8 Simple Steps: A Practical Guide to Slowing Down the Aging Process from the Inside Out* (Harry). *LivingHealthyLookingYounger.com*

•**Grape juice or red wine.** These contain flavonoids known as *proanthocyanidins* and proteins called *tenascins*—both help make the skin smoother and more elastic.

My advice: Enjoy a daily glass of grape juice—or red wine if your doctor says daily alcohol consumption is appropriate for you. Both are high in proanthocyanidins.

In addition, a grape seed extract supplement (typical dose 200 mg once a day) is beneficial, but check first with your doctor if you take medication, especially a blood thinner—the supplement may interact with certain drugs.

•**Soy foods.** Tofu, soy milk and other foods derived from soy can make skin appear significantly younger. This is mainly due to genistein, an antioxidant in soy that slows skin aging and increases collagen. Genistein and other compounds are linked to increased skin elasticity and plumpness. These compounds give the skin a "glow" that makes it appear younger.

My advice: Have one or more daily servings of soy foods.

Good choices: Edamame (steamed soy beans) and miso (a fermented paste used in cooking). Check first with your doctor if you have breast cancer or kidney disease or take any medication. Soy may be harmful for some breast cancer and kidney disease patients…it may also interact with certain drugs, including blood thinners and some antidepressants.

Also: To help keep skin hydrated, drink eight eight-ounce glasses of water each day.

STEP 2: USE THE RIGHT SKIN-CARE PRODUCTS

Skin-care products can help smooth wrinkles and provide other benefits, but there are so many on the market that most people are confused about which to use. *Best choices for younger-looking skin…*

•**Topical vitamin C.** About 80% of the dermis (the second layer of skin) consists of that all important protein collagen. Because collagen production declines with age, it's a good idea to promote collagen production any way you can.

That's where vitamin C enters the picture. The body uses vitamin C to produce collagen, but whatever is consumed orally doesn't reach adequate concentrations in the skin to boost collagen. That's why you need to apply it topically.

My advice: Use skin-care products (such as lotions and sunscreens) that have ascorbic acid (vitamin C)—the best form of the vitamin for absorption as well as collagen production and sun protection. Studies show that topical vitamin C can reduce the appearance of fine lines and wrinkles in as little as three months.

To save money: Buy powdered vitamin C at a health-food store, and mix in a small pinch each time you use a moisturizer/sunscreen that does not contain the vitamin.

•**Retinoic acid.** This is a form of vitamin A that is added to hundreds of over-the-counter (OTC) skin-care products. It is also available by prescription. Retinoic acid increases cellular turnover, the rate at which cells divide. This makes the skin appear brighter, smoother and plumper.

My advice: Use OTC retinol cream once daily. Apply it at night because it temporarily increases the skin's sensitivity to sun. Most products have a concentration of 1% or less. Prescription-strength retinoic acid usually is not necessary.

•**Moisturizer.** Everyone should use this as they age. Adding moisture to skin cells makes them expand, which improves skin volume and texture. Moisturizers protect the skin from environmental factors (heat, dryness and pollution) that undermine skin health.

My advice: Use moisturizer with sunscreen at least twice a day. I advise a vitamin C–enhanced moisturizer that includes green-tea extract. Both ingredients improve the skin's ability to absorb the moisturizer. Compounds in green tea also reduce skin inflammation and sun-related skin damage. Soy moisturizers may provide similar benefits.

Also important: Exfoliation, an effective form of controlled trauma that stimulates the skin to produce more collagen. Every week or two, use a gentle facial scrub with fine grains and a soft facial brush. This practice also removes the dead skin cells that dull your complexion.

Sensitive skin sometimes cannot tolerate even a mild scrub. An ultrasonic brush, such as Clarisonic ($100 to $200 at department stores and online), with a hydrating cleanser is a good alternative.

A chemical peel once or twice a year is another good way to remove dead skin cells. OTC peels contain glycolic acid, lactic acid or salicylic acid, usually in a concentration of about 5% to 10%. Peels should also contain moisturizing ingredients to minimize irritation. If you're new to chemical peels, talk with your dermatologist before using one of these products, since they can irritate skin, especially sensitive skin.

---

12 Things That Make You Look Older

Kim Johnson Gross, cocreator of the Chic Simple book series and author of *What to Wear for the Rest of Your Life* (Grand Central Life & Style) and *Chic Simple Dress Smart: Men* (Grand Central). Based in New York City, she is a former Ford model and has been fashion editor at *Town & Country* and *Esquire* magazines and a columnist for *More* and *InStyle*. *KimJohnsonGross.com*

As you get older, wardrobe and style choices that worked when you were younger may no longer be serving you well. This goes for both men and women. Without knowing it, you may be looking older than you are. This could cause others to treat you as older and potentially hold you back from employment opportunities and advancements. This also can make you feel like you are not up to your game or comfortable in your skin. When you are not style confident, you are less body confident, which makes you feel less life confident.

Helpful: Seek out style mentors—people who look elegant and modern without chasing youth-oriented trends. Observe them carefully, and adapt elements of their style to your own. TV newscasters make good style mentors because they are required to look contemporary while also projecting dignity and authority.

Give yourself a good, hard look, and ask yourself whether you are looking older than your actual age with any of these common signals…

1. Sneakers for everyday wear. Your feet should be comfortable, but sneakers outside the gym just look sloppy and careless. Young people get away with it—but there are more stylish options when you're older. These include loafers or driving moccasins for men and low-heeled pumps with cushioned soles for women. Wedge-soled shoes are a comfortable alternative to high heels.

2. Baggy pants. Although young men may look trendy in high-waisted, loose-fitting jeans, this style screams old on anyone else. For women, the rear end tends to flatten with age, causing pants to fit loosely in the rear. And front-pleated pants for women generally are unflattering and unstylish.

Better: Spend the time to find pants that fit well—or figure a tailor into your wardrobe budget. Baggy is dowdy, but overly tight makes you look heavier. Well-fitting clothes make you look slimmer and younger.

3. Boring colors. Skin tone gets duller with age, so the colors you wear should bring light to your face. If you are a woman who has worn black for years, it may be too harsh for you now. Brown makes men fade into the woodwork.

Better: Stand in front of a mirror, and experiment with colors that you never thought you could wear—you may be surprised at what flatters you. Avoid neon brights, which make older skin look sallow, but be open to the rest of the color spectrum. Try contemporary patterns and prints. For neutrals, gray and navy are softer alternatives to black for women, and any shade of blue is a good bet for men.

4. Boring glasses and jewelry. Men and women should have some fun with glasses. It's a great way to update your look and make it more modern. Tell your optician what you're looking for, or bring a stylish friend with you.

As for jewelry for women, wearing a large piece of fab faux jewelry (earrings, necklace, ring) or multiple bracelets adds great style and youth to your look.

5. Turtlenecks. You may think a turtleneck hides a sagging neck and chin, but it is more likely to draw attention to jowls.

Better: A cowl neckline for women, or a loosely draped scarf. A scarf is the single best item to help a woman look thinner, taller, prettier and more chic. For a video on how to tie a scarf, go to NYCityWoman.com and type "Six Ways to Wear a Scarf" in the search box. For a man, an oblong scarf, looped, is a stylish European look that adds a welcome shot of color.

6. Stiff or one-tone hair. An overly styled helmet of hair looks old-fashioned. Hair that's a solid block of color looks unnatural and harsh.

Better: Whether hair is short or shoulder-length, women need layers around the face for softness. As for color, opt for subtle highlights in front and a slightly darker tone toward the back.

Keep in mind that gray hair can be beautiful, modern and sexy. You need a plan to go gray, though, which means a flattering cut and using hair products that enhance the gray. Ask your stylist for recommendations. Also, if your hair is a dull gray, consider getting silver highlights around your face to bring light and "energy" to your hair.

Men who dye their hair should allow a bit of gray at the temples—it looks more natural than monochrome hair. But avoid a comb-over or a toupee. A man who attempts to hide a receding hairline isn't fooling anyone—he just looks insecure.

Better: Treat your thinning hair as a badge of honor. Either keep it neatly trimmed or shave your head.

7. Missing (or bushy) eyebrows. Women's eyebrows tend to disappear with age. Men's are more likely to grow wild.

Better: Women should use eyebrow pencil, powder or both to fill in fading brows. Visit a high-end cosmetics counter, and ask the stylist to show you how. You may need to try several products to find out what works best. Men, make sure that your barber or hair stylist trims your eyebrows regularly.

Also: Women tend not to notice increased facial hair (especially stray hairs) on the chin and upper lip—a result of hormonal change. Pluck!

8. Deeply tanned skin. Baby boomers grew up actively developing suntans using baby oil and sun reflectors. Now pale is the norm. A dark tan not only dates you, it increases your risk for skin cancer and worsens wrinkling.

Better: Wear a hat and sunscreen to shield your skin from sun damage.

9. Less-than-white teeth. Yellowing teeth add decades to your appearance. Everyone's teeth get yellower with age, but with so many teeth-whitening products available, there is no excuse to live with off-color teeth.

Better: Ask your dentist which whitening technique he/she recommends based on the condition of your teeth—over-the-counter whitening strips, bleaching in the dentist's office or a custom bleaching kit you can use at home.

10. Women: Nude or beige hose. Nude stockings on women look hopelessly out-of-date. Bare legs are the norm now for young women, but they are not a good option for older women who have dark veins.

Better: In winter, wear dark stockings or opaque tights. In summer, use spray-on tanner for a light tan...or wear nude fishnet stockings or slacks or capris.

11. Poor-fitting bra. Get a bra that fits. Most women don't know that bra size changes as your body does. Giving your breasts a lift will make you look younger and trimmer.

12. Excess makeup. Thick foundation, heavy eyeliner, bright blusher and red lipstick all add years to your face.

Better: Use a moisturizing (not matte) foundation, and dab it only where needed to even out skin tone. To add color to cheeks, use a small amount of tinted moisturizer, bronzer or cream blush. Use liquid eyeliner in soft shades such as deep blue or brown, and blend it well. For lips, choose soft pinks and mauves, depending on your skin tone.

Bottom line: The idea is to have fun putting yourself together. That inner spark and personal style will show that you are getting better with age.

Stay Sharp As You Age—Surprising Causes of Memory Loss

Pamela W. Smith, MD, MPH, MS, founder and director of The Fellowship in Metabolic, Anti-Aging and Functional Medicine, Boca Raton, Florida, and codirector of the master's program in medical sciences with a concentration in metabolic and nutritional medicine, University of South Florida College of Medicine, Tampa. She is author of *What You Must Know About Memory Loss & How to Stop It* (Square One).

It is no secret that age and memory are intertwined. But age itself is not the sole reason that we forget things. Memory loss often can be traced to specific factors, including hormonal changes, inflammation and exposure to mercury and other toxins.

Common causes of memory loss—and what you can do to control them...

LOW TESTOSTERONE

After a man reaches age 30, his testosterone goes into free fall. Levels drop by about 1% a year. At least 30% of men in their 70s are hypogonadal, with very low testosterone.

Low testosterone increases the death of brain cells. It also has been linked to an increase in amyloid-B, proteins that are associated with Alzheimer's disease and other forms of dementia.

What to do: If a saliva test shows low testosterone, your doctor may recommend creams, injections or other forms of testosterone replacement. Men who supplement with testosterone have been shown to have improvements in verbal memory (the recall of verbal information) and spatial memory (the part of the memory responsible for recording information about one's environment and spatial orientation).

Important: Women need testosterone, too, and should get tested. Testosterone replacement in women with low levels can help preserve memory.

LOW ESTROGEN

Women often refer to the "brain fog" that occurs during menopause. It's a real phenomenon that is caused in part by declining levels of estrogen. Every brain cell is affected by estrogen, which conducts chemical signals through the hippocampus and other areas of the brain.

Low-dose estrogen replacement can improve brain circulation and reduce the risk for Alzheimer's disease by up to 54%.

Men also depend on estrogen for brain function, although they require smaller amounts than women.

What to do: Both men and women should ask their doctors for a saliva-estrogen test. It measures "free" levels of the three different forms of estrogen (estrone, estradiol and estriol). Free estrogen is the form that is active and available for immediate use in the body.

If your estrogen is low, your doctor may prescribe supplemental hormones. I advise patients to use bioidentical hormones that are made from natural substances. They may be more effective—and cause fewer side effects—than synthetic forms of estrogen.

LOW THYROID

People with low levels of thyroid hormone (hypothyroidism) often experience memory loss. Unfortunately, doctors don't routinely test for it. They mistakenly attribute the symptoms—such as memory loss, fatigue, increased sensitivity to cold, apathy or weight gain—to other conditions, including depression.

What to do: Get a thyroid test if you have any of the above symptoms. A diet high in B vitamins (from meats, whole grains and fortified cereals) and vitamin A (from brightly colored produce) can help improve thyroid function. An adequate intake of iodine (iodized salt is a source) also is important.

If your level of thyroid hormones is too low, your doctor probably will prescribe a thyroid replacement, such as *levothyroxine* (Synthroid) or Armour Thyroid.

IMPAIRED CIRCULATION

If you have high cholesterol or other cardiovascular risk factors—you smoke, have high blood pressure, are sedentary, overweight, etc.—you probably have at least some atherosclerosis, fatty plaques in the arteries that reduce the flow of blood and oxygen to the brain.

What to do: In addition to the obvious—more exercise, weight loss, not smoking—I strongly advise patients to eat a Mediterranean-style diet. This features lots of fruits, vegetables and grains along with healthy amounts of olive oil and fish. A recent study found that people who closely followed this diet were 28% less likely to develop mild cognitive impairment and 48% less likely to get Alzheimer's disease.

Also helpful: Eating more soluble fiber (such as that found in oatmeal, beans, fruit and nuts) or taking a fiber supplement has been shown in both men and women to decrease hardening of the arteries and improve circulation.

EXPOSURE TO MERCURY

Americans are exposed to mercury all the time. It is present in soil, the water supply and some foods, including many fish. It also is used in many dental fillings. Over time, the mercury from fillings and other sources can cause inflammation and oxidative stress in the brain, both of which can damage the neurotransmitters that are essential for memory and other brain functions.

What to do: You can get tested for mercury and other heavy metals, but the tests will be positive only after long-term exposure. I advise patients to reduce their exposure long before it will show up on any test.

If you have dental fillings made of amalgam (an alloy of mercury and other metals), consider replacing them with fillings made from plastics or other materials. The work should be done by an environmental dentist who specializes in the safe removal of mercury.

Also important: Avoid eating shark, swordfish, king mackerel, marlin, orange roughy, ahi tuna and tilefish, which tend to accumulate mercury. Limit canned albacore tuna to three servings or less per month and canned light tuna to six servings or less per month.

Best: Cold-water salmon.

6 Herbs That Slow Aging

Donald R. Yance, CN, MH, RH (AHG), clinical master herbalist and certified nutritionist. He is medical director at the Mederi Foundation's Centre for Natural Healing in Ashland, Oregon. He is author of *Adaptogens in Medical Herbalism* (Healing Arts) and *Herbal Medicine, Healing & Cancer* (Keats). *DonnieYance.com*

You can't escape aging. But many Americans are aging prematurely.

Surprising fact: The US ranks 42nd out of 191 countries in life expectancy, according to the Census Bureau and the National Center for Health Statistics.

The leading cause of this rapid, premature aging is chronic stress. Stress is any factor, positive or negative, that requires the body to make a response or change to adapt. It can be psychological stress, including the modern addiction to nonstop stimulation and speed. Or it can be physiological stress—such as eating a highly processed diet...sitting for hours every day...absorbing toxins from food, water and air...and spending time in artificial light.

Chronic stress overwhelms the body's homeostasis, its inborn ability to adapt to stress and stay balanced, strong and healthy. The result?

Your hormonal and immune systems are weakened. Inflammation flares up, damaging cells. Daily energy decreases, fatigue increases and you can't manage life as effectively. You suffer from one or more illnesses, take several medications and find yourself in a downward spiral of worsening health. Even though you might live to be 75 or older, you're surviving, not thriving.

We can reduce stress by making lifestyle changes such as eating better and exercising. You also can help beat stress and slow aging with adaptogens. These powerful herbs balance and strengthen the hormonal and immune systems...give you more energy...and repair cellular damage—thereby boosting your body's ability to adapt to chronic stress.

Important: Adaptogens are generally safe, but always talk with your doctor before taking any supplement.

Omega-3s Help You Live Longer

People over age 65 with the highest blood levels of omega-3 fatty acids were 27% less likely to die of any cause during the study period...40% less likely to die of coronary heart disease...and 45% less likely to die of an arrhythmia than people with the lowest levels of omega-3s. Overall, those with the highest omega-3 levels lived an average of 2.2 years longer than those with the lowest levels.

Study of 2,692 people, average age 74, by researchers at Harvard School of Public Health, Boston, published in *Annals of Internal Medicine.*

Here are six of the most powerful adaptogens...

ASHWAGANDHA

This adaptogen from Ayurveda (the ancient system of natural healing from India) can help with a wide range of conditions.

Main actions: It is energizing and improves sleep, and it can help with arthritis, anxiety, depression, dementia and respiratory disorders, such as asthma, bronchitis and emphysema.

Important benefit: It is uniquely useful for cancer—it can help kill cancer cells...reduce the toxicity of chemotherapy (and prevent resistance to chemotherapeutic drugs)...relieve cancer-caused fatigue...and prevent recurrence.

ELEUTHERO

This is the most well-researched adaptogen (with more than 3,000 published studies). It often is called the "king" of adaptogens. (It was introduced in the US as "Siberian ginseng," but it is not a ginseng.)

Main actions: Along with providing energy and vitality, eleuthero protects the body against the ill effects of any kind of stress, such as extremes of heat or cold, excessive exercise and radiation. More than any other adaptogen, it helps normalize any type of physiological abnormality—including high or low blood pressure...and high or low blood sugar.

Important benefit: Eleuthero is a superb "ergogenic" (performance-enhancing) aid that can help anyone involved in sports improve strength and endurance and recover from injury.

GINSENG

Used as a traditional medicine in Asia for more than 5,000 years and the subject of more than 500 scientific papers, ginseng has two primary species—Panax ginseng (Korean or Asian ginseng) and Panax quinquefolius (American ginseng).

Main actions: Ginseng is antifatigue and antiaging. It increases muscle strength and endurance and improves reaction times. It also strengthens the immune system and the heart and helps regulate blood sugar.

Important benefits: American ginseng can be beneficial for recovering from the common cold, pneumonia or bronchitis (particularly with a dry cough)...and chronic stress accompanied by depression or anxiety.

Korean or Asian ginseng is helpful for increasing physical performance, especially endurance and energy. It is effective for restoring adrenal function and neurological health such as learning and memory.

RHAPONTICUM

This herb contains more anabolic (strengthening and muscle-building) compounds than any other plant. It is my number-one favorite herb for increasing stamina and strength.

Main actions: It normalizes the central nervous and cardiovascular systems...improves sleep, appetite and mood...and increases the ability to work and function under stressful conditions.

Important benefit: This herb is wonderful for anyone recovering from injury, trauma or surgery.

RHODIOLA

Rhodiola has gained popularity over the past few years as studies show that it rivals eleuthero and ginseng as an adaptogen. It is widely used by Russian athletes to increase energy.

Main actions: Rhodiola increases blood supply to the muscles and the brain, enhancing physical and mental performance, including memory. It normalizes the cardiovascular system and protects the heart from stress. It also strengthens immunity.

Red flag: Don't use rhodiola alone—it is extremely astringent and drying. It is best used along with other adaptogens in a formula.

SCHISANDRA

This herb has a long history of use as an adaptogen in China, Russia, Japan, Korea and Tibet. The fruit is commonly used, but the seed is more powerful.

Main actions: Schisandra can treat stress-induced fatigue...protect and detoxify the liver...treat insomnia, depression and vision problems...and enhance athletic performance.

Important benefit: This adaptogen may help night vision—one study showed it improved adaptation to darkness by 90%.

COMBINATIONS ARE BEST

Any one herb has limitations in its healing power. But a combination or formula of adaptogenic herbs overcomes those limitations—because the adaptogens act in concert, making them more powerful.

This concept of synergy—multiple herbs acting together are more effective than one herb acting alone—is key to the effectiveness of the herbal formulas of traditional Chinese medicine (TCM) and Ayurveda. Both these ancient forms of medicine often employ a dozen or more herbs in their formulas.

But it's not only the combination of herbs that makes them effective—it's also the quality of the herbs. There are many more poor-quality adaptogens on the market than high-quality (or even mediocre-quality).

My advice: Look for an herbalist or herbal company that knows all about the source and content of the herbs it uses.

Example: Herbalist & Alchemist, a company that grows most of the herbs used in its products.

Or find a product sold to health practitioners, who then sell it to their patients—this type of product is more likely to be high-quality.

Example: MediHerb, from Standard Process.

Herbal formulas from my company, Natura Health Products, also meet these criteria for high quality.

The Secret Thief of Good Health

Michael J. Grossman, MD, a specialist in antiaging and regenerative medicine. He is medical director of BodyLogicMD of Irvine, California, which focuses on bioidentical hormones, nutritional support and stress reduction. He is author of *The Vitality Connection: Ten Practical Ways to Optimize Health and Reverse the Aging Process* (Vitality). *DrMichaelGrossman.com*

You probably know all about osteoporosis, the gradual, age-related loss of bone.

What you may not know: There also is an age-related loss of muscle mass, strength and function—a condition called sarcopenia. And it is a problem for all of us as we age.

Sarcopenia generally starts at age 40. By the time you're 50, you're losing 1% to 2% of your muscle mass every year. And as you lose muscle, you lose strength.

Example: Starting in your 40s, leg strength typically drops by 10% to 15% per decade until you're 70, after which it declines by 25% to 40% per decade.

But you don't have to become physically debilitated to suffer the devastating effects of muscle loss. When you have less muscle, you have more fat—and fat cells produce inflammatory compounds that drive many deadly chronic diseases, such as heart disease and cancer.

The good news: Starting today, there are many actions you can take to slow, stop and even reverse sarcopenia...

WHAT YOU NEED TO KNOW

When sarcopenia is at its worst—what some experts call pathological sarcopenia—you become weak, walk slowly, fall easily, are less likely to recover from an illness and are more likely to die from any cause. That degree of sarcopenia afflicts 14% of people ages 65 to 75 and 45% of those 85 and older.

Sarcopenia is linked to a 77% increased risk for cardiovascular disease. It's also linked to higher death rates in breast cancer survivors and older people with lymphoma.

With less muscle, you burn less glucose (blood sugar), so it becomes harder to prevent, control or reverse type 2 diabetes, a disease of chronically high blood sugar that can plague your life with complications such as vision loss, nerve pain and kidney failure. Diabetes also doubles your risk for heart attack, stroke and Alzheimer's disease.

Studies also link sarcopenia to triple the risk for osteoporosis, a fourfold increase in post-operative infections and severe menopausal symptoms.

NUTRITION

The right diet and supplements can fight muscle loss...

- **Eat protein-rich food daily.** Increasing the amount of protein in your diet not only can help stop the breakdown of muscle, but it also helps build new muscle.

Scientific evidence: In a three-year study, published in *The American Journal of Clinical Nutrition*, older people who ate the most protein lost 40% less muscle compared with people who ate the least.

My advice: Every day, eat at least four ounces of protein-rich food, such as lean beef, fish, chicken or turkey. A four-ounce serving is about the size of a deck of cards.

Helpful: Whey protein, from milk, is rich in branched-chain amino acids. These three amino acids (leucine, isoleucine and valine) comprise 35% of muscle protein and are uniquely effective in building muscle. Look for a protein powder derived from whey protein, and use at least one scoop daily in a smoothie or shake. You also can get some of these amino acids by eating Greek yogurt, nuts, seeds, cheese and hard-boiled eggs.

- **Take vitamin D.** Vitamin D is widely known to stop bone loss, but it also stops muscle loss.

Scientific evidence: A study published in *Journal of Internal Medicine* linked low blood levels of vitamin D to a four-fold increase in the risk for frailty, a problem of old age that includes pathological sarcopenia.

Vitamin D works to protect muscle by decreasing chronic, low-grade inflammation, which contributes to the breakdown and loss of muscle protein.

Consuming Olive Oil Can Protect Your Skin

According to a recent study, men who consumed more than two teaspoons of olive oil daily showed fewer signs of sun-related aging than men who consumed smaller amounts.

Possible reason: The monounsaturated fatty acids in olive oil may protect the body against damage by free radicals.

Study by researchers at University of Paris and Research Center on Human Skin, founded by Chanel, Neuilly sur Seine, France, published in *PLOS One*.

Annals of Internal Medicine

Unfortunately, an estimated nine out of 10 Americans have suboptimal blood levels of vitamin D, below 30 nanograms per milliliter (ng/ml). A simple blood test can reveal your vitamin D level. Research shows that people with a blood level of 55 ng/ml or higher of vitamin D have 50% less heart disease and cancer than people with a blood level of 20 ng/ml or below. It also reduces the risk of falling by 19%.

My advice: I recommend the same 55 ng/ml level to control muscle loss. To achieve that level, most people need to take a daily vitamin D supplement that supplies 3,000 international units (IU) to 5,000 IU.

- **Take fish oil.** Like vitamin D, fish oil works to protect muscle by reducing the chronic inflammation that damages muscle cells.

Scientific evidence: In a study in *The American Journal of Clinical Nutrition*, women who participated in strength-training and also took fish oil had much stronger muscles after three months than women who did only strength-training.

My advice: To protect and build muscle, I recommend a supplement containing 1,000 milligrams (mg) of omega-3 fatty acids, with 400 mg of EPA and 300 mg of DHA. Take it twice daily.

- **Consider creatine.** Creatine is an amino acid–like compound found mostly in red meat, pork and fish, such as salmon, tuna and herring. More than 70 clinical studies show that regularly taking a creatine supplement can help build muscle and increase strength.

However: The nutrient works to build muscle only if you are exercising—without that regular challenge to the muscles, supplemental creatine has no effect.

My advice: If you're exercising regularly, take three grams of creatine daily.

EXERCISE

Regular exercise is one of the best ways to stop or reverse muscle loss. You need both aerobic exercise and resistance exercise (which stresses the muscles, causing them to get stronger). *My advice...*

- **For aerobics, use your lower and upper body.** Walking is a good exercise, but it builds only lower-body strength. Also include aerobic exercise that uses the lower and upper body, such as tennis, ballroom dancing or working out on an elliptical machine. Try to participate in 30 to 60 minutes of aerobic exercise five or more days a week.
- **For resistance training, work all your muscles.** I recommend resistance exercise three times a week, concentrating on the different muscle groups at each session—chest and triceps...back and biceps...and legs and shoulders. If you don't like weight-lifting, try another form of resistance exercise, such as resistance bands.

Calcium Supplements Reduce Mortality Rates

Contrary to recent research finding that calcium supplements increase risk for heart disease, a more recent study found that women who took up to 1,000 milligrams of calcium a day were 22% less likely to die over a 10-year period than women who didn't take the supplements. Calcium supplements had no statistically significant effect on men.

Study of 9,033 people by researchers from the Canadian Multicentre Osteoporosis Study Research Group, published in *The Journal of Clinical Endocrinology & Metabolism.*

HORMONES

As you age, you lose bone, muscle—and hormones. And many of those hormones, particularly testosterone, are crucial for building muscle in both men and women. (Women manufacture testosterone in the ovaries and adrenal glands.) Estrogen and dehydroepiandrosterone (DHEA) also play a role in creating and maintaining muscle.

My advice: Find a doctor trained in antiaging medicine and bioidentical hormone replacement therapy (BHRT), which uses compounds that are identical to the hormones that your body manufactures rather than synthetics. Ask the doctor to test your hormone levels and determine if BHRT is right for you.

Say "No!" to a Nursing Home

Wendy A. Jordan, a Certified Aging in Place Specialist (CAPS), designated by the National Association of Home Builders. Based in Washington, DC, Ms. Jordan is author of numerous books on residential design and remodeling, including *Universal Design for the Home: Great-Looking, Great-Living Design for All Ages, Abilities, and Circumstances* (Quarry). She also writes for various trade and consumer magazines.

Wouldn't you love to stay in your own home as you get older? Well, thanks to a new trend called "aging in place" (AIP), thousands of aging baby boomers and older people are comfortably, economically and safely remaining at home—avoiding the high cost and upheaval of moving to assisted-living facilities or nursing homes.

What's involved: Homes are now being cost-effectively and stylishly modified for individuals living with vision, balance, mobility or other health concerns. Renovations are done so that the space doesn't feel sterile and the home is functional for anyone, regardless of age or health condition. For example, an able-bodied person can be comfortable in the same environment as a spouse in a wheelchair...and children can spend time at their grandparents' home without ever noticing anything "different" about the space.

Most Americans Don't Want to Live Beyond 100

Of the people recently surveyed, 69% said that they want to live to between the ages of 70 and 100, with the ideal age cited as 90. More than half of those surveyed would not want medical treatment that would extend their lives to 120 years. The current US average life span is 78.7 years.

Survey of 2,012 adults by Pew Research Center, Religion & Public Life Project, Washington, DC.

AIP features include skylights and well-placed task lighting for people with diminished vision...open showers for individuals in wheelchairs...easy-to-turn lever doorknobs and faucets for arthritis sufferers and much more. People needn't wait to renovate until they have retired or been diagnosed with a chronic condition—many home owners are proactively retrofitting their living spaces.

Bonus: AIP saves money. The average cost of a nursing home is currently about $6,700 a month or $80,400 a year. Of course renovations cost money as well, but while some are more involved and costly, many are fairly simple and inexpensive. Plus, making a home more comfortable, functional and safe adds to its resale value, especially when modifications are done stylishly.

Products to check out now...*

• **Better lighting.** Vision inevitably deteriorates with age. Adequate lighting throughout the house helps prevent falls and run-ins with walls, corners and doors. Central ceiling fixtures, wall sconces with translucent shades and skylights are all good choices. Motion-activated lighting is helpful during middle-of-the-night trips to the bathroom. Task lighting in the bathroom, kitchen and reading nooks should be directed from the side, versus overhead, to avoid glare. Rocker light switches are easier to use than traditional flip switches, and when positioned 42 to 48 inches above the floor, they are accessible to everyone, including someone in a wheelchair.

• **Easy-to-reach cabinets and drawers.** Vision difficulties, limited range of motion or the constraints of a wheelchair make it extremely difficult to locate and reach items in the back of a typical pantry, cabinet or drawer. Customized shelving and ready-made inserts (these can be cut to fit a drawer) that easily pull out bring items in the deeper parts of cabinets, drawers and pantries within reach with a minimum of bending and lifting. Pop-up shelves work well for heavy items such as kitchen mixers or blenders—a lift mechanism does all the work.

Check: Rev-A-Shelf.com...ShelfGenie.com.

• **Accessible sinks.** Wheelchair users require ample clearance below sinks (typical sinks might have a vanity or pipes underneath). They also need sinks that are a minimum of 27 to 29 inches and a maximum of 34 inches off the floor so that faucets are within reach. Since standard counter height is 36 inches, the slightly shorter height often works fine for non-wheelchair users.

Rear-mounted pipes, four-legged consoles and wall-mounted sinks are all good alternatives. There are many stylish sinks that meet these requirements. Faucets installed on the side of the sink enhance accessibility, and lever-style handles offer better grip than knobs (the same goes for doorknobs).

• **Elevated toilets.** At 17 to 19 inches high (a few inches higher than a standard toilet), "comfort height" or "chair height" toilets are often more comfortable for anyone to use, regardless of health condition. For people with painful joints or arthritis, they require less bending at the knee, and wheelchair users find them easier to get on and off of. They come in a range of designs, from utilitarian to trendy, and need not cost more than standard-height models.

• **Grab bars.** Used to maintain balance or offer something to grasp in case of a slip, grab bars have traditionally had an institutional look. But today's grab bars come in beautiful finishes,

*Most of these items are widely available at home-improvement and plumbing-supply stores. For proper installation, consult an occupational therapist or Certified Aging in Place Specialist (CAPS)—architects, designers, contractors and health-care consultants with special training in modifying homes for older individuals. To find a CAPS in your area, go to *NAHB.org/directory.*

Best Age Ever

Did you know that 55 is the age most baby boomers (ages 49 to 67) want to be? A survey asked American adults what age they would pick if they could live forever in good health at that age. People ages 68 and older picked age 67.

Survey of 2,252 American adults by Harris Interactive, reported in *Prevention*.

such as brushed nickel and bronze. They can be installed next to the toilet and inside and outside the tub and shower area but also in the kitchen, hallways, entryways and other living spaces.

Note: A towel bar is not the same thing as a grab bar—the latter is designed to be weight bearing and must be anchored into blocking (a secure mount). If they are in the right location, your contractor can attach grab bars to wall studs. Otherwise, a contractor can open the wall and install mounts for grab bars.

- **Open showers.** Wheelchair users need a wide entry and turnaround space in the shower. A flat entry promotes safe access for anyone who has balance, vision or mobility concerns. With no raised threshold to avoid overflow, the floor of the shower should be gently angled toward the drain. To guard against slipping, the floor should have a nonskid surface. Honed-finish ceramic tiles and tiles with nonslip coating are good choices. Small tiles (four inches or smaller) are preferred—the extra grout lines also help prevent skids.

An AIP shower needs a bench or seat...and multiple showerheads (an overhead fixture plus a handheld), ideally with heat-control function to avoid accidental burns. The faucet, handheld showerhead and grab bar should be reachable from the seat. These accessories come in a range of prices and styles and don't take up as much room as you would think.

For people who prefer baths, wide, flat tub ledges provide seating for safe transfer into the tub. And faucets can be offset for easier transition in and out of the tub. Another option is a walk-in tub, with a hinged door for easy, safe entry. Walk-in tubs come in a variety of sizes—compact, standard and oversized. Prices vary widely.

Video Game May Erase Effects of Aging on the Brain

Adam Gazzaley, MD, PhD, associate professor, neurology, physiology and psychiatry, and director, Neuroscience Imaging Center, University of California, San Francisco.

John Krakauer, MD, director, the Brain, Learning, Animation and Movement (BLAM) Lab, Johns Hopkins University School of Medicine, Baltimore.

Nature

A specially designed video game may help sharpen mental skills that fade with age, a recent study shows.

The study, which was published in the journal *Nature*, tested a video game that was created by brain scientists and dubbed NeuroRacer.

The game requires players to multitask, rapidly switching attention between multiple tasks, back and forth, so that various duties are accomplished in tandem.

People had to keep a car centered in its lane and moving at a certain speed while they also tried to quickly and correctly identify signs that flashed onto the screen, distracting them from their driving.

In a series of related experiments, researchers from the University of California, San Francisco, showed that the ability to multitask suffers with age. But healthy seniors who regularly played the game were able to turn back the clock. After a month of practice, they were able to multitask even more effectively, on average, than younger adults.

"It would be a medical diagnostic and therapeutic, potentially even going the route of FDA approval," said Adam Gazzaley, MD, PhD, director of the Neuroscience Imaging Center at the University of California, San Francisco. Dr. Gazzaley is a cofounder of the company that is developing the next generation of the video game. The study was funded by Health Games Research, a program of the Robert Wood Johnson Foundation and the U.S. National Institute on Aging.

STUDY DETAILS

For the research, scientists recruited 174 healthy adults aged 20 to 80. About 30 people from each decade of life were asked to play the NeuroRacer game to see how well they were able to multitask. These first tests showed that the ability to multitask gets worse with age. Adults in their 20s saw a 28% drop in performance when they were doing two things at once, while those in their 30s saw their performance drop about 39%.

Next, they wanted to see whether people could get better at multitasking with practice. For these experiments, they picked 46 healthy seniors who were between the ages of 60 and 85 and assigned them to one of three groups: 16 were asked to play the NeuroRacer game for an hour a day three times a week, 15 played a version of the game that required them to do only a single task at a time and 15 others didn't play the game at all.

After a month, seniors who had practiced multitasking with NeuroRacer showed big gains compared to their peers in the other two groups.

The drop in performance that everyone experiences when they try to do two things at once "improved dramatically from 65% to 16%, and even reached a level better than 20-year-olds," who had only played the game once, Dr. Gazzaley said.

What's more, seniors who played for an hour a day three days a week saw improvements in other mental skills that weren't directly trained by the game. Working memory, or "the ability to hold information in mind, as people do when they're participating in a conversation and they have to think about what they want to say and remember it while they wait their turn to speak" got better, Dr. Gazzaley said, as did their visual attention (the ability to sustain focus on a task in a boring environment).

Additional tests, which measured the brain's electrical activity, showed a boost in areas responsible for cognitive control, the skill that helps the brain switch back and forth between activities.

The improvements in mental function lasted for about six months after seniors stopped playing, the researchers said.

IMPLICATIONS

The study suggests that the value of video games might extend beyond entertainment. Experts say video games may not only stave off the mental deficits that come with age, but could also help in the diagnosis and treatment of mental problems.

The study was conducted in healthy adults who were able to think and remember normally for their age. But researchers have already begun to test NeuroRacer to see if it might benefit people with ADHD or depression, two conditions that hamper the ability to pay attention and stay on task.

They said they're also developing four other games that will challenge different mental skills.

These games aren't likely to be sold in stores, but if further testing proves them to be valuable, researchers think they may one day make their way to doctors' offices.

EXPERTS COMMENT

What remains to be seen, experts said, is whether these improvements will help people in real life.

"I think people are soon going to use video games to collect data and to train [the brain]," said John Krakauer, MD, director of the Brain, Learning, Animation and Movement Lab at Johns Hopkins University School of Medicine in Baltimore. "I think it's very promising. I think it's going to happen."

"They could argue that if you got better at this game then maybe you would be a safer driver when you're elderly," Dr. Krakauer said. "You

Best Season for Longevity

A recent study of centenarians born in the 1800s found that people born in September, October or November were more likely to live to be 100 years old than people born in other months.

Study of 1,574 people who were born in the US between 1800 and 1895 who lived to be 100 or older by researchers at University of Chicago, published in *Journal of Aging Research.*

may be able to look for what exit you need to take and stick to the road."

"[But] they haven't tested that," he said. "We don't know the answer to that."

The researchers agreed.

"In order to see improvement in daily life, you need larger numbers of people" who are studied for a longer period of time, Dr. Gazzaley said. Planning for those studies is currently in the works.

info For more ways to prevent aging, visit the U.S. National Institute on Aging website at *http://www.nia.nih.gov/health/publication/can-we-prevent-aging.*

Is the Way You Walk Giving You a Warning?

Mary Harward, MD, a geriatrician in private practice in Orange, California. She specializes in the diagnosis and treatment of gait disorders and other diseases affecting older adults. She is editor of *Medical Secrets* (fifth edition, Mosby Elsevier).

Have you surprised yourself recently with a stumble or a fall? If you blamed it on your shoes...your eyesight...or an obstacle, such as a throw rug, you may not be getting at the root cause of why you stumbled or fell. The fact is, the real reason many people fall (and sometimes die from it) is the way that they walk.

A problem that goes undetected: Most people who have treatable abnormalities in their gait (the way in which a person walks) never even discuss it with their doctors.

Here's why: When you go to the doctor, odds are that you are taken to an exam room and asked to "have a seat" until the doctor arrives. The problem is, you'll probably stay seated during the entire visit, and your doctor may miss a symptom—a dangerous gait—that's just as important as abnormal X-rays or blood tests.

TAKE IT SERIOUSLY

It's never normal to shuffle, be off-balance or have an unusual posture. A gait disorder always means that something—or, in most cases, a combination of factors—is awry.

Problems with gait affect about 15% of adults age 60 and older and more than 80% of those age 85 and older. Gait disorders, which interfere with stability and balance, are not only among the most common causes of falls and subsequent hospitalizations, but also can be one of the first health problems that eventually leads to nursing home care.

My advice: Doctors should ask every patient if he/she has fallen in the last year. In addition, if you're age 65 or older, you should ask your doctor to check your gait at least once a year.

WHAT'S BEHIND IT?

Patients often assume that problems with one's gait are due to neurological disorders, such as Parkinson's disease or multiple sclerosis (MS). With Parkinson's disease, patients also experience a resting tremor or shaking of one hand, muscle rigidity and slow movements, while MS typically is accompanied by vision problems, dizziness and trouble speaking. *But there are other possible causes of gait problems...*

- **Arthritis.** Gait problems are common in patients with arthritis, particularly osteoarthritis of the knee or hip. If you have knee or hip pain, you may favor that side and use other muscles to compensate. This throws off your posture and body mechanics, which may cause you to limp or take tentative steps.

Helpful: Ask your doctor if it's appropriate to see a physical therapist for advice on exercises to strengthen the muscles around the arthritic joint—this will help you walk normally and with less pain.

Pain control is also very important. Apart from making you more comfortable, it will help you do the exercises that you need for a better gait. If you don't get adequate relief from over-the-counter pain relievers, talk to your doctor about stronger forms of pain control. Stretching, massage, heating pads, cold packs and/or acupuncture are helpful to some people.

- **Back problems.** A gait problem often is due to a painful back. Patients with lumbar stenosis, for example, will frequently experience nerve pressure from damaged vertebrae in the spine, affecting their ability to walk. Patients with sciatica (nerve pain that often accompanies lower-back problems) will have difficulty walking or standing. Suspect nerve problems if you have back or leg pain that gets worse when you walk or stand for more than a few minutes and gets better when you're off your feet. See your doctor for treatment advice.

•**Balance disorders.** If you sometimes feel as though you're about to fall (even when you're not), see a doctor right away. Problems with balance—often accompanied by dizziness, spinning sensations, etc.—are a major cause of falls. Potential causes include ear infections, inner-ear disorders, neuropathy (nerve damage) and circulatory problems.

Also: Ask your doctor to test your vitamin B-12 level. Older adults often have low levels of intrinsic factor, a protein that's needed for B-12 absorption. It's also common for vegetarians to be deficient in this vitamin because meat is a major source of B-12. Low B-12 can make you feel light-headed, cause numbness and/or tingling in the feet and make it difficult to walk.

Similar foot and leg symptoms are caused by diabetic neuropathy, nerve damage that may occur in patients with poorly managed (or undiagnosed) diabetes. Bunions and other foot conditions also can contribute to gait disorders.

•**Drug side effects.** It's not surprising that sedating medications such as *diazepam* (Valium) can increase fall risk. What many people don't realize is that nonsedating medications also can be an issue.

Example: Medications that lower blood pressure, such as diuretics, can cause orthostatic hypotension, a sudden drop in blood pressure that can make you dizzy or light-headed. Some blood pressure drugs also decrease magnesium, which can cause leg weakness or cramps. Your doctor might advise changing medications. Alcohol or drugs that lower blood sugar or affect mood or sleep also can change one's gait.

Important: Be especially careful after eating. Studies have shown that dizziness and gait problems tend to get worse about 30 minutes after meals—blood travels to the digestive tract after meals, sometimes lowering blood pressure.

•**Reduced brain circulation.** Gait disorders are often the first sign of infarcts, areas of brain damage caused by impaired circulation. Infarcts occur in patients who have had a stroke or other problems that affect blood vessels in the brain, such as hypertension or high cholesterol.

A patient who has multiple infarcts might walk very slowly...take short steps...stand with his feet wider apart than usual...and/or hesitate when starting to walk or have trouble slowing momentum when stopping.

HOW'S YOUR GAIT?

If you've noticed changes in the ways in which you move, see your doctor for an evaluation. *He/she will give you tests that may include...*

•**The timed get-up-and-go test.** This measures the time it takes you to get up from a chair (without using your hands to push off from the armrests), walk 10 feet, turn around and walk back to the chair. You should be able to complete the sequence safely in 14 seconds or less. If it takes longer than 20 seconds, your gait is seriously impaired.

How to Fall Down Without Getting Hurt—Tricks from a Stuntman

Hal Needham, a stuntman who appeared in more than 4,000 television episodes and more than 300 feature films. He also directed movies including *The Cannonball Run*. In 2012, he became only the second stunt performer to receive an honorary Oscar for his work. He is author of *Stuntman! My Car-Crashing, Plane-Jumping, Bone-Breaking, Death-Defying Hollywood Life* (Little, Brown).

When we fall, our natural instinct is to reach out for the ground with our hands. Unfortunately, that only increases our odds of injury—our hands, wrists and arms are

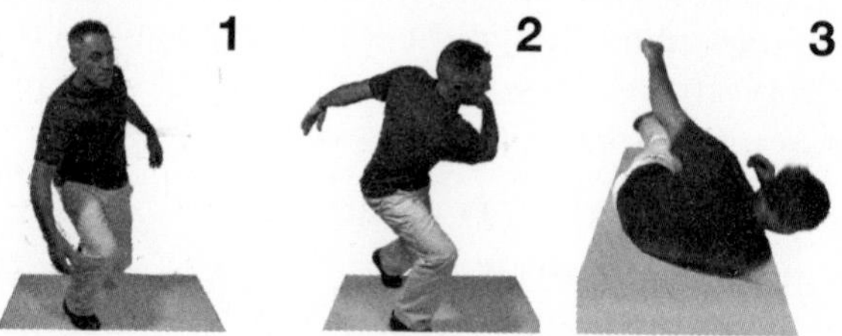

full of small bones that are easily broken. *Instead, when you realize you are falling...*

1. Buckle your knees. This can in essence lower the height that your upper body falls by as much as a foot or two, significantly reducing the impact when you hit the ground. In a forward fall, it might result in bruised knees, but that's better than a broken bone in the upper body.

Helpful: In a backward fall, tuck your head into your chest as you buckle your knees—try to turn yourself into a ball.

2. Throw one arm across your chest whether you're falling forward or backward. Do this with enough force that it turns your body to one side. It doesn't matter which arm you use.

3. Rotate the rest of your body in the direction that you threw your arm, increasing your spin. If you can rotate enough, you can come down mainly on your backside, a well-padded part of the body unlikely to experience a serious injury.

Trouble is, while stuntmen know exactly when and where they're going to fall, real-world falls usually take people by surprise. It can be difficult to overcome instinct and put this falling strategy into action in the split second before hitting the ground.

Practice can help. If you have access to a thick gym mat and you don't have health issues that make it risky, try out this falling technique until it feels natural.

Strengthen Your Feet for Better Balance

Without shoes, move your foot in circles, first one way and then the other, then side to side, moving only your foot and ankle, not your leg. Do toe curls—flex toes as much as possible and then uncurl them. With your foot flat on the floor, lift your big toe without lifting the other toes, then try lifting the others without lifting the big toe. Use your feet to pick up items such as marbles or pencils. Spread your toes apart like a fan. Roll a small rubber ball or golf ball under the sole of your foot to massage it.

UC Berkeley Wellness Letter. BerkeleyWellness.com

Don't Let Your Bladder Run Your Life!

Holly Lucille, ND, RN, a naturopathic doctor based in West Hollywood, California. She is author of *Creating and Maintaining Balance: A Woman's Guide to Safe, Natural Hormone Health* (Impakt Health) and serves on the Institute for Natural Medicine Board of Directors. *DrHollyLucille.com*

Women and men who scout out restrooms wherever they are may think that others don't have to worry so much about their bladders. But that's not true.

Eye-opening statistic: One in every five adults over age 40 has overactive bladder...and after the age of 65, a whopping one in every three adults is affected. If you regularly have a strong and sudden urge to urinate and/or need to hit the john eight or more times a day (or more than once at night), chances are you have the condition, too.

Men with prostate enlargement and postmenopausal women (due to their low estrogen levels) are at increased risk of having overactive bladder. Urinary tract infections, use of certain medications (such as antidepressants and drugs to treat high blood pressure and insomnia) and even constipation also can cause or worsen the condition.

But there is a bright side. Research is now uncovering several surprisingly simple natural approaches that are highly effective for many people with overactive bladder. *Among the best...**

START WITH YOUR DIET

Most people don't connect a bladder problem to their diets. But there is a strong link. *My advice...*

• **Take a hard line with irritants.** Alcohol, caffeine and artificial sweeteners can exacerbate the feeling of urgency caused by overactive

*Talk to your doctor before trying any of these herbal remedies, especially if you take medication or have a chronic health condition. You may want to consult a naturopathic doctor. To find one near you, check *Naturopathic.org.*

bladder. Cutting back on these items is a good first step, but they often creep back into one's diet over time.

What helps: Keep it simple—completely avoid alcohol, caffeine (all forms, including coffee, tea and caffeine-containing foods such as chocolate) and artificial sweeteners. Stick to decaffeinated herbal teas and coffee, and use agave and stevia as sweeteners.

Many individuals also are sensitive to certain foods, such as corn, wheat, dairy, eggs and peanuts. They often trigger an immune reaction that contributes to overall inflammation in the body, including in the bladder. If your symptoms of urinary urgency and/or frequency increase after eating one of these (or any other) foods, your body may be having an inflammatory response that is also affecting your bladder. Eliminate these foods from your diet.

•**Keep your gut healthy.** The scientific evidence is still in the early stages, but research now suggests that leaky gut syndrome, in which excess bacterial or fungal growth harms the mucosal membrane in the intestines, is at the root of several health problems, including overactive bladder.

The theory is that an imbalance of microbes, a condition known as dysbiosis, can irritate the walls of the bladder just as it does in the gut.

What helps: Probiotics and oregano oil capsules. Probiotics replenish "good" bacteria, and oregano oil has antibacterial properties that help cleanse "bad" bacteria and fungi from the gut.

•**Drink up!** People with overactive bladder often cut way back on their fluid intake because they already make so many trips to the bathroom. But when you don't drink enough fluids, urine tends to have an irritating effect because it becomes more concentrated. This increases urgency.

What helps: Drink half your body weight in ounces of water or herbal tea daily. Do not drink any fluids after 5 pm to help prevent bathroom runs during the night.

THE RIGHT SUPPLEMENTS

Cranberry supplements (or unsweetened cranberry juice) can be helpful for bladder infections, but they're usually not the best choice for overactive bladder. *My advice...*

•**Try pumpkin seed extract.** These capsules help tone and strengthen the tissue of your pelvic-floor muscles, which gives you better bladder control.

Typical dosage: 500 mg daily.

•**Consider Angelica archangelica extract.** This herb has gotten positive reviews from researchers who have investigated it as a therapy for overactive bladder.

Recent finding: When 43 men with overactive bladder took 300 mg of the herb daily, they had increased bladder capacity and made fewer trips to the bathroom.

Typical dosage: 100 mg daily.

OTHER WAYS TO KEEP YOUR BLADDER HEALTHY

•**Kegel exercises,** which help strengthen the pelvic-floor muscles, are essential for getting control of overactive bladder symptoms. Unfortunately, most people who try doing Kegels end up doing them the wrong way.

How to do Kegels: Three to five times a day, contract your pelvic-floor muscles (the ones you use to stop and start the flow of urine), hold for a count of 10, then relax completely for a count of 10. Repeat 10 times. If you're a woman and aren't sure if you're contracting the right muscles, there is a possible solution.

New option for women: A medical device called Apex acts as an automatic Kegel exerciser. It is inserted into the vagina and electrically stimulates the correct muscles ($299 at PourMoi.com—cost may be covered by some insurance plans). Check with your doctor to see if this would be an appropriate aid for you.

Even though there's no handy device to help men do Kegels, the exercises usually reduce urgency when they're performed regularly.

Kegels can easily be part of anyone's daily routine—do them while waiting at a red light, after going to the bathroom or while watching TV.

•**Try acupuncture.** An increasing body of evidence shows that this therapy helps relieve overactive bladder symptoms. For example, in a study of 74 women with the condition, bladder capacity, urgency and frequency of urination significantly improved after four weekly bladder-specific acupuncture sessions.

•**Go for biofeedback.** Small electrodes are used to monitor the muscles involved in bladder control so that an individualized exercise program can be created. Biofeedback is noninvasive and is most effective when used along with other treatments. To find a board-certified provider, consult the Biofeedback Certification International Alliance, *BCIA.org*.

Hearing Loss Is Linked to Memory Loss

Older adults with even mild-to-moderate hearing loss may experience a decline in brain function up to 41% faster—or three years sooner—than those who have not become hearing impaired.

Reasons: When people are faced with hearing loss, the brain works harder to process sounds rather than dedicating energy to memory and thinking. And the social isolation that occurs among people with poor hearing may result in cognitive decline.

Study of 1,984 people, ages 75 to 84, by researchers at The Johns Hopkins University School of Medicine, Baltimore, published in *JAMA Internal Medicine*.

Keep Your Bladder Healthy

Jamison Starbuck, ND, a naturopathic physician in family practice and a guest lecturer at the University of Montana, both in Missoula. She is past president of the American Association of Naturopathic Physicians and a contributing editor to *The Alternative Advisor: The Complete Guide to Natural Therapies and Alternative Treatments.*

If you're age 50 or older and haven't had a bladder infection, count yourself lucky. The reality is that these infections are among the most common complaints of the AARP crowd.

Here's why: With age, women—and men—are at increased risk because tissues in the bladder weaken, making it more difficult for it to fully empty...so bacteria have more time to proliferate and cause a urinary tract infection (UTI). As we age, our immune systems also don't work as well.

Interestingly, the symptoms of bladder infection become less apparent with age. Instead of the burning, cramping pain and bloody urine that generally accompany a UTI in younger people, only a modest increase in urinary frequency and a dark urine color may indicate a bladder infection once you're middle-aged or older. After about age 70, confusion, agitation, balance problems and falling may be a physician's only clues of a bladder infection.

Fortunately, there are some highly effective natural approaches to help prevent UTIs. *My favorite UTI-fighting strategies...*

•**Stay hydrated.** You must drink a minimum of two quarts of plain water daily—no matter what other beverages you consume. If you take a prescription medication, you may need even more water. Diuretics and some other drugs will make you lose water, so you'll need to drink more than usual. Discuss this with your pharmacist.

•**Use good hygiene.** OK, you might find this is a little embarrassing, but make sure that you wipe from front to back after a bowel movement...wash your genitals before and after sex...and change your undergarments regularly, particularly if you have incontinence or are sedentary (small amounts of stool on a person's underwear can increase infection risk).

•**Load up on cranberry.** Everyone knows that cranberry is supposed to be good for the bladder, but recent research made some people doubt its effectiveness. One study found that cranberry may not be very effective at preventing UTIs. But don't write off cranberry. The same research showed that compounds in cranberry do prevent infections by making it difficult for bacteria to stick to the walls of the bladder. Because most brands of cranberry juice (perhaps the most convenient form of the fruit) have added sugar to make them less tart, I usually advise people who develop more than one bladder infection a year to take 600 mg of a freeze-dried cranberry extract daily.

Caution: People with a history of calcium oxalate kidney stones or who take *warfarin* (Coumadin) or regularly use aspirin should avoid cranberry—it can increase stone risk and interact with these medications.

• **Get more probiotics.** The beneficial bacteria found in yogurt and other cultured foods, such as kefir and miso, reduce risk for bladder infection. Eat one cup of plain yogurt, kefir or miso soup daily or take a probiotic supplement.

• **Do Kegel exercises.** Women—and men—listen up! Strong pelvic muscles allow for more complete bladder emptying and reduce infection risk.

What to do: At least once daily, contract and release the muscles of your pelvic floor (the ones that stop urine flow) 10 times while seated or standing.

Don't Feel Ready for a Hearing Aid?

Barbara E. Weinstein, PhD, a professor of audiology and head of the Audiology Program at The City University of New York Graduate Center, where she specializes in hearing loss in older adults, hearing screening, disability assessment and evidence-based practice. She is author of the textbook *Geriatric Audiology* (Thieme).

If you are reluctant (or can't afford) to use a hearing aid, there are dozens of personal sound amplification products (PSAPs), over-the-counter devices that can help you hear a little better but don't cost as much as hearing aids, which run up to $3,000 each.

NOT QUITE A HEARING AID

Hearing aids are recommended for those who have been diagnosed with hearing loss by an audiologist. PSAPs, which come in many shapes and sizes, often resembling a Bluetooth headset, are meant to amplify sounds in situations where hearing is difficult, such as large gatherings or noisy restaurants.

In reality, it's not an either-or choice. Only 20% to 25% of people who could benefit from a hearing aid actually use one. PSAPs, with their lower price and availability on the Internet, in pharmacies and in stores such as RadioShack, can serve as "training wheels" for people who want to hear better but hesitate to shell out big bucks for a hearing aid.

Important: The hearing aids sold by audiologists are approved by the FDA as medical devices and must meet certain standards related, for example, to frequency ranges and distortion. PSAPs, on the other hand, are classified as electronic products. They aren't subject to FDA review, so you can't assume that they'll work for you. However, some PSAPs already rival the quality of "official" hearing aids and will keep getting better as technology improves.

KNOW WHAT YOU NEED

Before you look into PSAPs, get tested by an audiologist. About 14% of adults in their 50s, one-quarter in their 60s and more than one-third of those age 65 and older have some degree of age-related hearing loss. But do not assume that your hearing is normal—or that hearing loss is inevitable.

You may think that your hearing is becoming impaired because of your age when, in fact, it may be due to a medical issue, such as infection, abnormal bone growth, an inner-ear tumor or even earwax—all of which can be treated and sometimes reversed.

If your hearing loss is not related to a medical issue, a PSAP may be appropriate in the following situations...

• **You have trouble hearing the TV.** It is a common complaint but fairly easy to overcome. Inexpensive earbuds or a headset that merely amplifies the sound may be all that you need. Some products are wireless or have long cords that plug directly into the TV.

• **You have trouble hearing in quiet environments.** Speech can sound muffled or be entirely unintelligible if you have age-related hearing loss. Even if you can easily hear

Hope for Hearing Loss

According to a recent finding, loud noises damage nerve and hair cells in the inner ear, not the cochlea itself. Early treatments could reduce further damage.

Stanford University School of Medicine

background sounds (such as music), you might struggle with the high-frequency sounds that are characteristic of speech.

If you plan to use a PSAP mainly at home or in other quiet settings (such as a museum or a hushed restaurant), look for a device that amplifies high frequencies more than low ones. You'll hear voices more clearly without being overwhelmed by the volume of sounds.

Warning: Some inexpensive products boost both high and low frequencies indiscriminately—avoid them. Your best choice will be a product that allows you to make adjustments and fine-tune it in different settings.

- **You have trouble hearing in noisy environments.** Even mild hearing loss can make it hard to hear voices over the din of clattering plates, a chattering crowd and background music. A simple amplifier won't work because it will make all of the sounds louder.

Better: A device that amplifies the sounds you want to hear while filtering out the rest. Look for a PSAP that has a directional microphone that will pick up speech while muting noise...noise cancellation to filter out low-frequency background sounds...volume control...and multiple channels that are suitable for different sound environments.

- **You're on the fence.** It's common for people to put off getting a hearing aid because of embarrassment or cost. (Hearing aids aren't covered by Medicare or most insurance plans.) You might be telling yourself, "Maybe I'll get one when I'm a lot older."

Important: Don't wait too long. The parts of the brain associated with hearing become less active when they aren't used. You need to hear sounds to keep this brain circuitry working and actively processing speech.

You might want to use a PSAP while you're making up your mind about hearing aids. Even if you get a PSAP that just boosts volume, it will keep the brain signals firing. In my opinion, it's reasonable to use one of these devices for a few months or even a few years. You can always buy a hearing aid later.

GREAT PSAP MODELS

Personal sound-amplification products you may want to consider...

- **For TV listening.** Sennheiser Wireless RS Headphones look like old-fashioned stereo headsets, but they let you turn up the sound. $100 to $600, Sennheiser.com.

- **For more volume in loud environments.** Able Planet Personal Sound 2500 AMP is packed with high-end electronics to reduce background noise while amplifying sounds you want to hear (such as voices). $900 a pair, $500 for one, HearingHealth.AblePlanet.com.

- **For more volume in both loud and quiet places.** The Bean Quiet Sound Amplifier by Etymotic provides amplification of soft speech without distorting sounds. $700 a pair, $375 for one, QSABean.com.

- **For more volume at a low cost.** Dozens of affordable products mainly increase volume without other features.

Example: Sonic SE4000X SuperEar Personal Sound Amplifier, a handheld amplifier you can attach to a pocket, belt, hat or purse strap. About $40, SonicTechnology.com.

All of the PSAP manufacturers listed here offer a money-back guarantee if the product is returned within 30 days.

The Dry-Eye Epidemic—Remedies That Really Work

Robert Latkany, MD, ophthalmologist and founder and director of the Dry Eye Clinic at The New York Eye and Ear Infirmary and the Dry Eye Center at Physician Eyecare of NY, both in New York City. He is actively involved in dry-eye research and author of *The Dry Eye Remedy: The Complete Guide to Restoring the Health and Beauty of Your Eyes* (Hatherleigh). *DryEyeDoctor.com*

It's an epidemic—as many as 25 million Americans are suffering from dry-eye syndrome. They're complaining to their doctors of irritated and burning eyes. In fact, it's the second-most-common eye complaint after vision problems.

One reason dry eyes are so common is that the mucous membranes that produce a key component of tears get drier as we age. About one-third of adults ages 65 and older suffer from dry eyes.

Another key factor is that electronics aren't kind to eyes. If you spend a good part of your day in front of a computer or squinting at your smartphone or watching TV, you "forget" to blink. Your blink rate, as well as how completely you blink, affects eye moisture.

That's because tears consist of oil as well as water. The oil is squeezed from the meibomian glands in the upper and lower eyelids when you blink. It allows tears to cling to the surfaces of the eyes and also slows their evaporation. If you aren't blinking enough and, as a result, secreting little or no oil, the tears evaporate quickly. This condition, known as evaporative dry eye, is the most common cause of dryness.

Other conditions that can lead to eye dryness include medication side effects (from some antihistamines and antidepressants, for example) ...autoimmune diseases, such as Sjögren's syndrome, lupus and rheumatoid arthritis...and vision-correcting surgery (such as LASIK). Diabetes, too, can contribute to eye dryness by causing a decreased sensation of dryness, thus reducing your blink rate.

Before recommending a treatment, your doctor will want to know why your eyes are dry. Once the underlying cause—for example, medication use, autoimmune disease or diabetes—is identified and treated, the dryness may start to improve.

But even if medication use or a chronic illness is not to blame, you don't have to suffer from dry eye. There are steps you can take to relieve the discomfort...

WHAT YOU CAN DO

If your symptoms are mild, the following steps that you can take on your own may be enough to relieve dry eye. *If your symptoms are more severe, these steps can augment other treatments (see below) that your doctor may suggest...*

- **Blink better.** People normally blink between six and 15 times a minute. (You blink less when you're reading or concentrating and more when your eyes are relaxed.)

If you watch a lot of TV or use a computer for more than an hour at a time, your eyes probably are drier than they should be. This also happens to long-distance drivers (such as truckers) or people who stare at anything for long periods of time.

Important: Remind yourself to blink even when you don't feel that you need to.

Also helpful: Take a "blink break" at least twice an hour. Shut your eyes for 10 seconds, and move your eyeballs under the closed lids to bathe and lubricate them.

- **Try omega-3 fatty acids.** These healthful fats, found in walnuts, flaxseed oil and fish, can help reduce gland inflammation and improve the quality of your tears. Fish-oil supplements—a typical dose is 1,000 milligrams (mg) daily—aren't a replacement for other treatments, but they can slightly improve dryness.

Oily, cold-water fish, such as tuna and salmon, may be even better. A study at Harvard's Brigham and Women's Hospital found that patients who ate tuna five to six times a week had a 68% reduced risk of developing dry eye, compared with those who had only one serving a week.

- **Use warm compresses to unclog tear glands.** Use them two to four times a day for five minutes at a time.

- **Try artificial tears.** Sold over the counter, products such as Blink and TheraTears are very helpful for short-term relief. They work quickly and are soothing, particularly if you keep them chilled in the refrigerator. The liquid drops are mainly used for mild cases of dryness. Gel-containing drops are recommended for more severe dryness. If you use drops more than three or four times a day, get a product without preservatives, which can cause some discomfort.

- **Avoid foods high in omega-6 fatty acids,** such as margarine, mayonnaise and oils made from corn and soybeans. Also, reduce the salt in your diet and avoid alcohol.

DOCTOR HELP

If the steps above don't help you, see your ophthalmologist. *He/she may recommend the following...*

•**Restasis** (cyclosporine ophthalmic emulsion) is the only FDA-approved medication for increasing tear production. This prescription eyedrop reduces inflammation and helps prevent blockages in the tear-secreting ducts. It's a good choice for dryness that's caused by vision-correcting surgery, cataract surgery or postmenopausal declines in estrogen, among other conditions.

•**Punctal plugs.** After tears wash across the eyeballs, they drain into small openings. These tear duct openings, or puncta, are located on the inner corners of the eyelids. Their job is to divert "used" tears into nasal cavities and from there to the back of the throat. Your doctor might recommend that you block these openings to keep more of your tears in your eyes.

It's a simple office procedure that takes less than an hour. Your doctor might recommend that you start with temporary plugs. Made from collagen, they last about three months and then dissolve. If you're satisfied with the improvement, you can get another set of temporary plugs.

Another option: Permanent punctal plugs. If you get nondissolvable, silicone plugs, you won't have to replace them. However, they stick out a little more than temporary plugs. You might not see them, but you will feel them with your finger when you touch the eye.

•**Gland expression.** Blockages in the oil-producing meibomian glands will decrease the quality of your tears and lead to dryness. You can express (empty) the glands by using a cotton-tipped swab to push the lower edges of the eyelids against the eyeballs. It's like popping a pimple. The pressure pushes the oil out. Don't try this unless your doctor shows you how—you don't want to injure your eye.

You might have to do this every day—preferably after a shower, when heat and steam have softened the accumulated oil.

If you are considering vision-correcting surgery: Millions of Americans have had LASIK, one of the less expensive forms of vision-correcting surgery. It is a generally safe procedure, but it can reduce the frequency of your blinks for several years. In the meantime, many patients will have dry eyes as a side effect.

Ask your doctor about other forms of corrective surgery, such as PRK or LASEK. They are less likely to cause blink problems, so you have less chance of developing dry eye.

Cataract Fix Extends Life

In a study of more than 350 people with cataracts, those who had cataract surgery were 40% less likely to die from any cause within a 15-year period than those whose cataracts went untreated.

Possible explanation: The better eyesight that results from cataract surgery can increase a person's optimism and motivation to pursue a healthy lifestyle.

Jie Jin Wang, PhD, senior research fellow, Westmead Millennium Institute, The University of Sydney, Australia.

Beware of Eye Floaters

Adam Wenick, MD, PhD, assistant professor of ophthalmology in the Retina Division at the Wilmer Eye Institute at The Johns Hopkins School of Medicine in Baltimore. He is board-certified by the American Board of Ophthalmology, with special expertise in retinal tears and detachment as well as other diseases of the retina.

If you have ever noticed a few tiny dots, blobs, squiggly lines or cobweb-like images drifting across your field of vision, you are not alone. These visual disturbances, called floaters, are common, and most people simply dismiss them as a normal part of growing older. But that's not always the case.

When it could be serious: In about 15% of cases, floaters are a symptom of a harmful condition known as a retinal tear, which can, in turn, lead to a vision-robbing retinal detachment in a matter of hours to days.

HOW DOES THIS HAPPEN?

The retina, which is an extremely thin, delicate membrane that lines the inside of the back of the eye, converts light into signals that your brain recognizes as images. However, with age, a jelly-like material called the vitreous that fills much of the eyeball commonly shrinks a bit and separates from the retina. If the shrinkage

or some other injury exerts enough force, the retina can actually tear.

You might notice a sudden shower of new floaters or flashes of light that look like shooting stars or lightning bolts. What you're seeing when this occurs are actually shadows that are being cast on the retina by the tiny clumps of collagen fibers that comprise the floaters. The flashes of light are caused by the tugging of the vitreous on the retina, which stimulates the photoreceptors that sense light.

Why floaters and/or flashes are a red flag: The retina lacks nerves that signal pain, so these visual disturbances are the only way you will be alerted to a tear. Left untreated, fluid can leak through the retinal tear, and the retina can detach like wallpaper peeling off a wall. A retinal detachment is an emergency—if it's not treated promptly, it can lead to a complete loss of vision in the affected eye.

ARE YOU AT RISK?

Changes in the eye that increase risk for a retinal tear or detachment begin primarily in your 50s and 60s—and continue to increase as you grow older.

In addition to age, you can also be at increased risk for a retinal tear or detachment due to...

• **Nearsightedness.** People of any age with nearsightedness greater than six diopters (requiring eyeglasses or contact lenses with a vision correction of more than minus six) are five to six times more likely to develop a retinal tear or detachment. That's because nearsighted eyeballs are larger than normal. Therefore, the retina is spread thinner, making it more prone to tearing.

Important: If you're nearsighted, don't assume that corrective eyewear or LASIK surgery decreases your risk for a retinal tear or detachment. Neither does.

• **Cataract surgery.** This surgery alters the vitreous jelly, increasing the risk that the vitreous will pull away from the retina, possibly giving way to a retinal detachment.

Cataract surgery has been known to double one's detachment risk, but a recent Australian study suggests that improvements in technology, such as phacoemulsification, which uses an ultrasonic device to break up and remove the cloudy lens, have cut the risk from one in 100 to one in 400.

• **Diabetes.** Because it impairs circulation to the retina over time, diabetes leads to a higher risk for a severe type of retinal detachment that is not associated with floaters and flashes and can be initially asymptomatic.

Individuals who have diabetes should be sure to have annual eye exams with dilation of the pupils to check for this and other ocular complications of diabetes. The Optomap test provides a wide view of the retina, but you also need pupil dilation for a thorough screening.

THE DANGER OF A RETINAL TEAR

Anyone who experiences a sudden burst of floaters or flashes, especially if they are large or appear in any way different from how they have in the past, should contact an ophthalmologist right away for advice.

If an eye exam confirms a retinal tear, it can be treated in an eye doctor's office, using either lasers or freezing equipment to "spot-weld" the area surrounding the tear. (Anesthetic eyedrops are used to numb the eye, but the procedure can still be uncomfortable.)

The resulting scar tissue will seal off the tear so the fluid doesn't leak behind the retina and pull it away. The good news is that both laser photocoagulation and freezing are more than 90% effective in preventing detachment. There is a small risk for tiny blind spots.

WHEN A DETACHMENT OCCURS

If you suffer a retinal tear but don't get treatment within a day or two, the fluid can seep through the tear, detaching the retina.

Red flag for detachment: A gradual shading in your vision, like a curtain being drawn on the sides or top or bottom of your eye, means that a retinal detachment may have occurred. If your central vision rapidly changes, this also may signal a retinal detachment or even a stroke.

Retinal detachment is an emergency! When your doctor examines you, he/she will be able to see whether the center of your retina is detached. When the center is involved, vision often cannot be fully restored.

If you have suffered a retinal detachment, your doctor will help you decide among the following treatments…

•Vitrectomy. This one- to three-hour surgery is performed in a hospital operating room, usually with sedation anesthesia plus localized numbing of the eye. The vitreous is removed, tears are treated with lasers or freezing, and a bubble (typically gas) is injected to replace the missing gel and hold the retina in place until the spot-welding treatment can take effect. (The bubble will gradually disappear.)

Important: It is necessary to keep your head in the same position for seven to 14 days in order to "keep the bubble on the trouble," as doctors say. Therefore, you will need a week or two of bed rest at home. You may have to keep your head facedown or on one side.

•Scleral buckle. With this procedure, a clear band of silicone is placed around the outside of the eyeball, where it acts like a belt, holding the retina against the wall of the eyeball.

Also performed in a hospital operating room, scleral buckle involves freezing the retina or treating it with a laser to create localized inflammation that forms a seal, securing the retina and keeping fluid out.

Scleral buckle takes from one to two hours and is sometimes combined with vitrectomy to improve the outcome. It is frequently used for younger patients and those who have not had cataract surgery.

•Pneumatic retinopexy. Depending on where the retinal detachment is located, a 20-minute, in-office procedure called a pneumatic retinopexy is an option for patients with smaller tears. With this procedure, a gas bubble is injected, and retinal tears are frozen or treated with a laser.

This is followed by up to two weeks of bed rest. Your head may need to be held in a certain position, such as upright at an angle, depending on the location of your tear.

With pneumatic retinopexy, the reattachment success rate is lower than that of scleral buckle or vitrectomy (70% versus 90%), but it is less invasive and no hospital visit is required. In addition, pneumatic retinopexy costs less than a hospital-based procedure, which could range from $5,000 to $10,000.

Even with a successful procedure, 40% of patients who suffer retinal detachments see 20/50 or worse afterward even when using glasses. The remainder have better vision.

No-Stitch Cataract Surgery

The FDA recently approved the first gel sealant for the corneal incision that's required after cataract surgery. In clinical studies, ReSure was more effective than a single suture in preventing eye fluid from leaking through the incision. There were no significant differences between the gel sealant and suture in eye pain, corneal swelling or inflammation.

James J. Salz, MD, eye surgeon in private practice in Los Angeles.

"Body Clock" May Explain Why Some Body Parts Age Faster Than Others

University of California, Los Angeles, news release.

Scientists who say they discovered a "body clock" that can reveal the biological age of most human tissues suggest that their findings may help shed light on why people's bodies age and how to slow the process.

Their results also provide important insights into cancer and stem cell research, the researchers said.

"To fight aging, we first need an objective way of measuring it," Steve Horvath, PhD, ScD, a professor of human genetics and of biostatistics at the University of California, Los Angeles, said in a university news release. "Pinpointing a set of biomarkers that keeps time throughout the body has been a four-year challenge."

"I've pursued this clock to help improve understanding of what speeds up and slows down the aging process," Dr. Horvath said.

Dr. Horvath and his team are believed to be the first to identify a mechanism in the body that enables scientists to measure accurately the biological age of different tissues, organs and cell types. Using this newly discovered biological clock, the researchers said they were surprised to find that some parts of the body, such as a woman's breast tissue, appear to age faster than the rest of the body.

"Healthy breast tissue is about two to three years older than the rest of a woman's body," Dr. Horvath said. "If a woman has breast cancer, the healthy tissue next to the tumor is an average of 12 years older than the rest of her body."

The results may explain why breast cancer is the most common cancer in women, according to the news release.

The researchers also found that the biological clock ranked tumor tissue an average of 36 years older than healthy tissue.

RESEARCH DETAILS

For his research, Dr. Horvath focused on methylation, a naturally occurring process that alters DNA. Using nearly 8,000 samples of 51 tissue types and cells taken from throughout the body, he charted how age affects DNA methylation levels from before birth through age 101.

Dr. Horvath tested the bio clock's effectiveness by comparing a tissue's biological age to its chronological age and found that the clock repeatedly proved accurate.

"It's surprising that one could develop a clock that reliably keeps time across the human anatomy," he said. "My approach really compared apples and oranges or, in this case, very different parts of the body: the brain, heart, lungs, liver, kidney and cartilage."

The study was published in the journal *Genome Biology*.

info The U.S. Centers for Disease Control and Prevention offers advice about healthy aging at its website, *http://www.cdc.gov/aging/*.

Medical Newsmakers

What Your Height Says About Your Health

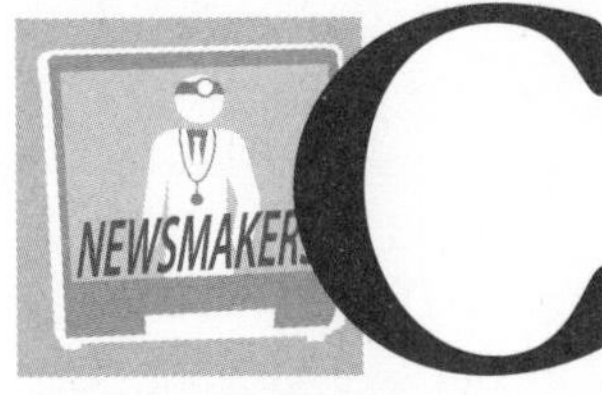

Common disease risk factors, such as family history, smoking, obesity and not getting enough exercise, are well-known. But researchers are now investigating another —and somewhat mysterious—risk factor that could be playing a role in a variety of chronic illnesses.

In both men and women, studies are increasingly linking stature to a number of very serious diseases. What scientists do not know is why.

To learn more, we spoke with Tim Byers, MD, MPH, a professor at the Colorado School of Public Health who has examined the relationship between height and disease.

What chronic illnesses are now being linked to height?

Cancer is one. A number of studies have shown that tall people are more likely to get certain types of cancer, including malignancies of the colon, kidney and breast, than shorter people.

For example, when scientists recently analyzed data on more than 20,000 postmenopausal women, they discovered that for every four-inch increase in height above 5' 1", there was a 13% to 29% increased risk for 19 types of cancer.

Although this study involved only women, previous research has shown that height is associated with pancreatic and colorectal cancers among men.

Conversely, people of smaller stature are more likely to suffer from stroke and cardiovascular disease.

And with Alzheimer's disease, one study found that men who were taller than 5' 10" were 59% less likely to develop the disease than men who were shorter than 5' 6".

Tim Byers, MD, MPH, a professor and associate dean for Public Health Practice at the Colorado School of Public Health in Aurora. He is the associate director for Cancer Prevention and Control at the University of Colorado Cancer Center, also in Aurora.

How important is height believed to be in the development of these diseases?

There is no question that height is somehow associated with risk for chronic diseases. Both the duration and degree, however, depend on the disease.

When researchers combined the data from previous scientific studies involving a total of more than three million people, they found that individuals of smaller stature (defined as 5' 3" or shorter) were 50% more likely to develop serious heart disease than taller people. This analysis was published in the *European Heart Journal.*

Stroke is another example. A study published in the journal *Stroke,* which looked at more than 10,000 men, discovered that those who were shorter (5' 3" or less) were 54% more likely to have a fatal stroke than those who were taller.

With regard to cancer, the risk for a tall person can be significant. For example, a woman who is 6' tall has about a 16% higher risk of getting cancer (such as colorectal, breast or ovarian) than a woman who is four inches shorter, according to research published in *The Lancet.*

Does this mean that height (tall or short) causes disease?

No, that has not been proven. In all previous research, height is associated with certain diseases.

It might be more accurate to say that height is a risk factor for disease. There could be other factors that influence both your height and your risk for certain diseases.

The scientific studies that have linked height and disease are primarily observational. In this type of study, scientists collect information—frequently from surveys or medical records—in order to identify common factors that influence health. Observational studies generate provocative ideas, but they cannot prove cause and effect.

So even though we know from these studies that a tall person is more likely to get cancer than someone who is short and that a short person has a higher risk for heart disease, we don't know that height itself is the reason.

What factors are likely to influence both disease and height?

Genetics is an obvious one. It's possible that some of the same genetic factors that make you tall or short also could produce changes in the body that increase the risk for certain diseases.

It's also likely that lifestyle factors, particularly those that occur early in life, are involved. Suppose that a child gets inadequate amounts of certain nutrients. He/she might not grow as tall as a child who eats greater amounts of nutritious foods. The same nutritional shortfalls could potentially lead to diseases later in life.

Meanwhile, high levels of insulin-like growth factor (a protein made by the body that stimulates the growth of many types of cells)—caused by such factors as diet, obesity and exercise habits—could trigger cell changes that eventually could lead to cancer.

Additionally, taller individuals tend to have larger organs and larger skin surface areas—this, of course, potentially increases the number of cells that could become malignant.

What should tall/short people do differently?

You shouldn't be particularly nervous about your disease risk if you're tall or short. In either case, you should be following the same prevention and screening recommendations as everyone else.

Your doctor will continue to focus on the risk factors that are known to cause disease, such as high blood pressure, elevated cholesterol, smoking and so on.

It is important to keep this research in perspective. For now, it's mainly of interest to scientists, who will use the association between height and health to gain a better understanding of the underlying causes of disease and the time in life when those causes might be acting.

In the future, doctors could potentially take height into consideration when assessing disease risk and giving health advice. The best advice, of course, is for everyone, tall or short, to do everything he/she can to stay healthy.

Advance Seen in Turning Adult Cells into Stem Cells

Jacob Hanna, MD, PhD, principle investigator, Laboratory for Pluripotent Cell Studies, Weizmann Institute of Science, Rehovot, Israel.

Konrad Hochedlinger, PhD, professor, medicine, Harvard Medical School, and researcher, Massachusetts General Hospital, Center for Regenerative Medicine, Boston.

Juan Dominguez-Bendala, PhD, director, Pancreatic Development and Stem Cell Laboratory, Diabetes Research Institute, University of Miami Miller School of Medicine.

Nature, online

Scientists have figured out a way to more readily turn adult skin cells into primitive stem cells that could potentially be used to treat a variety of chronic diseases.

In a study published in *Nature*, Israeli researchers reported that they identified the key molecule that stops adult cells from transforming into so-called induced pluripotent stem (iPS) cells. Those stem cells are similar to the primitive cells found in embryos, and have the potential to generate any type of body tissue, scientists believe.

Ultimately, the hope is to use iPS cells to treat damaged tissue in a range of chronic ills—from heart disease and diabetes, to arthritis, and spinal cord injuries and Alzheimer's disease.

That's still some years away, according to the experts, but the recent findings are a step forward.

"We've already known how to create these cells, but it's an inefficient process," said Konrad Hochedlinger, PhD, a stem cell researcher at Massachusetts General Hospital in Boston who was not involved in the study.

Right now, it could take weeks to months to coax human skin cells to transform into iPS cells. And even then, only a fraction of the cells are actually successfully "reprogrammed," Dr. Hochedlinger explained.

In the recent study, researchers reprogrammed in the space of one week nearly all of the mouse and human skin cells they studied.

HOW TO MAKE A STEM CELL

They did it by identifying a molecule that normally acts as a "roadblock" to keep adult cells from reverting back to infancy.

"We uncovered a new major pathway that prevents skin cells from converting back to an embryonic state," said senior researcher Jacob Hanna, MD, of the Weizmann Institute of Science in Rehovot, Israel.

"If we block this pathway, we increase current methods of making iPS cells up to 100% (efficiency), and eliminate the randomness and protracted nature of the process," he added.

Stem cells have been a hot topic in scientific research for years, with controversy swirling around the study of embryonic stem cells—because that requires an embryo to be destroyed in the process. But in 2007, researchers had their first success with reprogramming adult human cells to become embryonic-like stem cells.

It's done by activating just a few key genes that override the identity of an adult cell and send it back to an embryonic-like state. But the process has been hampered by inefficiency, and, Dr. Hochedlinger said, "we didn't know why that was."

The recent findings center on a molecule called Mbd3. Dr. Hanna's team found that blocking its action allowed human skin cells to be transformed into iPS cells almost 100% of the time.

Right now, Dr. Hochedlinger noted, the most efficient way to convert adult cells into pluripotent stem cells is through a viral vector—through which a virus is used to transport the necessary "reprogramming factors" into the cell.

The limitation is, the virus genetically alters the cell. And in animal research, that has been shown to sometimes cause cancer, according to the U.S. National Institutes of Health.

But this new process, Dr. Hochedlinger said, could make it easier for researchers to efficiently generate human iPS cells using virus-free techniques (which already exist).

Dr. Hanna stressed that point. "This is a major advance toward making safer iPS cells, without genetic modifications, at high efficiency," he said.

TOO SOON TO RATE SUCCESS, SAYS ONE EXPERT

But another stem cell researcher said it remains to be seen whether iPS cells created this way really do have a low rate of "reprogramming errors"—including activation of genes that could promote cancer.

It's not only viral vectors that introduce those errors into cells. The reprogramming process itself can do it, said Juan Dominguez-Bendala, PhD, of the Diabetes Research Institute at the University of Miami Miller School of Medicine.

"When a cell that has a specific function is forced to wipe out its memory and act as a stem cell, it has to activate genes that normally remain silent in adult cells," Dr. Dominguez-Bendala explained. Some of those genes, he said, are involved in controlling cell replication—and cancer is essentially out-of-control cell growth.

"Since there is a very thin line between a stem cell and a cancer cell," Dr. Dominguez-Bendala added, "you want the (reprogramming) process to be as clean as possible."

The new method may indeed be "cleaner," he said, but that's just conjecture for now.

Still, both he and Dr. Hochedlinger said that for researchers, these findings will help in sorting out exactly what goes on during cell reprogramming—which will be important if iPS cells are to be used to treat diseases.

Recently, Japanese researchers received approval for the world's first clinical trial of iPS cell therapy—to treat the age-related eye disease macular degeneration.

Dr. Hochedlinger said his guess is the therapy could become a reality for certain diseases within the next five to 10 years.

info The U.S. National Institutes of Health has a primer on stem cells at its website, *http://stemcells.nih.gov/info/basics/pages/basics10.aspx.*

This Mineral Prevents Headaches, Heart Disease, More—But 80% of Us Don't Get Enough

Dennis Goodman, MD, board-certified cardiologist, clinical associate professor of medicine at New York University School of Medicine and director of Integrative Medicine at New York Medical Associates, both in New York City. He is author of *Magnificent Magnesium: Your Essential Key to a Healthy Heart and More* (SquareOne). *DennisGoodmanMD.com*

At least 80% of Americans are deficient in magnesium. It's a serious problem because low magnesium has been linked to heart disease, stroke, hypertension and other chronic conditions, including headaches and depression.

Magnesium used to be plentiful in fruits, vegetables and grains, but decades of industrial-scale farming have stripped the soil of minerals. One study found that the nutrient content of crops has declined by as much as 40% since the 1950s. It now is almost impossible to get adequate amounts of magnesium from food.

What you need to know about magnesium now...

DANGEROUS DEFICIENCY

Magnesium is an essential component in many of your body's metabolic processes and involved in about 350 enzyme systems.

What happens when you don't get enough magnesium?

• **More heart disease.** Studies have shown that people with low levels of magnesium are more likely to die from heart disease than those with normal levels. The heart requires large amounts of magnesium to generate the energy needed to function normally. Heart cells that are deprived of energy begin to deteriorate. This can lead to inflammation, a known risk factor for heart disease.

A study published in *American Heart Journal* found that the risk for sudden death from heart disease was higher in areas of the country with low levels of magnesium in the water. Researchers found that the people who died tended to have lower-than-expected amounts of magnesium in their heart cells.

•**Higher blood pressure.** If you have hypertension, you might be taking a calcium-channel blocker, one of the medications that lowers blood pressure by relaxing blood vessels. Magnesium has a similar effect. It slows the passage of calcium into cells and can lower blood pressure by about 10 points. People with low levels of magnesium tend to have higher blood pressure than those who have higher levels.

•**Diabetes.** Research has shown that about 90% of people with diabetes are deficient in magnesium. Magnesium deficiency also has been linked to diabetes symptoms and complications, including diabetic retinopathy (damage to the blood vessels in the retina), hypertension and insulin resistance (a decline in the body's ability to respond to insulin).

•**Headaches.** The same blood vessel changes that increase the risk for hypertension also can lead to headaches. It's estimated that a majority of tension headaches are partly due to low magnesium.

The same is true of migraines. If you don't get enough magnesium, the blood vessels in the brain may expand and contract more than they should. This can lead to pain and other migraine symptoms.

Personal story: I suffered terrible migraines for much of my life. I got relief only when I started taking extra magnesium.

•**Depression.** Magnesium isn't the only factor involved in mood disorders, but it's more important than you might think. Low levels of magnesium cause a buildup of calcium and glutamate, which then overstimulate the N-methyl-D-aspartate (NMDA) brain receptor. Excessive stimulation of this receptor can lead to anxiety as well as depression.

WHO'S AT RISK?

If you have a lot of stress in your life or if you're taking calcium supplements, assume that you need more magnesium.

•**Calcium is an important mineral for bone health.** What people don't realize—and doctors rarely mention—is that high doses of calcium prevent magnesium from being absorbed. If you're supplementing with calcium, you have to get more magnesium.

The ideal ratio of calcium-to-magnesium intake is 1:1. For example, most people who take a daily 500-milligram (mg) calcium supplement also should take an equal amount of magnesium. But if you take very high doses of calcium, limit magnesium to 1,000 mg—more can cause diarrhea (and cut back if 1,000 mg causes problems).

Important: Patients with kidney disease should never take a magnesium supplement without checking with their doctor.

•**Stress is another leading risk factor.** If you have a lot of stress in your life, your body overproduces cortisol and other stress hormones. These hormones deplete magnesium from the body. Low magnesium also can cause stress by sapping your energy.

SUPPLEMENT SAFELY

Because a majority of Americans don't get enough magnesium from their diets, it makes sense to take a daily supplement, but always check with your doctor before taking any supplements.

If you decide to get your magnesium level checked, ask your doctor for a magnesium red blood cell (RBC-Mg) test. It measures the magnesium that is inside cells. It's a more accurate measure of magnesium than the standard serum magnesium test. An optimal RBC-Mg level is more than 5.5 mg/dL.

The test isn't essential. If you generally are healthy, you can't go wrong with extra magnesium. The Institute of Medicine advises women 31 years old and older to get 320 mg of magnesium daily. For men, the recommended amount is 420 mg. These are conservative estimates based on your minimal needs. *What I recommend...*

Multiply your weight in pounds by 3 mg to determine the optimal dose.

Example: A 140-pound woman would take 420 mg of magnesium. During times of stress, when your need for magnesium is higher, multiply your weight by five instead of three. Keep taking the higher dose until things calm down again. You will start to feel the benefits within a few days.

When you're shopping for supplements, look for products that end with "ate"—magnesium glycinate, taurate, malate, etc. These forms are readily absorbed into the bloodstream and less likely to cause diarrhea.

New Kind of Therapy Shows Early Promise in MS Patients

Stephen Miller, PhD, Judy Gugenheim Research Professor of Microbiology-Immunology, Feinberg School of Medicine, Northwestern University, Chicago.
Lawrence Steinman, MD, professor, neurology and neurological sciences, pediatrics and genetics, Stanford University, Stanford, California.
Science Translational Medicine

A new therapy for multiple sclerosis that teaches the body to recognize and then ignore its own nerve tissue appears to be safe and well-tolerated in humans, a small recent study shows.

If larger studies prove the technique can slow or stop the disease, the therapy would be a completely new way to treat autoimmune diseases such as multiple sclerosis (MS) and type 1 diabetes.

Most treatments for MS and other autoimmune diseases work by broadly suppressing immune function, leaving patients vulnerable to infections and cancers.

The new treatment targets only the proteins that come under attack when the immune system fails to recognize them as a normal part of the body. By creating tolerance to only a select few proteins, researchers hope they will be able to cure the disease but leave the rest of the body's defenses on guard.

"This is important work," said Lawrence Steinman, MD, a professor of neurology at Stanford University who was not involved with the study.

"Very few investigators are trying therapies in humans aimed at simply turning off unwanted immune responses and leaving the rest of the immune system intact to fight infections—to do surveillance against cancer," Dr. Steinman said. "The early results show encouragement."

STUDY DETAILS

For the study, published in the journal *Science Translational Medicine*, researchers in the United States and Germany recruited nine patients with MS. Seven had the relapsing-remitting form of the disease, while two others had secondary progressive MS (a more advanced phase). All were between the ages of 18 and 55, and were in good health except for their MS.

Blood tests conducted before the treatments showed that each patient had an immune reaction against at least one of seven myelin proteins.

Myelin is a white tissue made of fats and proteins that wraps nerve fibers, allowing them to conduct electrical signals through the body. In MS, the body attacks and gradually destroys these myelin sheaths. The damage disrupts nerve signals and leads to myriad symptoms, including numbness, tingling, weakness, loss of balance and disrupted muscle coordination.

Six patients in the study had low disease activity, while three others had a history of more active disease. Most were not experiencing symptoms at the time of their treatment.

On the day of the treatments, patients spent about two hours hooked up to a machine that filtered their blood, harvesting white cells while returning red cells and plasma to the body.

After the white cells were collected, they were washed and then combined with seven proteins that make up myelin tissue. A chemical was used to link the proteins to the white blood cells, which were dying.

In addition to fighting germs, another important role of the immune system is to get rid of dead and dying tissues. When these tissues are collected by the spleen, it sends out a signal to the rest of the immune system that the dying tissues are just harmless waste.

The new treatment aims to take advantage of the body's waste disposal system. In attaching the myelin proteins to dying white blood cells, the idea is to get the body to also recognize those proteins as harmless and hopefully leave them alone.

In animal models of MS, the same group of researchers has shown that using this system to

New Hope for MS Prevention

In a study of 73 people with early signs of multiple sclerosis, 58% of those given a vaccine that is used to prevent tuberculosis in other parts of the world did not develop MS by the end of the five-year study, compared with 30% of those in a placebo group. More study is under way.

Neurology

induce immune tolerance can stop the progression of disease.

This was the first test of this kind of therapy in humans, and although the study was too small to show whether the treatment changed the course of the disease, researchers did see some promising signs.

Blood tests taken before and after the treatment showed that the infusions turned down immune reactivity to myelin proteins, but didn't affect the immune response to potential infections, like tetanus.

"We were only trying to turn down the myelin responses, which we did," said study researcher Stephen Miller, PhD, a professor of microbiology and immunology at the Northwestern University Feinberg School of Medicine, in Chicago. "And we didn't turn down the response to tetanus. That suggests...that this therapy, just like in mice, can induce tolerance in humans."

Patients reported mild and moderate side effects during their treatments. Nearly all these problems, except for a metallic taste in the mouth, were judged to be unrelated to the study treatment.

The six patients with mild disease activity showed no new symptoms or worsening in their conditions three months after the infusions. What's more, MRI scans showed no new areas of inflammation after their treatments.

Two of the three patients with more active disease had worsening symptoms within two weeks of treatment. Those symptoms cleared up with steroid treatments. MRI scans showed all three patients developed new lesions that indicated a worsening of inflammation.

None of the patients lost neurologic function during the six months they were followed after their treatments.

"Whether it's going to have a long-standing effect, or an effect in locking down the disease symptoms in MS patients, is going to take a phase 2 or phase 3 trial," said Dr. Miller, who disclosed that he shares rights to a patent on the technique.

The study was supported by private grants from foundations in Germany and the United States, and by funding from the German government.

info For more information on immune tolerance therapies, head to the U.S. National Institute of Allergy and Infectious Diseases website at *http://www.niaid.nih.gov/topics/immunetolerance/pages/default.aspx.*

You Might Have Deadly Kidney Disease and Not Know It

Robert C. Stanton, MD, principal investigator in the section on vascular cell biology and chief of the nephrology section at Joslin Diabetes Center and Joslin Clinic. He is associate professor of medicine at Harvard Medical School and a staff member at Beth Israel Deaconess Medical Center, all in Boston.

Even if you feel fine right at this moment, your kidneys could be gradually failing. Nearly six in 10 Americans will develop kidney disease in their lifetimes, according to a recent analysis published in *American Journal of Kidney Disease.* In comparison, lifetime risk for diabetes, heart attack and invasive cancer is approximately four in 10.

As a result of this and other findings, the National Kidney Foundation recently called for health-care professionals to screen patients in specific high-risk groups for chronic kidney disease (CKD)—those age 60 or older and those with high blood pressure or diabetes—by adding a simple urine albumin test for kidney damage to annual physical examinations.

My advice: Get checked even sooner, at about age 50, and then yearly after that. If you have been diagnosed with diabetes or hypertension, then you should get tested annually regardless of your age. If your doctor finds any sign of impairment, get a referral to a nephrologist to see if anything should be done.

Here's what else you need to know now about CKD...

A DISEASE ON THE RISE

CKD is the result of damage to the kidney's one million-plus filtering units (kidney nephrons). This damage impairs the body's ability to remove wastes as well as to do many other functions that the kidney does, such as regulating the amount of fluid in your body and the amount of critical chemicals, including sodium, potassium, calcium, phosphate and more. Typically there are no symptoms until 75% to 80% of kidney function is lost. At that point, eventual kidney failure is likely, with dialysis and/or a transplant being the only treatment options.

Unfortunately, kidney disease is on the rise. In the mid-1980s, about 70,000 Americans were getting dialysis for kidney disease. In the years since, the number has risen to about 450,000, a sixfold increase. And millions of people with CKD aren't even aware that they have it.

The number of people with kidney disease is rising partly because the American population is aging, and older people get more chronic diseases, including CKD. There also has been an enormous increase in diabetes, which is the leading cause of CKD, followed by high blood pressure. More than one-third of people with diabetes and more than 20% of patients with high blood pressure show signs of kidney damage.

Smoking, obesity and high cholesterol also increase the risk.

You can reduce damage and slow the progression of CKD with medications and by treating the conditions that cause it. Once the disease has progressed, your options are limited—and the risks are high. Among dialysis patients, there is a 15%-to-20% death rate every year. Worsening kidney function increases the risk of dying from cardiovascular disease. It also can lead to bone weakness, anemia and other complications.

It's critical to get diagnosed while the kidneys still are working well.

SIMPLE TESTS

Most cases of CKD can be detected with a few basic (and inexpensive) tests. If your doctor finds any sign of impairment, a referral to a nephrologist is a good idea to determine what is causing the kidney disease.

- **Serum albumin.** This is the test that the National Kidney Foundation recommends be added to the annual physical for anyone over age 60. Serum albumin is a protein found in the urine of patients with CKD. The most commonly used way to measure urine albumin is by dipping a test strip in the urine. Although this is a good screen, it does not pick up a low-level increase in the urine albumin level.

A better test is the microalbumin test (also called the albumin/creatinine ratio test). It can be done on a single urine specimen sent to any laboratory. This is the best test to determine the urine albumin level. The presence of albumin in the urine usually indicates kidney damage. An increase in the urine albumin level often is the first sign of kidney damage from diabetes. It also can be due to hypertension and other conditions. A reading of more than 30 milligrams (mg) of albumin per 1 gram (g) of creatinine is a sign of CKD.

- **Serum creatinine.** A product of normal muscle metabolism is creatinine. Because your creatinine is produced at about the same level every day and filtered by the kidneys, it has been used to estimate kidney function. Elevated levels might mean that you have kidney disease. In young men up to age 40, normal levels are 0.6 mg per deciliter (dL) of blood to 1.2 mg/dL. In young women up to age 40, 0.5 to 1.1 mg/dL is the normal range. Normal serum creatinine values decline as we age.

Caution: Creatinine alone is not a perfect measure of kidney health. If your creatinine is elevated, you will need additional tests to confirm—or rule out—CKD. For example, your creatinine can rise due to dehydration.

- **Glomerular filtration rate (GFR).** This is a measure of kidney function estimated from your creatinine level and other factors, including age, sex and race. The GFR gives a more accurate reflection of kidney function than the serum creatinine test alone. A healthy 50-year-old typically will have a GFR of about 80 milliliters per minute (mL/min) to 100 mL/min. A reading of 60 mL/min or lower that persists for at least three months is a sign of CKD.

NEXT STEPS

There isn't a cure for CKD, and the damage can't be reversed. However, you can slow the rate at which the disease progresses and possibly avoid dialysis/transplantation. *Important...*

- **Strict glucose control.** Since most cases of CKD are caused by diabetes, it's essential to maintain healthy blood sugar levels. Elevated glucose damages the blood vessels that are used by the kidneys to filter wastes. If you have diabetes, follow your doctor's instructions about when and how often to test your blood sugar. Eat a healthy diet...exercise most days of the week...and take medications as instructed.

- **Better blood pressure.** The same factors that are good for diabetes (and your heart) also will improve your blood pressure.

Important: Even if your blood pressure is normal or just slightly elevated, your doctor still might prescribe a drug called an ACE inhibitor (such as Capoten or Vasotec) or an angiotensin II receptor blocker (such as Cozaar or Diovan) if you have elevated urine albumin levels. Blood pressure–lowering medications can slow the progression of CKD by lowering urine albumin levels, even if your blood pressure is normal.

Skin Symptom for Kidney Disease

People with psoriasis should be screened for kidney disease if the condition covers 3% or more of the body, advises Joel M. Gelfand, MD. (The palm of the hand is about 1% of body surface area.) People who have moderate-to-severe psoriasis have a higher risk for chronic kidney disease.

Joel M. Gelfand, MD, associate professor of dermatology and associate professor of epidemiology at Perelman School of Medicine at University of Pennsylvania, Philadelphia. He led a seven-year study of nearly 144,000 people with psoriasis, published in *BMJ*.

- **Less salt.** Limit your daily salt consumption to 1,500 mg (about two-thirds of a teaspoon) or less if you have high blood pressure, take a diuretic or have swelling in your legs.

- **Not too much protein.** Animal studies indicate that a high-protein diet causes more serious illness in those with kidney disease. It's not clear whether it has the same effect in humans—but moderation makes sense.

You don't have to follow a very-low-protein diet—you just don't want too much protein. In my view, if you have CKD, it is likely that a protein intake of up to 56 g/day for men and 46 g/day for women is safe. Ask your doctor for a referral to a dietitian. He/she will help you calculate how much protein you need.

- **Be careful with painkillers.** People who regularly take large doses of painkillers—such as aspirin, *ibuprofen* or *acetaminophen*—have an elevated risk for CKD. If you depend on these medications—to control arthritis, for example—talk to your doctor. This is particularly important if you already have been diagnosed with CKD.

Annual Dental Cleaning May Be Enough for Some

University of Michigan, news release.

For many people, once-a-year dental cleaning may be enough to prevent gum disease that leads to tooth loss, according to a recent study.

"Twice-yearly cleanings have been recommended for over 50 years without supporting evidence," study author William Giannobile, DDS, a professor of dentistry and biomedical engineering at the University of Michigan, said in a university news release.

But the results of this study "showed that one yearly cleaning is likely to be enough for patients with no risk factors," he said. "Patients with one or more risk factors, which represent over half of the population, should visit at least twice a year and likely more in some cases."

Scientists Can "See" Dreams

Brain scans can reveal some of what a person is seeing in a dream, such as streets or cars. This is possible because of recent advances in decoding brain signals that correspond with what patients see while they are awake. The process cannot reveal a dream's story line, but its ability to observe detail likely will improve in time.

Study by researchers at ATR Computational Laboratories, Kyoto, Japan, published in *Science*.

STUDY DETAILS

For the study, which was published online in the *Journal of Dental Research*, Dr. Giannobile and colleagues looked at data from more than 5,100 adults who visited the dentist regularly for 16 straight years, had no history of gum disease and received one or two cleanings each year.

The researchers examined the link between the frequency of teeth cleanings and long-term tooth loss in the participants, as well as three key gum disease risk factors: smoking, diabetes and genetics.

Two dental cleanings a year provided significant benefits to people with one or more of the three risk factors, while people with two or three of the risk factors may require more than two cleanings a year. But one cleaning per year appears sufficient for people with none of the risk factors, according to the study.

"The future of health care is personalized medicine," Dr. Giannobile said. "This study represents an important step toward making it a reality, and in a disease that is widespread, costly and preventable."

"We have long known that some individuals are at greater risk of [gum] disease, but tools haven't been available to adequately identify those at increased risk and prevent disease progression," he said.

info The U.S. National Institutes of Health has more about preventing gum disease at its website, ***http://newsinhealth.nih.gov/issue/jul2010/feature2***.

A Toothache Can Turn Deadly—Even Mild Pain Should Never Be Ignored

Samuel O. Dorn, DDS, chair of the department of endodontics and program director at The University of Texas Health Science Center at Houston, where he holds the Frank B. Trice, DDS, Professorship in Endodontics. He is the president-elect of the International Federation

It's hard to imagine how a toothache could turn deadly—but it can. Even mild or moderate discomfort (for example, pain while chewing...sensitivity to hot and cold...and/or redness and swelling of the gums) can quickly turn into a potentially serious condition, known as an abscess, a pus-filled infection inside the tooth or between a tooth and the gum. Though the pain may be merely annoying in the beginning, within a day or so, it can turn into the intense, throbbing pain or sharp, shooting pain that is the telltale sign of an abscess.

Dangerous trend: The number of Americans hospitalized for dental abscesses is on the rise. Over a recent eight-year period, hospitalizations for periapical abscesses (infections at the tip of the tooth root) increased by more than 40%.

No one has a precise explanation for the trend, but some experts speculate that the high cost of dental insurance is preventing many people from seeking routine dental care and perhaps delaying treatment when a problem occurs. Medicare does not cover routine dental care, and many private health insurance plans offer very limited coverage.

WHAT GOES WRONG

If there's a breach in a tooth's protective enamel—from tooth decay, a chip or even gum disease, for example—you're at risk for an abscess. Some cracks can be taken care of with bonding or a crown. Some don't need treatment at all because they don't go through to the tooth pulp (the soft tissue inside the tooth). But if bacteria get inside the tooth, an abscess can form.

Other signs to watch for: In addition to the symptoms described earlier, other red flags of a dental abscess may include persistent foul breath, a swollen face, jaw and/or neck glands and a fever.

Once the pain kicks in, people who have dental abscesses will often describe it as the worst they've ever experienced. If you've ever had a root canal (see below), you might have had an abscess.

• **Get help immediately.** An abscess will not go away on its own. Worse, the infection can spread as quickly as overnight (in some cases, however, it can take years to spread). An abscess can cause death when the infection spreads to the brain or heart or when swelling cuts off the airway.

When to be especially suspicious: If you have pain in one of your back teeth. They're the ones that do most of the chewing, and they're also the ones that are harder to reach with dental floss and a toothbrush. If you crunch something hard, such as a popcorn kernel, piece of ice or even an almond, a back tooth is the one most likely to be cracked.

GETTING PROMPT TREATMENT

Your dentist can diagnose an abscess in just a few minutes. All he/she has to do is gently tap on the suspected tooth with a small metal device and see if you wince. A tooth abscess will be very sensitive to pressure. An X-ray will confirm if there's a pus-filled pocket near the tooth root.

You might be given penicillin or another antibiotic if the infection has spread beyond the tooth. *In addition, your dentist will treat the abscess in one of three ways...*

• **Incision and draining.** If the abscess is between the tooth and the gum, your dentist will make a small incision, drain out the pus and clean the area with saline. The pain will start to diminish almost immediately. Your dentist also can drain an abscess that occurs inside a tooth, but this won't cure it—the infection will probably come back.

• **Root canal.** This is the most widely used treatment for an abscess near the tooth root. Your dentist will drill into the infected area, scrape away damaged tissue and drain the pus. After that, the canal will be filled with sealant, and the tooth will be crowned (a porcelain or metal cap is put over the tooth).

If you get a root canal, there's a good chance that the tooth will survive. The drawback is cost. Root canals usually are done by an endodontist (a dentist with advanced training). Expect to pay from $300 (for a front tooth) to $2,000 for a molar. The crown is an additional $500 to $3,000 (prices depend on where you live and whether you go to a specialist or your regular dentist).

• **Extraction.** This is the most permanent treatment for a deep abscess. It costs about $75 to $300 to remove a tooth—and once the tooth is gone, the abscess goes away with it.

Some patients save money by choosing not to replace an extracted tooth. But there are health risks associated with not replacing a tooth, such as increased chance of additional decay and infection, bone loss, poor chewing function and speech disturbances.

Better: Replace the tooth with an implant (at least $2,400) or a bridge (at least $1,100).

If you can't see a dentist immediately: Consider going to an ER if you have severe pain and/or swelling. If you are having trouble breathing, go to an ER right away.

PREVENTING AN ABSCESS

If you take care of your teeth, there's a good chance that you'll never have an abscess.

In addition to regular brushing and flossing and avoiding a lot of sugar-filled foods and drinks...

• **Use fluoride toothpaste.** It remineralizes tooth enamel and makes it stronger. This is particularly important for older adults, whose receding gums can expose parts of the tooth and leave it vulnerable to decay.

Patch Replaces Bone for New Teeth

A new "bio patch" may help those who need a dental implant but don't have enough bone to anchor it. The patch, seeded with DNA, sends genetic instructions that cause cells to produce new bone.

Biomaterials

Also helpful: A fluoride mouth rinse. There are many brands in drugstores. They strengthen the enamel and reduce tooth decay.

•**Don't slack off on dental visits.** Most people should have dental checkups and cleanings every six months. If you smoke or have gum disease, diabetes or any other condition that increases your risk for dental problems, it's usually a good idea to schedule even more frequent dental visits.

FDA Starts Regulating Compounding Pharmacies

Margaret Hamburg, MD, commissioner, U.S. Food and Drug Administration

Janet Woodcock, .MD, director, Center for Drug Evaluation and Research, U.S. Food and Drug Administration.

The U.S. Food and Drug Administration is now regulating compounding pharmacies, which create new drug combinations or alter drugs to suit individual patient needs.

Under the Drug Quality and Security Act, signed into law November 27, 2013, by President Barack Obama, compounding pharmacies are being encouraged to register with the FDA. The agency will then classify them as outsourcing pharmacies, enabling them to sell bulk drugs to hospitals and other health-care facilities.

The law was prompted by the deaths in 2012 of 64 people who received fungus-contaminated steroid medications that were given in injections to treat back and joint pain. An additional 750 people in 20 states were sickened by the contaminated drug. The medication was made by the now-shuttered New England Compounding Center, in Framingham, Massachusetts, according to federal health officials.

"The part of the law related to compounding is a step forward by creating a new pathway in which compounders register with FDA as an outsourcing facility," said FDA commissioner Margaret Hamburg, MD, during a press briefing.

If a compounding pharmacy registers with the agency, hospitals and other health-care providers will be able to buy products compounded by companies that are subject to FDA oversight, she said.

FACILITIES WILL BE INSPECTED

The oversight includes inspections and adherence to "good manufacturing practices," Dr. Hamburg said. To get compounding pharmacies to register, the FDA will encourage hospitals and other health-care providers to buy their compounded products only from FDA-registered companies, she added.

"This will be a critical step they can take to protect the health and safety of their patients," Dr. Hamburg said.

UNREGISTERED COMPANIES CAN STILL OPERATE

One of the loopholes in the new law: Since pharmacy registration is voluntary, unregistered compounding companies that ship products will only be caught if a problem like contamination arises and is reported.

"We will need to work closely with the states," Dr. Hamburg said. "They will have to provide us with ongoing information about the facilities they are overseeing."

The FDA doesn't know just how many compounding pharmacies exist in the United States. Janet Woodcock, MD, director of the FDA's Center for Drug Evaluation and Research, said there may be as many as 1,000 such businesses.

"While the new law doesn't provide the FDA with all the additional authority it sought, these provisions are definitely progress," Dr. Woodcock said. "The FDA is committed and stands ready to implement this new law immediately."

In addition to revised regulations for compounding pharmacies, the new law also authorizes the FDA to develop a national track-and-trace system. This system should reduce chances for contamination, adulteration or counterfeiting of drugs, Dr. Hamburg said.

info For more on compounding pharmacies, visit the U.S. Food and Drug Administration at its website, *http://www.fda.gov/drugs/GuidanceComplianceRegulatoryInformation/Pharmacy Compounding/.*

Nail Fungus Drug Might Help Against HIV, Study Suggests

Rutgers New Jersey Medical School, news release.

A common drug used to treat nail fungus may hold promise against HIV, the virus that causes AIDS, according to a recent study.

In laboratory research, the anti-fungal drug *ciclopirox* enabled the killing of HIV-infected cells by blocking the cells' mitochondria—their powerhouse. In addition, ciclopirox eliminated HIV from cell cultures, and the virus did not return when the anti-fungal drug was stopped, the study authors said.

This does not occur with currently available anti-HIV drugs, which must be taken for the rest of a patient's life, said study leaders Michael Mathews and Hartmut Hanauske-Abel, of the Rutgers New Jersey Medical School.

The effectiveness of ciclopirox against HIV needs to be confirmed in human clinical trials. But because the drug is already approved by the U.S. Food and Drug Administration for treatment of fungal infection and is considered safe, the clinical trial process for this treatment could be quicker and less costly than usual, the researchers said.

The study was published in the journal *PLoS One*.

The use of combination antiretroviral drugs has vastly improved HIV treatment, the study authors said in a Rutgers news release. These so-called drug cocktails are effective at keeping HIV under control, but they never completely eradicate the infection.

info The U.S. National Institute of Allergy and Infectious Diseases has more about HIV treatment at its website, *http://www.niaid.nih.gov/topics/hivaids/understanding/treatment/pages/default.aspx*.

Trees May Save a Life Each Year in Big Cities

David J. Nowak, PhD, urban forests, human health, and environmental quality unit, U.S. Forest Service, Syracuse, New York.

Janice Nolen, assistant vice president, national policy, American Lung Association.

Washington Post; *Environmental Pollution*

Parks and tree-lined streets may give city dwellers more than shade. They may also save some lives, a recent study from the U.S. Forest Service suggests.

Researchers estimate that across 10 US cities, "urban forests" prevent an average of one death per year, by helping to clear the air of fine particulate matter released when fossil fuels are burned. Those particles (from car exhaust and industrial sources) are a particular concern when it comes to people's health, said David Nowak, PhD, a Forest Service researcher who led the study.

The particles are thought to cause inflammation in the blood vessels and airways, which can be dangerous for people with existing heart or lung disease. The recent findings, reported in the journal *Environmental Pollution*, suggest that trees play a role in protecting urban dwellers from the health effects of air pollution.

But, Dr. Nowak said, it's not just a simple matter of "let's plant more trees."

This study shows a "large-scale" correlation between tree coverage and human health. But researchers still have to figure out the nitty-gritty, Dr. Nowak said. "How do we best design to protect people from [fine particle pollution]? What configuration of plants do we need? What species of tree?" he said.

And all of that, Dr. Nowak added, has to be figured out at the local and regional levels.

Trees, he noted, do a lot more than clear fine particles from the air. They have many beneficial effects—including reducing other air pollutants such as ozone, and keeping the temperature down during the summer. But certain other effects are not so good for human health: Trees release pollen, for example, which can exacerbate allergies and asthma.

RESEARCH DETAILS

The findings are based on daily air-quality data from 10 U.S. cities, along with information on the cities' tree coverage. To gauge how trees might be affecting city residents' health, Dr. Nowak's team used a computer program from the U.S. Environmental Protection Agency (EPA) that estimates the health impact of changes in air quality.

Overall, Atlanta was number one when it came to the amount of fine particle pollution removed by trees, at 64.5 metric tons—owing to the city's relatively dense urban forest.

But as far as lives saved, New York City came in on top, with an average of eight lives saved per year. That, Dr. Nowak said, was partly due to the city's large population, but also to the "moderately high" removal of fine particles from the air—thanks to trees.

DO CITIES NEED MORE TREES?

No one is claiming that trees are the main answer to air pollution, though.

Trees may be a smaller-scale way to give people extra protection from pollution, said Janice Nolen, assistant vice president of national policy for the American Lung Association.

"But they're not going to be the solution," Nolen said. The "big tools," she said, are measures to reduce emissions from power plants, cars and other sources of pollutants.

info The US Environmental Protection Agency has more on fine particle air pollution at its website, *http://www.epa.gov/pm/*.

Scope of Ebola Outbreak May Be Greater Than Statistics Show

World Health Organization; Associated Press

The magnitude of the Ebola outbreak in West Africa may be far greater than some current statistics indicate, according to officials from the World Health Organization.

Patients flooded treatment centers, and the recorded case and death tolls may "vastly underestimate the magnitude of the outbreak," said WHO spokesman Gregory Hartl, the Associated Press reported.

For example, an 80-bed treatment center that opened in Liberia's capital filled up immediately, Hartl noted, and dozens of people lined up the next day to be treated for Ebola.

WHO figures (as of late September 2014) peg the death toll at 3,090, with 3,626 confirmed cases. At this point, Ebola cases have been reported in Guinea, Liberia, Sierra Leone and Nigeria.

The CDC is also providing computer software and hardware to the countries hit hardest by Ebola, so officials there can track and analyze the outbreak's spread in real time, WHO added.

info Visit the U.S. Centers for Disease Control and Prevention website *http://www.cdc.gov/vhf/ebola/* for more on the Ebola outbreak.

Medication Smarts

Is the Drug You're Taking Triggering a Disease?

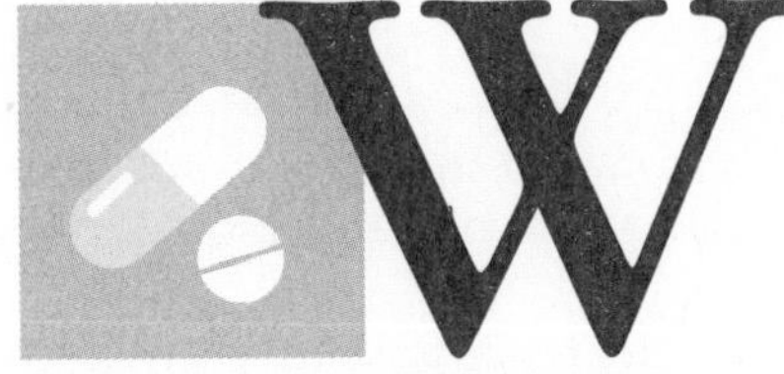

When your doctor pulls out his/her prescription pad, you probably assume that your health problem will soon be improving. Sure, there may be a side effect or two—perhaps an occasional upset stomach or a mild headache. But overall you will be better off, right?

Not necessarily. While it's true that many drugs can help relieve symptoms and sometimes even cure certain medical conditions, a number of popular medications actually cause disease—not simply side effects—while treating the original problem.

Here's what happens: Your kidney and liver are the main organs that break down drugs and eliminate them from your body. But these organs weaken as you age. Starting as early as your 20s and 30s, you lose 1% of liver and kidney function every year. As a result, drugs can build up in your body (particularly if you take more than one), become toxic, damage crucial organs such as the heart and brain—and trigger disease.

Older adults are at greatest risk for this problem because the body becomes increasingly less efficient at metabolizing drugs with age. But no one is exempt from the risk.

To protect yourself—or a loved one...

DEMENTIA

Many drugs can cause symptoms, such as short-term memory loss, confusion and agitation, that patients (and physicians) frequently

Armon B. Neel, Jr., PharmD, a certified geriatric pharmacist, founder of the Georgia-based MedicationXpert, LLC, a private practice focused on pharmaceutical care for outpatients and institutional geriatric patients. Dr. Neel is also coauthor of *Are Your Prescriptions Killing You? How to Prevent Dangerous Interactions, Avoid Deadly Side Effects, and Be Healthier with Fewer Drugs* (Atria). *MedicationXpert.com* mistake for dementia. The main offenders are anticholinergic medications, which treat a variety of conditions by blocking the activity of the neurotransmitter acetylcholine.

Hundreds of medications are anticholinergic, and it's likely that any class of drugs beginning with anti- is in this category—for example, antihistamines and antispasmodics. Cholesterol-lowering statins also can cause dementia-like symptoms.

Other offenders: Beta-blockers (for high blood pressure or cardiac arrhythmias)...benzodiazepines (for anxiety)...narcotics...tricyclic antidepressants...anticonvulsants...muscle relaxants...sleeping pills...fluoroquinolone antibiotics...heartburn drugs (H2 receptor antagonists and proton-pump inhibitors)...antipsychotics...nitrates (for heart disease)...and sulfonylurea derivatives (for diabetes).

My advice: If you or a loved one has been diagnosed with dementia, the patient should immediately undergo a comprehensive medication review—drug-induced dementia usually can be reversed by stopping the offending drug (or drugs). A competent physician or consultant pharmacist can always find an alternative drug to use.

Surprising threat: Even general anesthesia can cause weeks or months of dementia-like confusion (and an incorrect diagnosis of Alzheimer's) in an older person, as the drug slowly leaves the body.

The anesthesia is collected in the fat cells in the body, and normal cognition may take months to return. The longer a person is under anesthesia, the longer it takes to recover.

CANCER

Medications known as biologics are frequently used to treat autoimmune diseases such as inflammatory bowel disease, or IBD (including Crohn's disease and ulcerative colitis), and rheumatoid arthritis.

This class of drugs includes *adalimumab* (Humira), *certolizumab* (Cimzia), *etanercept* (Enbrel), *golimumab* (Simponi) and *infliximab* (Remicade).

Important finding: The use of biologics was linked to more than triple the risk for lymphoma, breast, pancreatic and other cancers in a study that was published in *The Journal of the American Medical Association.*

The danger: While these medications may have a role in the treatment of autoimmune diseases, they often are carelessly prescribed by primary care physicians. For example, a biologic that is intended for IBD may be mistakenly prescribed for irritable bowel syndrome (IBS), a far less serious digestive disorder.

If you are prescribed a biologic for IBD: Before starting the drug, ask for a comprehensive workup to confirm the diagnosis. This may include lab tests, imaging tests (ultrasound, CT or MRI), a biopsy and a stool analysis (to rule out C. difficile and other bowel infections that would require an antibiotic). Do not take a biologic for IBS.

If you are prescribed a biologic for rheumatoid arthritis: Before starting the medication, ask your doctor for a comprehensive workup to confirm the diagnosis, including lab tests and imaging tests (X-ray, ultrasound or MRI). Do not take a biologic for osteoarthritis. Besides increasing cancer risk, the suppression of the immune system opens the door for serious bacterial and viral infections.

DIABETES

Many commonly prescribed drugs increase risk for type 2 diabetes. These medications include statins...beta-blockers...antidepressants...antipsychotics...steroids...and alpha-blockers prescribed for prostate problems and high blood pressure.

Safer alternatives to discuss with your doctor, consultant pharmacist or other health-care professional...

If you're prescribed a beta-blocker: Ask about using a calcium-channel blocker instead. *Diltiazem* (Tiazac) has the fewest side effects. The 24-hour sustained-release dose provides the best control.

If you're prescribed an antidepressant: Ask about *venlafaxine* (Effexor), a selective serotonin and norepinephrine reuptake inhibitor (SSNRI) antidepressant that treats depression and anxiety and has been shown to cause fewer problems for diabetic patients than any of the older selective serotonin reuptake inhibitor (SSRI) drugs.

If you're prescribed an alpha-blocker: For prostate problems, rather than taking the alpha-blocker *tamsulosin* (Flomax), ask about using *dutasteride* (Avodart) or *finasteride* (Proscar). For high blood pressure, ask about a calcium-channel blocker drug.

HEART DISEASE

Pain relievers called nonsteroidal anti-inflammatory drugs (NSAIDs), frequently taken to ease pain due to arthritis, other joint problems or headaches, are widely known to damage the digestive tract. What's less well-known is that NSAIDs have been found to increase the risk for cardiovascular disease.

My advice: No one over the age of 50 with mild-to-moderate pain should use an NSAID.

Fortunately, there is an excellent alternative. A daily dose of 50 mg of the prescription non-narcotic pain reliever *tramadol* (Ultracet, Ultram) and/or 325 mg of *acetaminophen* (Tylenol) works well and has less risk for adverse effects. Acetaminophen, taken in appropriate doses (less than 3,000 mg daily) without alcohol use, is safe and effective. I also recommend 3 g to 4 g of fish oil daily—it has been shown to effectively treat joint pain. Talk to your doctor first because fish oil may increase risk for bleeding.

5 Medication Mistakes You Never Want to Make

Albert W. Wu, MD, MPH, an internist and professor of medicine, surgery and health policy & management at The Johns Hopkins Bloomberg School of Public Health and the director of the Center for Health Services and Outcomes Research, both in Baltimore. He was a member of the committee formed by the Institute of Medicine to identify and prevent medication errors.

Chewing a pill when it is meant to be swallowed might taste pretty bad, but it wouldn't necessarily be dangerous, right? Wrong—it can be fatal if too much of the active ingredient is released at one time.

This is just one of the preventable medication errors that occurs regularly in our country—in fact, at least 100,000 Americans are hospitalized from such mistakes every year. How could something as simple as taking a medication go so wrong?

Here's how some of the most common medication mistakes can occur—and how to avoid them...

***Mistake #1:* Not verifying the instructions on e-prescriptions**. Prescription pads are quickly becoming a thing of the past. Instead, your doctor now may enter your prescription into a computer, which electronically transmits it to your pharmacy. The good news is, e-prescriptions solve the problem of illegible handwriting and help stop errors. For example, if your doctor enters a dose of a drug that is

The Very Best Drug Self-Defense

If you're over age 60—especially if you take more than one medication or suffer drug side effects—it's a good idea to ask your physician to work with a consulting pharmacist who is skilled in medication management. A consulting pharmacist has been trained in drug therapy management and will work with your physician to develop a drug management plan that will avoid harmful drugs. These services are relatively new and may not be covered by insurance, so be sure to check with your provider.

To find a consulting pharmacist in your area, go to the website of the American Society of Consultant Pharmacists, *www.ASCP.com*, and click on "Find a Senior Care Pharmacist."

Also helpful: Make sure that a drug you've been prescribed does not appear on the "Beers Criteria for Potentially Inappropriate Medication Use in Older Adults." Originally developed by Mark Beers, editor of *The Merck Manual of Medical Information,* the list has been recently updated by The American Geriatrics Society. To download the list for free, go to *AmericanGeriatrics.org/files/documents/beers/PrintableBeersPocketCard.pdf.*

too low or too high for any patient, the computer will flag it. In hospitals, computerized prescribing has reduced medication errors by up to 85%. But mistakes still happen.

How errors can occur: Let's say that your doctor wants you to take a long-acting diabetes medication only once a day, but the computer's default setting, which comes up automatically, calls for twice-daily dosing. If he/she does not notice, the computer will send that information to the pharmacy. The level of medication in your body could become too high, and blood sugar could drop dangerously low.

My advice: Always ask your doctor how to take medication—how much...how frequently...what time of day...and with or without food. Write all this information down. Then check this information on the drug label when you pick up the prescription. If there's any discrepancy between what the doctor told you and what the label says, the pharmacist should contact your doctor.

Vital Questions for Your Pharmacist

Do yourself a favor—the next time you pick up a prescription talk to your pharmacist. This is one of the best ways to avoid medication errors. *Key questions to ask your pharmacist...*

- **What is the active ingredient in this medicine?**
- **Should I avoid any other medicines, supplements, foods or drinks when taking this drug?***
- **Is there anything I should watch for—such as allergic reactions or other side effects?**
- **Should I take this medication on an empty stomach or with food?**
- **What should I do if I miss a dose...or use too much?**
- **Will I need any tests to check on the medicine's effectiveness—such as blood tests?**
- **How and where should I store this medicine?**

**You also can check for interactions at PDRHealth.com.*

Mistake #2: **Not discussing the name of the drug with the doctor.** There are more than 10,000 prescription drugs and some 300,000 over-the-counter (OTC) medications. Many have similar-sounding—and similarly spelled—names that are easily confused.

How errors can occur: Your doctor might inadvertently key in *clonazepam* (an antianxiety drug) instead of *clonidine* (for high blood pressure). Or he might mix up Flomax (for prostate problems) and *Volmax* (for lung problems). A computer would not pick up this error.

My advice: Ask your doctor to pronounce and/or write down for you the name of the drug he is prescribing. Repeat the name to make sure you have it right. When you pick up the drug, say the name aloud to the pharmacist and/or show him the paper so you can double-check that you're getting the right medication.

Mistake #3: **Accepting an "average" dose.** When prescribing a drug, most doctors choose an average dose that would cover people of various sizes and ages. It's approximate, not precise.

How errors can occur: Suppose that you need a 10-mg dose of Lasix (a diuretic), based on your body weight, gender and age. If the lowest dose from the manufacturer is 20 mg, that's probably what you'll get (you could be instructed to cut the pill in half, but that may not happen). Too-high doses increase the risk for side effects and other complications.

My advice: Tell your doctor that you'd like to start low. Ask for the lowest possible effective dose. You and your doctor can increase it later.

Mistake #4: **Splitting pills that should never be split.** Some people split their pills in half to save money. But some pills can be safely split...others can't.

How errors can occur: Splitting a time-released medication could cause all of the active ingredient to be released at once. Or the pill's protective coating may be damaged, causing the drug to be broken down in the stomach rather than in the intestine, so it is not properly absorbed.

My advice: If cost is an issue, tell your doctor. There might be a lower-priced medication that will work as well. For example, a generic antiviral can cost $9, while a brand-name option could be as much as $65.

Mistake #5: Taking double doses. This happens a lot—mainly because people don't realize what the active ingredients are in the various drugs they're taking.

How errors can occur: Let's say that you take OTC *acetaminophen* for joint pain. But maybe you are taking a cold medicine that also contains acetaminophen. Then your doctor or dentist gives you a prescription for Tylenol with codeine (which contains even more acetaminophen). You could wind up getting a double or even triple dose.

Too much acetaminophen can cause liver damage, particularly when combined with alcohol.

My advice: Even though the active ingredients are listed on package inserts or packaging for all drugs, ask your pharmacist about this when you pick up a medication (see the box on page 286). If any active ingredients are found in more than one of the drugs you take, ask your pharmacist and/or doctor if the combined dosage is safe.

When Is the Best Time to Take Your Meds? Follow Your Body Clocks...

Georgios Paschos, PhD, research assistant professor of pharmacology at the Smilow Center for Translational Research at the Perelman School of Medicine at the University of Pennsylvania in Philadelphia. His research focuses on biochemistry, molecular biology and chronobiology, the study of the physical, mental and behavioral changes that occur in 24-hour cycles.

If you have asthma, have you ever noticed that it tends to flare up early in the morning? Or maybe you have arthritis and have wondered why your pain often gets worse in the morning...or the evening. What you might not know is that your body's internal rhythms are behind the curious patterns that occur for many health conditions...and that these cycles can be a key to optimizing medical treatment and reducing side effects.

Until recently, it was believed that there was one "body clock" that controlled our internal rhythms. Now, research shows that we all have numerous body clocks that regulate how our bodies operate over a 24-hour cycle. Your body clocks trigger daily changes in body temperature, hormones, sleepiness and wakefulness, digestive efficiency and more. These fluctuations influence the time of day when you're more likely to have symptoms and when treatments, such as medications, can be more effective.

How to use your body clocks to get the best treatment for common health conditions...

ARTHRITIS: NIGHT OR MORNING PAIN?

If you have osteoarthritis, you probably have more pain late in the day, while if you have rheumatoid arthritis, pain and stiffness will often peak in the morning.

What to do: It is generally best to take your pain medication two to four hours before the pain usually starts. If your pain is worst first thing in the morning, talk to your physician about taking a delayed-release pain reliever at bedtime.

BETTER ASTHMA CONTROL

Asthma flare-ups tend to occur more often in the early morning than at other times of day.

Why: The lungs are less active during sleep, which can cause lung congestion when you first wake up.

What to do: If you use an oral steroid for long-term asthma control, ask your doctor about taking it around 3 pm. It will reach its

---

Daily Blister Packs Can Save Your Life

Can't remember if you took your medicines? Ask your pharmacist to make daily blister packs containing all your medicines. Not all pharmacies can make the packs—and the ones that do probably will charge extra for them, and that cost will not be reimbursed by insurance. But it may be a worthwhile expense if you want to be sure that you take all prescribed medicines every day and don't accidentally take any pill more than once.

(*Editor's note*: You also can buy a plastic pill organizer at most pharmacies that has compartments for daily pills.)

Consumer Reports on Health. *ConsumerReports.org*

---

peak effectiveness after six to 12 hours—while you are sleeping. However, a short-acting bronchodilator such as albuterol typically should be taken a bit later, usually around 6 pm, because it reaches its peak effectiveness four to six hours later.

BEST TIME TO TAKE BLOOD PRESSURE MEDICATION

Your blood pressure naturally fluctuates over 24 hours. It reaches its highest level at about midday...declines somewhat in the evening... and reaches its lowest level while you sleep. It starts climbing again in the hour before you wake up. When you first get out of bed in the morning, you can expect up to a 25-point increase in systolic (top number) blood pressure. There also appears to be an early-morning increase in the tendency of blood to clot. These factors could explain why about half of all heart attacks and other cardiovascular events occur between 6 am and noon.

What to do: If you are on blood pressure–lowering medication, ask your doctor if you should take it at night. A recent Spanish study found that people who took at least one of their blood pressure drugs at night had better overall blood pressure control. They also were about one-third less likely to have a heart attack or stroke than those who took their pills in the morning.

Also: If you take a daily low-dose aspirin to prevent a heart attack, talk to your doctor about taking it at night so that it will be absorbed in time to counteract the tendency of blood to clot early in the day. Night is also a good time to take cholesterol-lowering drugs—the amount of cholesterol produced by the liver is highest in the middle of the night.

MORE EFFECTIVE CHEMOTHERAPY

Cancer cells divide, multiply and die at predictable times of the day (timing depends on the type of cancer). By giving chemotherapy at specific times, oncologists can target cancer cells when they're most vulnerable—and when healthy cells are more resistant to a drug's toxic effects. Proper timing also can help minimize side effects from chemo.

Night Shift Alert

Night workers are more likely to be obese than people who work days, studies have shown. They're also more prone to diabetes and high blood pressure, among many other health problems.

Reason: Your internal clocks expect you to be active during the day and to sleep at night. People who work at night often consume most of their calories during the night, which can cause weight gain even when their total daily calories are the same as for people who eat at more conventional times and don't gain weight.

Additionally, people who are active at night have a rise in blood pressure and changes in hormone output, which can contribute to health problems.

What to do: Avoid getting most of your calories at night. For example, if you work the 8 pm to 4 am shift, have your main meal around 7 pm. Drinking plenty of water also can help prevent overeating during the shift.

People who don't work nights should avoid eating at night as well.

Best: Eat dinner at least three hours before bedtime.

Also: No matter what time you go to bed, try not to eat any snacks two hours beforehand. A before-sleep snack produces energy that's not needed—the excess calories get stored as fat.

Example: Recent lab research has found that the self-repair mechanisms of some cancer cells work six to seven times faster during the day than at night. This suggests that late-day or evening chemotherapy might be more effective than treatments given earlier.

What to do: If you need chemotherapy, ask your oncologist about the timing. There may be times of day when the treatment is more likely to work—and less likely to cause side effects.

YOUR BODY CLOCKS

It used to be thought that the body had just one "master clock"—a tiny group of cells in the suprachiasmatic nuclei part of the brain. Scientists have since learned that every cell in the body has an individual clock that controls how that cell behaves at different times of day.

The Hidden Danger of Medications—These Popular Drugs Can Steal Crucial Nutrients from Your Body

Suzy Cohen, RPh, a licensed pharmacist based in Boulder, Colorado. She is the author of the syndicated column *"Dear Pharmacist"* and numerous books, including *Drug Muggers: Which Medications Are Robbing Your Body of Essential Nutrients—and Natural Ways to Restore Them* (Rodale).

Chances are, you have a thief living in your home. This thief comes in the form of medication that can rob your body of a variety of essential nutrients.

It's true that many drugs on the market today effectively treat health problems. But if you're taking one of the thousands of over-the-counter (OTC) and prescription drugs that steals nutrients from your body, it's crucial that you know what to do to protect yourself. Here are some of the worst "drug muggers"—along with supplements you may be able to take to counteract their nutrient-depleting effects...*

NONSTEROIDAL ANTI-INFLAMMATORY DRUGS (NSAIDS)

Nutrient robbed: Folate. It can be depleted by aspirin, *ibuprofen* (Motrin) and prescription NSAIDs, such as *diclofenac* (Voltaren). This B vitamin, which is vital for the production of the mood-regulating neurotransmitter dopamine, also helps maintain DNA and build red blood cells.

Low folate levels are associated with elevated levels of the amino acid homocysteine, which has been linked to an increased risk for heart attack, stroke, Alzheimer's disease and cancer.

When to be concerned: Taking NSAIDs, at recommended doses, for a few consecutive days isn't a problem, but daily use for more than two weeks (which often occurs with such conditions as back pain and tendinitis) may compromise folate levels enough to dampen your mood.

Simple blood tests can detect dangerously elevated homocysteine levels and/or low folate levels.

Supplement to consider: If your homocysteine level is elevated or your folate level is too low, you may benefit from an activated folic acid supplement (folic acid is the synthetic form of folate, and "activated" means that it's easily absorbed by the body).

Typical dosage: 1 mg daily.

Good products: Seeking Health L-5-MTHF Lozenges, $17.95 for 60 lozenges...and Thorne Research 5-MTHF, $18.65 for 60 capsules, both at Amazon.com.

STATINS

Nutrient robbed: Coenzyme Q10, also known as CoQ10 or "Q." This nutrient can be depleted by cholesterol-lowering statins, such as *atorvastatin* (Lipitor) and *rosuvastatin* (Crestor). A vitamin-like substance that acts as a powerful antioxidant, Q supports healthy brain, heart and muscle function.

Statin drugs work by suppressing an enzyme called HMG-CoA Reductase, which the body requires to produce cholesterol. But this action also depletes Q levels.

When to be concerned: Because *Q* (ubiquinol is its active form) supports healthy muscle

*Never stop taking a prescription drug without talking to your doctor. Also, check with your doctor before trying these supplements if you take any medications or have a chronic medical condition.

Common Antibiotics Can Cause Serious Nerve Damage

Fluoroquinolones, such as *ciprofloxacin* (Cipro), *levofloxacin* (Levaquin), moxifloxacin (Avelox), *norfloxacin* (Noroxin) and others, often are used to treat respiratory, bladder and sinus infections. The nerve damage, peripheral neuropathy, is not common, but it can be severe when it does occur. If you take a fluoroquinolone and start having any symptoms—such as nerve tingling, burning or weakness—immediately contact your doctor.

Jay S. Cohen, MD, adjunct associate professor of psychiatry and family and preventive medicine at University of California-San Diego and author of *Prostate Cancer Breakthroughs* (Oceansong).

function, symptoms often strike the heart muscle first, in the form of palpitations. You might also experience overall muscle aches and weakness. If such changes occur, it may be within weeks of starting a statin or not until a year later.

Supplement to consider: In a study published in *The American Journal of Cardiology*, CoQ10 supplements reduced muscle pain severity by 40% over a 30-day period in people taking statins.

Typical dosage: 100 mg of CoQ10 daily—it's best taken in the morning because of its energizing effect, while a statin is usually taken in the evening when cholesterol production peaks.

Good products: Healthy Origins Ubiquinol, $56.24 for 150 softgels, Amazon.com...and Nature Made CoQ10 Liquid Softgels, $23.99 for 40, *Walgreens.com*.

ACID BLOCKERS

Nutrients robbed: B vitamins, minerals such as calcium, magnesium and zinc, and other nutrients. They can be depleted by acid blockers and antacids used to treat heartburn and reflux.

These drugs reduce stomach acid production, which raises pH level. But while less stomach acid means less painful heartburn, it also means less acid to break down the food you eat, compromising your body's absorption of important nutrients.

For example, when used for a year or more, proton pump inhibitor (PPI) acid blockers, such as *omeprazole* (Prilosec) and *esomeprazole* (Nexium), may double risk for hip fracture in adults over age 50—likely due to the sharp drop in calcium and vitamin D absorption.

Less acid also can increase one's risk of developing adult-onset food sensitivities—for example, even if you've never been bothered by dairy or wheat products, you might have stomach problems when you eat these foods after three to six months of daily PPI use. Long-term use of PPIs also has been shown to deplete magnesium enough to cause irregular heartbeat and seizures. For this reason, your doctor should monitor your magnesium level every four to six months if you take a PPI.

When to be concerned: Restless legs syndrome, elevated blood sugar and unexplained digestive complaints may be due to a PPI-induced magnesium deficiency.

Supplements to consider: Spirulina and chlorophyll, two natural types of algae, are the most effective and convenient ways to restore the nutrients depleted by acid blockers. Follow label instructions.

Good products: Nutrex Hawaii Spirulina Pacifica, $29.99 for 180 tablets, Nutrex-Hawaii.com...and Sun Chlorella, $27.19 for 300 tablets, Amazon.com.

ANTIDEPRESSANTS

Nutrient robbed: Iodine, a mineral required for healthy cell metabolism and thyroid function. It can be depleted by selective serotonin reuptake inhibitors (SSRIs), the most widely prescribed antidepressants in the US.

When to be concerned: If you're low on iodine (urine testing is available), you may experience hair loss, weight gain, depressed mood and lowered immunity—all due to sluggish thyroid function.

Supplements to consider: For low iodine, consider kelp or iodine supplements. Follow label instructions.

Good products: Solgar North Atlantic Kelp, $12.36 for 250 tablets, iHerb.com...ThyroScript (a product I helped formulate), $29.95 for 60 capsules, ScriptEssentials.com.

Do You Really Need an Antibiotic?

Joseph Kellerstein, DC, ND, a chiropractor and naturopathic and homeopathic physician who lectures at the Canadian College of Homeopathic Medicine and internationally. He has private practices in Toronto and Oshawa, Ontario, Canada. *DrJoeND.com*

Most likely you've been taught that if you have any type of bacterial infection, you must take an antibiotic. But overuse of antibiotics is increasingly rendering them ineffective and contributing to the rise of

Homeopathy for Skin Infections

Silica, a homeopathic remedy, helps treat painful skin infections—such as boils, inflamed acne and skin wounds—that seem to take forever to heal.

Natural approach: Take one pellet (6C concentration) every day for seven to 14 days until the area is about 80% healed. After that, watch the area for a few days to make sure it finishes healing.

Caution: If, at any point, the wound gets very red and inflamed...if redness spreads quickly...or if you have a high fever and/or chills, see your doctor immediately. Also, see your doctor if the wound does not finish healing after using the silica. These are signs that you may need an antibiotic.

deadly drug-resistant superbugs. Not only are new strains of MRSA now emerging, but other types of bacteria, including Clostridium difficile and Salmonella, are becoming increasingly difficult to treat.

What's more: Antibiotics inhibit the growth of nearly all bacteria in the body that they come into contact with (good and bad), often causing annoying side effects such as diarrhea and yeast and intestinal infections.

Time to change your thinking: For many minor infections, natural antibiotics found in foods, supplements and herbs can eliminate harmful microbes just as well as prescription antibiotics—without side effects. Plus, if you do need a prescription antibiotic, natural products can often help these medications work more effectively.

If you think you have an infection: See your doctor.* He/she can tell you whether antibiotics are necessary or if it is safe to try natural products—some may interact with medications you are taking. (A high fever—with or without chills—is one sign you may need an antibiotic.) If you are cleared to try a natural regimen, check back with your doctor if the infection does not improve within 48 hours.

*To find a naturopathic or homeopathic doctor near you, go to *Naturopathic.org* or *HomeopathyUSA.org*.

PROBIOTICS FOR RESPIRATORY INFECTIONS

You probably already know to take probiotics or eat yogurt to reduce the chance of side effects when you are on antibiotics. What you might not know is that probiotics also can help prevent and treat infections. And yogurt isn't the only food source. Little-known probiotic-rich alternatives include fermented vegetables (such as sauerkraut and kimchi)...fermented soy foods (such as miso and tempeh)...and kefir, a fermented milk product. When you eat these foods, their beneficial bacteria displace some of the disease-causing bacteria and secrete substances that inhibit or kill harmful germs.

A study found that individuals who took daily supplements of Lactobacillus reuteri (a common probiotic) were less than half as likely to take sick days for upper-respiratory or gastrointestinal illnesses than those who took placebos.

Natural approach: Regularly consuming probiotic foods helps prevent and treat infections. If you get recurrent infections and/or frequently use antibiotics, a probiotic supplement may be advised as well. Check with your doctor for the best probiotic and dosage for you.

COLLOIDAL SILVER FOR EAR INFECTIONS, MORE

The antibiotic properties of colloidal silver were first described nearly 2,000 years ago. It comes as a suspension—microscopic bits of silver are suspended in water or a gel-like substance—and can be used for ear, nose, throat and eye infections. Another silver product, silver sulfadiazine cream, is used to prevent and treat skin and wound infections.

Natural approach: Colloidal silver can be used orally or topically, depending on the condition being treated. Use a product that contains "true silver particles" rather than "ionic silver," which may be less effective at killing pathogens.

Caution: Colloidal silver can cause argyria, a grayish or bluish skin discoloration that may be permanent if you take massive doses (38 g per day). A standard colloidal silver product has less than 1 mg of silver per dose.

OIL OF OREGANO FOR THROAT AND BLADDER INFECTIONS

Oregano contains carvacrol, a powerful antimicrobial chemical compound. In a lab study, even low doses of oregano oil inhibited the growth of staph (Staphylococcus aureus) as effectively as streptomycin and other antibiotics. I recommend this oil for throat and bladder infections.

Natural approach: Add one or two drops of concentrated oregano oil to one teaspoon of olive or coconut oil to avoid burning your mouth. Take once a day during an infection.

GARLIC FOR DIARRHEA, MORE

Garlic has allicin, a broad-spectrum antimicrobial agent that fights a variety of bacteria, viruses and fungi. It's been found to be effective against Helicobacter pylori, a bacterium linked to stomach ulcers and cancer, and against certain bacteria that cause diarrhea.** Even some antibiotic-resistant strains of H. pylori responded to garlic in studies. And in both World Wars, garlic was used to prevent wound infections.

Natural approach: For prevention and treatment of the infections above, take deodorized garlic capsules (such as Vitacost Deodorized Garlic Ultra). They're more convenient—and less smelly—than eating lots of fresh garlic. Follow label directions. For a topical solution for wounds, mix one part garlic juice (found in health-food stores) with three parts water. Apply to gauze and place on skin. Never put garlic juice or crushed garlic directly on the skin—it can cause irritation.

****Caution*: If diarrhea lasts for more than 24 hours in a child or more than two days in an adult, see a doctor. Also, see a doctor if diarrhea is accompanied by blood in your stool, severe abdominal pain or signs of dehydration, such as dry mouth and/or low urine output.

High Doses of Common Pain Relievers Raise Risk for Heart Disease

According to recent research, people who take more than 400 milligrams (mg)/day of *celecoxib* (Celebrex) have one-third higher risk for cardiovascular disease than people who take less.

Garret A. FitzGerald, MD, professor at the Institute for Translational Medicine and Therapeutics, Perelman School of Medicine, University of Pennsylvania, Philadelphia, and a participant in an analysis of studies published in *The Lancet.*

Painkillers Can Harm Your Hearing

Women who regularly took *ibuprofen* (such as Advil or Motrin) or *acetaminophen* (Tylenol) at least twice a week had up to a 24% higher risk for hearing loss than women who used the painkillers infrequently. Other studies have found similar effects in men. These pain relievers may damage the cochlea in the inner ear by reducing blood flow or depleting antioxidants.

Self-defense: Limit painkillers to occasional short-term use—but talk to your doctor before making any changes in your medications.

Study of more than 62,000 women by researchers at Harvard Medical School, Boston, published in *American Journal of Epidemiology.*

ER Visits Tied to Ambien On the Rise

U.S. Substance Abuse and Mental Health Services Administration, news release.

There has been a dramatic increase in the number of emergency-room visits related to sleep medications such as Ambien, according to a recent US study by the U.S. Substance Abuse and Mental Health Services Administration (SAMHSA).

Adverse reactions to *zolpidem*—the active ingredient in the sleep aids Ambien, Ambien CR, Edluar and Zolpimist—rose almost 220% between 2005 and 2010, researchers found.

STUDY DETAILS

After analyzing findings from a public health surveillance system that monitors drug-related illnesses and deaths, the researchers found that emergency-room cases involving medications such as Ambien increased sharply from about 6,000 in 2005 to more than 19,000 in 2010.

The study authors concluded that use of these drugs for the short-term treatment of insomnia should be carefully monitored. Zolpidem, which has been approved by the U.S. Food and Drug Administration, has been used safely and effectively by millions of Americans, but adverse reactions to the medication have increased. Most of these cases involved people aged 45 and older, the researchers said.

"Although short-term sleeping medications can help patients, it is exceedingly important that they be carefully used and monitored," SAMHSA administrator Pamela Hyde said in an agency news release. "Physicians and patients need to be aware of the potential adverse reactions associated with any medication, and work closely together to prevent or quickly address any problems that may arise."

WOMEN AFFECTED MORE

Women were more often affected than men. The findings revealed that during the study time frame, there was a 274% increase in the number of women who went to the emergency room due to a reaction involving zolpidem, compared with a 144% increase among men. In 2010 alone, women accounted for 68% of all trips to the emergency room for an adverse reaction related to zolpidem, the researchers said.

Possible adverse reactions from medications containing zolpidem include:

- **Daytime drowsiness**
- **Dizziness**
- **Hallucinations**
- **Agitation**
- **Sleep-walking**
- **Drowsiness while driving**

In response to the increase in adverse reactions, in January 2013 the FDA required drug manufacturers to cut the recommended dose for women in half. The FDA also recommended that drug companies reduce the dosage for men.

SLEEP AIDS AND OTHER DRUGS DON'T MIX

The study authors also noted that adverse reactions to these sleep aids could be worsened when the medication is taken with other substances, such as certain antianxiety drugs and narcotic pain relievers.

The SAMHSA report said that in 2010, half of all emergency-room visits related to zolpidem involved its interaction with other drugs. Moreover, 37% of all emergency visits resulted from the combination of these sleep aids and drugs that depress the central nervous system.

info For more information on zolpidem, visit the U.S. National Institutes of Health website, *http://www.nlm.nih.gov/medlineplus/druginfo/meds/a693025.html.*

Heartburn Drugs May Lead to Vitamin B-12 Deficiency

According to recent research, people who took proton-pump inhibitors, such as *lansoprazole* (Prevacid), *omeprazole* (Prilosec) and *esomeprazole magnesium* (Nexium), for two years or longer were 65% more likely to have a vitamin B-12 deficiency. Those who took histamine 2 receptor antagonists, such as *ranitidine hcl* (Zantac), were 25% more likely. B-12 deficiency can lead to anemia, neurological problems and/or dementia.

Douglas A. Corley, MD, PhD, MPH, a research scientist at Kaiser Permanente, Oakland, California. He is lead author of a study published in *The Journal of the American Medical Association.*

New Drug May Help Immune System Fight Cancer

Roy Herbst, MD, PhD, chief, medical oncology, Yale University, New Haven, Connecticut.

Drew Pardoll, MD, PhD, codirector, cancer immunology, Johns Hopkins Sidney Kimmel Comprehensive Cancer Center, Baltimore.

Press briefing, American Society of Clinical Oncology.

An experimental drug that taps the power of the body's immune system to fight cancer is shrinking tumors in patients for whom other treatments have failed, an early study shows.

The drug binds to a protein called PD-L1 that sits on the surface of cancer cells and makes them invisible to the immune system, almost like a cloaking device.

"That [the protein] allows the tumor cell to grow unchecked and cause harm to the patient," said study author Roy Herbst, MD, PhD, chief of medical oncology at Yale University.

But with the protein blocked, the immune system can see and destroy cancer cells.

DRUG STUDY RESULTS

Of 140 patients in the pilot safety study, 29 (or 21%) initially saw significant tumor shrinkage after at least three months on the medication. Researchers say 26 patients have continued to respond over time, including some who have been on the drug for more than a year. One patient saw tumors disappear completely.

The drug also seems to work on a wide range of cancers, including some of the toughest to treat, including non-small cell lung cancer, melanoma skin cancer, colorectal cancer, kidney cancer and stomach cancer.

"This has all the characteristics of a really amazing drug," said Dr. Herbst, who has been testing new cancer medications for two decades. "I can count on one hand the number of times I've seen response rates like this."

The study was funded by Genentech/Roche, the company that is developing the drug. The results were presented by the American Society of Clinical Oncology in advance of its annual meeting.

Study results presented at medical meetings are considered preliminary because they have not been subjected to the rigorous scrutiny required for publication in a medical journal.

SIMILAR DRUGS IN DEVELOPMENT

At least four other companies—Merck, Bristol-Meyers Squibb, MedImmune and Amplimmune—also are racing to develop drugs that target PD-L1 or the molecule that binds to it (PD-1).

"I don't think in the history of cancer therapy have you had five or more companies virtually simultaneously developing antibodies targeted at the same pathway," said Drew Pardoll, MD, PhD, codirector of cancer immunology at the Johns Hopkins Sidney Kimmel Comprehensive Cancer Center, in Baltimore.

Dr. Pardoll is testing a drug that targets PD-1 for Bristol-Myers Squibb. He was not involved in the above study.

The drugs are part of a wave of new treatments that work by spurring the immune system to take on tumors. These drugs are building on the successes of medications like Provenge, the first cancer immunotherapy, which was approved in 2010 to treat prostate tumors, and Yervoy, which was approved in 2011 to treat metastatic melanoma.

Yervoy works early in the immune reaction to wake up T-cells that are essentially napping on the job, Dr. Pardoll said. The PD-1 and PD-L1 drugs work later, at the cellular level.

"This is a whole new kind of treatment, and the early data has looked so impressive," Dr. Pardoll said. "I think this just reflects the excitement among biotechnology companies and big pharma in this field."

Researchers are excited because most cancer drugs perform poorly in early trials. A study published in the journal *Clinical Cancer Research* in August 2005 found that middle-of-the-road response rates for cancer drugs in early trials was just 3%, with the best response rate topping out at 18%.

Response rates are so dismal in part because doctors usually don't try unproven drugs in cancer patients until they have run out of other op-

Painkillers Can Cause Severe Liver Damage

Several prescription painkillers contain 325 mg of *acetaminophen* or more.

Example: Percocet contains *oxycodone* and acetaminophen. The most severe liver damage occurred in patients who took more than the prescribed dose or took more than one product containing acetaminophen. OTC products that contain acetaminophen include Excedrin, NyQuil and Sudafed—and Tylenol's only ingredient is acetaminophen.

Jane C. Ballantyne, MD, FRCA, a professor of anesthesiology and pain medicine at University of Washington School of Medicine, Seattle.

tions. All the patients in this study had seen their cancer progress despite several prior treatments. Most had seen their cancer spread beyond its original site.

Dr. Pardoll said he also has been impressed with the length of time that patients continue to see benefits from the medications in the recent study.

"Among the patients that did respond to anti-PD-1, who had been followed for more than a year, roughly two-thirds were still in a response a year out," he said. "That's something you don't see with chemotherapy; you don't see it with current targeted therapies.

"We think this is because the immune system is being re-educated," Dr. Pardoll continued. "If that's the case, will we be able to discontinue the antibody and have the patient's immune system take over and keep the cancer at bay?"

DOWNSIDE OF NEW TREATMENT

PD stands for programmed death, and together the two molecules work to switch off the body's immune response. Blocking one or the other keeps the immune system active, which is good for fighting cancer, but there are also early signs that manipulating this response may have a downside.

Although the drugs have great promise, the researchers said they also were keeping an eye on the adverse side effects, some of which have been very serious. Those side effects include lung and liver inflammation, rashes and hypoglycemia (low blood sugar), perhaps because of a problem with the thyroid gland. Researchers believe these reactions are caused by autoimmunity—the body mistakenly attacking its own organs and tissues.

In a study published the *New England Journal of Medicine*, three patients who were taking an anti-PD-1 drug died from pneumonitis, or inflammation of the lungs.

The researchers said they're working to understand why the drugs seem to be particularly toxic to the lungs and to mitigate their adverse effects.

"We need to be cautious about the toxicities," Dr. Herbst said. "It's great that we're making progress, and now we need to go to randomized trials."

info To find clinical trials that are testing immunotherapy drugs, visit the website of the Cancer Immunotherapy Trials Network at *http://citninfo.org/index.html.*

Oral Zinc Shortens Colds

Using oral zinc lozenges or syrup can end a cold a day and a half sooner than not using zinc. Larger doses bring greater benefits, primarily for adults. But zinc users often report nausea and a bad taste in the mouth.

Meta-analysis of 17 trials, including a total of 2,121 participants, by researchers at The Hospital for Sick Children, Toronto, Canada, and McMaster University, Hamilton, Canada, published in *Canadian Medical Association Journal.*

Watch Out for TV Drug Ads: 67% of Claims Are Not True

Adrienne E. Faerber, PhD, fellow, Center for Medicine and the Media, The Dartmouth Institute for Health Policy and Clinical Practice, Lebanon, New Hampshire. Her study was published in *Journal of General Internal Medicine.*

Remember the TV ads for certain sneakers that claimed to tone your legs and butt as you walked? Those ads don't air anymore because the Federal Trade Commission said that the manufacturers' claims were bunk...and Reebok and Skechers shelled out millions of dollars in settlements for making the claims.

Now, why does the sneaker industry get such scrutiny—while the drug industry makes loads of false or misleading claims and yet hears hardly a peep from regulators? And meanwhile, drugs can really hurt you...or kill you...which you can't say about sneakers!

Now there's additional statistical backup on the hype made by pharmaceutical companies. According to a recent study, two-thirds of claims made in TV commercials about drugs are misleading or simply not true.

Drug ads are meant to persuade consumers to take medicines.

Alarming: When ads persuade with falsehoods, people could end up being convinced to take drugs that they may not need. Given that all drugs carry a risk for side effects, some of which can be terribly severe, this is outrageous. Can you spot the half-truths, exaggerations, unproven claims and even falsehoods in drug ads? *Here's what to watch out for...*

JUDGMENT DAY FOR DRUG ADS

For the recent study, researchers at Dartmouth selected 168 television ads that ran during nightly news broadcasts on four major networks between 2008 and 2010. Then they determined the advertisements' major claims—the points that were most emphasized based on repetition, placement of the claim in the ad, duration of the claim, etc. For example, a claim that was said out loud more than once and also appeared in text was given more weight than a claim that was only presented orally.

Three analysts, all trained in how drugs work and in evaluating drug literature, reviewed these major claims and classified them as to their veracity. The researchers had access to each drug's technical information, an authoritative review of comparative effectiveness for each drug class and other pertinent facts. *What they found...*

- **Only a paltry 33% of major claims were considered completely true.** Examples of true statements included, "Lyrica is the only approved treatment for fibromyalgia," because at the time the commercial was aired, other products were used off-label to treat fibromyalgia, but only Lyrica had obtained FDA approval... and "Just two Aleve have the strength to relieve arthritis pain all day," because there was substantial, high-quality evidence to show that the two-pill dose relieves arthritis pain for 12 hours.

- **Another 10% of major claims were false.** Ads for nonprescription drugs were worst in this regard, with 17% of claims being false...by comparison, in prescription drug ads, 2% of claims were false.

Example: An ad claimed, "Alka-Seltzer crystal packs are a taste-free powder"—yet inspection of the label showed that the product included both flavoring and sucrose. The researchers also included unsubstantiated claims in the false category. For instance, "The difference between Advil PM and Tylenol PM is a better night's sleep," was rated as false because the specificity of this claim implied that specific head-to-head comparative evidence was available—yet no studies had been published comparing Advil PM (*ibuprofen* with *diphenhydramine*) versus Tylenol PM (*acetaminophen* with *diphenhydramine*), only studies comparing ibuprofen with acetaminophen.

The remaining 57% of major claims were potentially misleading. Prescription and nonprescription drug ads were about equally guilty of this advertising trick. *There were several different reasons why a claim might fall into the misleading category...*

- **Omission of important information.** This "cherry-picking" occurred in 11% of claims. The ads presented only certain favorable facts while omitting other relevant facts that consumers would need to fully evaluate the attribute. For example, a heartburn treatment that had recently switched from prescription to over-the-counter claimed that it was "the same medicine, [but with a] new location—the store shelf." While this claim was factually true, it failed to mention that stronger doses of the drug continued to be available only by prescription—which meant that, for some consumers, the same medicine was not available on the store shelf.

- **Exaggeration.** About 20% of claims fit into this category. For instance, the claim that "nothing works better than Prevacid" implies that Prevacid is superior to other heartburn remedies—but what the statement really means is that Prevacid is no worse than other drugs. Another example is the claim that Bayer Quick Release Crystals are "ready to work faster than caplets or tablets." This is misleading because, although the formulation may dissolve more quickly, it is not taken up by the body any more quickly, nor does it relieve pain any more quickly than other formulations.

- **Nonfactual claims.** These claims typically are opinions or statements about intangible characteristics that can be misinterpreted by consumers as objective product evaluations. They are the most common type of potentially misleading claim, representing 26% of claims—so it's especially important for consumers to learn to spot them, the researchers noted. Examples of nonfactual claims include, "Levitra works for me. Maybe it will work for you"...and "I'm doing my best to build strong healthy bones [with Boniva]."

Be a smart consumer: Simply being aware of the types of misleading and false claims pharmaceutical companies make—and how common they are!—can help keep you from falling for false advertising.

Sleeping Pills Dangerous for Hospital Patients

The fall rate in hospital patients given the sleep medication *zolpidem* (Ambien) was more than four times higher than in patients who didn't take the drug. Zolpidem posed greater susceptibility for falls than other risk factors, such as age or cognitive impairment, regardless of the dose.

If you're having trouble sleeping in the hospital: Ask that nighttime interruptions and noise be kept to a minimum and/or bring earplugs.

Timothy I. Morgenthaler, MD, professor of medicine, Center for Sleep Medicine, Mayo Clinic, Rochester, Minnesota.

Common Anesthesia Drug Linked to Higher Risk of Dying

Study titled "Anesthetic Induction with *Etomidate*, Rather than *Propofol*, Is Associated with Increased 30-Day Mortality and Cardiovascular Morbidity After Noncardiac Surgery," published in *Anesthesia & Analgesia*.

A patient anticipating surgery usually doesn't have much say about which anesthesia drug is used. Most of the time, a patient meets with the anesthesiologist just moments before the procedure, and he's asked only whether he has had any problems with anesthesia in the past. From there, the anesthesiologist decides what to use.

But we urge you to speak up before you're put under! That's because, according to a large recent study, people who receive one particular anesthesia drug are more likely to die or suffer serious complications in the weeks following surgery than those who get a different drug.

The study: Researchers at the Cleveland Clinic searched the medical records of more than 100,000 patients who had operations requiring general anesthesia at their facility between 2005 and 2009. In 84% of cases, patients got an anesthesia drug called *propofol* (Diprivan)...8% were given a drug called *etomidate* (Amidate)...the rest got other drugs or a combination of drugs. The patients who got etomidate were generally older and sicker, so—to level the playing field—the researchers matched each patient who received etomidate with up to three other patients with similar medical profiles who received propofol for the same surgical procedure.

Worrisome findings: Compared with patients who received propofol, those who got etomidate were 2.5 times as likely to die from any cause within 30 days after surgery. They also had a 50% higher risk of experiencing major cardiovascular problems—even though the study included only patients who were having noncardiac surgery. The findings did not vary regardless of the dose of etomidate, meaning that even the smallest amount was associated with increased risk.

Researchers aren't sure how etomidate, which is a short-acting drug, could affect patients several weeks after surgery. One possible explanation is that even a small dose of etomidate interferes with the function of the adrenal glands, which normally release the hormone cortisol in response to stressful situations (including surgery)—and this suppression increases the risk for shock, seizures, coma and death. Propofol also suppresses cortisol production, but etomidate's effect in this regard is 1,500 times greater.

Caveat: The researchers were limited to information gleaned from medical records, which did not necessarily include detailed explanations of the factors that led anesthesiologists to choose one drug over another...so there may have been good reasons why certain patients got etomidate. For instance, etomidate has the advantage of working very fast and minimizing the dangerous drop in blood pressure—and accompanying risk for abnormal heart rhythms or cardiac arrest during surgery—that can occur with general anesthesia. This is thought to be particularly important when dealing with critically ill patients. Still, this short-term advantage looks less attractive when you factor in etomidate's newly discovered longer-term risks...especially considering the fact that the drug's adrenal-suppressing effects last longer in critically ill patients than in healthier ones.

Self-defense: If you are anticipating surgery that requires general anesthesia, ask your anesthesiologist what type of drug will be used and why...and bring up the concerns about etomidate. Until additional studies shed more light on etidomate's safety or lack thereof, it's only prudent to consider using an alternative anesthesia drug.

Men's Health

To Test or Not? Smart New Thinking on PSA Screening

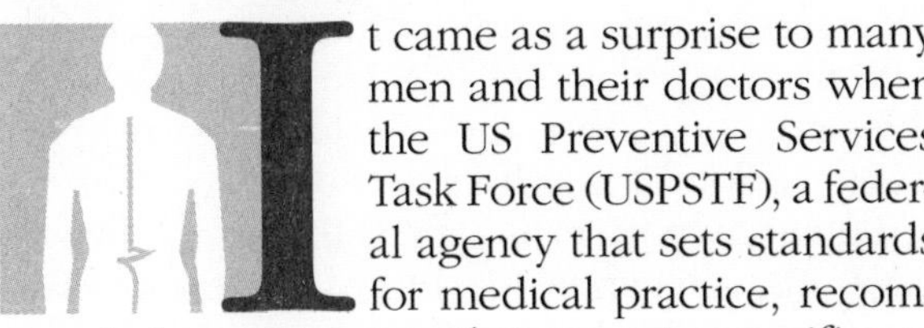

It came as a surprise to many men and their doctors when the US Preventive Services Task Force (USPSTF), a federal agency that sets standards for medical practice, recommended two years ago that prostate-specific antigen (PSA) screening be stopped. Altogether. For all men. The test, the USPSTF concluded, was causing more harm than good.

Since then, many experts and professional groups, including the American Urological Association and American Cancer Society, have sharply disagreed with that recommendation, arguing that PSA testing is too valuable to give up.

So what is the best approach for men? For the latest thinking on PSA screening—and details on important new tests that help prevent unnecessary biopsies—we turned to Peter T. Scardino, MD, a renowned authority on prostate cancer.

His advice: Don't throw out the PSA altogether—but rather screen smarter to maximize the good and minimize the harm associated with the test. *Here's how...*

WHAT'S WRONG WITH PSA TESTING?

Prior to the USPSTF recommendation, the PSA was typically given every year to men ages 50 and up. Results above a certain threshold—3 nanograms per milliliter (ng/mL) or 4 ng/mL, depending on how cautious the doctor was in his/her treatment approach—automatically led to a biopsy. If the biopsy found any cancer at all, surgery and/or radiation were usually recommended.

However, there were three problems with this approach...

Peter T. Scardino, MD, chairman of the department of surgery at Memorial Sloan-Kettering Cancer Center in New York City. He is coauthor of *Dr. Peter Scardino's Prostate Book: The Complete Guide to Overcoming Prostate Cancer, Prostatitis, and BPH* (Avery).

•**A rise in PSA usually doesn't mean cancer.** Many things can affect a man's PSA level, including benign prostate enlargement...inflammation of the prostate...and a urinary tract infection. Even use of aspirin, statins, diuretics and other medications has been found to have an effect.

Result: A lot of men were receiving unnecessary biopsies. Up to one-third who were biopsied experienced such adverse effects as pain, fever, bleeding or serious infection.

•**Most prostate cancer isn't deadly.** An estimated one out of three men ages 50 to 70—and nearly three-fourths of those over age 70—have some malignant cells in their prostates, which may sit harmlessly for years. But once cancer is found, it's hard not to take action.

Result: A lot of men have been treated for a disease that would have never caused trouble in their lifetimes.

•**Prostate cancer treatment can have lasting effects.** Surgery to remove the prostate and radiation to destroy prostate cancer cells carry a high risk for very unpleasant consequences. Up to 40% of men who receive prostate surgery and/or radiation suffer erectile dysfunction. Problems with urinary function were reported in 7% of men who had surgery. Among those who had radiation, 18% experienced urinary difficulties and 9% had problems with bowel function.

THERE IS A BETTER WAY

The question of PSA screening is a personal decision that each man needs to make with the help of his doctor. To provide guidance, doctors at Memorial Sloan-Kettering Cancer Center evaluated all the research on PSA to come up with an approach that gives men the greatest possible benefits of PSA testing while minimizing the potential dangers.

Our approach: Men should begin PSA testing at age 45 (or even younger if there's a family history of prostate cancer or the man is African-American). If the level is under 1 ng/mL, the test should be repeated every five years until age 60. If it's still under 1 ng/mL at that time, PSA screening can stop—the man's risk of ever dying of prostate cancer is negligible.

If PSA at age 45 is between 1 ng/mL and 3 ng/mL, repeat the test every two to four years, until age 70. If it's still normal, then testing stops. Even if you develop prostate cancer at this point, odds are you'll die of something else before the malignancy causes you trouble. If you're age 70 or older and have never been screened, check your PSA once or twice—if it's under 3 ng/mL, no further testing is needed.

Better Prostate Cancer Screening

Two new tests help men avoid unnecessary treatments. The PCA3 test measures urinary levels of prostate cancer gene 3, found only in cancerous prostate cells. Men with higher-than-normal PSA levels should ask for a PCA3 test before getting a biopsy. A PCA3 score of 25 or lower means that a biopsy likely is not needed. The Prolaris test uses cancer cells taken during a biopsy to determine how aggressive a tumor is. This helps doctors pursue the best course of treatment.

Prevention. Prevention.com

WHEN PSA IS HIGH

Most doctors who treat prostate cancer agree that PSA over 3 ng/mL suggests a possibility of a prostate malignancy that should be investigated. But it's crucial to remember that a single PSA reading often means nothing—transient elevations as high as 6 ng/mL are not unusual. In this situation, check the PSA level again in six to 12 weeks...if it's on its way down, repeat the test again two months later. If PSA remains over 3 ng/mL, you can have a biopsy or consider further testing (see below) that can analyze blood proteins in more detail.

New testing options: Ask your doctor about the Prostate Health Index, a new test that measures levels of PSA subtypes. In clinical trials, it reduced the number of men who were biopsied by 50% but still found almost all the cancers that required treatment. The test is now available from Beckman Coulter. A similar test, the 4Kscore (or 4 kallikrein score), showed good or better results in recent trials.* The 4Kscore blood test is available from Opko Health.

*Dr. Scardino is on the scientific advisory board of the company that developed the 4Kscore.

WHEN IT'S CANCER

If a man's prostate biopsy is positive for cancer, doctors usually analyze the cancerous tissue to determine his Gleason score, which indicates how likely the malignancy is to spread. A score of 7 means a medium risk of spreading...8 or above means the risk is high. The Gleason score isn't a perfect predictor of how a cancer will behave. But several new tests have recently become available to give patients and doctors additional valuable clues about a man's prostate cancer.

New tests all men should know about: The Prolaris (Myriad) and Oncotype DX (Genomic Health) assays analyze molecules that are produced by certain genes that regulate how rapidly cancer cells multiply (the tests are similar, so a man would have one or the other). Use of one of these tests helps determine whether a tumor with a Gleason score of 6 or even 7 must be treated aggressively or can safely be left alone and monitored.

Prostate Cancer Breakthroughs...a Doctor With the Disease Shares His Experience

Jay S. Cohen, MD, a nationally recognized expert on medications and side effects. He is author of *Prostate Cancer Breakthroughs* (Oceansong) and *Over Dose: The Case Against the Drug Companies* (Tarcher). He is a faculty member at University of California–San Diego and has lectured at the FDA and major medical conferences. *MedicationSense.com*

There are good reasons why men worry about prostate cancer. According to the American Cancer Society, it is the second-most-frequently diagnosed cancer (after skin cancer) in American men and the second-leading cause of cancer deaths (after lung cancer). One in every six men will ultimately be diagnosed with prostate cancer—about 240,000 each year, resulting in close to 30,000 deaths.

Sometimes the treatment is worse than the cure. In their zeal to prevent prostate cancer deaths, doctors send thousands of men for prostate-removal surgery or radiation, and more than half sustain sometimes lifelong impairments of their sexual functioning and/or bladder control. And surgery or radiation isn't always curative—about 25% of men relapse.

What's particularly alarming is that of the nearly 100,000 men who receive these treatments each year, 85% don't need them. This massive overtreatment has led expert government panels and medical associations to recommend discontinuing prostate specific antigen (PSA) testing, our most reliable early-warning test for prostate cancer—as if not diagnosing prostate cancer early will make the problem go away.

I was diagnosed with prostate cancer two years ago. *Here's what I learned—and what every man should know...*

DANGERS OF HALTING PSA TESTING

Use of PSA screening began around 1990. It worked, and annual deaths from prostate cancer dropped by 40%, from 50,000 to 30,000 a year. But it is a nonspecific test that can signal many prostate problems. An elevated PSA test does not always mean prostate cancer, but that is how some doctors interpret it. The solution to overtreatment is not to tell men to forgo the PSA test. The solution is to modernize our approach to better differentiate the men who need treatment from those who don't.

How to react to abnormal PSA results? An elevated PSA result can be caused by many factors such as prostate infection, an enlarged prostate gland, laboratory error, even recent sex. An elevated PSA test always should be repeated.

My advice: Begin annual PSA testing at age 50. If a blood relative has had prostate cancer or you are African-American, the risk for prostate cancer is higher, so begin PSA testing at age 40.

THE NEW, TARGETED BIOPSY

If your PSA test has risen above 4 ng/mL on repeated tests, your doctor may recommend a prostate biopsy, an invasive, outpatient test in which fine needles are inserted through the rectal wall into the prostate. A biopsy is the only way to confirm that prostate cancer is present and to determine its level of aggressiveness (Gleason score). A biopsy is an important test, yet of the 1.2 million performed each year, about half are unnecessary.

The vast majority of prostate biopsies are blind. The doctor takes 10 to 12 samples (cores) from diverse areas of the prostate gland, but there's no guarantee that he/she will hit the right spot. Blind biopsies miss at least 20% of prostate cancers.

A growing number of top-notch cancer centers now are using the new dynamic, contrast-enhanced MRI (DCE-MRI) that, for the first time, can identify prostate cancer within the gland (see below for more on this important test). If the DCE-MRI does not show areas suspicious for cancer, a biopsy may not be necessary. Moreover, approximately 40 doctors in the US perform an in-office test called color Doppler ultrasound that also can identify cancer within the prostate.

With DCE-MRI guidance or color Doppler ultrasound, the doctor can aim the biopsy needles at the targeted areas. Guided biopsies typically require fewer tissue samples, so there is less damage to the prostate gland and a lower risk of bleeding or infection. This is important because 4% of men undergoing blind biopsies require hospitalization for serious infection. Moreover, when blind biopsies do not obtain evidence of cancer, the biopsies may have to be repeated.

The New Test for Prostate Cancer

The following medical centers offer the DCE-MRI, which can identify cancer within the prostate gland.

- **California** Sharp Hospital and Medical Center, San Diego... University of California–Los Angeles(UCLA)...University of California–San Francisco (UCSF)
- **Illinois** University of Chicago Medical Center
- **Maryland** The Johns Hopkins Hospital, Baltimore
- **Massachusetts** General Hospital, Boston
- **Minnesota** Mayo Clinic, Rochester
- **New York** Memorial Sloan-Kettering Cancer Center, New York City...NYU Langone Medical Center, New York City
- **Pennsylvania** Jefferson Prostate Diagnostic Center, Philadelphia...University of Pittsburgh Medical Center
- **Texas** MD Anderson Cancer Center, Houston
- **Canada** Sunnybrook Research Institute, University of Toronto

ADVANCED PROSTATE MRI

Although doctors have been using MRIs for virtually every other part of the human body for 25 years, the technology had not existed to differentiate normal prostate tissue from prostate cancer. Now that the DCE-MRI can accurately identify prostate cancers, diagnostic methods and treatment options are taking a giant leap forward. But this is being done today at only 13 major cancer centers in the US.

With the DCE-MRI, the patient is injected with a gandolinium-based contrast agent that is absorbed more readily by cancerous tissue than by healthy prostate cells. This makes the cancerous tissue clearly visible if you have a high-powered MRI machine and the necessary software.

I was told by four prostate surgeons that I must have prostate surgery or radiation, but my DCE-MRI clearly showed that my cancer was limited and well-contained. This test was a game-changer for me—and for many others.

FOCAL THERAPY

With the new technology, we now can see that many cancers are present in only a part of the prostate gland. With this information, some doctors are recommending focal therapy—that is, treatment that removes only half of the prostate gland or just the area around the tumor. This approach is similar to the lumpectomies that some women elect to have for localized breast cancer.

These focal therapies do not cause nearly as much damage as prostatectomy or radiation, so adverse effects are far fewer and less severe. Cryotherapy, a freezing technique, is available in the US. Focal laser ablation, which employs a thin probe to burn the cancer, is in the latter stages of study here, and you can sign up for treatment at certain cancer centers. High-intensity focused ultrasound (HIFU), which heats the cancer to nearly 212°F, is available in Canada and overseas and is in FDA-approved clinical trials in the US. These therapies are performed in outpatient centers.

ACTIVE SURVEILLANCE

The majority of prostate cancers are low risk—the risk for death from this type of prostate cancer is only 2% over 10 years. So active surveillance sometimes is a good option. In active surveillance, your PSA levels are drawn regularly (every three months at the start) and a DCE-MRI is performed annually. Biopsy may be needed but not in every case. The key is that with the new tests, your prostate cancer can be tracked. Treatment can be delayed (or avoided) if the cancer doesn't change. With these methods, a man will know quickly if his cancer is getting more dangerous, and treatment can be started promptly.

It can be difficult for men to choose active surveillance. They often are so acutely stressed that they lapse into what I call the "get-it-out-now!" syndrome. This is another reason that there is so much overtreatment. Yet most prostate cancers grow slowly, so there usually is time to obtain a full diagnostic evaluation and to consider all of the options appropriate for your risk level. For example, you can consider active surveillance if you fit all of the following low-risk criteria—you have a normal digital rectal exam...your PSA is less than 10...your Gleason score is 6 or less...you have two or fewer positive biopsy cores out of the 12 samples taken...and none of the cores is more than 50% cancer.

After considering many options, I chose active surveillance and have done well for a year and a half.

High Doses of Selenium Double Risk for Prostate Cancer

Alan Kristal, DrPH, associate program head of the Cancer Prevention Program at Fred Hutchinson Cancer Research Center, Seattle, and leader of a study published in *Journal of the National Cancer Institute.*

In a recent study, men who had moderate or high levels of the antioxidant selenium at the start of the study and who then took daily supplements of 200 mcg of selenium doubled their prostate cancer risk.

What to do: Limit your selenium intake to no more than the recommended daily intake (RDI) of 55 mcg.

Allspice May Combat Prostate Cancer

Bal Lokeshwar, PhD, professor of urology and radiation oncology, Miller School of Medicine, University of Miami, Florida. His study was published in *Carcinogenesis.*

An aromatic flavoring that's familiar on the Thanksgiving buffet has a health benefit that men will be grateful for. That flavoring is allspice, which comes from the dried unripe berry of the tropical Pimenta dioica plant.

With a taste reminiscent of cinnamon, cloves, nutmeg and pepper all mixed into one savory little package, allspice is best known as the flavor powerhouse in pumpkin pie—but researchers recently discovered that it also may have the power to shrink prostate cancers. But then the question is...how would a man use it for health?

ALL-POWERFUL ALLSPICE

To understand why allspice might protect the prostate, you must start with the fact that most forms of prostate cancer thrive on androgens (male hormones, such as testosterone). That's why doctors treat prostate cancer with powerful drugs that either stop the production of androgens or block them from being used by the body. But the medications' side effects—severe hot flashes, decreased libido and increased risk for osteoporosis, diabetes and coronary artery disease—can be so difficult to tolerate that many men don't remain on the drugs long enough to reap the full benefits.

The recent study shows that allspice can block androgen receptor molecules that are vital to the growth and spread of prostate cancer—at least in mice. Though preliminary, this research is so encouraging that all men should take note.

Part of the study took place in test tubes. The researchers prepared an allspice extract from the crushed berries and distilled water, then mixed the extract with human prostate cancer cells. Using several different methods, they determined that the allspice extract slowed the growth of prostate cancer cells by half in just 48 hours...blocked the progression of the cancer cell cycle...and induced cancer cell death.

Next, the researchers tested allspice in animals. First, mice were injected with human prostate cancer cells to make tumors grow. Then, one group of mice was given allspice extract to drink every day...a second group was injected with the extract three times per week. Other mice, serving as controls, were not given any of the extract.

Six weeks later: Compared with prostate tumors in the control mice, tumors in the mice that were injected with the allspice extract were 58% smaller. Drinking the extract seemed even more beneficial, with tumors in that group of mice being 62% smaller than those in the control group. There were no apparent adverse effects from the allspice.

After some trial-and-error testing, the researchers determined that the compound in allspice responsible for the slower tumor growth was ericifolin. Rather than affecting androgens themselves (as anti-androgen drugs do), ericifolin prevents the androgen receptor from being synthesized in the cancer cells. Because it gets to the root cause of the trouble, the researchers said, this mechanism potentially makes ericifolin particularly useful in fighting a deadlier, advanced form of the disease (called hormone refractory prostate cancer) in which the receptor works autonomously, without the androgens.

Bonus: Ericifolin also has been shown to have antioxidant, antibacterial and pain-relieving effects.

Obviously, since this study was performed in test tubes and mice, it is way too early to suggest that allspice can prevent or cure prostate cancer in men—but the researchers did call it "potentially a unique dietary chemopreventive agent" in the fight against the number-two cause of cancer deaths among men.

Allspice generally is considered safe when consumed in amounts typically used to season foods, but not enough is known about its safety in medicinal amounts...and there is some concern that it may slow down blood clotting or interfere with medications that reduce blood clotting. Clearly, future studies are needed to test allspice's safety and efficacy in reducing prostate tumor size and/or preventing prostate cancer and to determine the most appropriate medicinal dosage. In the meantime, it's worth talking to your doctor about the possibility of adding more allspice to your diet.

Adding more allspice to your diet: To receive a dose of allspice equivalent to that which the mice received, a man would have to consume about two teaspoons of powdered allspice per day. You're probably not going to eat enough pumpkin pie daily to get that much allspice (though you might enjoy trying), but there are lots of other ways to get allspice into your diet. For instance, allspice is frequently used in Asian, Middle Eastern and Caribbean cuisine, especially Jamaican jerk seasoning and spiced teas. You can use allspice by sprinkling it on green beans, carrots, sweet potatoes or scrambled eggs...using it to season braised or barbequed meats after cooking...or adding it to ground coffee before brewing. Experiment to see what tastes good to you.

Prostate Device Gets Nod

Sheldon Marks, MD, associate clinical professor of urology, The University of Arizona College of Medicine, Tucson.

UroLift, a small, permanent implant designed for men with benign prostatic hyperplasia (BPH), now is available in the US. Less invasive than traditional BPH surgery, the tiny device pulls prostate tissue away from the urethra, relieving pressure and improving blocked urine flow. Men who received the device had an average 30% increase in urine flow and a decrease in other symptoms, such as frequency and urgency of urination. Side effects may include pain or burning during urination. UroLift may be covered by insurance.

Gene Test May Help Predict Prostate Cancer Aggressiveness

Columbia University, news release.
Louis Kavoussi, MD, chairman of urology, North Shore-LIJ's Arthur Smith Institute for Urology, New Hyde Park, New York.
Aaron Katz, MD, chairman of urology, Winthrop-University Hospital, Mineola, New York.

A new gene test may help identify slow-growing prostate cancers that will require treatment, a recent study suggests.

The test revealed the levels of "expression" of three aging-related genes within low-risk cancerous tumors and could be used to predict whether seemingly slow-growing prostate cancer will remain slow-growing, according to Columbia University Medical Center researchers.

Using the three-gene test along with existing cancer-staging tests could help doctors better determine which men with early prostate cancer can be safely monitored and spared the potential risks of prostate removal or other invasive treatments, the study authors suggested.

The investigators assessed the test in 43 prostate cancer patients who had been monitored for at least 10 years. All of the men had initially been diagnosed with low-risk cancer, but 14 eventually developed advanced prostate cancer. All 14 of those patients were correctly identified by the three-gene test, according to the study, which was published online in the journal *Science Translational Medicine.*

The researchers plan to conduct a larger study to assess the test's accuracy.

"Most of the 200,000 prostate cancers diagnosed each year in the US are slow-growing and will remain so, but the three-gene biomarker could take much of the guesswork out of the diagnostic process and ensure that patients are neither overtreated nor undertreated," study leader Cory Abate-Shen, a professor of urological oncology at Columbia University Medical Center, said in a university news release.

And, as study coauthor Dr. Mitchell Benson, chairman and professor of urology at the medical center, explained in the news release: "The problem with existing tests is that we cannot identify the small percentage of slow-growing tumors that will eventually become aggressive and spread beyond the prostate."

Currently, men diagnosed with low-risk prostate cancer can choose either active surveillance, which includes regular testing and monitoring but risks missing the window when the disease is localized and potentially curable, or aggressive treatment, which can cause serious side effects such as urinary incontinence and impotence.

EXPERTS COMMENT

Louis Kavoussi, MD, is chairman of urology at North Shore-LIJ's Arthur Smith Institute for Urology in New Hyde Park, New York. He said: "Men getting a diagnosis of prostate cancer are initially shocked and begin conjuring images of themselves as desperate, dying patients. In reality, the majority of patients with prostate cancer do not die of the disease, and a large portion can be managed with observation. This study looks at novel molecular tools to help define which patients can be managed conservatively, and avoid potential side effects and expensive treatments."

Aaron Katz, MD, chairman of urology at Winthrop-University Hospital in Mineola, New York, said: "In the current era, it is clear that PSA screening has detected many men with prostate cancer. In the years past, we believed that all men needed to be treated. The good news is that many men who are found to have these abnormal cells in their prostate may not need any treatment. With advances in genomics and DNA testing, we are now able to stratify those men with indolent disease, and prevent unnecessary treatment."

info The U.S. National Cancer Institute has more about prostate cancer at its website, *http://www.cancer.gov/cancertopics/wyntk/prostate.*

Radiation Therapy Overused in Advanced Prostate Cancer, Study Says

Justin Bekelman, MD, assistant professor, University of Pennsylvania Perelman School of Medicine, Philadelphia.
Colleen Lawton, MD, professor, radiation oncology, Medical College of Wisconsin, Milwaukee.
Journal of the American Medical Association

Most men given radiation to control pain from advanced prostate cancer undergo more treatments than they really need, a new study suggests.

Once cancer advances to invade the bones, radiation therapy is usually used to ease the pain it causes. And in the past decade, studies have shown that one treatment is enough for most patients.

But those findings have not made it into practice—at least for older US men with prostate cancer, researchers report in the *Journal of the American Medical Association.*

Looking at Medicare claims data, the investigators found that single-session treatments were done in only about 3% of men receiving radiation for prostate cancer that had spread to the bones. What's more, half of the patients went through more than 10 treatments.

The low rate of single treatment is surprising, said Colleen Lawton, MD, a radiation oncologist who was not involved in the study.

"But it's just as surprising that so many patients had more than 10 fractions," said Dr. Lawton, who chairs the board of directors for the American Society for Radiation Oncology.

"Fraction" refers to a session of radiation treatment. Studies have found that one treatment, at a relatively larger dose of 8 Gy (a unit of radiation dosage), is as effective for pain relief as 20 Gy given over five treatments, or 30 Gy given over 10 treatments.

And that data started emerging in the late 1990s. So it's not clear why so few prostate cancer patients get a single treatment, said lead researcher Justin Bekelman, MD, of the University of Pennsylvania Perelman School of Medicine in Philadelphia.

"We know that it takes time for clinical trial evidence to get into routine practice. But these findings are nonetheless surprising," Dr. Bekelman said.

"The fact is, this is a good treatment that's better for patients," he added. "It's effective, it's more convenient, and better for their quality of life. Single-fraction treatment should be the standard of care."

Dr. Lawton said there are some cases where patients might need 10 or more treatments—such as when the cancer has spread not only to the bones but also to the nearby soft tissue. But that would be only about 10% of patients.

"That would not explain the 50% in this study," Dr. Lawton said.

So what would explain the others? "It's likely a combination of factors," Dr. Bekelman said. Some doctors might worry about a recurrence after a single treatment, or the potential need for repeat radiation therapy later on, he noted.

On top of that, Dr. Bekelman said, "there's the reimbursement."

Doctors get paid per treatment, so there is a potential financial motivation, Dr. Lawton agreed. "I would hope that isn't an impetus," she said, "but it's possible that's part of it."

In this study of men aged 65 and older, the cost of radiation-related therapy averaged just under $1,900 for men who had one session, but about $5,000 for men who had 10 or more treatments.

"To give doctors the benefit of the doubt," Dr. Lawton said, "they may not have been aware of the research (supporting single treatments)."

Although the evidence started coming in more than a decade ago, it was in 2005 that a large US clinical trial showed that a single radiation treatment was just as good as multiple treatments for patients whose cancer had spread to the bones.

The current findings are based on Medicare data for 3,050 US men treated between 2006 and 2009, which might help explain why so few received a single treatment, Dr. Lawton said.

But whatever the reasons, she agreed that most patients should get a single session of radiation. Some may then need another treatment after about a year, Dr. Lawton noted. "But that's still a lot better than going in for multiple treatments," she said.

And the cost savings are not the primary reason to promote single treatment, Dr. Bekelman stressed. "This is a treatment that is just as effective, and shorter, and less expensive. It just makes sense," he said.

WHAT PATIENTS CAN DO

He and Dr. Lawton said patients should feel free to question their doctor if multiple radiation treatments are recommended for bone pain. "The question should be, 'Am I a candidate for single treatment?' And if not, why not?" Dr. Bekelman said.

He added that patients need not worry that doing one radiation treatment instead of several will affect their cancer survival. "The goal with this treatment is to treat pain. It has nothing to do with survival," Dr. Bekelman pointed out.

Other types of cancer, such as breast and lung cancers, commonly spread to the bones at advanced stages. And a single radiation treatment is effective at treating pain in those patients as well, Dr. Lawton said.

It's not clear whether single treatments are also underused in those patients. But, Dr. Lawton said, "I would guess that they are."

info The Choosing Wisely campaign has more on reducing unnecessary radiation therapy at the website *http://www.choosingwisely.org/doctor-patient-lists/american-society-for-radiation-oncology/.*

The Truth About Fish Oil

Geovanni Espinosa, ND, LAc, CNS, director, Integrative Urology Center, New York University Langone Medical Center, New York City.

A controversial bit of research concludes that eating a lot of oily fish or taking potent fish oil supplements may increase a man's risk of developing prostate cancer.

Moreover, marine sources of omega-3 fatty acids may also raise the risk for aggressive prostate cancer, according to a recent study by scientists at the Fred Hutchinson Cancer Research Center in Seattle.

So...should men stop taking fish oil?

In my opinion, this latest research on fish oil is weak. First, the study does not show that fish oil causes prostate cancer. The finding suggests only an association—in analyzing reams of health data on a group of men, the researchers found that men with prostate cancer were more likely to have high blood levels of the omega-3 fatty acids found in fish oil. But just why this might be the case isn't known.

Interestingly, in the media coverage, it wasn't widely reported that the same researchers inexplicably found a reduced risk for prostate cancer in men whose diets included more trans fats (the harmful type found in margarine) and omega-6 fatty acids (another dangerous fat, which is implicated in some cancers)!

It's crucial to be skeptical of new, headline-grabbing studies and to look at the preponderance of evidence. Clearly, there are multiple, high-quality studies showing that fish oil (from one's diet and supplements) has a wide range of health benefits, such as reducing risk for heart disease, stroke—and prostate cancer. I take fish oil—and will continue to do so. My suggestion to you is to be sure to discuss any supplement you take with a nutritionally oriented doctor, but don't make any changes based on this study alone.

"Low T" Therapy: Is It for You?

Ryan Terlecki, MD, urologist, Wake Forest Baptist Medical Center, Winston-Salem, North Carolina.

Steven Canfield, MD, chief, division of urology, University of Texas Health Science Center at Houston

When men are young, testosterone tends to get a bad rap, often blamed for aggressive and overly competitive behavior. But as men get older, the bad rap continues, though for a different reason.

In older men, it's low testosterone that has captured attention.

Testosterone, the male hormone, plays a vital role in many body functions, and low testosterone levels can leave men tired, uninterested in sex, infertile and with thinning bones, according to the US National Library of Medicine.

It's also a fairly common problem in older men. As many as four in 10 men older than 45 have lower than normal levels of testosterone, according to the American Urological Association.

But, replacing lost testosterone isn't a panacea, despite what you might have seen on TV.

"There's been a lot of advertising, and every guy that comes in now asks about testosterone," said Ryan Terlecki, MD, a urologist at Wake Forest Baptist Medical Center in Winston-Salem, NC. "They've been led to believe that it's a fountain of youth, but it's not a cure-all."

For example, many men hope that testosterone therapy will help treat erectile dysfunction. But, Dr. Terlecki said that though testosterone is a treatment for low libido and taking replacement testosterone may increase a man's sex drive, it's not a direct treatment for erectile dysfunction.

Testosterone replacement also isn't an option for men who want to preserve their fertility. That's because when a man takes testosterone therapy, the testosterone receptors in the body tell the brain that there's enough testosterone, and, in turn, the brain signals the testes to stop producing sperm.

Dr. Terlecki said it's possible that sperm production could return to normal levels after testosterone therapy is stopped. But there's no solid evidence that it will, so doctors prefer to err on the side of caution if a man believes he might still want to have children.

Men who have active prostate cancer or male breast cancer also aren't candidates for testosterone therapy.

However, other men with symptoms of low testosterone may want to consider it. For starters, that includes men who "might notice a drop in energy and low libido," Dr. Terlecki said.

Steven Canfield, MD, chief of urology at the University of Texas Health Science Center at Houston, said that symptoms of low testosterone that men might notice also include "the development of breast tissue, a loss of body hair, small or shrinking testicles, no need for shaving, flushing, sweats and bone loss."

But, he said, there are less specific symptoms, too. Men with low testosterone might also notice "a decrease in self-confidence, feeling sad or depressed, problems with sleeping, memory problems, reduction in body mass, and a decrease in work performance," Dr. Canfield said.

All it takes to tell if a man's testosterone level is low, he said, is a simple blood test.

Although low testosterone is common in older men, it's not necessarily a normal part of aging. Other conditions that are common with aging, such as obesity or depression, can cause lower levels of testosterone, according to research presented at the Endocrine Society meeting in Houston this year.

Dr. Canfield said that testosterone levels can drop if testicular tissue is lost, which can happen with age. And Dr. Terlecki said that prior testicular trauma, undescended testicles and radiation treatment to the testicles also can cause lower testosterone levels. Testosterone levels can drop because of a pituitary tumor, though that's rare, he said. And some medications, such as narcotics, can also lower testosterone levels.

Testosterone Therapy Caution

According to a recent study, prescriptions for testosterone increased threefold from 2001 to 2011, according to health data from more than 10 million men age 40 and older.

However: Only about half the men taking testosterone had been diagnosed as having hypogonadism (the inability to produce a sufficient amount of the hormone).

If you're a man considering testosterone replacement: Make sure your testosterone levels are below 350 ng/dL before beginning therapy. Possible side effects of testosterone replacement include worsening sleep apnea and mood swings.

Jacques Baillargeon, PhD, associate professor in preventive medicine and community health, The University of Texas Medical Branch at Galveston.

OPTIONS AVAILABLE FOR LOW T

Several options exist for treating low testosterone. For men who want to keep their fertility,

Dr. Terlecki said, the drug *clomiphene* can be prescribed. In men for whom that's no longer an issue, testosterone replacement therapy can boost testosterone levels.

Options for testosterone replacement, Dr. Canfield said, include injections, patches, a gel and implantable pellets. He said that a pill form of testosterone is available in other parts of the world, but not in the United States.

Injections are given once every two weeks, Dr. Terlecki said. The downside to this option is that injections provide a large dose of testosterone in the beginning but it drops fairly quickly.

Topical formulations, such as testosterone gel, are put on in the morning and absorbed within two to six hours and, if used consistently, provide a steady consistent dose of testosterone. "But, men have to remember to do it," Dr. Terlecki said. "And, they have to wait while the gel dries. It may leave the area feeling a little tacky."

Also, it's important not to expose children, pregnant women or women who may become pregnant to the testosterone on the skin because it can alter their hormonal balance.

Patches can provide a longer-term steady dose of testosterone, but they may cause irritation, Dr. Terlecki said. And implantable pellets, according to Dr. Canfield, can provide a steady, long-acting dose of testosterone. They're injected just underneath the skin on your backside during an outpatient office procedure.

This option is becoming increasingly popular because it lasts for four months and generally is inexpensive, Dr. Terlecki said.

RISKS AND MISCONCEPTIONS OF TESTOSTERONE THERAPY

Risks of testosterone therapy include an increase in the size of the prostate, water retention, worsening sleep apnea, a lower sperm count and an increase in the platelet count, which could increase the risk for blood clots, according to Dr. Canfield.

Both men agreed that testosterone therapy won't solve all of a man's health issues.

"The most important thing men need to know is that testosterone therapy isn't a substitute for taking care of overall health," Dr. Terlecki said. "A lot of men come in obese, with a poor diet and no exercise, and they want to blame low testosterone. While testosterone may play a role in their overall health, it needs to be viewed in context with these other factors."

info The Urology Care Foundation has more about low testosterone at its website, *http://www.urologyhealth.org.*

Hormone Troubles in Men

Jamison Starbuck, ND, a naturopathic physician in family practice and a guest lecturer at the University of Montana, both in Missoula. She is past president of the American Association of Naturopathic Physicians and a contributing editor to *The Alternative Advisor: The Complete Guide to Natural Therapies and Alternative Treatments.*

Out-of-whack hormones can turn women's lives upside down. But hormones are just as important to men's health as they are to women's. You see, a man's hormones—cortisol, DHEA, norepinephrine, testosterone and, yes, even estrogen and progesterone—affect everything from mood, sleep and memory to inflammation, heart disease risk and overall energy levels. Both men and women have the same hormones. It's just that the levels vary depending on your gender, and they often change significantly throughout life. So if you are a middle-aged or older man and aren't satisfied with your overall health, your hormones may be the culprit.

Start by asking yourself some basic questions: How well do you sleep? Do you eat well and get enough fluids? How often do you exercise? Do you have any chronic pain? How often are you happy? How do you feel about your sex life? If your assessment comes up short in any of these areas, consider the following suggestions, which I've found to be quite helpful with my middle-aged male patients...*

•**Keep your liver healthy.** Your liver is vital to your hormone health because steroid

*If you have any chronic health conditions or take medications, talk to your doctor before trying the herbs in this article.

T level "Sweet Spot"

An analysis of the health records of 3,690 men ages 70 to 89 found that those with the lowest testosterone levels had the highest risk for death. And those with the highest levels of testosterone had the next highest death risk. Men who had testosterone levels in the middle range (9.8 nmol/L to 15.8 nmol/L) tended to live the longest.

Bu Beng Yeap, MD, PhD, endocrinologist and professor in medicine, The University of Western Australia, Perth.

hormones (reproductive and adrenal) are made from cholesterol, which is produced primarily in the liver. For that reason, I advise most men (there are some exceptions, such as men who have had heart attacks) to avoid statin drugs if at all possible. One reason for this advice is that statins can drive cholesterol too low for adequate hormone production, and studies show that cholesterol that's too low is as dangerous to long-term health as elevated cholesterol.

If possible, get your total cholesterol under 200 mg/dL with diet and exercise (see below). To promote the health of your liver, eat lots of leafy greens...root vegetables, such as beets and carrots...healthy oils (two tablespoons daily), such as olive, coconut and fish oils...fresh fruit...and some lean meats.

•**Don't shirk exercise.** It's simply a fact that adrenal and reproductive hormone levels are improved with regular, moderate exercise. I recommend one hour of brisk walking daily. If you're unable to do this, consider swimming, pilates or hiking.

•**Try botanicals.** Urtica dioica (also known as stinging nettle) has a long history of use as an anti-inflammatory for the male urinary tract and as a treatment for prostate enlargement. I usually recommend 250 mg of Urtica dioica root a day.

Caution: If you have prostate cancer, talk to your doctor before taking Urtica to ensure that the herb is safe for you. Eleutherococcus senticosus (sometimes found labeled as Siberian ginseng) helps the body adapt to stress and is useful in treating fatigue, concentration problems and mild depression. This herb is best absorbed in tincture form, typically one-quarter teaspoon in water, 15 minutes before or after meals, twice daily for three months.

If these simple changes aren't enough, get help. You may not need an endocrinologist—many naturopathic physicians and conventional family doctors are skilled at hormone evaluation and treatment. Just be sure to inquire about experience, training and treatment style.

Testosterone Not the Whole Story in "Male Menopause"

Joel Finkelstein, MD, associate director, Bone Density Center, Massachusetts General Hospital, Boston.
John Amory, MD, MPH, professor, medicine, University of Washington, Seattle.
New England Journal of Medicine

Symptoms of so-called "andropause"—the male equivalent of menopause—may be triggered not only by declines in testosterone, but in the "female" hormone estrogen as well, a recent study suggests.

Experts said the study, published recently in the *New England Journal of Medicine*, deepens researchers' understanding of the hormonal shifts that occur as men age.

And it's more complicated than those ads about "low T" and testosterone supplements might lead men to believe.

Instead, researchers found, there is no black-and-white cutoff for "low" or "suboptimal" testosterone. Different symptoms crop up at different testosterone thresholds: Muscle mass and strength do not decline until testosterone drops quite low, whereas libido may dampen with relatively small dips in the hormone.

"The question that patients always have is, 'What's a normal testosterone level?'" said John Amory, MD, MPH, professor of medicine at the University of Washington in Seattle, who was not involved in the study.

"Well, now I'm going to ask, 'What endpoint are you talking about?'" Dr. Amory said. "Different functions of testosterone start to deteriorate at different levels."

What's more, the study shows that men's functioning can be impaired not only by a loss of testosterone, but estrogen as well, according to lead researcher Joel Finkelstein, MD, associate director of the Bone Density Center at Massachusetts General Hospital in Boston.

A small amount of the testosterone men produce is converted into estrogen in the body, so that hormone also declines as men get older.

And in this study, estrogen and testosterone loss both affected men's libido and erectile function. And it was the loss of estrogen, in particular, that appeared to promote body fat gain.

That might sound surprising, since women—who produce much more estrogen than men do—typically have more body fat. But Dr. Finkelstein said it's known from lab research that when male rodents' estrogen receptors are "knocked out," the animals "get fat."

STUDY DETAILS

To dig deeper, Dr. Finkelstein's team recruited 400 healthy men between the ages of 20 and 50. All of them took a drug that suppresses natural testosterone and estrogen production. Then, half of them used different doses of testosterone gel or an inactive placebo gel for 16 weeks. The other half used those gels plus a medication that blocked their testosterone from being converted into estrogen.

That way, the researchers were able to pinpoint the levels at which testosterone loss spurred particular symptoms—and whether estrogen played a key role in any of those problems.

In general, they found, increases in body fat and a waning interest in sex started to emerge at mild levels of testosterone deficiency. But muscle loss and erectile dysfunction were not seen until testosterone dropped lower—around 200 ng/dL or below.

Dr. Finkelstein agreed that none of this answers the big question of whether testosterone replacement is a good thing. And the researchers still need to see whether their findings hold true in men older than 50 as well.

WHAT IT ALL MEANS FOR MEN

So what does this all mean to men? Dr. Amory said that the "elephant in the room" remains: Doctors still don't know whether testosterone supplements actually do more harm than good.

And that's a major issue, both Dr. Amory and Dr. Finkelstein said. Testosterone deficiency is diagnosed in millions of men each year, and in the United States, prescriptions for testosterone shot up 500% between 1993 and 2000 alone.

Right now, the definition of "low" varies, depending on the lab doing the testing, according to Dr. Amory.

But on average, testosterone levels below 300 nanograms per deciliter (ng/dL) are considered low, Dr. Finkelstein said—and it's a sort of one-size-fits-all definition. "One of the goals of this study was to do better than that," he said.

"This study is a step along the way in our understanding," Dr. Finkelstein said. "I would tell men to stay cautious and conservative" about testosterone therapy.

Dr. Amory said there are some men who benefit from testosterone therapy, which comes in the form of topical gels, patches and injections, and can cost up to $300 a month.

But they are the men whose testosterone levels are clearly low and causing problems. The difficulty, according to Dr. Amory, is when a man has a moderately low testosterone level and a vague symptom such as fatigue—which can have many causes.

Testosterone Supplements Decrease Male Fertility

According to recent research, testosterone supplements, often taken by men to improve their sex drive or fuel muscle growth, can impede sperm production. But the effect is not permanent. Most men who stopped taking testosterone supplements saw a jump in their sperm count. Average sperm concentration in semen went from 1.8 million per milliliter to 34 million per milliliter within one to six months.

Study of 1,500 men, average age 35, by researchers at University of Alabama, Birmingham, presented at the annual meeting of the American Urological Association in San Diego.

Testosterone supplements have potential side effects, including acne and prostate enlargement. But maybe the biggest worry is that the long-range health effects are unknown.

"If a man asks me if this will raise his risk of heart disease 10 years from now, all I can say is, 'I don't know,'" Dr. Amory said. "We're flying a bit blind on this."

He and Dr. Finkelstein both pointed to the story of hormone replacement in women as a cautionary tale. Doctors once widely prescribed estrogen and progesterone to women as a way to ward off heart disease—until a large US trial found that older women given the hormones actually faced increased risks of blood clots, heart attack, stroke and breast cancer.

"We haven't had an analogous study in men yet," Dr. Amory said.

info The Urology Care Foundation has more on low testosterone at its website, *http://www.urologyhealth.org/urology/index.cfm?article=132.*

Low Testosterone Linked to Rheumatoid Arthritis (RA)

According to a recent finding, men with low testosterone were more likely to be diagnosed with RA from one to 28 years after their testosterone level was measured. The average time to diagnosis was 13 years. The study does not show that low testosterone causes RA—only that low levels of the hormone make a diagnosis of the condition more likely for both men and women.

Study of 278 men by researchers at Lund University, Malmö, Sweden, published online in *Annals of the Rheumatic Diseases.*

Lack of Sperm Linked to Increased Cancer Risk

Michael Eisenberg, MD, assistant professor and director, male reproductive medicine and surgery program, Stanford University School of Medicine, and physician, Stanford Hospital and Clinics, Stanford, California. His research was published in *Fertility and Sterility.*

When someone mentions male infertility, you probably think about the huge disappointment a couple may face when the man is unable to father a child…and that is upsetting, indeed. But male infertility is linked to another concern that has nothing to do with having a baby. It's a cancer problem—that's right, cancer. For men with fertility problems (and the women who love them), this newly discovered risk is very important to know about.

There are many different reasons why a man could be infertile. For instance, he might produce sperm that are misshapen or immobile and so are unable to fertilize a woman's egg…he might produce normal sperm, but these sperm never reach the semen…he might have a problem with ejaculation…or he might produce too few sperm or none at all. It is this last condition that is of concern when it comes to cancer risk, a recent study shows.

MISSING SPERM

About 15% of infertile men have a condition called azoospermia, meaning a complete absence of sperm in the semen. For some such men, normal sperm are produced in the testes but some obstruction prevents them from reaching the semen. The majority of these men, however, have nonobstructive azoospermia—in which the testes don't produce enough sperm for any to reach the semen.

A previous study noted increased rates of testicular and prostate cancers among men with fertility problems. So for this recent study, researchers set out to shed additional light on this link. They used semen analyses from men who had been evaluated for infertility at a large Texas medical center. To limit the possibility that the cancer came first and was causing any participant's infertility—rather than that the infertility came first and was a risk factor for cancer—the researchers excluded samples from men who were diagnosed with cancer within six months of their initial semen analysis.

Next, the researchers searched the Texas Cancer Registry (which records information about all cases of confirmed cancer in Texas residents) to see which of the infertile participants ended up developing some type of cancer during the study follow-up period, which lasted about six years, on average, after the semen analyses. Then they compared the cancer rates among infertile men with the cancer rates in the general population.

THE CANCER CONNECTION

What the researchers found was both reassuring and disturbing. The reassuring part was that men whose infertility was caused by something other than azoospermia had rates of cancer similar to that of the general population. The disturbing part was that men whose infertility was due specifically to azoospermia had a cancer risk that was nearly triple that of the general population. Even worse, within the group of men with azoospermia, those under age 30 had a cancer risk more than eight times higher than normal for men of that age.

Finally, to be even more certain that it wasn't the cancer itself that was causing infertility, researchers removed from their analysis all men who were diagnosed with cancer up to three years after their semen tests, then recrunched the numbers. Again, the same risks were found.

Surprisingly, the risk was not limited only to testicular or prostate cancer. In fact, the types of cancers seen in men with azoospermia also included cancers of the stomach, brain and small intestine, as well as melanoma and lymphoma.

Explanation: DNA probably holds the key to the azoospermia/cancer connection. Studies have shown high rates of defects in DNA repair mechanisms and abnormalities in life cycles of cells among men with azoospermia—and these same genetic defects may increase the likelihood of cancer, researchers suspect.

Self-defense: Men with azoospermia have approximately the same cancer risk as their peers who are about a decade older, researchers estimate. If you have azoospermia, it would be wise to talk with your doctor about the healthful diet and lifestyle choices that can help reduce your cancer risk...about cancer warning signs to watch for...and about when you should start getting regular cancer screenings.

Joyful news: If you and your partner want to have children, also ask your doctor about surgical testicular sperm extraction followed by in vitro fertilization. According to the study researchers, this type of assisted reproductive technology can help about half of azoospermic men to father children.

Urinary Tract Infections in Men: New Advice on Antibiotics

Dimitri Drekonja, MD, staff physician, Infectious Disease Section, Minneapolis Veterans Affairs Health Care System, and assistant professor of medicine, University of Minnesota, Minneapolis.

Andrew L. Rubman, ND, founder and medical director, Southbury Clinic for Traditional Medicines, Southbury, Connecticut. *SouthburyClinic.com*

Burning pain, frequent trips to the toilet, urine that's cloudy and strong-smelling—such symptoms suggest a urinary tract infection (UTI). If you're a man, when you go to your doctor for antibiotics, there's almost no way of knowing how many days' worth of pills you'll be prescribed...because chances are that your doctor doesn't know what's best.

That's a problem. Treat a UTI too briefly, and there's a risk that the bacteria may survive to invade your kidneys and do serious damage. Treat the infection too long, and you're more

Peyronie's Drug Gets FDA Nod

Men with Peyronie's disease develop a lump in the penis that causes abnormal curvature and pain upon erection and difficulty with intercourse. *Collagenase clostridium histolyticum* (Xiaflex) recently became the first FDA-approved nonsurgical treatment for Peyronie's disease. The drug, prescribed for men whose curvature is at least 30 degrees upon erection, is believed to break down the collagen that causes the penile curvature. Consult a health-care professional who has been trained to administer the drug—it can cause adverse effects such as injury to the penis.

Andrea Fischer, spokesperson, FDA, Silver Spring, Maryland.

likely to experience side effects from the drugs (including severe dizziness and even ruptured tendons)...and, according to a recent study, you also encourage your UTI to return and boost your odds of developing a nasty colon infection as well.

Why all the confusion? Because there is scant research into the optimal length of time to treat men who have UTIs. Up to about age 50, UTIs are so much more common in women than men that the research has focused mostly on women. Based on numerous studies of women, the Infectious Diseases Society of America concluded that the optimal length of antibiotic therapy for women with UTIs is usually three days.

There is no similar research-based guideline for men, so doctors often make the assumption that, because men's urethras are longer than women's, their treatment time should be longer, too. Yet the actual number of days prescribed varies widely from doctor to doctor. For instance, the recent study found that treatment times often ranged anywhere from three days to 30 days—and "there didn't seem to be much rhyme or reason as to why," said lead author Dimitri Drekonja, MD, a staff physician at the Minneapolis Veterans Affairs (VA) Health Care System. That's why he and his colleagues set out to study the situation.

THE BIG VA DATABASE

Dr. Drekonja's team sifted through data on 33,336 male VA patients nationwide who had developed one or more UTIs, comparing recurrence rates and complications for patients who received shorter-duration antibiotic treatment (seven days or less) with those who received longer treatment (more than seven days). *What they found...*

• **UTIs recurred after 30 or more days in 11% of men given the longer treatment,** but in just 8% of those given the shorter treatment. (Recurrence rates prior to 30 days were similar in both groups.)

• **Men who received the longer treatment were nearly twice as likely as those treated for less time to develop an infection of Clostridium difficile** (C. difficile). This bacterium can take hold when antibiotics wipe out beneficial bacteria in the gut, leading to inflammation of the colon, severe diarrhea, abdominal pain and/or fever.

Of course, it's possible that some of the patients who were given the longer course of treatment also had the most severe UTIs, in which case it makes sense that they would be at highest risk for recurrence. Still, the study does suggest that many men are being treated for longer than is ideal—and that such extended treatment has serious side effects.

Unfortunately, the confusion about optimal UTI treatment duration will continue until additional research provides insights on which to base more specific guidelines. *In the meantime, though, men do have another option...*

AN ALTERNATIVE APPROACH TO UTI

If you're a guy with a UTI, you may be able to avoid antibiotics altogether by taking a more natural approach to treatment that includes the use of supplements, said Andrew Rubman, ND, medical director of the Southbury Clinic for Traditional Medicines in Southbury, Connecticut. You would need to consult a naturopathic

Diet and Exercise Can Boost Sperm Health

Diet and exercise can boost sperm health. Walnuts improve sperm quality in younger men. Men ages 21 to 35 who ate 2.5 ounces of walnuts daily for 12 weeks had improvements in sperm motility. A diet rich in antioxidants helps preserve sperm quality in middle-aged and older men.

Men over age 44 who had higher intakes of vitamins C and E and the mineral zinc produced sperm with less DNA damage than men with lower intakes of these substances. Physically active men had better-formed and faster-swimming sperm than sedentary men. And men who watched TV for more than 20 hours a week had lower sperm concentration than men who watched none.

Roundup of studies from UCLA and UC Berkeley, and studies published in *European Journal of Applied Physiology* and *British Journal of Sports Medicine*, reported in *University of California, Berkeley Wellness Letter*.

physician to confirm your diagnosis and determine appropriate dosages.

With his own patients, Dr. Rubman explained, an important step is to make the environment of the urinary tract more acidic so that E. coli (the bacterium most commonly associated with UTIs) cannot thrive. With that goal in mind, he often prescribes a concentrated cranberry extract. Cranberry not only makes urine more acidic, but it also contains substances called proanthocyanidins that keep the bacteria from binding to the urinary tract. Another acidity booster is powdered vitamin C (ascorbic acid). Dark berry extracts, as a broad-based proanthocyanidins source, may also be prescribed. (Dr. Rubman's favorite is Nutrigenomic Berry POW-der from Eclectic Institute, *EclecticHerb.com.*) In addition, patients may be advised to drink more water to help flush out the urinary tract.

Even if natural therapies don't cure you and you do end up needing an antibiotic, your naturopathic doctor will want to do a urine test to determine which specific organisms are causing you trouble. Dr. Rubman said, "Another bacterial infection in your body could be what made you vulnerable to a UTI in the first place, so that should be addressed. Plus, it's helpful to identify the UTI organism in order to know which antibiotic will work best and to gauge the most appropriate length of treatment."

Walking May Help Older Men Sidestep Hip Fractures

Diane Feskanich, ScD, assistant professor, Harvard Medical School, and associate epidemiologist, department of medicine, Brigham and Women's Hospital, Boston.

Neil S. Roth, MD, attending orthopedic surgeon and sports medicine specialist, Lenox Hill Hospital, New York City.

American Journal of Public Health

Even a little walking each week appears to lower the risk of hip fractures in men over age 50, a recent long-term study suggests.

THE STUDY

Researchers from Brigham and Women's Hospital mined data from a large study, collecting information on the activity and sitting habits of nearly 36,000 men over 24 years.

Their study relied on answers on questionnaires that the men filled out every two years about how vigorously they walked—at an easy, average or brisk pace—as well as their time spent sitting and performing other activities, including tennis, lap swimming and outdoor work.

During the 24-year follow-up period, 546 hip fractures were reported, not including fractures due to cancer or a traumatic event, such as a fall during skiing or a car accident. "Low-trauma" events, such as slipping, tripping or falling from a chair, were responsible for 85% of the fractures.

The results suggest that the more a man walked, and the more vigorously he walked, the lower his risk for hip fracture as he aged, the authors reported. For men whose primary activity was walking, doing so at least four hours a week was associated with a significant drop in hip fractures—a 43% lower risk than walking less than one hour a week.

The study was published in the *American Journal of Public Health.*

GOOD NEWS: MILD EXERCISE WORKS

"It's well known that physical activity helps to prevent hip fractures, that it helps to build bone and muscle tone. It can help with balance, too," said study author Diane Feskanich, ScD, an assistant professor at Harvard Medical School and an associate epidemiologist in the department of medicine at Brigham and Women's Hospital in Boston.

"One thing we're pointing out here is that it doesn't necessarily have to be strenuous activity," Dr. Feskanich said. "A lot of studies have focused on the benefits of strenuous activity, but we found walking alone helped to prevent hip fractures, and when you come down to it, older people are often more comfortable with walking."

EXPERT COMMENTARY

Neil S. Roth, MD, an attending orthopedic surgeon at Lenox Hill Hospital in New York City, and a specialist in sports medicine, said bones are not static organs—they're fluid. "The cells are constantly breaking down bone and making new bone," he said.

The way to keep bones healthy and strong is by increasing stress on the bone through activity, but not to overdo it, either, he said. "You want to stay below the threshold that becomes dangerous but also push it to the point that builds bone mass—find the sweet spot—but that will be different for everybody," Dr. Roth said.

An obese 75-year-old man will not be able to do the same activity as a 65-year-old who is in good shape, Dr. Roth noted. He also said that while walking may help with some balance and cardiovascular issues, it may not fully address those and other health issues.

"Balance in the elderly is a very complicated situation. If someone has better balance, they're much less likely to fall and the majority of hip fractures occur from a fall. But all sorts of things can affect balance in elderly—inner ear issues, or vertigo," he said, as well as poor eyesight and medications. But he said a walker or cane can help people maintain a healthy walking routine.

Dr. Roth advises that men get cleared by their internist or cardiologist, though, before starting an exercise routine, and that they listen to their bodies during physical activity, especially if they experience bone pain.

SIMILAR RESULTS IN WOMEN

Dr. Feskanich said she and colleagues performed a similar earlier study in women and the results almost mirrored this study: "We found almost the exact same results in women and men, about the same numbers."

She said the recent findings may boost recommendations for more walking. "But a good clinician is already telling their older patients to be walking and active," she added.

info For more on exercise and bone health, visit the U.S. National Institute of Arthritis and Musculoskeletal and Skin Diseases website, *www.niams.nih.gov,* and search "exercise and bone health."

Pain Relief

The Power of Energy Healing—It Works…and Anyone Can Do It

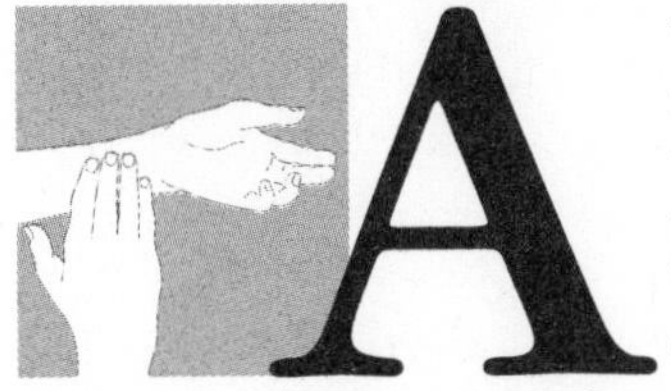

A woman with rheumatoid arthritis was told by her doctor that she would be confined to a wheelchair within the year—but a year after that diagnosis, she's taking her dog for long walks. A person with nonstop sciatica for 30 years achieved relief in one hour—and the pain never returned. A woman with skin ulcers from severe circulatory problems was scheduled for surgery to amputate her leg—but after four months, her wounds were completely healed and the surgery was canceled.*

What happened: All these people were treated with a simple form of energy healing that you can learn quickly and use to treat yourself, your family, your friends, even your pet.

How it works: Using deep breathing, steady attention and touch, energy healing enlivens and directs the life force, the fundamental energy that animates the body and the mind. The practitioner raises his/her energy level…that energy level then is matched by the recipient…and the life force does the healing. Scientists call this *resonance* and *entrainment*—similar to when a motionless tuning fork starts to vibrate at the frequency of an already-vibrating tuning fork.

Many ancient cultures discovered and used the life force in their healing modalities. For example, in China, it is called qi (or chi) and used in Qiqong (pronounced "chee-gong"), the therapeutic exercises of Traditional Chinese Medicine. In India, it is called prana and is used

*You can see these and other testimonials at *YouTube.com/QuantumTouch.*

Richard Gordon, a pioneer of energy healing and founder of Quantum-Touch, a method of natural healing that works with the life-force energy of the body. Based in Santa Monica, California, he is author of several books, including *The New Human: Quantum-Touch 2.0* and *Quantum-Touch: The Power to Heal* (both from North Atlantic). Quantum-Touch has 300 certified instructors in 50 countries. *QuantumTouch.com* in pranayama, yogic breathing techniques for self-healing and spiritual development.

And there's scientific evidence that energy healing works...

Standout research: In a study by researchers at University of Granada, Spain, energy healing calmed the parasympathetic nervous system (activated during the "fight-or-flight" response) of nurses suffering from burnout. In a study published in *Journal of Alternative and Complementary Medicine*, researchers at University of Arizona found that laboratory rats subjected to daily noise stress had far less stress-caused damage to their circulatory systems when they received energy healing—and with rats, there is no placebo effect involved!

There are many modern forms of energy healing, such as therapeutic touch, polarity therapy and Reiki. I have developed a method of energy healing that I call Quantum-Touch. It simplifies the principles of energy healing, making the process so straightforward that anyone can become an effective energy healer.

I have created a condensed yet effective form of the technique...

THREE STEPS TO ENERGY HEALING

1. Breathe deeply. Conscious, deep breathing amplifies the life force. Try a simple "4 x 4" breath—inhale while you mentally count to four, and exhale doing the same. Continue to breathe deeply for the entire healing session.

2. Feel your love. I am not speaking of the love a mother has for a child or a husband for a wife. I mean giving your attention as an act of loving. I call this steady, focused attention on another person preconditional love—an instinctive, basic energy that has nothing to do with your background, race, religion, politics or belief. Like deep breathing, love amplifies energy—and that energy can move through your hands, regardless of your mood.

3. Put your hands on the area of pain or disease in the person's body. As you do this, keep your hands relaxed (before you start, give them a bit of a light shake to let go of any tension), and don't use any force or pressure—let the energy do the work. Most important, feel your hands (the literal physical sensation in your hands), feel your love coming through your hands as steady attention and feel your intention to heal. While continuing to breathe deeply and feel steadily, leave your hands on the painful or ailing area for five to 10 minutes. (Use common sense, of course. Don't put your hands into a wound or touch a burn.)

Glucosamine Supplement Alert!

According to a recent study, when 17 adults began taking about 1,000 mg daily of glucosamine for arthritis, the fluid inside their eyes built up, leading to elevated intraocular pressure (IOP)—a known risk factor for glaucoma. When the study participants stopped taking the supplement, their IOP readings dropped.

Theory: Glucosamine blocks spaces between tiny fibers in the eye, decreasing its ability to drain fluid.

If you take glucosamine: An ophthalmologist should regularly monitor your IOP.

Edward Jaccoma, MD, clinical associate professor of ophthalmology, University of New England College of Osteopathic Medicine, Portland, Maine.

HEALING SPECIFIC HEALTH PROBLEMS

You can use energy healing for a wide range of health problems. For best results, the recipient should be either seated or lying down, and you also should be comfortable. Don't hold your body or your hands in an awkward position.

•**Pain relief.** I tested energy healing on the men's basketball team at the University of California-Santa Cruz and discovered that it provided an average of 50% pain reduction. Sandwiching a painful spot between your hands is an excellent way to enhance energy in that area, because having two points of contact creates a stronger energy field between you and the person you are working on.

Examples: For lower-back pain, put your hands on either side of the spine. For a headache on the top of the head, put one hand on the forehead and the other on the back of the head.

Don't make assumptions about where the pain is—ask the person in pain to point to exactly where he/she is hurting.

The pain may move around during the session of energy healing. Before you start, ask the person you are working on to tell you if the pain shifts or moves. If it does, move your hands to the new area of pain.

• **Specific organs and glands.** I have found that you can use energy healing for problems with any organ or gland. Putting your hands over the heart, for example, may improve blood pressure and heart arrhythmia. Putting your hands over the pancreas (toward the back of the left side of the body, behind and below the stomach) may help lower blood sugar in people with prediabetes and type 2 diabetes.

• **Self-healing.** Use energy healing on yourself regularly and often. Just as when you use energy healing on a family member or friend, sandwich any part of your body that you can reach comfortably. (Of course, if you're treating a problem such as tennis elbow, you will be able to use only one hand, which still is effective.)

• **Ailing animals.** Energy healing has worked wonderfully on all sorts of animals, including dogs, cats, horses, rabbits—even turtles. As with people, sandwich with your hands any area that you think needs healing. (A diagnosis from a veterinarian may help you pinpoint the problem.)

DEALING WITH SKEPTICISM

If you're a skeptic about energy healing, you're not alone. Many people I work with started as skeptics, including Chris Duffield, PhD, a former visiting scholar at Stanford University. He became one of the coauthors of my book *The New Human: Quantum-Touch 2.0. Chris's advice...*

Simply suspend your disbelief, and try it out. Don't think about how energy healing is impossible. Act as though it were possible, which creates an opportunity for it to work if it's going to work. Think of the skeptics who doubted Galileo and refused to look through the telescope. Those who did look saw the craters on the moon, the rings of Saturn and four moons around Jupiter—a new universe.

Energy healing is a view into the capabilities for healing that science has yet to fully confirm, but my work with thousands of people has shown it to be very real.

Headaches That Stump Doctors and How to Finally Get Relief

Alan M. Rapoport, MD, a clinical professor of neurology at The David Geffen School of Medicine at the University of California in Los Angeles and president of the International Headache Society. He has authored more than 275 articles, book chapters and posters on headache. Dr. Rapoport created *ProMyHealth.org*, an online resource to help doctors (and patients) evaluate headaches.

When you are in the throes of a headache, you do not care what is causing the pain. You just want relief. But not all headaches or migraines respond to the same treatment—and the wrong approach can keep you locked in your misery or even worsen the pain.

Should you take a migraine pill or a powerful pain reliever? Or would it be better to lie down in a cool, dark room or even go for a run? The answer depends on what is really causing your headache.

The problem is, there are more than 300 different causes of headaches, and just over half of people who have severe headaches are properly diagnosed.

The Fruit That Gives Muscle Aches the Boot

Muscle soreness is the big downside of working out.

Good news: When athletes drank 16 ounces of watermelon juice an hour before exercise, they had less muscle soreness than when they did not drink it.

Theory: Watermelon contains L-citrulline, an amino acid that boosts blood flow and oxygen in muscles, reducing pain.

To ease sore muscles: Try eating some watermelon (or drinking the juice if you have a juicer).

Encarna Aguayo, PhD, associate professor of food technology, Technical University of Cartagena, Spain.

What makes a difference: The more you know about symptoms associated with different types of headaches, the better equipped you'll be to help your doctor pinpoint the underlying cause of your pain. Unusual symptoms, which often occur with headaches, are easily misinterpreted.

THE HEADACHE MYSTERY

Surprisingly, these common types of headaches can be difficult for some doctors to diagnose. *For example...*

•**Migraine with aura.** The main symptom is throbbing or pounding head pain that occurs during or shortly after an aura (visual disturbances such as blurred vision...white, black or colored dots...flashing light...or blind spots). Nausea and, less frequently, vomiting may also occur. Severe migraines may develop without an aura, too.

Symptoms that can be misdiagnosed: Numbness or tingling or even weakness on one side of the face or body and/or speech difficulties—all of which may be misdiagnosed as stroke—and increased sensitivity to touch (called allodynia) can be symptoms of migraine with aura. So can dizziness, a runny nose or tearing eyes.

Important: Most "sinus" headaches are really migraines.

Best treatment: Most individuals diagnosed with migraine are aware of lifestyle changes that can help—this includes avoiding triggers such as caffeine, certain odors and the artificial sweetener aspartame...eating a healthful diet...and exercising regularly. Most important, do not miss or delay meals—this commonly triggers migraines.

Medication also may be needed but should be taken promptly for the best results. For example, if a triptan migraine drug, such as *sumatriptan* (Imitrex), or similar medication is prescribed, be sure to take it within the first 60 minutes of the migraine (the sooner, the better).

Supplements, including vitamin B-2, magnesium and coenzyme Q10, may be taken daily as a preventive. They may help by increasing energy in the nerve cells.

•**Episodic cluster headache.** Unlike most headaches, cluster headaches strike more men than women, with excruciating and sudden daily headaches one to three times per day, always on one side of the head, in or around an eye. The headaches can last from 15 minutes to three hours and often persist for one to three months, about once a year.

While a migraine sufferer's pain may improve when relaxing in a cool, dark room, a cluster headache patient may get some relief from walking or even running.

Symptoms that can be misdiagnosed: Doctors may misdiagnose cluster headaches as sinusitis or a tooth problem because the pain extends to the sinuses, upper teeth, back of the head or even the neck.

Best treatment: To treat cluster headaches, steroid pills may be taken daily for a week or two. An injection of sumatriptan may be given for each headache. Nasal spray triptans such as *zolmitriptan* (Zomig) also may be tried, and breathing pure oxygen via a mask may help. If cluster headaches persist, the calcium channel blocker *verapamil* (Verelan) is usually prescribed. If these therapies fail, patients may need a nerve block—an injection of anesthetics and steroids in the occipital nerve, which immediately numbs the pain. A tiny electrical device also can be implanted to stimulate the nerve.

•**Episodic tension-type headache.** Most adults get these headaches occasionally. They cause squeezing or pressing (nonthrobbing) pain, often on both sides of the head. Stress is the usual trigger. Muscles in the back of the neck and scalp tighten, which may cause headache pain.

Symptoms that can be misdiagnosed: Some tension-type headaches are so severe that they are misdiagnosed as migraines, and patients are prescribed migraine medication that is not always helpful.

Best treatment: Most people with tension-type headaches get some relief from over-the-counter drugs, such as aspirin, *naproxen* (Aleve) or *acetaminophen* (Tylenol). There are two other effective but underused treatments—

removing yourself from the stressful situation and getting any kind of aerobic exercise.

GETTING THE HELP YOU NEED

To properly diagnose your headaches, your physician should review your medical history and your family's medical history, conduct a physical examination and rule out other possible causes of head pain, such as an aneurysm or a congenital malformation. Be sure that you thoroughly describe your symptoms to your doctor.

What helps most: Keeping a headache diary, either in a notebook or on a computer or tablet, is crucial to getting the right diagnosis. This diary should include such information as the time of day your headaches occur...the specific location and type of pain (for example, throbbing, pressing or piercing)...other symptoms (such as nausea, light sensitivity or dizziness)...food you ate before the headache...and activities before the headache developed. For a free chart you can use as a headache diary, go to *AmericanHeadacheSociety.org* and click on "Tools for Patients."

If you don't get relief after working with your physician for a few months, consider consulting a headache specialist or neurologist. Board-certified headache specialists are the best qualified to treat headaches. To find one near you, consult *ProMyHealth.org.*

Neck Pain Could Indicate a Serious Problem

Seek medical attention if neck pain precedes or accompanies a headache—it could indicate an impending stroke...when the pain radiates to your shoulders or arm or is accompanied by leg weakness or difficulty walking—this may be a sign of a herniated disk...if the pain worsens at night or is accompanied by fever or weight loss—this may indicate an infection or another serious condition.

Mayo Clinic Health Letter. HealthLetter.MayoClinic.com

First Device to Treat Migraine With Aura Approved

Food and Drug Administration, news release.

The first device to treat migraine pain when the headache is preceded by an often-visual disturbance called an aura has been approved by the U.S. Food and Drug Administration (FDA).

HOW THE DEVICE WORKS

The Cerena Transcranial Magnetic Stimulator (TMS) is held to the back of the head and the user presses a button to release a pulse of magnetic energy. This stimulates the brain's occipital cortex, which may reduce or eliminate migraine-associated pain, according to the FDA.

STUDY DETAILS

The device was tested in a clinical trial of 201 people with mostly moderate-to-strong migraines. Nearly 38% of people with migraine pain were pain-free two hours after use, compared with 17% of people who didn't use the device, the FDA said. The device was not evaluated among people with headaches other than those with migraines preceded by aura, the agency said.

Among the rare side effects reported were sinusitis and dizziness. The device shouldn't be used by people with metals in the head, neck or upper body, or by people with an implanted medical device such as a pacemaker or deep brain stimulator, the FDA said.

The Cerena TMS is produced by eNeura Therapeutics, based in Sunnyvale, California.

info For more information about the TMS device, visit the FDA website at *www.fda.gov/NewsEvents/Newsroom/PressAnnouncements/ucm378608.htm.*

Behavioral Therapy Might Ease Kids' Migraine Symptoms

Journal of the American Medical Association, news release

A specific type of therapy helps reduce the number of migraines and migraine-related disabilities in children and teens, according to a recent study.

The findings provide strong evidence for the use of cognitive behavioral therapy—which includes training in coping with pain—in managing chronic migraines in children and teens, said study leader Scott Powers, PhD, codirector of the headache center at Cincinnati Children's Hospital Medical Center, and colleagues.

The therapy should be routinely offered as a first-line treatment, along with medications, he said.

MIGRAINE IN CHILDREN

More than 2% of adults and about 1.75% of children have chronic migraines, according to the study, which was published in the *Journal of the American Medical Association*. But there are no treatments approved by the U.S. Food and Drug Administration to quell these debilitating headaches in young people, the researchers said.

RECENT STUDY

The study included 135 youngsters, ages 10 to 17, who had migraines 15 or more days a month. They were assigned to receive either 10 cognitive behavioral therapy sessions or 10 headache education sessions.

Patients in both groups were treated with the drug *amitriptyline* (Elavil).

At the start of the study, patients averaged migraines on 21 of 28 days, and had a severe level of migraine-related disability. Immediately after treatment, those in the cognitive-therapy group had 11.5 fewer days with migraines, compared with 6.8 fewer days for those in the headache-education group.

Twelve months after treatment, 86% of those who received cognitive therapy had a 50% or more reduction in days with migraines, compared with 69% of those in the headache-education group. In addition, 88% of patients in the cognitive-therapy group had mild or no migraine-related disability, compared with 76% of those in the other group.

TREATING MIGRAINE WITH COGNITIVE BEHAVIORAL THERAPY

Cognitive therapy should not be offered only as an add-on treatment if medications aren't working well, the researchers said. It also should be covered by health insurance, they said.

However, use of cognitive therapy as a first-line treatment for chronic migraines in children and teens faces a number of barriers, according to an accompanying editorial by Mark Connelly, PhD, of Children's Mercy Hospitals and Clinics in Kansas City.

Having behavioral health consultants in primary-care offices is one possible way to overcome these barriers, he said. Telephone- or Internet-based programs might also be effective, he said.

info The U.S. National Institute of Neurological Disorders and Stroke has more information about migraine at *www.ninds.nih.gov/disorders/migraine/migraine.htm*.

How to Wreck Your Back—6 Little Mistakes That Cause Big Pain

David Borenstein, MD, clinical professor of medicine at The George Washington University Medical Center in Washington, DC, and a partner at Arthritis and Rheumatism Associates, the largest rheumatology practice based in Washington/Maryland. He is host of Speaking of Health with Dr. B, a weekly radio program and author of *Heal Your Back* (M. Evans & Company). *DrBHealth.com*

As many as 80% of Americans will suffer an episode of back pain at some time in their lives. Back problems are among the main reasons for doctor visits, and they can be excruciatingly slow to heal.

What people don't realize is that most back injuries are predictable and how to avoid them might surprise you. *Here are the six worst mistakes that people make that hurt their backs...*

WEIGHT AND EFFORT MISMATCH

I see this all the time. Suppose you lift a box that is heavier than you expected. You get it a few inches off the floor and then realize that it's really heavy. It's going to crash back down if you don't bring all of your strength into play. The sudden contraction of unprepared back muscles can cause an instant strain.

Or maybe you're lifting a box that you think is heavy but turns out to be as light as a feather. All of the muscle force that you generated causes a "snap" in the muscles (and the box goes flying).

Self-protection: Before you lift something, test the weight. Slide it a few inches, or lift just a corner. You have to know what you're dealing with. If it's heavy, get your legs under you...use the muscles in your legs more than the muscles in your back. If it's light, lift with a smooth motion—you won't need that initial hard jerk to get it moving.

OVERHEAD BIN REACH

If you think that the cramped, knees-to-chest seating in today's airplanes is hard on your back, wait until you use the overhead bins. You will pay in pain what you saved on checked luggage.

Travelers often overstuff their carry-ons. A 20-pound bag that's easy to carry (or wheel) can feel like 50 pounds when you're off-balance and reaching overhead. Unloading also is a hazard. You probably had to angle, wedge and stuff your bag to get it to fit. You will have to give it a hard yank to get it out, a motion that is very hard on the back.

Self-protection: Pack light. If you're in reasonable shape, you probably can manage, say, a 10-pound bag when your arms are extended and you're standing on tiptoe. Use both hands to place the bag in the bin...don't swing it up with one arm. Store it with the handle facing out. That way, you can grip the handle with one hand and use your other hand for support. For anything much heavier, put it in checked baggage—it's worth it even if you have to pay.

SUPER-SOFT CHAIR RECLINE

It feels good to sink into a soft chair or sofa—but it is hard to extricate yourself from the pillowy depths.

Surprising fact: Sitting in a soft chair is hard work.

When you sit in a firm chair, your back is supported, so it relaxes. But a soft chair doesn't provide the same sensory input, so the muscles stay contracted. After an hour or so, you might notice that your back is hurting even though you haven't done anything more strenuous than read a book or work the TV remote.

Self-protection: When you're settling in, choose a chair that provides a decent amount of back support. It doesn't have to be hard, but it should be firm.

Also helpful: If you have a history of back problems, you probably will do better if you stand up for one to two minutes now and then—say, every 15 or 20 minutes.

THE CAR TRUNK LEAN

How many times have you felt a "pinch" when you lift a suitcase or a sack of groceries from a car's trunk or cargo area? It's not so much the weight that causes problems but your position. When you bend over and lift, you are at a mechanical disadvantage. You are not using the big muscles in your legs. Your back muscles aren't very strong. Their job is to stabilize your spine, not help with heavy lifting.

Self-protection: Get as close to the vehicle as you can before pulling the item to the front of the trunk and taking it out. This allows you to bring your leg muscles into play. Most people stand back from the rear of the car because they don't want to get their clothes dirty. Step in closer. It's easier to clean your clothes than to deal with a month or two of back pain.

TWIST AND SHOUT

"Twist and shout" is what I call the stab of pain that occurs when people use a twisting motion to bend over. Suppose that you're picking something up off the floor that's a little bit off to your side. You might pivot at the hips and swing one hand down to snag it. Don't! This is an unnatural motion because the spinal joints are designed to shift from front to back, not side to side. Twisting strains the soft tissues and can lead to sprains and spasms.

Self-protection: Before you pick something up, take a fraction of a second to move into a position of strength. With both feet facing the object, squat down and pick it up. Face it square, and use your legs more and your back less.

SHOVELING ANYTHING HEAVY

Back specialists see a lot of new patients in the spring after they have been working in the yard shoveling mulch, dirt or gravel. The same is true after snowstorms. Even when snow looks light and fluffy, each shovelful packs a lot of weight—and you never move just one shovelful.

Self-protection: Warm up before picking up the shovel. Walk around the house for a few minutes. Stretch out the muscles in your back, legs and arms.

Once you're outside, let your legs do the work. Bend your knees when you load the shovel, then straighten them when you lift. Don't bend your back any more than you have to. And don't take the heaviest shovelfuls that you can manage—if you're grunting, it's too much.

Also helpful: Home-supply stores stock a variety of ergonomic shovels that make it easier to stand upright when you're shoveling.

Stop Chronic Back Pain Without Surgery

David Hanscom, MD, board-certified orthopedic spine surgeon, Swedish Medical Center, Seattle. He is author of *Back In Control: A Spine Surgeon's Roadmap Out of Chronic Pain* (Vertus). *DrDavidHanscom.com*

Every year, Americans spend an estimated $86 billion on back pain treatments, including pain pills, injections and surgery. And although about 800,000 surgical procedures are performed each year for back pain, in about 75% of those cases, the surgery doesn't help.

That's why David Hanscom, MD, an orthopedic spine surgeon at Swedish Medical Center in Seattle, does something that few surgeons would dream of—he talks most of his patients out of having surgery. Instead, he recommends a new six-step approach to treating chronic back pain that he finds far more effective than surgery for most people.

AN OLD PROBLEM

In this current environment of health-care reform, expensive yet ineffectual spine surgeries are a hot topic—but even decades ago, questions were being asked about whether too many were being performed. For example, back in 1989, *Iowa Orthopaedic Journal* published "Are We Performing Too Much Spinal Surgery?"...and the 2001 American Academy of Pain Medicine annual meeting presented the session "Failed Back Syndrome: The Disturbing Statistics." New research continues to raise questions about the associated dangers, including a recent Stanford University study that linked spinal fusion surgery with a higher risk for stroke.

Dr. Hanscom acknowledged that overzealous surgeons and hospitals looking to maximize profits play a role in how many spine surgeries are performed. However, he said, it's also important to realize that many surgeons are loath to turn away desperate patients who are begging for help. "These patients can't work, they can't sleep, they're miserable—so they're willing to try anything, even if there's no guarantee that surgery will get rid of their pain," he said.

WHY SURGERY USUALLY WON'T HELP

The main reason why spine surgery so often doesn't work, Dr. Hanscom said, is that an operation can relieve back pain only if there is a structural abnormality, such as a ruptured disk or pinched nerve. But the vast majority of chronic, severe back problems don't fall into that category. Instead, the back pain is nonspecific, rooted in inflammation in the body's soft tissues (ligaments, tendons, fascia, muscles). "These types of problems cannot be seen on imaging tests—and if you can't see it, the best surgeon in the world won't be able to fix it," said Dr. Hanscom.

So when the problem is a soft-tissue issue, whether or not the patient undergoes surgery, his pain is likely to go on and on. Understandably, this leads to a lot of frustration (because nothing is helping) and fatigue (because pain is exhausting). A vicious cycle is created—pain leads to frustration and fatigue, and frustration and fatigue exacerbate pain.

The longer the pain continues, the worse the situation gets. "Long-lasting pain creates neurologic pathways that outlast the root cause," Dr. Hanscom explained. "Once these pain pathways are formed and remembered, the cycle is established and the pain becomes chronic. So even after the soft-tissue problems are gone, the pain often isn't. The only way to fix this type of chronic pain is to tackle the central nervous system's response to pain."

TAKING CONTROL

Dr. Hanscom knows firsthand whereof he speaks. His book *Back In Control: A Spine Surgeon's Roadmap Out of Chronic Pain* describes his own battle with chronic pain—from tennis elbow, migraine headaches, burning feet syndrome and more—and the surprising strategy that he used to overcome it. Based on his personal and professional experience, he has developed a program—called Defined, Organized, Comprehensive Care (DOCC)—that he uses in treating his own patients and in training other surgeons. Its premise is that pain is a perception...and that understanding it gives you greater power to gain control over it. "Freedom from pain is not only possible, with the right tools it is probable," he said.

Basically, the DOCC approach works by calming down the nervous system and allowing it to heal while also laying down new neurological pathways so the nervous system isn't trapped in the endless loop of pain signals. Dr. Hanscom explained, "It's not that you simply learn to live with the pain. Instead, your brain stops responding to the pain—so you literally do not feel it." *The DOCC program involves six basic steps...*

• **Sleep.** Getting at least eight hours of sleep per night is a cornerstone of the program. "If sleep issues aren't addressed, nothing else will work," Dr. Hanscom said. For people who have trouble sleeping due to their pain, prescription sleep medications are an option.

• **Stress management.** Chronic stress creates a cascade of biological events that exacerbate inflammation and sleeplessness, which in turn perpetuate chronic pain. Managing stress requires a two-pronged approach—making time for activities that build up your energy reserves (exercise, hobbies, socializing, spending time alone)...and learning to deal more effectively with aspects of your life that drain your energy (things that make you anxious, angry or unhappy).

• **Pain medication.** If you (or your doctor) have been leery of using pain medication for fear of its potential side effects, it is worth reconsidering this issue. Taking pain medication to achieve short-term relief while you work to resolve your chronic pain problem can help you halt that vicious cycle through which pain begets more pain, Dr. Hanscom said.

• **Physical therapy.** Rehabilitation of soft tissues soothes inflammation and facilitates true healing.

• **Goal setting.** Creating a detailed picture of what you are trying to achieve and devising a plan to work toward that goal helps you decrease anxiety, frustration and depression. This, in turn, calms the central nervous system and eases physical pain.

• **Retraining the brain.** The DOCC program moves people from being reactive to being creative in their lives. Meditation, visualization and creative play are among the primary tools Dr. Hanscom recommends. Particularly helpful is writing, he said.

Example: Write down a situation that bothers you (for instance, "My spouse is always late and it stresses me out"). Then, on paper, examine your thought processes about this situation (such as, "When she's late, I imagine that she's been in a terrible accident...or that she just doesn't care enough about me to be on time"). Next, look for errors in your thinking ("It's highly unlikely that she's had an accident...and she shows me in many ways every day that she loves me"). Finally, write about more rational ways in which to view the situation ("She's just not good at budgeting her time. I'll ask her to meet me 15 minutes earlier than necessary so that, by the time she arrives, we'll be right on schedule"). Even though the problem or problems you write about might not seem to be related to your back pain, the writing exercises essentially help reprogram your nervous system to undo the old pain pathways, allowing your brain to lay down new, positive, pain-free neural pathways.

A Surprising Cause of Back Pain

R. Douglas Orr, MD, director of the Cleveland Clinic Spine Institute at Lutheran Hospital and staff physician at the Cleveland Clinic Center for Spine Health. An orthopedic surgeon, Dr. Orr specializes in adult spinal surgery and deformity surgery. His research interests include spinal biomechanics and biomaterials.

It may have been years since you've heard anyone mention scoliosis. We tend to think of it as an ailment that strikes only children and adolescents.

What most people don't realize: Scoliosis, marked by an abnormal curvature of the spine, also affects adults, including those who have no history of the condition.

Why this is important: For adults, in particular, scoliosis can be an undiagnosed cause of pain in the back, legs or buttocks. Numbness or weakness in a leg or foot also may occur.

And these symptoms can go on for years without scoliosis being discovered as the culprit! In fact, the telltale "S" curve of adult scoliosis is sometimes severe enough that it's quite easy to see when the person is unclothed and viewed from behind, but in other cases, the curve is barely noticeable to the untrained eye.

WHAT HAPPENS TO THE SPINE

When scoliosis is discovered in an adult, it could have started in childhood but was never diagnosed…or the condition may have first developed in adulthood. If you're over age 40 and develop scoliosis for the first time, then you probably have degenerative scoliosis.

Here's what happens: As we grow older, the disks and facet joints (located between the vertebrae) of our spines degenerate. Over time, the degeneration can lead to scoliosis.

Important: If you have osteoporosis (bone thinning that is worse than the degeneration that naturally occurs with age) and develop scoliosis, the scoliosis will progress more rapidly than it would in a person without osteoporosis.

In some adults who had scoliosis as children, the degenerative process can cause the condition to worsen with age. If this occurs, the curve generally progresses by about one degree per year (scoliosis is diagnosed when the spine is curved vertically by more than 10 degrees).

In addition to the degenerative process that puts adults at increased risk for scoliosis, genetics may also play a role. The condition tends to run in families. The good news is that most adults with scoliosis have no symptoms.

HOW TO HAVE A HEALTHY SPINE

If you know that you had scoliosis as a child or think that you may have it as an adult, see your doctor for advice. If your childhood curvature was more than 30 degrees, you should go to a spine specialist every three to five years to monitor whether the curve is progressing.*

If you suspect that you have adult scoliosis, there are red flags that may signal the condition (see page 327). Scoliosis is relatively easy for a spine specialist to diagnose with a physical exam and spine imaging tests, such as X-rays and/or CT or MRI scans.

It's important for anyone who has scoliosis to keep a close eye on his/her body weight (being overweight puts additional stress on your spine)…and to stay physically active (inactivity can worsen symptoms by allowing trunk muscles to weaken, which can increase the muscle pain associated with scoliosis).

EASY WAYS TO HELP YOURSELF

Once you have scoliosis, exercise won't straighten your spine—nor will it stop the disorder from progressing. But it will help you keep your spine as supported as possible, reduce pain and keep you feeling strong.

While cardiovascular exercise (such as walking, swimming and biking) is a good idea for most people, a core-strengthening program is crucial for anyone with scoliosis. If you think of your spine as a flagpole with the muscles as guy wires, it's easy to visualize how the muscles

*For a referral to a spine specialist or a scoliosis support group near you, contact the National Scoliosis Foundation, *Scoliosis.org*.

help support the spine. The goal of core exercises is to strengthen the muscles of the abdomen, back and pelvis.

Depending on your overall fitness and agility, a core workout might include abdominal exercises as well as an exercise called the plank, which strengthens the abdominal and back muscles.

How to do the plank: Start in a raised push-up position with your toes perpendicular to the floor, then bend your elbows and rest your weight on your forearms. Keep your body in a straight line from your shoulders to your ankles. Stay still in this position—that is the exercise. If you can, begin by doing the plank for about 20 seconds and work up to about a minute daily. Because scoliosis can limit movement of the spine, stretching also can help ease stiffness.

Helpful: Many people with scoliosis are able to curb pain if they work with a physical therapist, who can help them design an exercise program that targets their specific issues.

IF YOU NEED MORE HELP

Because the severity of adult scoliosis varies so much from person to person, there is no one-size-fits-all treatment for the condition.

In addition to exercise, here's what often helps...

•**Nondrug therapies.** Chiropractic care (especially for acute episodes of pain), massage and acupuncture seem to help some people with scoliosis.

Note: Bracing, which is often prescribed for young scoliosis patients (whose skeletons are still growing), is rarely offered to adults, since it weakens the core muscles and can increase symptoms.

•**Medication.** A nonsteroidal anti-inflammatory drug (NSAID), such as *ibuprofen* (Motrin), sometimes helps control pain.

Note: If you take an NSAID for long periods, be sure that your doctor supervises your use to help you avoid side effects such as stomach irritation.

If your scoliosis pain is caused or worsened by narrowing or pressure on nerve roots, you may benefit from a steroid injection. The frequency and timing will depend on symptoms, but you should get no more than a few injections per year.

•**Surgery.** Contrary to what you might assume, the degree of your spinal curve is not used to determine whether surgery is needed. Instead, surgery is an option when pain—regardless of the severity of the curve—interferes with your ability to go about your daily activities.

Decompression surgery helps ease the pressure that is placed on nerves where the spine has weakened. This type of surgery usually involves removing (totally or partially) a bony structure or ligament that is applying pressure.

Another option is spine-stabilization surgery, which is performed to help straighten the spine. With this procedure, bones of the spine are fused together with bone grafts to stabilize the spine and eliminate as much of the spinal curve as possible. In most cases, a combination of both surgeries may be needed. The extent of surgery also varies. Major surgery is sometimes done to correct and stabilize the spine. In other cases, a small part of the curve can be addressed with a less extensive, lower-risk surgery.

The risk for complications, such as subsequent pain, increases with the magnitude of the surgery and can be as high as 30% in major reconstructions. There is a small (one in 3,000) risk for paralysis with major spine surgery. The patient's age and the presence of other conditions (such as diabetes) also affect risk for complications. Recovery times range from six weeks up to a year. A spine surgeon is best qualified to perform these procedures.

DO YOU HAVE SCOLIOSIS?

Signs that you may have scoliosis...

•**You have lost more than one inch of height.**

•**One shoulder appears higher than the other.**

•**One hip is higher than the other.**

•**If you find it more comfortable to stand or walk leaning forward,** or if you like to lean on a shopping cart in the grocery store, you may have spinal stenosis (a condition that causes narrowing in the spine), which is associated with adult scoliosis.

Help for Spinal Arthritis

Harris McIlwain, MD, rheumatologist in private practice in Tampa, and coauthor of *Diet for a Pain-Free Life* (Da Capo).

What helps to ease the pain and stiffness that accompanies arthritis in the spine?

You should walk, bike or swim every day. You can do it for just a few minutes if you're in pain, but gradually work up to 20 or 30 minutes daily. Tai chi and yoga are also good for all forms of arthritis.

An anti-inflammatory diet can help relieve pain as well. Cruciferous vegetables—broccoli, cauliflower, Brussels sprouts, kale, cabbage and bok choy—provide the antioxidant sulforaphane, which has been shown to slow the destruction of cartilage. Other anti-inflammatory foods include grapes, green and black tea, pineapple, blueberries, spinach, plums and those high in omega-3s, such as salmon. Avoid inflammatory foods, such as baked goods, which often contain trans fats.

Massage, acupuncture and meditation also may be helpful.

5 Myths About Arthritis—Plus Ways to Ease the Aches

C. Thomas Vangsness, Jr., MD, professor of orthopaedic surgery and chief of sports medicine at Keck School of Medicine at University of Southern California, Los Angeles. He is author, with Greg Ptacek, of *The New Science of Overcoming Arthritis: Prevent or Reverse Your Pain, Discomfort and Limitations* (Da Capo Lifelong).

About one in six Americans will have to cope with osteoarthritis* during their lifetimes. But even though so many people have it, there's still a lot of misinformation about it. *What's true about osteoarthritis—and what's not...*

***Myth*: Running causes arthritis.**

It would seem likely that the pounding the body receives during running could damage cartilage and increase the risk for arthritis. Not true.

A study that followed nearly 75,000 people for seven years found that those who ran 1.2 miles a day were 15% less likely to develop osteoarthritis and 35% less likely to need a hip replacement than those who merely walked.

Even though runners strike the ground with a force that equals eight times their body weight, they take longer strides (and require fewer steps) than walkers. The cumulative jolts caused by running actually appear to be similar to the slower-speed impacts among walkers.

That said, if you have, say, an arthritic knee, you should consult with a medical professional before beginning a running program. The joint stress from running could increase the progression in an already-damaged joint.

***Myth*: Don't move when you're hurting.**

The traditional arthritis advice is to give your joints total rest during flare-ups. Don't believe it.

You obviously don't want to overdo it when a joint is inflamed. But gentle movements keep joints mobile, flush out inflammatory chemicals and improve the flow of oxygen and nutrients to damaged tissues.

On "good" days, you could swim, lift weights, jog, etc. Yoga is an excellent exercise because it strengthens muscles and joints in a controlled

*The advice in this article may help with rheumatoid arthritis, too. Talk ot your doctor.

Antibiotics May Relieve Chronic Low-Back Pain

Nearly half the people whose pain is caused by a herniated disk later develop a bacterial infection. For those people, a 100-day course of the antibiotic *amoxicillin* reduced pain by up to 80% in a recent study. If you have had severe low-back pain for at least three months...have a damaged vertebra and swelling...and other treatment options have failed, ask your doctor whether an extended course of antibiotics is worth trying.

Study of 61 people with back pain by researchers at University of Southern Denmark, Odense, published in *European Spine Journal*.

Injections Don't Have to Contain Steroids

Recent research shows that injecting a nonsteroidal liquid into the area around the spinal cord—even a simple saline solution—relieved back pain as much as steroids.

Meta-analysis of 43 studies involving more than 3,600 patients by researchers at The Johns Hopkins University School of Medicine, Baltimore, published in *Anesthesiology.*

fashion. Tai chi is another excellent form of gentle exercise.

Important: If you have more pain than usual, talk to your doctor or physical therapist before starting—or continuing—exercise. You might need to adjust your workouts, including stopping/starting particular exercises.

***Myth*: It's an age-related disease.**

This is one of the most pervasive myths. Over the last few decades, people have begun to get osteoarthritis at younger and younger ages. Today, the average age at which symptoms start is 45—and the downward trend is likely to continue.

Experts aren't sure how to explain the increase in younger adults. Americans are heavier than they used to be, and obesity is strongly associated with arthritis. Also, injuries to joints during sports can lead to joint pain down the road. Ongoing inflammation increases cartilage destruction in the joint.

Important: If you have had a joint injury—a torn meniscus in the knee, for example—at any age, there's a good chance that you eventually will develop arthritis in the same joint. Work with a physical therapist to strengthen the muscles and tendons that surround the joint before symptoms start.

***Myth*: A little extra weight is OK.**

Studies have shown that people who are obese have more inflammation, less joint mobility and more cartilage damage than those who are lean. But what if you're just a few pounds overweight?

It's still a problem. People tend to exercise less when they're overweight. Reduced movement leads to less joint mobility—and more pain. Also, even a small amount of extra weight increases pressure on the joints. Every 10 pounds that you add above the waist generates an extra 70 to 100 pounds of pressure on the knees when you walk.

Research has shown that women who lose about 11 pounds can reduce their risk of developing arthritis symptoms by more than 50%.

***Myth*: You can't stop it.**

Arthritis may be persistent, but it's rarely hard to treat. Most patients get good relief without high-tech treatments or expensive medications.

Though the American College of Rheumatology advises patients with knee and/or hip arthritis to start with *acetaminophen* (Tylenol), I tell my patients that acetaminophen is an effective painkiller, but it doesn't help with inflammation.

My advice: Take one of the NSAIDs (nonsteroidal anti-inflammatory drugs) such as aspirin, *ibuprofen* or *naproxen.* They reduce pain as well as inflammation. Follow the dosing directions on the label, or ask your doctor for advice.

Helpful: To reduce stomach irritation (a common side effect of all the NSAIDs), take an antiulcer medication, such as *cimetidine* (Tagamet). I also have been prescribing a newer medication, *misoprostol* (Cytotec), for stomach irritation. Ask your doctor whether either of these might help you.

Quick Yoga Cures for Arthritis and Foot Cramps

Tara Stiles, the founder and owner of Strala Yoga in New York City. She is author of two books, *Yoga Cures* (Harmony) and *Slim Calm Sexy Yoga* (Rodale). Stiles has also created several yoga DVDs with Jane Fonda, Deepak Chopra and others. *TaraStiles.com*

Yoga aficionados know that this ancient practice can tone muscles and calm the mind. But few people are aware of yoga's ability to cure everyday ailments that can cause pain and sap our energy.

As a low-impact exercise that focuses on physical postures (asanas) and breathing techniques, yoga helps relieve a number of chronic conditions—by increasing blood flow, for example, and improving range of motion.

And even though regular yoga practice offers the broadest range of health benefits, doing targeted yoga moves, as needed, can often help you feel better within minutes. Do not worry about doing the move perfectly—simply breathe deeply while gently moving your body into position.

If you suffer from one of the following conditions, consider trying the single, carefully chosen yoga pose described here. This can help other treatments, such as medication, work more effectively—or, in some cases, the pose alone may alleviate the problem. *Best single-pose yoga cures (stay in each pose for five to 10 deep, long breaths)...**

ARTHRITIS

Pose to try: "Hands and knees fist release." For many people, this pose helps the swelling, joint pain, stiffness and limited range of motion that accompanies rheumatoid arthritis and osteoarthritis—especially in the hands.

What to do: Gently, get on your hands and knees. Make tight fists with both hands. Bend your elbows out to your sides, and place the tops of your hands on the ground, with your knuckles facing each other. Begin to straighten your elbows, but keep your fists tight and only do as much as you can without causing pain. You should feel a stretch on the tops of your wrists.

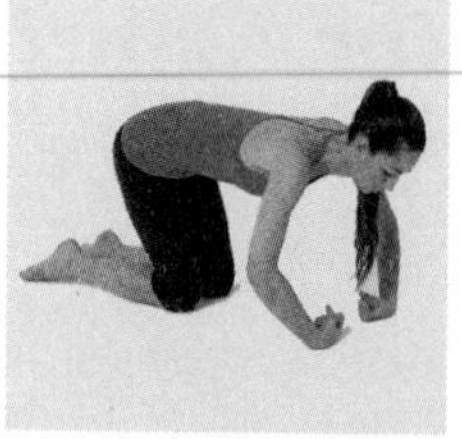

How it works: Whether you have arthritis or just sit at a desk all day, which dramatically limits your range of motion, this move increases flexibility in the wrists, hands, arms and back—important in easing arthritis pain.

FOOT CRAMPS

Pose to try: "Runner's stretch."

What to do: Gently, move into a low lunge with your right foot forward. Tuck the toes of your left foot so that they point forward and lower your back knee to the ground. Shift your hips back to sit on your back heel to stretch the arch of your foot. Relax your torso over your right leg. Stay in the pose for five long, deep breaths. Then do the pose with the other leg.

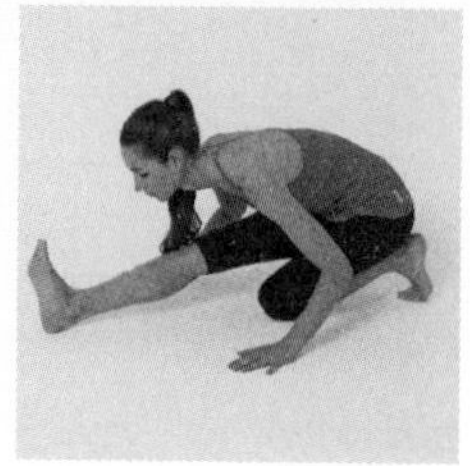

How it works: Foot cramps typically respond quickly to the even pressure this pose places on the foot and arch. This move also helps maintain the foot's flexibility, which is important for balance.

Photos of yoga poses: Thomas Hoeffgen

*If you have a chronic medical condition, check with your doctor before doing the poses, which should be done on a mat or carpeted floor.

Surprising Fixes for Common Foot Problems

Johanna S. Youner, DPM, a podiatric surgeon in private practice and attending physician at New York Downtown Hospital, both in New York City. Dr. Youner is a board-certified foot surgeon and a Fellow of the American College of Foot and Ankle Surgeons. *HealthyFeetNY.net*

When severe foot pain just won't go away, you may think that surgery is the only solution. Fortunately, that's not always true. There are several nonsurgical options available.

Here's the catch: Your podiatrist might not suggest these nonsurgical approaches—most doctors who treat foot disorders are used to patients demanding the "quick fix" of surgery (even though there's no guarantee of fast or lasting relief).

But in my experience, nonsurgical therapies such as those described here improve the pain by 60% to 80% in most cases—and completely eliminate it in some people—within six to eight weeks.

If your feet are affected by severe degenerative joint disease, surgery may be required.* *But most people are able to avoid the risks associated*

*If you have diabetes or smoke, you may not be a candidate for foot surgery due to poor circulation. Speak to your primary health-care provider for advice.

with foot surgery (such as pain and infection) with one of the innovative and effective options for the conditions listed below...

FOR MORTON'S NEUROMA

A neuroma is a benign tumor on a nerve. Morton's neuroma is a thickened area of nerve tissue that causes pain in the ball of the foot. Tight, pointy and/or high-heeled shoes can squeeze the toes together, causing the nerve leading to the toes to swell and thicken. Sometimes age alone causes this condition. People with flat feet or high arches are at increased risk—the nerve is more likely to get irritated.

Roomier footwear, orthotics (custom shoe inserts and pads), ice packs, anti-inflammatory drugs and cortisone injections are the standard recommendations. In people who opt for surgery, a small piece of the affected nerve is removed to release the pressure.

Surprising fix: Radiofrequency treatment, which is often used to treat back pain, can help. In a 2012 analysis of 29 patients who received this treatment for Morton's neuroma, 83% experienced complete relief of pain.

What happens: The foot is first numbed, then a thin needle attached to a small radiofrequency device is inserted into the neuroma, delivering a computer-generated signal that stuns and shrinks the nerve. The procedure is generally performed in a hospital operating room because the radiofrequency equipment is usually not available in podiatrists' offices.

Radiofrequency treatment of neuromas is still considered experimental, so check with your insurer to confirm coverage.

FOR HAMMERTOES

With this condition, one of your toes becomes permanently bent at the middle joint due to pressure on the toes' muscles and ligaments.

Hammertoes are mainly caused by shoes with a low toe box in which the toe joint presses into the top of the shoe. Arthritis, toe injuries and a family history of hammertoes also increase risk. Traditional treatments include padding the hammertoe with a silicone or gel pad.

Stretching exercises also may be useful.

What to do: Take hold of the tip of the toe and gently pull it out straight. Hold for five seconds. Repeat the exercise three times a day.

If these measures are not effective, a surgeon can make a small incision to straighten the tendon associated with the hammertoe and/or remove some of the affected bone.

Surprising fix: It sounds obvious, but the best solution is to look for a shoe with a roomy toe box and a heel of an inch to an inch-and-a-half—the range that supports your foot's natural curve. Contrary to what many people think, flats and very low heels do not give the most natural foot position.

If wearing different shoes doesn't give you adequate relief, an injection of a hyaluronic acid gel filler commonly used to help smooth wrinkles, such as Juvéderm Ultra 4 or Restylane, works well for reducing the pain of a hammertoe.

What happens: This 10-minute office procedure begins with an injection of *lidocaine* to numb the affected area. An injection of hyaluronic acid is then administered at the bony top of the bent toe. Hyaluronic acid for hammertoes is not covered by insurance—treatment for one hammertoe usually requires one syringe, which costs $700 to $1,000. The effect generally lasts for six to nine months.

Don't Rush to Have Surgery for a Torn Meniscus

People who had meniscal tears repaired surgically had almost exactly the same improvements in their knees as people who had a sham procedure. Both groups had chronic meniscal tears and did not have arthritis. Meniscal repair still may be needed for an acute tear, such as a sports injury...and for unstable tears that cause locking of the knee.

David T. Felson, MD, MPH, professor of medicine and epidemiology and chief of the Multidisciplinary Clinical Research Center Grant, Boston University School of Medicine.

Shoulder-Replacement Surgery Works for Arthritis

According to a recent finding, 93% of rheumatoid arthritis (RA) patients who had a total shoulder replacement...and 88% of those who had a partial replacement had pain relief and improved function. RA patients with severe shoulder pain and stiffness that are not relieved by medication or physical therapy should consider the surgery.

John Sperling, MD, an orthopedic surgeon at the Mayo Clinic, Rochester, Minnesota, and leader of a study published in *Journal of Shoulder and Elbow Surgery.*

FOR BUNIONS

A bunion is a bony bump that develops over the joint at the base of your big toe. Too-tight shoes are commonly the culprit, but bunions may also be inherited or can occur if you have arthritis.

Besides causing pain, bunions can create tingling from nerve compression. Orthotics and ice can help alleviate pain, and steroid injections can ease joint inflammation. But these treatments won't get rid of the bunion. If you do opt for surgery, a bunionectomy (a small incision is made so that the bunion can be removed and the big toe straightened) can be effective. Most individuals are back on their feet within three days, but full recovery can take up to eight weeks. Swelling may last for six months.

Surprising fix: Before resorting to surgery, start by loosening your shoelaces and/or buying slightly larger shoes. Your bunion may be taking up space in your shoes and compressing the nerves.

To ease pain in the big-toe joint, bunion sufferers should wear rigid shoes that provide extra support to the painful joint. (When shopping for a shoe, try to twist the sole...if you can twist it, put it back.)

Good brands for men: Rockport Dressports, Ecco and Allen Edmonds.

Good brands for women: Munro, Ariat and BeautiFeel. Avoid flip-flops—they provide no support, which worsens bunions.

In addition, consider wearing a night splint (available at drugstores and online), which can help stretch and straighten the joint.

Good product: The PediFix Nighttime Bunion Regulator, about $24.

Exercise will not change the bony overgrowth on the bunion but may help ease the pain.

What to do: While slightly lifting your foot off the ground, point it straight ahead and hold for five seconds. Then curl your toes under for five seconds. Repeat 10 times daily.

FOR WARTS

Plantar warts are noncancerous skin growths on the soles of the feet. The warts are caused by an infection with the human papillomavirus. You can catch the virus if you have a cut or scrape on your foot and walk barefoot in a public shower or gym locker room.

Some people try various over-the-counter products, such as salicylic acid. Others cover the wart with duct tape (with or without Aldara, a genital wart cream), and sometimes it falls off. However, these therapies aren't always successful, so some sufferers opt for surgical removal. Unfortunately, this can cause scarring that may lead to lifelong pain and discomfort.

Surprising fix: An injection of the chemotherapy drug *bleomycin sulfate.* Multiple studies have shown cure rates of 87% to 96% for plantar warts. Bleomycin sulfate is believed to kill the wart virus by stimulating the immune system to fight off the virus. The FDA has not approved the drug for plantar warts, but it can be used off-label for this purpose. When used in the small dose needed to treat plantar warts, common side effects of chemotherapy (such as hair loss and fatigue) do not occur.

Many insurance companies will cover this technique if it is preauthorized. Ask your podiatrist to inquire on your behalf. Be sure your podiatrist is experienced—permanent pain at the injection site can result if the drug is administered improperly.

Key to Fibromyalgia Pain Lies in the Skin of the Palms

Frank L. Rice, PhD, CEO and chief scientist, Integrated Tissue Dynamics, Rensselaer, New York, and former professor, Center for Neuropharmacology and Neuroscience, Albany Medical College, Albany, New York. His study was published in *Pain Medicine. intidyn.com*

People with fibromyalgia experience near-constant widespread pain, their hands and feet ache, and they often feel exhausted and foggy-brained. Yet because there is no blood test, lab test or scan that can confirm fibromyalgia, many doctors are skeptical about its very existence and suspect the problem is "all in the patient's head."

Finally, that's about to change—because researchers at last have discovered a surprising key to this confounding and debilitating condition. The problem isn't in patients' heads—it's in the skin of their hands.

BLOOD FLOW BASICS

To understand the recent research, you first need to understand some basics about circulation. After leaving the heart, oxygenated blood travels through arteries and then into arterioles (small arteries) before entering the tiny capillaries. Oxygen and nutrients leave the capillaries to get into the body's tissues and cells, and waste enters the capillaries. The blood then enters venules (small veins) and then larger veins, ultimately traveling to the lungs so it can be reoxygenated and filtered. And the cycle constantly repeats.

But not all blood enters the capillaries. Some blood flows directly from arteries into veins via arteriole-venule (AV) shunts, valves that open and close to control the passage of blood. The valves respond to cues from the nervous system, mainly to regulate body temperature. When a person is too hot, the shunts close, forcing the blood into the skin's capillaries, where the heat can leave the body. When a person is cold, the shunts open, allowing the blood to flow into the venules and conserving heat. The parts of the body where AV shunts are most plentiful are the cheeks, nose, soles of the feet and palms of the hands. The skin in those areas is different—smooth, hairless and noticeably more sensitive to heat and cold.

EXAMINING SHUNTS

For this recent study, researchers took small samples of skin from the palms of the hands of women with and without fibromyalgia. (Women are more than twice as likely to be diagnosed with fibromyalgia as men, and the hands are particularly painful in fibromyalgia sufferers.) Using special dyes, filters and lenses, the researchers closely examined many structures in the skin that are supplied by nerve fibers, including the AV shunts.

Startling finding: The number of AV shunts didn't differ between the two groups, but their size did. In fact, the AV shunts in women with fibromyalgia were nearly four times larger and had roughly two to eight times as many nerve fibers as those in women without fibromyalgia. This most likely explains why cold exacerbates fibromyalgia symptoms...and it also leads to a compelling theory about the development of fibromyalgia pain and fatigue.

As mentioned before, the AV shunts open and close in response to temperature—but they also regulate blood flow to other tissues, including muscles, when increased blood flow is needed, such as during movement and exercise. If the AV shunts are unable to function properly due to the presence of excessive nerve fibers, the mismanaged blood flow could be the source of the widespread muscle pain, achiness, fatigue and cognitive problems that plague fibromyalgia patients. The researchers are now investigating why there are excess nerve fibers around the shunts. Study leader Frank L. Rice, PhD, explained, "The AV shunts are sites where sensory nerve fibers are intermingled with nerve fibers of the sympathetic nervous system, which is activated by stress. The excess nerves involve mostly the sensory fibers that might be proliferating in response to stress activation of the sympathetic fibers."

GETTING HELP

Hopefully, this new information about fibromyalgia patients will lead to effective treatments...but in the meantime, it's reassuring to know that there is a real pathology involved in the disorder.

Dr. Rice's team is currently investigating whether men with fibromyalgia have a similar pathology to that discovered in women. Preliminary results indicate that women normally have more of the sensory fibers affiliated with the AV shunts, which may put them at greater risk of having excess fibers. Still, fibromyalgia is thought to be vastly underdiagnosed in men. According to recent research from the Mayo Clinic, 19 out of 20 men likely to have the disorder are not being properly diagnosed.

Bottom line: Male or female, if you have symptoms that suggest fibromyalgia and your doctor dismisses them, get a second opinion. To find a health-care provider who is experienced in detecting and treating this disorder, check the National Fibromyalgia Association online directory. For a wealth of information about fibromyalgia and Dr. Rice's ongoing research, visit the website of Integrated Tissue Dynamics at *intidyn.com.*

Reflexology Can Reduce Pain by 40% and May Be as Effective as Drugs

Reflexology involves applying pressure to specific points on the hands, feet or ears—that is believed to stimulate the body's production of pain-relieving endorphins in the brain and spinal cord.

Study of reflexology by researchers at University of Portsmouth, England, published in *Complementary Therapies in Clinical Practice.*

Nerve Stimulation Might Ease Fibromyalgia Pain

Mark Plazier, MD, neurosurgeon, University Hospital Antwerp, Belgium.
Patrick Wood, MD, director, fibromyalgia clinic, Madison River Oaks Medical Center, Canton, Mississippi.
International Neuromodulation Society meeting, Berlin.

An implanted device that zaps the nerves at the nape of the neck—shown effective in treating some people with migraines—may also help ease the ache of fibromyalgia, an ailment that causes widespread body pain and tenderness.

A Belgian scientist treated small numbers of fibromyalgia patients with "occipital nerve stimulation," which rouses the occipital nerves just beneath the skin at the back of the neck using an implanted device. Mark Plazier, MD, a neurosurgeon at University Hospital Antwerp, Belgium, found that pain scores dropped for 20 of 25 patients using this device over six months and their quality of life improved significantly.

"There are only a few treatment options [for fibromyalgia] right now and the response to treatment is far from 100%, which implies there are a lot of patients still looking for help to get a better life. This treatment might be an excellent option for them," said Dr. Plazier. But, "it is difficult to determine the impact of these findings on fibromyalgia patients, since larger trials...are necessary."

Dr. Plazier presented his research at a meeting of the International Neuromodulation Society, in Berlin. Research presented at scientific conferences has not typically been peer-reviewed or published and is considered preliminary.

BACKGROUND

Fibromyalgia is thought to affect about 5 million American adults—most of them women—according to the U.S. National Institutes of Health. The cause of the disorder, which can also involve sleep problems, anxiety and depression, is unknown and it can be difficult to treat.

Neuromodulation is a group of therapies that use medical devices to relieve symptoms or restore abilities by altering nerve system function.

ADDITIONAL STUDY AND PARTICIPANT RESPONSE

Dr. Plazier also presented a separate study on six fibromyalgia patients using PET scan images to visualize brain changes from occipital nerve stimulation treatment. It suggested that the nerve stimulation changes activity in the limbic system, a brain region that helps determine pain perception.

"In fibromyalgia, we see that there is a hypervigilance to pain, so patients are more sensitive to pain and more aware of it," Dr. Plazier said. "They also have high scores on questionnaires concerning catastrophizing behavior, which implies the high impact of pain on their lives."

"During [occipital nerve] stimulation we see differences in brain activity on PET scans in regions involved in pain," he added. "This all might suggest that we are influencing a cerebral system and might even turn it back to 'normal' perception."

Study participants didn't find the nerve-zapping treatment to be painful, Dr. Plazier noted. The occipital nerve stimulation device is implanted during a brief surgery using general anesthesia, he said, and postoperative pain is normal but not extreme.

EXPERT RESPONSE

Patrick Wood, MD, director of the fibromyalgia clinic at Madison River Oaks Medical Center in Canton, Mississippi, called the studies "interesting and promising," but said additional research is necessary before treatment with occipital nerve stimulation—which may cost around $10,000—could become mainstream for fibromyalgia patients.

"It's mostly used in headaches, and even in the headache realm it's still considered experimental," Dr. Wood said. "It would be nice to have expanded data here that would indicate there's something worth banking on and putting our hopes on. It's promising, but more work needs to be done before the average patient can consider it."

info For more information on fibromyalgia, visit the website of the U.S. National Institute of Arthritis and Musculoskeletal and Skin Diseases at *http://www.niams.nih.gov/Health_Info/Fibromyalgia/*.

Adjust the Lights, Hold the Morphine?

Journal of Advanced Nursing, news release

Changing lighting patterns in hospital rooms to more closely align with normal sleep-wake cycles may improve patients' health by reducing fatigue and pain, a recent study suggests.

The findings highlight a simple and inexpensive way to improve patient care, according to the researchers.

RECENT STUDY

The study was designed to determine if there were any links between hospital lighting, mood, sleep and pain in adult patients. Twenty-three women and 17 men in a large US hospital had their light exposure levels and sleep-wake cycles continuously monitored over 72 hours.

The patients' moods were checked daily through questionnaires, and their pain levels determined from medical records, according to the study published in the *Journal of Advanced Nursing*.

The patients were exposed mainly to low levels of light 24 hours a day and lacked the natural fluctuation between bright and low light required to help maintain normal sleep patterns.

PAIN LINKED TO LIGHT AND FATIGUE

The patients slept poorly, and the less light they were exposed to during the day, the greater their levels of fatigue. The more fatigued they felt, the more pain they had.

STUDIES ON LIGHT ENHANCEMENT NEEDED

"It is important to note that these findings were preliminary, and more research needs to be done to determine any possible clinical implications of enhancing the lighting environment for patients in the hospital," said study author Esther Bernhofer, PhD, RN, of the Cleveland Clinic in Ohio.

"Future intervention studies should include investigating different 'doses' of light exposure for medical inpatients," she added. "Such research would determine if lighting interventions could offer unique, cost-effective ways to more effectively address the problems of sleep-wake disturbances, distressed mood, and pain in hospitalized patients, providing for overall better patient outcomes."

info For more information on sleep, visit the U.S. National Institute of Neurological Disorders and Stroke website, *www.ninds.nih.gov/disorders/brain_basics/understanding_sleep.htm.*

Check That Implant

Hip and knee implants are sometimes recalled. If you are planning implant surgery, you should inquire about the track record of the device the surgeon intends to use. If you already have an implant, you can contact your physician's office for information on the type of implant and then access the FDA website (*FDA.gov*) to see if it has been recalled. If it has, talk to your surgeon about next steps, which could include further surgery, monitoring or simply reassurance that the device is unlikely to be problematic.

Douglas E. Padgett, MD, chief of adult reconstruction and joint replacement, Hospital for Special Surgery, New York City.

Music May Ease Pain for Kids During Hospital Procedure

University of Alberta, news release
Lisa Hartling, PhD, associate professor of pediatrics at the University of Alberta.

Music decreases children's pain when they're undergoing an uncomfortable medical procedure, according to a recent study.

STUDY FINDINGS

The study included 42 children, ages three to 11, who were treated at a pediatric emergency department and required an intravenous (IV) needle insertion. Some of the children listened to music while getting an IV.

Children who listened to music reported much less pain and some showed lower levels of distress than those who didn't listen to music. In addition, the parents of children who listened to music were more satisfied with their youngster's care.

Among health care providers, 76% of those who dealt with children who listened to music said the IVs were very easy to administer, compared with 38% of those who gave IVs to children who didn't listen to music, the investigators found.

The study was published in the journal *JAMA Pediatrics.*

IMPLICATIONS

"We did find a difference in the children's reported pain—the children in the music group had less pain immediately after the procedure," said study leader Lisa Hartling, PhD, associate professor of pediatrics at the University of Alberta. "The finding is clinically important and it's a simple intervention that can make a big difference. Playing music for kids during painful medical procedures would be an inexpensive and easy-to-use intervention in clinical settings," she added.

Dr. Hartling and her colleagues hope to investigate if music or other distractions can reduce pain and distress for children undergoing other painful medical procedures.

"There is growing scientific evidence showing that the brain responds to music and different types of music in very specific ways," Dr. Hartling said. "So additional research into how and why music may be a better distraction from pain could help advance this field."

info The Nemours Foundation explains how parents can prepare their children for a visit to the doctor at *http://kidshealth.org/parent/system/doctor/dr_visits.html.*

Women's Health

Natural Cures for Women's Vexing Health Problems

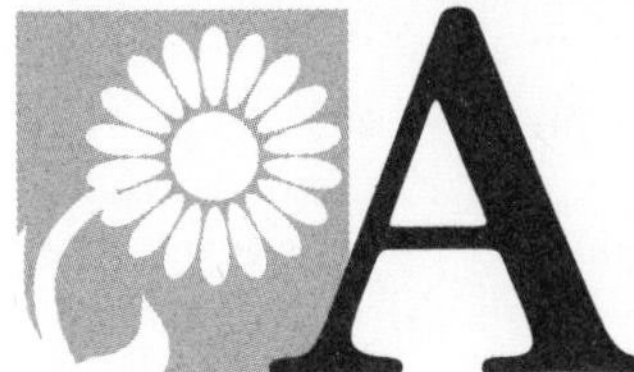

Across America, millions of women have been suffering for years from two common health problems that can be cured or at least dramatically improved.

If you're a woman with one of these conditions, you may mention it to your gynecologist, but chances are slim that you will get long-lasting relief from medication or other treatments prescribed by most MDs.

What I see in my practice: Every day, I treat women who are suffering unnecessarily from interstitial cystitis (also known as "painful bladder syndrome") and painful and/or lumpy breasts. Frequently, women actually give up on ever getting relief from these problems.

While anyone who has never endured these conditions may think that they are "not that big a deal," the truth is, these problems can greatly interfere with a woman's ability to go about her daily life and may even cause difficulties in her sexual relationship.

A natural approach: As a naturopathic physician, I look for the root cause of these conditions and help women use natural therapies that rely on the body's inherent ability to restore good health.

Here's how I treat my patients who have one of these vexing problems...

INTERSTITIAL CYSTITIS

Researchers are now finding that interstitial cystitis (IC) is much more prevalent than originally thought, affecting as many as eight million women in the US.

What it feels like: IC causes pelvic and/or perineal pain (the area between the anus and vagina). It can range from mild burning or discomfort to severe, debilitating pain that

---

Tori Hudson, ND, a naturopathic physician, medical director of A Woman's Time Health Clinic in Portland, Oregon, and program director of the Institute of Women's Health & Integrative Medicine. She is author of *Women's Encyclopedia of Natural Medicine* (McGraw-Hill).

can also affect the bladder, lower abdomen, low back and/or thighs.

Along with the pain there can be urinary problems including a constant urge to urinate…frequent urination (more than eight times a day)…and needing to urinate several times overnight.

What MDs typically prescribe: Drugs, including painkillers, antidepressants and the medication *pentosan* (Elmiron), which is FDA approved for IC. Pentosan may take up to four months to relieve pain and six months to improve urinary frequency.

Other procedures, such as stretching the bladder and administering medication directly into the bladder, are sometimes also used.

All of these approaches have potential side effects, including gastrointestinal damage and liver problems and, most importantly, work less than 50% of the time.

My natural approach: Using several of the following natural treatments at the same time, my patients find that their symptoms of pain and urinary urgency and/or frequency typically improve within about three months—sometimes even faster.

Here's what I recommend…

- **Avoid acidic foods and beverages.** In one study, 53% of IC patients linked a flare-up of their symptoms to specific foods, especially citrus fruits, tomatoes, chocolate and acidic beverages such as alcohol and coffee. To see whether this is true for you, avoid these foods for two weeks. If your symptoms improve, avoid these foods indefinitely.

If you need more relief, try adding the following supplements (you may be able to reduce the doses as your symptoms start to improve)…*

- **Glycosaminoglycans (GAGs).** These two related natural compounds strengthen the lining of the bladder (epithelium), which may be more permeable in people with IC, leading to irritation and pain.

Typical dose: N-acetyl glucosamine—500 mg, twice daily…glucosamine sulfate—750 mg, twice daily.

- **Vitamin A.** This nutrient can help IC by decreasing inflammation and stimulating epithelial repair.

Typical dose: 5,000 international units (IU) daily.

- **L-arginine.** This amino acid helps regulate levels of nitric oxide in the blood, relaxing the muscles of the bladder and improving circulation. It also improves urinary frequency and sometimes helps reduce the pain associated with IC.

Typical dose: 500 mg, twice daily.

- **Kava extract.** This herb from the South Pacific acts in several ways to relieve the symptoms of IC, including balancing potassium levels (high potassium can increase pain sensitivity).

Typical dose: One capsule, three times daily. Don't exceed 280 mg daily of kavalactones (an active ingredient).

PAINFUL AND/OR LUMPY BREASTS

Painful and/or lumpy breasts are one of the most common reasons women see a gynecologist. The good news is that this condition rarely accompanies breast cancer—cancer occurs as a painful, firm lump in only about 5% of cases.

What it feels like: Breasts that are painful and/or have one or more grape-size (or smaller) soft, rubbery lumps that can be moved are often due to hormonal changes during a woman's menstrual cycle. The breast pain can also be caused by an old injury or an acute infection (mastitis).

What MDs typically prescribe: When breasts are painful and/or lumpy due to hormonal changes, conventional doctors typically refer to it as fibrocystic breast disease.

Drug treatments that are frequently prescribed, such as birth control pills, can cause serious side effects, including headache, nausea and a slightly increased risk for stroke and deep vein thrombosis.

My natural approach: Because most women have some lumps or lumpy areas in their breasts all the time, as well as occasional pain, I don't consider this a disease.

*Check with your doctor before starting a new supplement regimen—especially if you have a chronic medical condition and/or take medication.

Here's what I recommend...

• **Start with your diet.** Though scientists aren't sure why, research shows that simply eating more fruits and vegetables and avoiding caffeine (in all forms, including food sources such as chocolate and certain over-the-counter medications such as Anacin) can help prevent lumpy breasts.

In a one-year study, increasing daily soy intake also reduced breast tenderness and fibrocystic changes. Soy does not increase breast cancer risk, as some researchers had theorized, or pose danger to women who have had or have the disease.

Recommendation: One to two servings daily (a serving equals one cup of soy milk, for example, or four ounces of tofu). Also, consider taking the following...

• **Vitamin E.** Two studies show that vitamin E relieves breast pain and tenderness regardless of whether they are linked to a woman's menstrual cycle.

Typical dose: 400 IU to 800 IU daily of the d-alpha tocopherol form of vitamin E.

• **Evening primrose oil.** The linoleic and gamma linolenic acid in the oil help the body produce compounds that reduce pain and balance hormones.

Typical dose: 1,500 mg, twice daily.

If your condition doesn't improve in two to three months, consider...

• **Iodine.** Studies suggest that iodine deficiency plays a role in fibrocystic breasts. Without an adequate amount of iodine, breast tissue becomes more sensitive to estrogen, producing lumps.

Typical dose: 3 mg to 6 mg daily of aqueous iodine (by prescription).

Also helpful: Consume more iodine-rich foods, such as shellfish, seaweed, Swiss chard and lima beans.

Don't forget: In addition to undergoing an annual breast exam by a physician and any imaging tests he/she recommends, every woman should conduct a monthly breast self-exam. If any new, unusual changes, thickenings or lumps are detected, they should be promptly evaluated by a physician.

New Analysis Confirms Hormone Therapy Won't Prevent Disease After Menopause

JoAnn Manson, MD, PhD, chief, preventive medicine, Brigham and Women's Hospital, Boston.

Elizabeth Nabel, MD, president, Brigham and Women's Hospital, Boston.

Journal of the American Medical Association

There is not enough evidence to support using hormone replacement therapy after menopause to prevent heart disease or other chronic ills, but short-term use for hot flashes should remain an option.

That's the conclusion of the latest analysis of the Women's Health Initiative (WHI), a group of major US trials set up to test the use of hormone replacement therapy for preventing chronic diseases in healthy, older women.

The WHI was launched in the 1990s, at a time when doctors were prescribing hormone replacement therapy to postmenopausal women to ward off heart disease. The results changed common practice, however.

In 2002, one of the trials was stopped early when researchers found that women taking the hormones—estrogen-plus-progestin pills—actually had higher risks of blood clots, heart attack, stroke and breast cancer than placebo users did.

A second trial, looking at estrogen therapy alone, was stopped two years later. Women on the hormone showed no lower risk of heart disease, but did have a slightly elevated rate of blood clots and stroke.

The recent findings, published in the *Journal of the American Medical Association*, do nothing to change the general advice on hormones, according to lead researcher JoAnn Manson, MD, PhD, chief of preventive medicine at Brigham and Women's Hospital in Boston.

"Hormone therapy is not indicated for long-term disease prevention," Dr. Manson said.

HORMONE THERAPY OK FOR THE SHORT TERM

On the other hand, for women who have recently gone through menopause and are suffering from severe hot flashes, hormone therapy is still the most effective remedy. So short-term use "may be appropriate" for those women, Dr. Manson said.

That's not a new recommendation; experts have long said that short-term hormone therapy should be an option for severe hot flashes. But these latest results bolster the belief that hormone therapy is safer for relatively younger women who use it for a finite time, Dr. Manson said.

She noted that some doctors seem to have had a "misunderstanding" regarding the original WHI findings, and are reluctant to use hormone therapy even for hot flashes.

"Many women have a hard time finding a doctor who'll prescribe it," Dr. Manson said. She added that these latest findings paint "a clearer picture of what the message should be."

RESEARCH DETAILS

The results are based on about 16,600 women who were randomly assigned to take either estrogen/progestin or placebo pills, and more than 10,700 who took either estrogen alone or a placebo. The women were on hormone therapy for about six to seven years before the WHI trials were stopped, and Dr. Manson's team followed them for six to eight years beyond that.

Over the longer term, most of the risks originally tied to hormone replacement therapy declined—and so did the benefits, such as lower risks of hip fractures and diabetes. The exception was breast cancer risk, which remained higher for women who used estrogen and progesterone. Across the study period, there were 434 cases of breast cancer among those women, versus 323 among placebo users.

The findings were "more favorable" among relatively younger women, aged 50 to 59, who used estrogen only, the researchers said. They actually had a slightly lower rate of heart attack and fewer deaths, versus women in their 50s who used placebo pills.

But those differences were small, and Dr. Manson said there are concerns about other hormone therapy risks, even in younger women—such as the risk of blood clots that could cause a stroke or travel to the lungs.

EXPERT COMMENTARY

So, no one should take hormones for the sake of cutting long-term disease risks, said Elizabeth Nabel, MD, who wrote an editorial published with the study.

"Even though short-term use of this therapy may be helpful in [menopause] symptom relief, this recent, 13-year follow-up study clearly does not support the long-term use of hormone therapy for the prevention of chronic diseases," said Dr. Nabel, president of Brigham and Women's Hospital.

MORE HORMONE OPTIONS BEING EXPLORED

For a drug to be used to prevent, rather than treat, disease, the benefits have to clearly be worth it, Dr. Manson noted. "We have to set the bar very high," she said.

Studies are still looking into whether hormone therapy might cut relatively younger women's disease risks—including whether lower doses or different "routes of delivery" might work better.

It's thought, Dr. Manson said, that hormone patches might be safer than pills, because they may not carry the same blood-clot risk. But there is no conclusive evidence that patches should be used for disease prevention either, she stressed.

info For more information on hormone replacement therapy, visit the website of the U.S. Department of Health at *http://www.womenshealth.gov/menopause/symptom-relief-treatment/menopausal-hormone-therapy.html.*

Dangers of Early Menopause

Machelle Seibel, MD, a professor of obstetrics and gynecology at the University of Massachusetts Medical School in Worcester. He is editor in chief of *My Menopause Magazine* and coauthor, with Karen Giblin, of *Eat to Defeat Menopause: The Essential Nutrition Guide for a Healthy Midlife* (Da Capo Lifelong).

For the average woman in the US, menopause occurs between the ages of 45 and 55. But what if it happens earlier than that?

Up to 5% of American women do reach menopause earlier than normal—due, for example, to genetics, chemotherapy, surgical removal of the ovaries or a seemingly unrelated condition such as an autoimmune disease (see details below).

What's new: A growing body of evidence is now uncovering dangers associated with early menopause. Fortunately, research is showing that there are steps that women can take to protect themselves.

WHY MENOPAUSE HAPPENS EARLY

A woman is said to have reached menopause when a year has passed since her last menstrual period. The same symptoms that occur with regular menopause usually are present with early menopause, such as hot flashes, decreased sex drive, vaginal dryness and sleep problems.

When menopause comes early because of genetics or an autoimmune disorder, it's a specific medical condition—doctors call it primary ovarian insufficiency. Decreased activity of the ovaries causes a drop in estrogen that leads to menopause. Autoimmune diseases that can trigger early menopause include thyroid disease, rheumatoid arthritis and lupus, among others.

Medical treatments also can cause early menopause. Women who undergo surgical removal of the ovaries experience menopause right away. Chemotherapy and pelvic radiation can damage the ovaries, resulting in menopause that occurs earlier than normal.

Early Menopause and Estrogen

It has been more than a decade since a high-profile study in *The Journal of the American Medical Association* (*JAMA*) reported that hormone-replacement therapy (HRT) increases risk for heart disease, stroke, breast cancer and blood clots in the lungs.

After the study was reported, prescriptions for HRT, commonly used to help ease menopausal symptoms, dropped by 50%—and today millions of women still refuse HRT.

What most people don't realize: Many women in the *JAMA* study began HRT 12 years after menopause. Also, the increased risks linked to HRT use have been shown to mainly occur in women who took the hormone progestin along with estrogen.

If women start estrogen soon after early (or regular) menopause, research shows that they'll have lower risk for heart disease, Alzheimer's disease and osteoporosis than those who take it later in life.

My advice for women with early menopause: Consider taking estrogen for at least 10 years, but talk to your doctor to be sure estrogen's benefits outweigh any potential risks (such as stroke). An estrogen patch may be safer than the oral form. If you've missed the window described in this article for estrogen therapy, consult your doctor.

Another area of study: Scientists also are learning more about a link between environmental toxins and early menopause. Smoking—and exposure to cigarette smoke—has been found to promote early menopause by damaging the ovarian cells that release estrogen. Women who smoke should do their best to stop. Research shows that female smokers start menopause an average of two years earlier than nonsmokers.

Talk to your doctor: If your periods have stopped and you're also experiencing weight loss, dizziness or low blood pressure, you may need a test for Addison's disease—a condition that affects the adrenal glands and is associated with about 3% of cases of primary ovarian insufficiency.

STAY SAFE AFTER MENOPAUSE

For the majority of women, the dangers of early menopause can be nearly eliminated with the use of supplemental estrogen, along with lifestyle approaches…

- **Heart attack and stroke.** Menopause that occurs even at a normal age increases heart disease risk—the decline in estrogen causes about a 10% boost in LDL "bad" cholesterol, reduces the ability of the coronary arteries to expand and contract and hastens the development of atherosclerosis.

Important study: Women who experienced early menopause were found to be twice as likely to suffer from a heart attack or stroke as those with a later menopause.

New Way to Predict a Woman's Final Menstrual Period

A formula based on changing levels of the hormones estradiol and follicle-stimulating hormone can predict when a woman's final period will occur. In the year before the final menstrual period, women experience accelerated bone loss and increased risk for heart disease. Knowing when the last period is due would allow doctors to prescribe medications or suggest other measures to reduce bone loss and maintain heart health.

Study by researchers at David Geffen School of Medicine, UCLA, published in *Journal of Clinical Epidemiology & Metabolism.*

My advice: Follow a cholesterol-lowering diet—include plenty of fish, vegetables and whole grains and limit red meat and other foods high in saturated fat. And exercise regularly (ideally, for at least 30 minutes, most days of the week).

Also: Be sure to get your cholesterol tested every one to two years. If it's high, your doctor may recommend niacin and/or a statin medication, such as *simvastatin* (Zocor).

• **Memory loss/dementia.** "Brain fog"—a common complaint among menopausal women of all ages—appears to be temporary, but there is another, more serious risk.

Important finding: Women who experience early menopause have nearly twice the risk of developing dementia as women whose menopause comes later.

My advice: Don't delay estrogen therapy. Research shows that women who start estrogen replacement within five years of menopause (the earlier the better), and continue to take it for 10 years or more, are about one-third less likely to get Alzheimer's than those who avoid estrogen until later in life. Despite well-publicized research that found dangers associated with hormone-replacement therapy (HRT) several years ago, there are safe ways for most women to use it (see box on page 341).

• **Osteoporosis.** Your risk of developing osteoporosis is roughly doubled if you have early menopause. When estrogen declines, the rate at which your bones break down outpaces your body's ability to build new bone.

My advice: After menopause, eat plenty of high-calcium foods, such as leafy greens and low-fat dairy. Postmenopausal women need a daily total of 1,200 mg of calcium (from food and supplements).

They should also get their vitamin D levels tested and take vitamin D supplements, if needed, as directed by their doctors. Vitamin D is just as important as calcium for healthy bones.

Remember: Weight-bearing exercises, such as walking, tennis and weight-training, are keys to building and maintaining bone density.

Free Yourself from Menopausal Fog

Miriam T. Weber, PhD, neuropsychologist, University of Rochester Medical Center, Rochester, New York. Her study was published in *Menopause: The Journal of The North American Menopause Society.*

Many women look forward to reaching menopause and being freed from monthly menstrual hassles and worries about unintended pregnancy.

But they're not so happy if they find themselves experiencing menopausal "brain fog"—including poor concentration...difficulty recalling where they put things...and/or trouble remembering names and phone numbers.

And they're really not happy when their husbands and others get frustrated and blame them for forgetting things and just seeming to be "not all there."

Up to two-thirds of women say they experience brain fog while going through the midlife transition. And while some studies support this, there is not much objective proof of the phenomenon—so some people claim that the menopausal brain drain is all in women's heads, so to speak.

Researchers decided to find out whether menopausal brain fog is real...and, if so, to pinpoint exactly when a woman can expect it to start. *What they found was fascinating...*

HEAD TEST

To go hunting for brain fog, the researchers gathered 117 women, average age 49, and, based on each woman's stage of menopause, split them into four groups...

1. Late reproductive stage—characterized by subtle changes in menstrual flow and/or the length of menstrual cycles.

2. Early menopausal transition—a woman's cycles become persistently irregular, varying in length by a week or more.

3. Late menopausal transition—periods come two months or more apart.

4. Early postmenopause—the first 12 months after a woman's final period.

For the study, the women answered questionnaires about their general health, quality of life and symptoms (if any) of depression or anxiety. And they completed a battery of tests designed to measure their cognitive function—including their attention level...short-term or "working" memory...verbal fluency...dexterity...visual/spatial skill (for instance, identifying objects that had been cut into pieces and rearranged)...and verbal learning (such as recalling lists of words).

Results: Surprisingly, women in the third stage did just as well on the cognitive tests as those in the first and second stages, according to the lead researcher, Miriam T. Weber, PhD. However, women in the fourth stage (the first year after the final menstrual period) were a different story—for the most part, they did significantly worse on tests of attention, verbal memory, dexterity and verbal learning. For instance, Dr. Weber said, they took an average of five to six seconds longer to complete the dexterity task of putting pegs into pegboards...and they remembered an average of two fewer words in tests measuring recall of 15-word lists.

In other words, brain fog in postmenopausal women is real—and it seems to begin shortly after the last menstrual period.

HELLO, BRAIN FOG—NOW GO AWAY

The good news is that the cognitive dip seems to be temporary. Though Dr. Weber's research wasn't focused on measuring how long these effects persisted past menopause, a national women's health study done a few years ago suggested that cognitive skills rebound to premenopausal levels once a woman is postmenopausal. That study didn't specify exactly when the rebound takes place—but "postmenopausal" by definition means that a woman's final menstrual period occurred at least 12 months earlier.

Now, what can women do about all this? If you're heading into menopause, you're probably hoping to cope well with brain lapses while you wait for things to get back to normal. *Dr. Weber offered these tips...*

- **Safeguard your overall health.** Eating right, exercising, maintaining an appropriate weight and keeping blood pressure and cholesterol under control will help your brain work optimally.
- **Keep a calendar handy.** Write frequent notes to keep track of appointments and other commitments.
- **Resist the urge to multitask.** Focusing on one task at a time optimizes brain power—so turn off your cell phone and disable e-mail pop-up windows when you're in the middle of an important task.
- **Relax and be patient.** As Dr. Weber said, "Just knowing that this is a normal part of life might reduce anxiety, and that helps your brain function better."

No More Hot Flashes!

In a study of more than 6,000 menopausal women, those who ate the most fruit and a Mediterranean-style diet with vegetables, whole grains, fish and healthy fats, such as olive oil, were less likely to experience hot flashes and night sweats than those who did not closely follow this diet.

Theory: Diets high in fat and sugar can increase blood sugar levels, which can trigger hot flashes.

Gerrie-Cor Herber-Gast, PhD, research fellow, School of Population Health, The University of Queensland, Australia.

Did Men Cause Menopause?

Rama Singh, PhD, professor, population genetics and evolution, department of biology, McMaster University, Hamilton, Ontario, Canada.
Lynnette Leidy Sievert, PhD, professor, University of Massachusetts Amherst, and trustee, North American Menopause Society.
PLOS Computational Biology, online

Can women blame men for menopause? They may have a case, according to recent research that suggests it was men's interest in mating with younger females that gave evolutionary rise to menopause by sidelining older women from reproduction.

Menopause—when a woman stops getting menstrual periods and can't become pregnant—is unique to humans and its cause is still unknown, explained study author and evolutionary biologist Rama Singh, PhD. "We accept as a given the idea that older women tend to be unable to reproduce," said Dr. Singh. "But this is actually an 'evolutionary puzzle.'"

It has long been thought that menopause is what causes women, primarily in their early 50s, to stop being able to get pregnant, but the researchers found evidence that things could actually have occurred the other way around. In other words, infertility may have been the cause, not the effect, of menopause in early humans.

There are at least 10 theories of why menopause occurs, according to the researchers, including ideas based on the fact that women are living longer and depleting the number of eggs in their ovaries, to what is called the "grandmother hypothesis." That idea holds that menopause allows older women to provide childcare that contributes to the survival of their grandchildren, making them more fit or valuable to the human tribe.

LATEST RESEARCH ON MENOPAUSE BLAMES MEN

But Dr. Singh's research, published online in the journal *PLOS Computational Biology*, suggests something altogether new.

The researchers used computational models and computer simulations to show how male mating preference for younger females could increase the number of mutations that stopped women's reproductive ability, creating menopause.

"This paper is saying that men have played the major or dominant part in choosing mates," said Dr. Singh, who is a professor of population genetics and evolution at McMaster University, in Canada. "Somewhere along the line in our evolutionary history, males did not mate randomly but preferred young women because they are more attractive."

Going way back in human history, people reproduced all their lives, explained Dr. Singh. While it's possible that some women may have experienced menopause 30,000 years ago, now 100% of women experience it. "Menopause is an evolutionary phenomenon," he said.

The scientists found that the development of menopause seems to have done nothing to improve the chances of human survival over time, but rather occurred because women of a certain age weren't finding mates, and thus reproductive ability was unnecessary for them.

Dr. Singh pointed out that if women long ago had been the ones choosing younger mates, older men would have been the ones losing their fertility, not women.

The process of natural selection favors the most fit, so women who are most likely to reproduce are protected, explained Dr. Singh. Natural selection is the gradual, non-random process through which biological traits become

Remedies for Uncomfortable Intercourse

To prevent dryness during intercourse, use a lubricant that mimics natural body fluids, such as Good Clean Love (*GoodCleanLove.com*) or Pre-Seed (available in drugstores).

Recent finding: 36% of women who used massage oil or baby oil as lubricants developed yeast infections...women who used petroleum jelly had twice the risk for bacterial infection.

Study of 141 women by researchers at David Geffen School of Medicine, University of California, Los Angeles, published in *Obstetrics & Gynecology*, with additional reporting from *Good Housekeeping*.

either more or less common, due to the way reproduction occurs, Dr. Singh explained.

IMPLICATION

Dr. Singh said his research suggests that it might be possible for women who delay childbearing to also postpone menopause, allowing them to have a longer window in which to conceive. "We might be able to extend the time period in which you can have children, rather than rush it," he said.

Dr. Singh said he's planning to do more simulations based on a Canadian long-term study of aging that is following 50,000 men and women. He is interested in learning more about the relationship between menopause, reproduction and genetic markers. "I really want to see if you can do something to delay menopause," he explained.

EXPERT RESPONSE

Lynnette Leidy Sievert, PhD, a biological anthropologist and a professor at the University of Massachusetts, Amherst, raised questions about the study.

"The study showed that by the age of 50 or 60, 50% of the population was still living, but that just doesn't match what we know about human evolution," she said. "By the age of 50, the skeletal evidence shows that only 10% of Neanderthals lived beyond 50. Our own homo sapiens [humans] had about 17% living past the age of 40."

Dr. Sievert, a member of the board of trustees of the North American Menopause Society, also questioned whether the concept of men mating with younger women fully explains menopause.

"Because it's a human and mammalian pattern for men to die younger [than women], you have a younger female with an older male who is going to die," she explained. "I get mixed up about how that pulls a woman's lifespan across menopause."

info To learn more about menopause, visit the website of the North American Menopause Society at *www.Menopause.org*.

Can Women Skip Antibiotics for Urinary Tract Infection?

Bart Knottnerus, MD, researcher, Academic Medical Center, University of Amsterdam, the Netherlands.

Jennifer Leighdon Wu, MD, obstetrician-gynecologist, Lenox Hill Hospital, New York City.

BMC Family Practice

Some women with symptoms of a urinary tract infection may be able to skip the antibiotics typically prescribed and have their symptoms improve or clear on their own, according to a recent Dutch study.

"In healthy people, many mild infections can be cured spontaneously," said study leader Bart Knottnerus, MD, a researcher at the Academic Medical Center of the University of Amsterdam.

A US expert, however, had a number of cautions about the findings, including the small number of women studied.

STUDY DETAILS

For the research, published in the journal *BMC Family Practice*, Dr. Knottnerus recruited women from 20 general medical practices in and around the Netherlands from 2006 to 2008. Women who

Standard Test for Urinary Tract Infection May Be Inaccurate

Nearly 25% of women who had signs of urinary tract infections (UTIs) had no evidence of bacteria in their urine when tested with the midstream urine culture, currently the standard test for detecting infection. E. coli, the most common bacteria that causes UTIs, often is present in such low amounts that they are missed by labs, which test only for high quantities.

If you think you have a UTI: Ask the doctor to request that the culture be tested for small amounts of E. coli.

Thomas M. Hooton, MD, professor of medicine at University of Miami Miller School of Medicine and lead author of a study published in *The New England Journal of Medicine*.

What Causes Recurring UTIs

Recurring urinary tract infections in women may be caused by a strain of E. coli that can flourish in both the gut and bladder. This strain can migrate back and forth despite repeated treatments—and even get stronger, causing recurring infections. This discovery may lead to new and better treatments for women who suffer recurrent infections.

Study of urinary tract infections by researchers at Washington University, St. Louis, published in *Science Translational Medicine.*

had contacted their doctor complaining of frequent urination, painful urination or both were asked if they would be willing to delay antibiotics—but only if their symptoms had been present for no longer than seven days.

Certain women were excluded, including those pregnant or breast-feeding or those whose immune systems were compromised.

In all, 176 women participated. Of those, 137 were asked to delay antibiotics and 51 agreed. All the women gave a urine sample to be analyzed and cultured. The women reported on their symptoms over the next week.

After a week, 28 of the 51 women willing to delay antibiotic use still had not used an antibiotic. Twenty of these women (71%) reported disappearance or improvement of their symptoms. Of these 20, more than a third had a positive culture result, indicating an infection. The researchers did not know the culture results at the start of the study.

Most of the women not willing to delay antibiotics had a positive culture.

The women who did agree to delay, Dr. Knottnerus said, might be aware of the bacterial resistance that can result from antibiotic use.

"Furthermore," he said, "in the Netherlands, other mild infections—like eye, ear, throat and respiratory infections—are usually not treated with antibiotics. Therefore, people might be more receptive to delayed antibiotic prescriptions."

Antibiotics for urinary tract infections usually work within two or three days. How would an infection clear on its own? "Our defense mechanisms are strong and often do not need any help from antibiotics," Dr. Knottnerus said. He studied only uncomplicated infections of the bladder—defined as those in healthy, nonpregnant women.

EXPERT WEIGHS IN

Jennifer Leighdon Wu, MD, a gynecologist at Lenox Hill Hospital in New York City, was cautious about the findings. "The number of women who agreed to delay was 51," she said. "Before changing my practice, I would like to see much larger numbers."

Checking in with your doctor might uncover some other problem, she said. "I can't tell you how many people have come in thinking it's a urinary tract infection and it's a yeast infection," she said.

In her practice, Dr. Wu will sometimes prescribe antibiotics right away, especially if a woman is in pain. For others, she may wait until the culture comes back, which usually takes about three days. "If you can wait until the culture comes back, the patient will probably receive more appropriate antibiotics," she said, as the doctor can then target the antibiotic to the organism found in the culture.

"You have to be really careful about who you are asking to forego antibiotic treatment," she said. It could be especially dangerous in older patients. The women in the study, on average, were in their early 40s.

Antibiotics are needed if a woman has symptoms such as fever, shivering and flank pain, Dr. Knottnerus said, as this may indicate the infection has progressed to the kidneys.

As for cranberry juice, which some women use to self-treat, Dr. Knottnerus said there is no hard evidence that it works to treat infections, but it may help prevent them.

info To learn more about urinary tract infections, visit the U.S. National Institute of Diabetes and Digestive and Kidney Diseases website at *http://kidney.niddk.nih.gov/Kudiseases/pubs/utiadult/.*

Probiotics for Vaginal Health

Laurie Cullen, ND, associate professor of clinical medicine and chair of the department of clinical sciences, Bastyr University, Kenmore, Washington, and core clinical faculty member, Bastyr Center for Natural Health, Seattle.

You know that helpful probiotics are good for your digestive health...but did you know that these beneficial bacteria also promote vaginal health?

Folk medicine has long recommended eating yogurt as a natural remedy for vaginal infections, and now studies are finding evidence that folk wisdom was on the right track. For instance, a recent study in *Journal of Family Practice* showed that the probiotics in yogurt and in certain vaginal suppositories may reduce the recurrence of bacterial vaginosis (BV), the most common type of vaginal infection among women of childbearing age.

Although we don't yet have a large body of peer-reviewed research proving that probiotics prevent various types of recurrent vaginal infections, it just makes sense to use beneficial bacteria to battle harmful bacteria.

The vaginal ecosystem is very sensitive. The beneficial Lactobacilli strains of bacteria that live in the vagina keep the pH around 4.2. Certain factors can raise the vaginal pH, leading to an overgrowth of various bacteria and causing BV. Situations that lower the vaginal pH can lead to an overgrowth of fungal organisms, such as Candida albicans, and cause a yeast infection.

Among the many factors that can affect vaginal pH are the use of antibiotics, oral steroid medications, spermicidal contraceptives or birth control pills...sexual intercourse, menstruation, tampon use, pregnancy or menopause...diabetes or obesity...cancer or cancer treatment...and conditions that compromise the immune system.

PROBIOTICS FOR PREVENTION

The following prevention strategies are appropriate for just about any woman who wants to keep her vagina as healthy as possible...and they're particularly helpful for those who have a history of vaginal infections.

Note: Whatever type of probiotic you use—be it in the form of yogurt, an oral supplement or a topical vaginal product—avoid brands that contain only the species of Lactobacillus called acidophilus. Acidophilus, which comes from cow's milk, is really good at populating a cow's vagina with cow-beneficial probiotics, but on its own it doesn't do much to help repopulate the human vagina with the various Lactobacilli species normally found there. Choose probiotics that contain a number of different Lactobacillus species in addition to acidophilus, such as Lactobacillus GG, rhamnosus, reuteri, plantarum and/or salvarius.

Try one, two or all three of the types of products below for two to six months to see if they help your vagina stay infection-free. If so, you can continue to use them indefinitely.

- **Cultured yogurt.** Eat at least one serving daily. For women who like dairy yogurt, consider the plain-flavored, American-style Stonyfield brand. For people who prefer a cultured soymilk yogurt alternative, try the Silk brand's Fruity & Creamy line. These brands are recommended because we can verify the cultures, meaning that we can grow in a lab the bacteria that they say are in their product.
- **Oral probiotics.** For my patients, I most often prescribe over-the-counter oral supplements such as Fem-Dophilus...FemEcology...or Pro-Flora Women's Probiotic by Integrative Therapeutics. Usually these are taken daily, following the guidelines on the product label.

Regular Pap Smears After Age 50 Are Vital

In a British study of 1,341 women, those who were not screened for cervical cancer after age 50 were six times more likely to be diagnosed with the disease later in life. Plus, women whose screening results were normal had a lower-than-average risk for cervical cancer into their 80s. Pap smears now are advised every three years until age 65 in the US.

Anne F. Rositch, PhD, MPH, assistant professor of epidemiology and public health, University of Maryland School of Medicine, Baltimore.

> **When Not to Wax**
>
> Don't get a "Brazilian" bikini wax before a gynecological appointment. Waxing a large part of the pubic area often causes redness and inflammation, which can make it harder for the doctor to provide an accurate exam.
>
> Hilda Hutcherson, MD, obstetrician and gynecologist, Columbia University Medical Center, New York City, writing in *Redbook*.

•**Vaginal moisturizers.** Sex affects the vaginal pH because men's semen has a pH of about 7.1 to 8.0. Spermicidal contraceptives also alter the pH of the vagina. A vaginal moisturizer helps keep the vaginal pH in balance, which is why it's a good idea to use one before and immediately after having sex. Also use it daily whenever you are taking antibiotics. Preferred brands include RepHresh Vaginal Gel...and Luvena Prebiotic Vaginal Moisturizer and Lubricant.

TREATING GYNO CONDITIONS WITH PROBIOTICS

If you develop any symptoms of a vaginal infection, such as itching, discharge, odor and/or pain, it's important to see a doctor who can diagnose the cause. Women who try self-treatment without first getting a diagnosis may end up making the problem worse. Treatment depends on the type of infection your doctor ends up diagnosing. The most common types are...

•**Yeast vaginitis.** Vaginal suppositories of boric acid (also called borax) are highly effective. Although such suppositories are available without a prescription, before using them, make sure that your doctor confirms the yeast diagnosis. If you are prone to recurrent yeast infections and your doctor is satisfied that you can recognize the symptoms, however, he/she may give you the go-ahead to self-treat. In such cases, I often prescribe a five-to-seven-day course of Yeast Arrest Suppositories, which contain several homeopathic anti-yeast ingredients in addition to boric acid.

After the boric acid treatment is done, it's a good idea to help restore vaginal health by inserting a probiotic product directly into the vagina once daily for one to two weeks. For this, I recommend capsules of Fem-Dophilus, Fem-Ecology or Pro-Flora Women's Probiotic—yes, the same oral probiotic supplements mentioned in the prevention section above also can be used as vaginal suppositories, she said.

•**Bacterial vaginosis.** Use Fem-Dophilus, Fem-Ecology or Pro-Flora Women's Probiotic both orally and vaginally—one oral and one vaginal capsule per day. Sometimes this strategy provides enough immune support to allow a woman's body to fight off the infection. However, if this approach doesn't work within three or four days, it may be necessary to use antibiotics to get rid of BV.

The Truth About "Designer Vagina" Cosmetic Surgery—Labiaplasty, Vaginal Tightening and More

Study titled, "An analysis of the content and clinical implications of online advertisements for female genital cosmetic surgery," published in *BMJ Open*.

Labiaplasty (when the labia minora, the inner "lips" surrounding the vaginal opening, are surgically trimmed and shaped) and other so-called "designer vagina" procedures, including vaginal tightening, have become increasingly popular—despite the fact that The American College of Obstetricians and Gynecologists (ACOG) issued a strongly worded statement to members noting that female genital cosmetic procedures are not medically indicated and that there is no documentation of their safety and effectiveness. ACOG even admonished, "It is deceptive to give the impression that...such procedures are accepted and routine surgical practices."

And now a recent study has raised some serious concerns about the quality of information on the websites of surgeons who perform genital cosmetic procedures. Even if you would never have such surgery yourself, you may have

Bras Cause Breasts to Sag More Over Time

The long-standing belief that bras keep breasts from sagging while preventing back pain and improving posture is incorrect.

Recent finding: Women ages 18 to 35 experienced about a one-quarter-inch lift in their nipples each year by not wearing a bra. Bras may discourage the growth of supporting breast tissue.

Study of 330 volunteers by researchers at Centre Hospitalier Universitaire, Besancon, France, reported online at *LiveScience.com*. This sample is not representative of the global population of women.

a loved one who would consider it...and who should be duly cautioned about the dangers of the procedures and the sneaky marketing tricks used to sell them.

MEDICINE'S "WILD WEST"

Various operations are offered under the umbrella term of female genital cosmetic surgery, including labiaplasty, clitoral hood reduction, vaginal tightening, hymen repair and more. Such procedures do not come cheap, typically running from $2,500 to $8,000, depending on the procedure and surgeon—costs generally not covered by insurance.

So why are women flocking to have their nether regions redesigned? The study authors cited direct-to-consumer Internet marketing as the force behind the growth in demand and noted that there is scant medical scrutiny of this kind of advertising. Even cosmetic surgeons themselves have said that the current marketing environment is like "the old Wild Wild West: wide open and unregulated."

To see what kind of information consumers typically get online, the study researchers Googled designer vagina (a familiar if erroneous term in popular culture), looking for private physicians who offer genital cosmetic surgery. Then they analyzed the top five websites that Google listed in the US plus the top five in the UK.

Results: The quality of information available for women considering such procedures was poor in most cases and downright inaccurate in some. *Examples...*

The websites often used terms that implied the existence of a medical abnormality needing treatment, even when there was no such abnormality. For instance, labial hypertrophy suggests that the labia are abnormally large—yet in the before-and-after photos, all of the "before" shots showed labia that were within the normal range.

All the sites claimed that surgery would have physical, psychological, social and/or sexual benefits (improved hygiene, restored confidence, enhanced sexual pleasure, improved relationships, even better career prospects!)—claims that are unsubstantiated by research.

Much of the information on the sites was "imbued with value judgment," the researchers noted. For instance, one site said that "you should bleed on your wedding night" and recommended surgical hymen repair (also called revirgination) as a way to "keep your head high."

There was no mention of less invasive ways of addressing concerns about body dissatisfaction, such as through psychotherapy.

The sites generally downplayed the risks of surgery, which include bleeding, infection, pain, scarring and/or altered sensation...and failed to mention that the long-term risks of the procedures are unknown.

Most sites gave no indication of success rates. Those that did claimed success rates of 95% to 100%—but offered no information on what constituted success or how the statistics were derived.

None of the sites gave a lower age limit for surgery, which the researchers deemed "most disturbing of all," especially given that anatomy changes throughout a woman's lifetime.

IF YOU ARE TEMPTED

Clear and detailed guidelines regarding genital cosmetic surgery are urgently needed, the researchers said, so that women can make fully informed choices. But until such guidelines exist, what should you do if you are interested in this type of surgery?

First, understand that there is wide variation in the appearance of normal female genitalia. Your gynecologist can tell you whether your genitals really do fall outside the normal range. It's also worthwhile to consult a psychologist trained in assessing and treating problems related to body image and sexuality—because surgery is unlikely to fix such problems. As the ACOG statement pointed out, "Patients who are anxious or insecure about their genital appearance or sexual function may be further traumatized by undergoing an unproven surgical procedure with obvious risks."

If you do decide to have an operation, understand that there are no specific training or licensing requirements for genital cosmetic surgery—so it is best to choose a board-certified plastic surgeon, board-certified gynecologist or board-certified urologist who has years of experience performing the specific procedure you're interested in. Have an in-depth discussion with any surgeon you're considering about his/her before-and-after photo gallery to satisfy yourself that the pictures are of procedures that this doctor actually performed...then ask for references from satisfied patients. With the doctor, discuss realistic expectations for results and review any possible risks and complications. If you perceive a patronizing or dismissive attitude ("Don't you worry, sweetie, everything will be fine"), go elsewhere.

Help for Hair Loss

Amy McMichael, MD, chair of dermatology, Wake Forest Baptist Medical Center, Winston-Salem, North Carolina.

Frontal fibrosing alopecia is a form of hair loss that occurs on the front hairline. It's a rare condition that usually affects postmenopausal women. The cause is not known, but it's an autoimmune condition—white blood cells attack the hair follicles, causing scarring and permanent damage.

There's no way to prevent frontal fibrosing alopecia. It is often treated with anti-inflammatory medications, such as topical corticosteroids or oral drugs.

In rare cases, follicles can grow hair again after the inflammation is decreased. *Minoxidil* (Rogaine) can be used to keep the hair in the growth phase longer.

If your hair follicles are indeed completely scarred, they won't ever grow hair again. The only option in this case (once your alopecia has gone into remission) would be a surgical restoration in which hair is removed from the back of your scalp and placed in the scarred area. This surgery should be performed by an experienced hair transplant surgeon to avoid complications, such as infection and poor hair growth.

Nosebleed Know-How

Murray Grossan, MD, Los Angeles–based otolaryngologist in private practice and author of *Free Yourself from Sinus and Allergy Problems Permanently* (Basic Health). *GrossanInstitute.com*

Fluctuating hormone levels in menstruating women can increase blood flow to the mucous membranes in the nose and trigger nosebleeds. After menopause, lower hormone levels can cause tissues in the nose to become drier, which can trigger bleeding.

Dry indoor air also can irritate and dry out the nasal tissues. A dab of a water-soluble gel, such as Breathe-ease XL Nasal Moisturizer Gel, twice a day will help heal nasal passages and keep them from getting dry.

In some instances, nosebleeds can be a sign that the nasal membranes have become too thin, which can happen when taking nonsteroidal anti-inflammatory drugs and other

One Dose Might Do It

A single dose of the HPV vaccine may be enough to protect women against cervical cancer. Officially, three doses of the vaccine are recommended. However, doctors have found antibodies to the human papillomavirus, which causes HPV, in women who received only two vaccinations six months apart...and in women who received only a single vaccination.

Mahboobeh Safaeian, PhD, investigator, division of cancer epidemiology and genetics, National Cancer Institute, Bethesda, Maryland, and leader of a study published in *Cancer Prevention Research*.

anticoagulant medications and/or blood-thinning supplements such as ginkgo biloba.

Daily Aspirin May Guard Against Ovarian Cancer

Britton Trabert, PhD, Hormonal and Reproductive Epidemiology Branch, National Cancer Institute division of cancer epidemiology and genetics, Rockville, MD.
U.S. National Institutes of Health, news release.

Taking aspirin every day might lower a woman's risk of developing ovarian cancer by one-fifth, a recent study suggests.

More than 20,000 women in the United States will be diagnosed with ovarian cancer this year, and more than 14,000 will die from the disease.

STUDY DETAILS

Researchers from the U.S. National Cancer Institute analyzed data from 12 studies that involved nearly 8,000 women with ovarian cancer and close to 12,000 women without the disease to determine how the use of aspirin, other nonsteroidal anti-inflammatory drugs (NSAIDs) and *acetaminophen* (Tylenol) affected the risk of ovarian cancer.

About 18% of the women used aspirin regularly, 24% used non-aspirin NSAIDs (which include drugs such as *ibuprofen* and *naproxen*) and 16% used acetaminophen. Those who used aspirin daily had a 20% lower risk of ovarian cancer than those who used aspirin less than once a week, the study found.

The risk of ovarian cancer was 10% lower in women who used non-aspirin NSAIDs at least once a week, compared with those who used them less often. However, this difference was not statistically significant, the researchers said.

There was no link between acetaminophen use and ovarian cancer risk, according to the study, which was published in the *Journal of the National Cancer Institute.*

IMPLICATIONS

The findings add to the growing list of cancers and other diseases aspirin might help protect against, the researchers said. Although the study showed an association between aspirin use and a lower risk of ovarian cancer, it did not prove a cause-and-effect link.

"Our study suggests that aspirin regimens, proven to protect against heart attack, may reduce the risk of ovarian cancer as well," said Britton Trabert, PhD, of the National Cancer Institute's division of cancer epidemiology and genetics.

"However intriguing our results are, they should not influence current clinical practice," Dr. Trabert said. "Additional studies are needed to explore the delicate balance of risk and benefit for this potential chemopreventive agent, as well as studies to identify [how] aspirin may reduce ovarian cancer risk."

ASPIRIN SIDE EFFECTS

Regular aspirin use can cause side effects, such as bleeding in the digestive tract or hemorrhagic (bleeding) stroke, the study authors said. Researchers advised getting a doctor's approval before starting to take aspirin daily.

info For more information about ovarian cancer, visit the American Cancer Society website, *cancer.org*, and search "ovarian cancer."

Glaucoma Risk for Women

According to recent research, women who took oral contraceptives for at least three years have twice the risk for glaucoma as women who took contraceptives for a shorter time or did not take them at all.

Possible reason: Birth control pills reduce estrogen—and estrogen is believed to protect the retina. Women who take or have taken birth control pills should consider getting an annual eye exam for glaucoma.

Shan Lin, MD, professor of clinical ophthalmology, University of California, San Francisco, School of Medicine, and leader of a study presented at the annual meeting of the American Academy of Ophthalmology in New Orleans.

Women Who Smoke Are At Greater Risk for Colon Cancer Than Men Who Smoke

According to a recent finding, women who smoke or who have ever smoked have nearly 20% higher risk for colon cancer than women who never smoked. Men who smoke have 8% higher risk for colon cancer than men who never smoked.

Study of data on more than 600,000 people ages 19 to 67 over 14 years by researchers in the department of community medicine, University of Tromsø, Norway, published in *Cancer Epidemiology, Biomarkers & Prevention*.

Cinnamon May Help Ease Common Cause of Infertility, Study Says

Daniel Kort, MD, postdoctoral fellow, reproductive endocrinology, Columbia University Medical Center, New York, New York.

Avner Hershlag, MD, chief, Center for Human Reproduction, North Shore University Hospital, Manhasset, New York.

International Federation of Fertility Societies and American Society for Reproductive Medicine, Boston, annual meeting.

Cinnamon has long been used to add flavor to sweet and savory foods. Now, preliminary research suggests the spice may also help jump-start irregular menstrual cycles in women affected by a common infertility disorder known as polycystic ovary syndrome.

"There is a lot of interest in homeopathic or natural remedies for this condition," said study author Daniel Kort, MD, a postdoctoral fellow in reproductive endocrinology at the medical center. "This may be something we can do using a totally natural substance that can help a large group of patients."

BACKGROUND ON POLYCYSTIC OVARY SYNDROME

An estimated 5% to 10% of women of childbearing age have polycystic ovary syndrome, with up to five million Americans affected. Polycystic ovary syndrome, which involves many of the body's systems, is thought to be caused by insensitivity to the hormone insulin. Typical symptoms include menstrual irregularity, infertility, acne, excess hair growth on the face or body, and thinning scalp hair.

Treatment for polycystic ovary syndrome currently includes weight loss, ovulation-inducing drugs such as *clomiphene* (brand name Clomid) and diabetes medications such as *metformin*, said Avner Hershlag, MD, chief of the Center for Human Reproduction at North Shore University Hospital in Manhasset, New York.

STUDY DETAILS

The small study by researchers from Columbia University Medical Center in New York City found that women with polycystic ovary syndrome who took inexpensive daily cinnamon supplements experienced nearly twice the menstrual cycles over a six-month period as women with the syndrome given an inactive placebo.

Of the 16 patients who completed Dr. Kort's trial, 11 were given daily 1,500-milligram cinnamon supplements and five were given placebo pills. Diet and activity levels were monitored, and patients completed monthly menstrual calendars.

After six months, women receiving cinnamon had significant improvement in menstrual cycle regularity, having an average of nearly four menstrual periods over that time compared with an average of 2.2 periods among the placebo group. Two women reported spontaneous pregnancies after three months of cinnamon treatment, meaning they became pregnant without additional help.

Dr. Kort said that it's not yet clear exactly why cinnamon may work to regulate menstrual cycles in those with polycystic ovary syndrome, but it may improve the body's ability to process glucose and insulin. Prior research among diabetic patients suggested the spice can reduce insulin resistance.

Polycystic ovary syndrome "is one of the most common causes why women don't have regular menstrual cycles," Dr. Kort said. "But the clinical consequences later in life are truly great—from an increased risk of diabetes and glucose intolerance to endometrial cancer. Many women can go their whole lives without regular menstrual cycles, and it doesn't necessarily bother them until they want to have children."

The 1,500-milligram cinnamon dose was chosen for this trial because it was between the 1,000 to 2,000 mg daily that seemed to have metabolic effects on diabetic patients in earlier research, Dr. Kort said. But all doses in that range are cheaply obtained, costing pennies per capsule.

"Compared to most medical therapies these days, the cost is very small," he said.

The study was presented at a meeting of the International Federation of Fertility Societies and American Society for Reproductive Medicine in Boston.

Although the study suggests a link between cinnamon and improvement of polycystic ovary syndrome, it doesn't establish a direct cause-and-effect relationship.

EXPERT COMMENTARY

Still, fertility specialist Dr. Hershlag called the study "welcome and interesting" and said he sees no reason women with polycystic ovary syndrome shouldn't use more cinnamon in their food or take cinnamon supplements.

"Any work that's something nutritional in nature and seems to affect the abnormal physiology of polycystic ovaries is welcome," Dr. Hershlag said. "If they want to spice up their life and take it, that's fine . . . but I think the best thing to do when you have polycystic ovaries is to be under the control of a physician."

Some women with polycystic ovary syndrome from Dr. Kort's clinic are already trying cinnamon supplementation at home in the hopes of regulating their own menstrual cycles, he said, although he acknowledged the spice wasn't likely to be a cure-all for the condition.

"It's unlikely to be the sole source of improvement or to change entire (treatment) protocols," he said. "It's not going to regulate every patient who takes it, but a good percentage who take it may experience some benefit, and the side effects are low. It's relatively cheap and well tolerated."

Some day, Dr. Kort added, he hopes to organize a larger trial examining the issue.

info The PCOS Foundation offers more information about polycystic ovary syndrome at its website, *http://www.pcosfoundation.org/about-pcos*

New Treatment for Advanced Ovarian Cancer

According to a recent study, ovarian cancer patients given the drug *pazopanib* (Votrient) stayed in remission almost six months longer than women who didn't receive the medication. Ovarian cancer has a current cure rate of only 20% to 25%, and two-thirds of patients will experience a relapse despite successful initial treatment and chemotherapy. Side effects of the drug include hypertension, diarrhea, nausea, headache and fatigue.

Study of 940 ovarian cancer patients over 24 months by researchers at Kliniken Essen-Mitte, Essen, Germany, presented at the American Society of Clinical Oncology annual meeting.

Young Women Less Healthy Than Men Before Heart Attack

American Heart Association, news release.

Among young heart attack victims, women often have more medical issues, more chest pain and worse quality of life before the event than men, a recent study reveals.

The researchers, from the Yale School of Medicine, said young women also tend to have worse mental health with more physical limitations prior to their heart attacks.

The findings could help explain why young women often have worse outcomes than their male peers after a heart attack, said the researchers, who concluded that doctors should regularly assess young women's heart attack risk.

"Compared with young men, women under 55 are less likely to have heart attacks," study author Rachel Dreyer, PhD, a research fellow in cardiovascular medicine at Yale, said in an American Heart Association news release. "But when they do occur, women are more likely to have medical problems, poorer physical and mental functioning, more chest pain and a poorer quality of life in the month leading up to their heart attack."

STUDY DETAILS

The study involved nearly 3,000 women and men, aged 18 to 55, who participated in an international study of heart attack patients. The researchers questioned the participants to assess their chest pain and quality of life before their heart attack.

The study also revealed that the women were more likely than the men to have other conditions linked to heart disease, such as diabetes: 40% of women compared with just 27% of the men. Moreover, 55% of the women were obese, compared with 48% of the men.

Of the women, 6% had a history of stroke and 6% had heart failure. In contrast, 3% of men had a history of stroke, and 2% had heart failure. Meanwhile, 13% of women had renal failure and 49% suffered from depression. The researchers said only 9% of men had renal failure and just 24% were depressed.

WHAT'S NEEDED TO PROTECT WOMEN

"We need to develop better methods for recognizing and treating young women with chest pain to optimize their quality of life and potentially even prevent a heart attack," Dr. Dreyer said in the news release.

"General health and disease-specific health-status assessments are valuable tools for health care providers to measure the burden of disease on patients," she said. "These should be standardized into clinical practice, much like assessments for other traditional heart disease risk factors."

The study findings were presented at the American Heart Association's annual meeting. The data and conclusions of research presented at medical meetings should be viewed as preliminary until published in a peer-reviewed journal.

info For more information about women and heart disease, visit the website of the U.S. Centers for Disease Control and Prevention at *http://www.cdc.gov/dhdsp/data_statistics/fact_sheets/fs_women_heart.htm.*

Incontinence Surgery Beats Physical Therapy in Trial

Julien Labrie, MD, gynecology resident, University Medical Center Utrecht, the Netherlands.

Benjamin Brucker, MD, assistant professor, female pelvic medicine and reconstructive surgery, department of urology, NYU Langone Medical Center, New York City.

New England Journal of Medicine

Stress urinary incontinence is a common problem among women, and recent research suggests that surgery might be a better first-line treatment than pelvic muscle strengthening.

In what is billed as a first comparison of the two therapies, Dutch researchers found that almost 91% of women who had midurethral-sling surgery reported improvement compared with 64% of women who had physical therapy for pelvic floor muscle training to correct the problem.

"The prevalence of stress urinary incontinence—leakage on physical exercise, laughing, coughing—is high, and the impact on daily life can be substantial," said study lead author Julien Labrie, MD, a gynecology resident at the University Medical Center Utrecht, in the Netherlands.

"Regardless of the severity of the incontinence, pelvic floor muscle training is the first-line treatment in most international guidelines," Dr. Labrie said. "With rapidly increasing evidence that [midurethral-sling surgery] is safe with lasting efficacy, we believed it was time to compare surgery with pelvic muscle floor training as a first-line treatment for women with moderate to severe stress urinary incontinence."

Results of the study were published in the *New England Journal of Medicine.*

BACKGROUND ON INCONTINENCE

Stress incontinence is a problem that affects many women as they age, and it has a negative effect on quality of life, according to the National Association for Continence.

The treatment options include pelvic muscle floor training, which involves exercises known as Kegels that help strengthen the pelvic muscles. The hope is that the stronger muscles can effectively close the urethra, holding back urine. The rates of subjective success vary greatly for pelvic muscle floor training—from 53% to 97%, according to background information in the study.

There also are several surgical options. One is the midurethral-sling surgery, which is a minimally invasive procedure that involves inserting a hammock-like device underneath the urethra to give it additional support and compression to help it stay closed. Subjective cure rates for this procedure vary from 75% to 94%, the study reported.

STUDY DETAILS

To see how these options compared, the researchers recruited 230 women for pelvic muscle floor training (physiotherapy) and another 230 for surgery. The researchers allowed the women in either group to switch if they were unhappy with their treatment.

Nearly half of the women in the physiotherapy group switched to the surgical group, while 11% of the women in the surgery group crossed over to physiotherapy during the study.

After a year, the researchers found that subjective improvement was reported by 90.8% of the women in the surgery group and 64.4% in the physiotherapy group. The rates of subjective cure were somewhat lower—85.2% for those in the surgical group and 53.4% for the physiotherapy group.

Risks of surgery include perforation, the need for reoperation, postoperative bleeding, blood loss and new urinary urge incontinence (the sudden need to urinate that is difficult to control), according to the study.

"We feel surgery and physiotherapy should both be offered as first-line treatment options," Dr. Labrie said. "The woman herself should be involved in deciding what, in her individual case, should be the treatment."

Dr. Labrie noted, however, that the trial did not include women with mild incontinence, so the results shouldn't be applied to women who have mild stress incontinence.

EXPERT RESPONSE

Benjamin Brucker, MD, assistant professor of female pelvic medicine and reconstructive surgery at the NYU Langone Medical Center in New York City, called the study "very well designed."

The data on surgical complications was reassuring because the complications were relatively minor, he said.

But where does all this leave women who have urinary incontinence? What option should they choose?

"Each woman is unique," Dr. Brucker said. "What works best for one woman isn't what would work best for every other woman."

"On an individual level, this study shows that if you want to be conservative, you don't lose anything by having physiotherapy first," he said. "But it also shows that depending on your embarrassment and emotional health scores, if you're a woman who says, 'I just want to put this behind me,' you're not doing yourself a disservice by having surgery first."

info Learn more about stress incontinence and treatment options from the National Association for Continence website at *http://www.nafc.org/index.php?page=what-every-woman-should-know.*

Viagra for Menstrual Cramps?

Jill Rabin, MD, chief of ambulatory care, obstetrics and gynecology, and head of urogynecology, Long Island Jewish Medical Center, New Hyde Park, New York.

Richard Legro, MD, professor of public health sciences and obstetrics and gynecology, Penn State College of Medicine, Hershey.

Penn State University, news release.

Human Reproduction

Women dealing with painful menstrual cramps may receive relief from an unexpected source—the erectile dysfunction medication normally found in their husbands' little blue pills.

Sildenafil, the active ingredient in Viagra, appears to help women who are suffering from moderate to severe menstrual cramps, according to a small study funded by the U.S. National Institutes of Health.

Researchers found that administering the medication vaginally provided nearly double the pain relief compared with receiving a placebo, or dummy drug.

STUDY DETAILS

The study focused on 25 women aged 18 to 35 who were suffering from primary dysmenorrhea (PD), the medical term for painful menstrual periods. PD accounts for 600 million lost work hours each year in the United States, according to background information from the study, which was published in the journal *Human Reproduction*.

Ibuprofen and other nonsteroidal anti-inflammatory drugs are the current first-line treatment for menstrual cramps, but they do not work well for all women and can cause ulcers and kidney damage through prolonged use.

The researchers thought Viagra could dilate blood vessels and increase blood flow to the uterus, which might help relieve pain.

"It certainly makes sense for some women with PD that increasing blood flow to the area would increase oxygen to the pelvic tissues and potentially alleviate pain," said Jill Rabin, MD, chief of ambulatory care, obstetrics and gynecology at the Long Island Jewish Medical Center in New Hyde Park, New York. Dr. Rabin was not involved with the recent study.

Earlier studies tested oral use of Viagra to treat menstrual cramps, and found that the drug can ease pelvic pain. However, the side effects from oral use—most often headaches—were such that doctors ruled out routine use.

This was the first test of vaginal application of Viagra to try to treat menstrual cramps, the researchers said.

"The vagina is an effective route for drug administration intended mainly for local action because delivering medication in close proximity to the target organ decreases the incidence of side effects," they said.

STUDY DETAILS

Researchers from the Penn State College of Medicine worked with researchers from Croatia, who recruited 25 women at the Nova Gradiska General Hospital to receive either a 100-milligram sildenafil tablet or a placebo. The patients then rated their pain over a four-hour period.

Sildenafil administered vaginally was able to significantly alleviate menstrual pain, and without the side effects that come with oral use, the researchers said.

Women reported pain relief about double that of those who received a placebo, based on a scale used to measure their pain.

The researchers were not able, however, to explain why this occurred. Uterine blood flow increased from both sildenafil and the placebo, which did not match their initial theory.

IMPLICATIONS

Study coauthor Richard Legro, MD, professor of public health sciences and obstetrics and gynecology at Penn State College of Medicine, said future studies will be required to verify the results of this small study and figure out how Viagra helps women with their cramps.

"If future studies confirm these findings, sildenafil may become a treatment option for patients with PD," said Dr. Legro. "Since PD is a condition that most women suffer from and seek treatment for at some point in their lives, the quest for new medication is justified."

Dr. Rabin agreed that the idea shows great promise and should be further studied.

"It's always heartening when you have a tested medication like Viagra and someone thinks of a potential new use for it," she said.

info For more on managing painful menstrual symptoms, visit the website of the U.S. National Library of Medicine, *www.nlm.nih.gov*, and search "painful menstrual periods."

Enormous Gaps Remain in Medical Research for Women

Paula Johnson, MD, executive director, the Connors Center for Women's Health, Brigham and Women's Hospital, and professor, medicine, Harvard Medical School, Boston.

Eve Higginbotham, MD, vice dean, Diversity and Inclusion, Perelman School of Medicine, University of Pennsylvania, Philadelphia.

Lynn Gordon, MD, PhD, associate dean, diversity affairs, and professor, ophthalmology, David Geffen School of Medicine, University of California, Los Angeles.

Charting the Course: A National Policy Summit on the Future of Women's Health.

Two decades after the passage of a landmark law mandating that women be represented in government-funded medical research, a new report reveals that the world of science is still ignoring women's unique health issues far more than it should.

"The science that informs medicine routinely fails to consider the impact of sex and gender, and this occurs at some of the earliest stages of research—from animal to human studies," said report author Paula Johnson, MD. The findings were released at a national summit on women's health issues in Boston in early March 2014.

While women are now more routinely included in clinical trials and an entire field of women's health has emerged beyond reproductive health, "there are still enormous gaps in the scientific process as it relates to women," said Dr. Johnson, who is executive director of The Connors Center for Women's Health at Brigham and Women's Hospital in Boston.

The latest statistics are indeed grim...

•**Less than one-third of cardiovascular clinical trial participants are women,** and only one-third of trials that include women report sex-specific outcomes. Yet, cardiovascular disease is the number one cause of death among US women.

•**Less than 45% of animal studies on anxiety and depression use female animals,** although depression is a leading cause of disease among women worldwide.

•**Lung cancer researchers often fail to include an analysis of data by sex or gender-specific factors,** despite the fact that lung cancer behaves differently in nonsmoking women than in nonsmoking men. This disease kills more women each year than breast, ovarian and uterine cancers combined.

•**A woman's overall lifetime risk of developing Alzheimer's disease is almost twice that of a man,** and it has been thought that this is simply because women live longer. However, hormones may play a role.

EXPERT COMMENTARY

One expert explained the importance of including women in medical research.

"Unless you study the populations that you're treating, you really don't know how that population is going to respond," said Lynn Gordon, MD, PhD, associate dean of diversity affairs, at the David Geffen School of Medicine at the University of California, Los Angeles.

However, Dr. Gordon said, a lot of researchers don't want to do studies on women of childbearing age due to their monthly hormonal fluctuations, for example.

"When you're doing animal studies, you want to make things as standardized as possible," she explained. "If you add in gender, how do you standardize, especially considering the hormone issues," but that doesn't excuse the disparity, Dr. Gordon noted.

Dr. Gordon said pregnancy and safety to unborn children are concerns, too. "Again, I'm not excusing it or saying it's an appropriate reason, but it is a concern investigators have," she pointed out.

Dr. Gordon added that more studies on the natural history of diseases in women could be conducted, too, because they only require following women, not exposing anyone to experimental therapy.

Dr. Johnson said there may be a need for more rigorous enforcement of the law. "The law's scope may be too limited to address all the dynamics of the problem," she said.

She called on political, scientific and business leaders to push efforts to apply sex differences to research.

"We really have to raise awareness," Dr. Johnson said. "There's an overall lack of awareness among our population."

The report also recommends more transparency in research on drugs and medical devices, and suggests that clinical trials should carry a disclaimer if a study has not included enough female participants. Dr. Johnson said another goal is to adopt clinical care practices that use a gender-based lens in health care and medical research.

Women need to drive the conversation, said Eve Higginbotham, MD, vice dean for diversity and inclusion at the Perelman School of Medicine at the University of Pennsylvania, in Philadelphia.

"We still have a lot of bias embedded in academic medicine, and certainly it comes down to the people actually doing the studies," said Dr. Higginbotham. "Women are still struggling to get to the highest levels of academic medicine. In many cases, women are not the primary drivers in many of these studies."

Dr. Higginbotham noted that the highest levels of academia in medical schools are still slim on women—women only represent 5% of medical professors in the United States.

"Change takes time, and it's going to take a number of factors to drive that," Dr. Higginbotham said. "Having the summit is a good first step in at least acknowledging the lack of progress that has been made and making people more aware."

info For more information on the women's health summit, visit the Brigham and Women's Hospital website at *http://www.brighamandwomens.org/Departments_and_Services/womenshealth/ConnorsCenter/Policy/summithome.aspx.*

Index

D

E

N